Theories of Psychopathology and Personality

ESSAYS AND CRITIQUES

Edited and Introduced by

THEODORE MILLON, Ph.D.

University of Illinois

SECOND EDITION

1973

W. B. SAUNDERS COMPANY

Philadelphia · London · Toronto

W. B. Saunders Company: West Washington Square
Philadelphia, PA 19105

12 Dyott Street
London, WC1A 1DB

833 Oxford Street
Toronto 18, Ontario

Theories of Psychopathology and Personality   ISBN 0-7216-6382-6

Print No.:   9   8   7   6   5   4   3   2   1

To my parents

ABNER AND MOLLIE MILLON

*who showed me how well
intelligence and compassion can blend*

CONTRIBUTORS

ALBERT BANDURA, Ph.D. Professor of Psychology, Stanford University

HOWARD S. BECKER, Ph.D. Professor of Sociology, Northwestern University

LUDWIG BINSWANGER, M.D.* Formerly Director, Bellevue Sanatorium, Kreuzlingen, Switzerland

EUGEN P. BLEULER, M.D.* Formerly Director, Burgholzli Clinic and Mental Hospital, Zurich, Switzerland

MEDARD BOSS, M.D. Professor of Psychoanalysis, University of Zurich School of Medicine

LOUIS BREGER, Ph.D. Associate Professor of Psychology and Psychiatry, University of California, Berkeley

JOHN DOLLARD, Ph.D. Professor of Psychology, Yale University

H. WARREN DUNHAM, Ph.D. Professor of Sociology, Wayne State University

ALBERT ELLIS, Ph.D. Director, Institute for Rational Therapy, New York

ERIK H. ERIKSON. Professor of Human Development, Harvard University

HANS J. EYSENCK, Ph.D. Professor of Psychology, University of London

VIKTOR E. FRANKL, M.D. Professor of Neuropsychiatry, University of Vienna Medical School

SIGMUND FREUD, M.D.* Founder of psychoanalysis

ERICH FROMM, Ph.D. Professor of Psychology, National University of Mexico

ERVING GOFFMAN, Ph.D. Professor of Sociology, University of Pennsylvania

KURT GOLDSTEIN, M.D.* Formerly Professor of Neuropsychiatry, University of Berlin and founder of organismic theory

ROY R. GRINKER, Sr., M.D. Director, Institute for Psychosomatic and Psychiatric Research, Michael Reese Hospital

ERNEST M. GRUENBERG, M.D. Professor of Psychiatry, College of Physicians and Surgeons, Columbia University

HEINZ HARTMANN, M.D. Former President, International Society for Psychoanalysis

HAROLD E. HIMWICH, M.D. Director, Galesburg State Research Hospital, Illinois

PAUL HOCH, M.D.* Formerly Clinical Professor of Psychiatry, College of Physicians and Surgeons, Columbia University

ROBERT R. HOLT, Ph.D. Professor of Psychology, New York University

*Deceased

KAREN HORNEY, M.D.* Formerly Dean, American Institute of Psychoanalysis

MAXWELL JONES, M.D. Director, Dingleton Mental Hospital, Melrose, Scotland

CARL G. JUNG, M.D.* Formerly Professor Medical Psychology, University of Basel and founder of analytic psychology

LOTHAR KALINOWSKY, M.D. Clinical Professor of Psychiatry, College of Physicians and Surgeons, Columbia University

FRANZ J. KALLMANN, M.D.* Formerly Professor of Psychiatry, College of Physicians and Surgeons, Columbia University

FREDERICK H. KANFER, Ph.D. Professor of Psychology, University of Cincinnati

GEORGE A. KELLY, Ph.D.* Formerly Professor of Psychology, Brandeis University

SEYMOUR S. KETY, M.D. Professor of Psychiatry, Harvard University School of Medicine

DONALD C. KLEIN, Ph.D. Program Director, National Institute of Applied Behavioral Sciences, Bethesda

EMIL KRAEPELIN, M.D.* Formerly Professor of Neuropsychiatry, University of Heidelberg Medical School, Germany

LEONARD KRASNER, Ph.D. Professor of Psychology, State University of New York, Stony Brook

LAWRENCE S. KUBIE, M.D. Professor of Psychiatry, University of Maryland School of Medicine

RONALD D. LAING, M.D. Private practice; formerly Psychiatrist, Tavistock Institute, London

NATHAN S. LEHRMAN, M.D. Clinical Associate, College of Physicians and Surgeons, Columbia University

ALEXANDER H. LEIGHTON, M.D. Professor of Behavioral Science, Harvard University School of Public Health

ERICH LINDEMANN, M.D. Professor of Psychiatry, Stanford University School of Medicine

ABRAHAM H. MASLOW, Ph.D.* Formerly Professor of Psychology, Brandeis University

ROLLO MAY, Ph.D. Training Analyst, William Alanson White Institute of Psychiatry, New York

JAMES L. MCGAUGH, Ph.D. Professor of Psychobiology, University of California, Irvine

PAUL E. MEEHL, Ph.D. Professor of Psychology and Psychiatry, University of Minnesota

ADOLF MEYER, M.D.* Formerly Professor of Psychiatry, Johns Hopkins School of Medicine

NEAL E. MILLER, Ph.D. Professor of Psychology, Rockefeller University

THEODORE MILLON, Ph.D. Professor of Psychology and Psychiatry, University of Illinois

DAVID RAPAPORT, Ph.D.* Formerly Director, Research Departments, Menninger and Austen Riggs Foundations

CARL R. ROGERS, Ph.D. Fellow, Western Behavioral Science Institute and formerly Professor, Universities of Chicago and Wisconsin

JULIAN B. ROTTER, Ph.D. Professor of Psychology, University of Connecticut

MELVIN SABSHIN, M.D. Professor and Head, Department of Psychiatry, University of Illinois College of Medicine

GEORGE SASLOW, M.D. Professor and Head, Department of Psychiatry, University of Oregon Medical School

THOMAS SCHEFF, Ph.D. Professor and Chairman, Department of Sociology, University of California, Santa Barbara

WILLIAM H. SHELDON, Ph.D., M.D. Professor and Director, Constitution Laboratory, College of Physicians and Surgeons, Columbia University

B. F. SKINNER, Ph.D. Professor of Psychology, Harvard University

M. BREWSTER SMITH, Ph.D. Provost, University of California, Santa Cruz

HARRY STACK SULLIVAN, M.D.* Formerly Director, Washington School of Psychiatry

THOMAS S. SZASZ, M.D. Professor of Psychiatry, Upstate Medical Center, State University of New York

LEONARD P. ULLMANN, Ph.D. Professor of Psychology, University of Hawaii

RICHARD H. WALTERS, Ph.D.* Formerly Professor of Psychology, University of Waterloo

ROGER J. WILLIAMS, Ph.D. Professor of Biochemistry, University of Texas

LEWIS R. WOLBERG, M.D. Director, Postgraduate Center for Mental Health, New York

JOSEPH WOLPE, M.D. Professor of Psychiatry, School of Medicine, Temple University, Philadelphia

PREFACE
TO THE SECOND EDITION

The first edition of this anthology has been extremely well received; in fact, it has become a sort of "classic" at the graduate level, as well as a frequently used supplement for undergraduates. Despite the many plaudits it evoked, the book had notable deficiencies, and these I have sought to remedy in the revision.

First, several articles assumed a level of technical sophistication in esoteric matters such as neurochemistry; papers faulted on these and similar grounds have been either deleted or edited to minimize difficulties. *Second,* several theorists, of both historical or contemporary significance, were omitted from the first edition (e.g., Kraepelin, Meyer, Goldstein, Rotter, Kelly, Frankl, Ellis); with an enlarged format to work with, we have been able to add them to our list of contributors. *Third,* numerous instructors and students felt the book would be strengthened by adding sections on "sociocultural" and "integrative" approaches. Although I hold to the view that the four basic orientations which comprised the first edition—biophysical, intrapsychic, phenomenological and behavioral—are, from a philosophical perspective, the major alternatives for a theory of man, the surge of recent interest and work representing these two additional approaches well justifies their inclusion. *Fourth,* the major theorists of psychopathology also are the prime theorists of personality. Most of them argue that their concepts and propositions apply with equal utility to the understanding of normal as well as abnormal processes. Moreover, on a purely empirical basis, I have observed that the first edition was adopted almost as frequently in "personality" as in "abnormal" courses; on both grounds, then, it seems appropriate that we change the title of the second edition to Theories of Psychopathology *and Personality.*

To those who aided me in preparing the first edition, I am pleased to add the names of several associates who were most helpful in the revision. Melvin Sabshin has not only provided me with intellectual stimulation and warm friendship in my post at the University of Illinois Neuropsychiatric Institute, but was instrumental in guiding me to several important papers included in the sociocultural section. Research colleagues, Leila Foster, Ruth Sosis, Terry Brown, Bruce Wilson, and Diane Millon, my daughter, have been and continue to be a constant source of ideas and encouragement. To my most able and efficient secretary, Luberta Shirley, my thanks for her many skills, patience and good spirits.

As a son of a much beloved father, I deeply mourn his recent death. He would have been pleased to know that this book, dedicated to him and my mother, was thought of well enough to be reprinted numerous times and, now, to be published in a second edition. In many ways the book is his as much as mine. *Zichrono l'vrocho;* may his memory be blessed.

Chicago   Theodore Millon
January, 1973

PREFACE
TO THE FIRST EDITION

Authors and editors feel called upon to present in the prefaces of their books well-reasoned justifications for their work; certainly there should be some sound rationale for contributing another volume to the surfeit of publications inundating the field. Typically, these rationales demonstrate the shortcomings of previous books and the clever manner in which the author has circumvented problems, brought matters up to date, and illuminated new directions for future work; the rationale for this present volume is no different. But it does have a less pretentious reason for its existence: no one has gathered the *diverse* viewpoints of the major theorists of psychopathology into one volume.

While researching the literature for another book, this writer was struck by the fact that no one text had been published dealing primarily with the different schools of psychopathological thought. Excellent works had been written and edited contrasting *personality* theories, but none focused specifically on theories of personality *pathology,* or *abnormal* behavior. Useful volumes appeared discussing critical issues, case reports, and research methods in psychopathology, but these topics relate only peripherally to the systematic theories that generated them. In short, it seemed time to fill an important gap in our academic library, one that should have been filled years before.

The task of writing an original work in this field could not be undertaken by the editor because of prior writing commitments. The decision to bring together original papers by the major theorists should not be viewed, however, as a second-rate compromise. Original sources not only provide us with a theorist's clearest statement of his own position, but they also convey the special logic and subtlety of language that characterize the thought of the man himself. The intensity, flavor, and persuasiveness found in the writings of a primary exponent of a theory can rarely be matched by second-hand summaries.

There must be justifications for doing a book other than the fact that it had not been done before; many things that have not been done are best left undone since they accomplish no useful purpose. But as noted in the introduction, there is considerable confusion in psychopathological theory today. A dazzling array of doctrinaire concepts, propositions, and theories vie to catch the eye of the beginning student. They do not illuminate his pathway; rather, this profusion of disconnected and seemingly contradictory thought only confounds him. The impression the student comes away with is that the data and propositions of each theoretical school are inconsistent with those of other schools, that only one of these approaches is "right," and that his task is to learn which one possesses the "truth." Such an attitude can only lead him further from the truth.

It is the contention of this book that each of the major theoretical approaches makes a distinctive contribution to our understanding of that multidimensional complex of behaviors we call psychopathology. If these alternate theories can be organized in terms of their different and distinctive areas of focus, the student may learn that they are complementary and *not* contradictory approaches to the subject.

How can this intrinsically complementary character of theories be demonstrated?

The book's introductory essay asserts that diverse theorists can be grouped together in terms of the particular class of psychopathological data they emphasize. The complex phenomena included under the label of psychopathology can be, and has been, divided fruitfully into several categories of data; no single category, however, encompasses all of the multidimensional features of psychopathology. If properly divided, each of these classes of data will be complementary to the others in that together they will comprise the total body of psychopathological phenomena.

Four such classes of data have been specified; these data levels— *biophysical, intrapsychic, phenomenological,* and *behavioral*—serve as the basis for the four major categories of theoretical investigation organized in the text. Each of these theoretical levels displays a characteristic and internally consistent series of propositions regarding the *etiology and development,* the *pathological patterns,* and the *therapy* of mental disorders. Stated differently, none of these levels has failed to provide hypotheses regarding the acquisition, clinical structure, or treatment of psychopathology. These hypotheses are interconnected, not by secondary philosophical or methodological predilections, but by the kind of data they focus upon; different data result in different hypotheses. No one expects the propositions of a physicist to be the same as those of a chemist; nor should we expect those of a behaviorist to be the same as those of a phenomenologist.

It is possible for the student to read the text profitably in either of two ways, given the format within which the book has been organized. He can progress through each theoretical level as a unit and thereby obtain a unified picture of the way in which theorists utilizing that class of data approach etiology, pathological patterns, and therapy. Equally useful is a procedure in which each of the four theoretical levels is compared section by section on each of the three major topics. Thus, he may prefer to concentrate on etiology first, comparing the biophysical, intrapsychic, phenomenological, and behavioral approaches to that topic, before progressing to comparisons among theories on the pathological pattern and therapy sections.

In addition to the three topical areas of etiology, patterns, and therapy, each theoretical level is prefaced by two *orientation* papers describing the class of data and the basic philosophy guiding theorists of that persuasion. Since few theories have escaped the scrutiny of dissident investigators, a set of two papers devoted to a *critique* of each school of thought concludes each of the four theoretical sections; controversy and dissent not only enliven the literature but alert the student to the logical and methodological shortcomings of alternate theoretical approaches.

This book may serve only to whet the appetite of the serious student, since it offers but a small sample of the myriad theories that have been propounded; we have selected what we believe to be those views that have exerted a substantial influence upon investigators at work today. No doubt, new theoretical formulations will emerge in so vital and growing a field as psychopathology. We hope, however, that the basic format organized for this book, in which the data levels for theories are stressed, will remain a useful framework for appraising new work.

Many authors and publishers have permitted us to include their work; we thank them for their generosity and cooperativeness. Margaret Caffrey, medical librarian of the Allentown State Mental Hospital, was most helpful in suggesting and tracking down several difficult-to-locate references. Ann Zarinsky, departmental secretary at Lehigh University, provided me with her usual highly competent assistance. To Sally Perlis goes my appreciation not only for her expert handling of correspondence, but for her ever-present and radiant good cheer.

Theodore Millon

CONTENTS

PART II   INTRAPSYCHIC THEORIES

Introduction

PART IV   BEHAVIORAL THEORIES

PART V   SOCIOCULTURAL THEORIES

PART VI   INTEGRATIVE THEORIES

Introduction

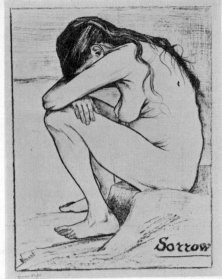

Vincent Van Gogh—*Sorrow* (1882). (The Museum of Modern Art, New York.)

Theory in Psychopathology and Personality

THEODORE MILLON

Nature was not made to suit our need for a tidy and well-ordered universe. The complexity and intricacy of the natural world make it difficult not only to establish clearcut relationships among phenomena, but to find simple ways in which these phenomena can be classified or grouped. In our desire to discover the essential order of nature we are forced to select only a few of the infinite number of elements which could be chosen; in this selection we narrow our choice only to those aspects of nature which we believe best enable us to answer the questions we pose. The elements we have chosen may be labeled, transformed, and reassembled in a variety of ways. But we must keep in mind that these labels and transformations are not "realities." The definitions, concepts, and theories scientists create are only optional tools to guide their observation and interpretation of the natural world; it is necessary to recognize, therefore, that different concepts and theories may coexist as alternative approaches to the same basic problem. An illustration in the field of bridge de-

sign may serve to clarify this point (Hebb, 1958):

The engineer who designs a bridge must think at different levels of complexity as he works. His overall plan is in terms of spans, piers, abutments; but when he turns to the design of a particular span, he starts to think in terms of lower-order units such as the I-beam. This latter unit, however, is still quite molar; an engineer is firmly convinced that an I-beam is just a special arrangement of certain molecules, the molecule in turn being a special arrangement of electrons, protons and so forth. Now note: At a microscopic level of analysis, a bridge is nothing but a complex constellation of atomic particles; and a steel I-beam is no more than a convenient fiction, a concession to the limitations of thought and the dullness of human conception.

At another level of analysis, of course, the I-beam is an elementary unit obviously real and no fiction. At this level electrons have a purely theoretical existence, which suggests that "reality" is meaningful as designating, not some ultimate mode of being about which there must be argument, but the mode of being which one takes for granted as the starting point of thought.

With this perspective in mind, let us look at the question, What is psychopathology? Clearly, mental disorders are ex-

Abridged from Chapter 2 of *Modern Psychopathology*, Philadelphia: W. B. Saunders Co., 1969.

pressed in a variety of ways; psychopathology is a complex phenomenon which can be approached at different levels and can be viewed from many angles. On a behavioral level, for example, disorders could be conceived of as a complicated pattern of responses to environmental stress. Phenomenologically, they could be seen as expressions of personal discomfort and anguish. Approached from a physiological viewpoint, they could be interpreted as sequences of complex neural and chemical activity. Intrapsychically, they could be organized into unconscious processes that defend against anxiety and conflict.

Given these diverse possibilities, we can readily understand why psychopathology may be approached and defined in terms of any of several levels we may wish to focus upon, and any of a variety of functions or processes we may wish to explain. Beyond this, each level or angle of approach lends itself to a number of specific theories and concepts, the usefulness of which must be gauged by their ability to help solve the particular problems and purposes for which they were created. That the subject matter of psychopathology is inherently diverse and complex is precisely the reason why we must not narrow our choice of approach to one level or one theory. Each has a legitimate and potentially fruitful contribution to make to our study. What should be clear, however, is that a theory is not "reality," that it is not an inevitable or predetermined representation of the objective world. Theories are merely optional instruments utilized in the early stages of knowledge. They serve to organize experience in a logical manner, and function as explanatory propositions by which experiences may be analyzed or inferences about them may be drawn. Their ultimate goal is the establishment of new empirical laws.

GOALS OF SCIENTIFIC SYSTEMS

Man acquired reliable and useful knowledge about his environment long before the advent of modern scientific thought. Information, skill and instrumentation were achieved without "science" and its methods of symbolic abstraction, research and analysis. If useful knowledge could be acquired by intelligent observation and common sense alone, what special values are derived by applying the complicated and rigorous procedures of the scientific method? Is rigor, clarity, precision and experimentation more than a compulsive and picayunish concern for details, more than the pursuit for the honorific title of "science"? Are the labors of coordinating knowledge and exploring unknown factors in a systematic fashion worth the time and effort involved? There is little question in our "age of science" that the answer would be yes! But why? What are the distinguishing virtues of scientific systems? What sets them apart from everyday common sense methods of acquiring knowledge? It is these questions to which we must turn next.

Since the number of ways we can observe, describe and organize the natural world is infinite, the terms and concepts we create to represent these activities are often confusing and obscure. For example, different words are used to describe the same behavior, and the same word is used for different behaviors. Some terms are narrow in focus, others are broad and many are difficult to define. Because of the variety of events that can be considered and the lack of precision in language, useful information gets scattered in hodgepodge fashion across the whole landscape of a scientific topic, and communication gets bogged down in terminological obscurities and semantic controversies.

One of the goals of scientific systems is to avoid this morass of confusion. Not all phenomena related to a subject are attended to at once. Certain elements are selected from the vast range of possibilities because they seem relevant to the solution of specific and important problems. To create a degree of consistency among scientists interested in a problem these elements are grouped or classified according to their similarities and differences and given specific labels which describe or define them. This process of classification is indispensable for systematizing observation and knowledge. But it is only a first step.

Classification of knowledge alone does not make a scientific system. The card catalog of a library or an accountant's ledger sheets are well organized classifications but hardly to be viewed as a system of science. The characteristic which distinquishes a scientific classification system from others is its attempt to group elements according to established or hypothesized explanatory propositions. These propositions are formed when certain properties which have been isolated and classified have been shown or have been hypothesized to be related to other classified properties or groupings. The groupings of a scientific system, therefore, are not mere collections of miscellaneous or random information, but a linked or unified pattern of known or presumed relationships. This pattern of relationships is the foundation of a scientific system.

Certain benefits derive from systematizing knowledge in this fashion. Given the countless ways of observing and analyzing a set of complex events, a system of explanatory propositions becomes a useful guide to the observer. Rather than shifting from one aspect of behavior to another, according to momentary impressions of importance, he is led to pursue in a logical and consistent manner only those aspects which are likely to be related.

In addition, a scientific system enables the perceptive scientist to generate hypotheses about relationships that have not been observed before. It enlarges the scope of knowledge by alerting the observer to possible new relationships among phenomena, and then ties these new observations into a coherent body of knowledge. Thus, from a small number of basic explanatory propositions, a scientific system develops broad applicability and subsumes a wide range of phenomena.

This generality or comprehensiveness leads to another important advantage. Because of the scope of the system, different observers are given an opportunity to check or verify the validity of its explanatory propositions. Thus, hasty generalizations, erroneous speculations and personal biases are readily exposed by systematic scrutiny. This exposure assures that propositions are supported by *shared* evidence and that the range of their validity is clearly delimited.

Bringing these points together then, we can see that a scientific system attempts to coordinate and seek relationships among a general but clearly delimited class of phenomena. The means by which a scientific system accomplishes these ends will be our next topic of discussion.

STRUCTURE AND ORIENTATION OF SCIENTIFIC THEORIES

Scientific endeavor consists of two types of activities. The *first* is the informal and systematic observation of empirical events and objects. The *second* involves the creation of abstract linguistic or mathematical symbols invented by the theorist to represent relationships among observable events, or relationships which be believes exist but have not been observed. This second, or symbolic and theoretical activity of science, will be our focus in this chapter.

As noted earlier, scientific systems consist of explanatory propositions which create order or render intelligible otherwise unrelated phenomena. There are two kinds of propositions in a scientific system, empirical laws and theories. An *empirical law* is a statement representing a universally established relationship observed among a group of empirical phenomena. A *theory*, in contrast, is composed of invented abstractions in the form of models, concepts, rules and hypotheses which function as provisional exploratory tools to aid the scientist in his search for empirical laws. Theories are subject to frequent change; empirical laws are durable.

Before we can discuss intelligently current theories of psychopathology we must examine the structural form into which theories are cast.

Formal Structure of Theories

Four major components of theory may be distinguished for our purposes: (1) an abstract *model* which serves as an analog or a visualizable pattern representing the overall structure of the theory; (2) a *conceptual terminology* by which various classes of phenomena relevant to the theory are symbolized or labeled; (3) a set of *correspondence rules* which coordinate relationships among the theoretical terms in accordance with the model; and (4) *hypotheses* which specify the manner in which these relationships may be tested in the empirical world.

Models. A model is an analogy which exploits certain aspects of a familiar or easily visualized system to guide the understanding of a less familiar or difficult subject. For example, theorists have utilized an electronic computer model to describe the processes and structure of psychopathology. Thus, human beings are likened to computers in that both receive complex information from the environment, integrate this information through devious circuits with prior information and emit relatively uncomplicated responses. More commonly, psychopathology has been organized in accordance with a biological disease model. In this format, psychopathology is conceived as if it stemmed from the intrusion of a foreign agent upon normal biological functioning; as in most physical ailments, symptoms are considered to be the organism's reaction to the intrusion.

Few theorists expect the models they adopt to represent accurately all of the features of psychopathology. Rather, the model is used merely as a way to visualize psychopathology "as if it worked like this."

Models pose a number of risks to the theorist. Certain features of a model which may have proved useful in its original setting are often assumed mistakenly to be appropriate elsewhere. Should such a model be adopted, the theorist will waste his time constructing erroneous hypotheses and pursuing unprofitable research. The adoption of the disease model in psychiatry, for example, has been viewed by many psychologists to have led to years of fruitless biochemical research. Similarly, the intrapsychic conflict model underlying psychoanalytic theory has been seen to have delayed the development of more effective psychotherapies. Unfortunately, there are no simple ways to tell beforehand whether a given model will prove to be fruitful or misguided. What should be kept clear in one's thinking is that the model adopted for a theory should not be confused with the theory itself.

Conceptual Terminology. The elements of a theory are represented by a set of concepts, that is, a language by which members of a scientific group communicate about a subject. Concepts may be seen as serving two functions. *First,* they possess a value in that they facilitate the *manipulation of theoretical ideas.* Concepts are systematically linked to other concepts; it is through the interplay of these concepts that meaningful ideas are formulated and deductive statements are made in the form of propositions and hypotheses. *Second,* most concepts possess an *empirical significance,* that is, they are linked in some explicit way to the observable world; although some concepts may represent processes or events which are not observable, they may be defined or anchored to observables. It is this translatability into the empirical domain that allows the theoretician to test his propositions in the world of "reality."

Ideally, all concepts of a scientific theory should be empirically anchored, that is, correspond to properties in the observable world. This would minimize confusion regarding the objects and events to which a term applies. Moreover, concepts should be more precise than words used in ordinary language; although everyday conversational language has relevance to significant events in the real world, it gives rise to ambiguity and confusion because of the varied uses to which conventional words are often put. Scientific concepts should be defined "precisely" in order to assure that their meaning is clear and specific.

Empirical precision, in the fullest sense of the term, can be achieved only if every concept in a theory is defined by a single observable phenomenon, that is, a different concept or label would be used for every difference that can be observed in the empirical world. This ideal simply is not feasible for reasons which will become apparent shortly. Psychological concepts do differ, however, in the degree to which they satisfy this criterion. A discussion of three types of concepts—operational definitions, intervening variables and hypothetical constructs—will be of value in noting these distinctions and their consequences.

OPERATIONAL DEFINITIONS. Certain concepts are defined literally by observable events and possess no meaning other than these events; they have been termed *operational definitions.* To paraphrase Bridgman (1927), the founder of "operationism," an operational definition is a concept that is defined by the procedure employed to measure the particular empirical event it represents; thus, the meaning of a concept is synonymous with how man measures it, not with what he says about it. For example, the concept "learning" would involve nothing more than the set of operations by which it is measured.

There would be a different concept for learning when it is measured by the number of errors a child makes on a task than when measured by the speed with which he completes the same task. The advantage of operational definitions is obvious; concepts are unambiguous, and propositions utilizing these concepts are translatable directly into the empirical phenomena they represent.

Useful as operational definitions may be, they present several problems. Theoretical concepts should be generalizable, that is, they should enable the theorist to include a variety of observations with his concept. Operational definitions are restrictive; they preclude predictions to new situations that are even slightly different from the original situation. Certainly, one of the primary goals of a theory is to integrate diverse observations with a minimum number of concepts; a strict operational approach would flood us with an infinite number of concepts and clutter thinking with irrelevant distinctions. The major value of operational definitions is cautionary; it alerts the theorist to the importance of conceptual precision and empirical relevance.

INTERVENING VARIABLES. Certain concepts cannot be measured by currently available techniques (e.g., the earth's core and biochemical processes in memory). Also, internal or organismic processes which connect observable phenomena may not themselves be observable and must be inferred or invented until such time as they can be observed. These unobservables, often referred to as mediating structures or processes, are necessary in all phases of theory construction. Two types of concepts, intervening variables and hypothetical constructs, deal with these mediating factors; their similarities and differences are worthy of note.

An *intervening variable* is a concept which represents a guess regarding an unobserved mediating process which may account for an observed event. Although they signify an unknown mediating process, intervening variables are defined by and entirely reducible to empirical events. For example, the concept "habit," formulated as an intervening variable, may be defined empirically by the number of trials an individual was given to learn a task, or by the demonstrated speed with which he performs it. Although the term "habit"

implies a residue of experience within the individual, which cannot be observed, its existence is inferred from a *variety of observables,* e.g., the number of opportunities to learn a task or the skill of performance.

There is a similarity between intervening variables and operational definitions in that both are defined by or anchored to empirical phenomena. But they differ in two important respects. First, a *variety* of empirical phenomena may be used to define an intervening variable; in this respect it is less precise than an operational definition. Second, although both intervening variables and operational definitions are anchored to observables, intervening variables always *imply* the existence of a mediating process whereas operational concepts need not.

HYPOTHETICAL CONSTRUCTS. The difference between an intervening variable and a hypothetical construct is largely a matter of degree. *Hypothetical constructs* are admittedly speculative concepts which are formulated without explicit reference to observable phenomena. Their freedom from specific empirical referents distinguishes them from intervening variables. Because they are not defined or anchored to observable events, their use in theory often is questioned. Clarity gets muddled and deductions often are tautological when psychological data are "explained" in terms of a series of hypothetical constructs. For example, statements such as "the mechanisms of the ego are blocked in the anal-character when libidinous energies are dammed up by super-ego introjections," are, at best, puzzling. Postulating connections between one set of hypothetical constructs and another leads to facile but often meaningless "explanations." Such use results in imprecise formulations which are difficult to decipher because we cannot specify observables by which they can be anchored or evaluated.

Vagueness and surplus-meaning are both the weakness and strength of the hypothetical construct. A theory is a human artifact; not every concept of a theory should be linked to empirical events since the purpose of a theory is to extend the range of our knowledge. Moreover, unrealistic standards of empirical anchorage in the early stages of theory construction may discourage the kind of imaginative speculation necessary to decipher elusive and obscure phenomena. Vague and risky as hypothetical constructs may be, they often are necessary tools in the development of a productive theory.

Correspondence Rules. Even if all the terms of a theory were empirically anchored and precise, something further would have to be added to indicate how these terms are combined and related to one another. Without a set of rules by which its concepts are integrated, a theory lacks internal coherence and its function as a tool for explaining and predicting empirical events is hampered markedly. Many labels have been coined for this linkage or correspondence system; it has often been referred to as the *syntax* of a theory because of its similarity to the rules of grammar.

These rules serve as deductive procedures by which theoretical concepts are arranged or combined to provide new inferences or insights about empirical relations. They give a theory a coherent system of interlocking channels through which diverse facts may be related and derived. For example, the calculational rules of mathematics are frequently used in science as inferential principles which guide the manipulation of concepts and their subsequent derivation into empirical hypotheses. When formulated logically and explicitly, correspondence rules provide tremendous power for systematizing experience and generating research hypotheses.

Hypotheses. Correspondence rules in psychopathological theories are usually loose and imprecise, if formulated at all. As a consequence, hypotheses, that is, provisional explanations which are stated as predictions about empirical relationships, are rarely derived rigorously from the correspondence rules of a theory. In most undeveloped sciences, hypotheses are formulated as a result of perceptive observations and intuitive hunches.

Whether hypotheses are rigorously derived or intuitively conjectured, it is important that their final form be translatable into empirical terms. We must recall that the ultimate goal of a theory is the development of empirical laws. Such laws develop not only through ingenious speculation or derivation, but also by factual *confirmation*. Unless a hypothesis can be translated into a specific empirical test, its validity cannot be confirmed.

Our discussion has presented a condensation of relatively conventional notions about the structure of theory as formulated by logicians and philosophers of science. Most students may be unacquainted with these terms and may have found them difficult to grasp or see in perspective. Greater clarity may be obtained by reference to Figure 1 which summarizes these notions and their interrelationships in pictorial fashion. Although the serious student would do well to obtain a thorough grounding in these fundamental elements of theory, a sophisticated understanding is not essential to follow the major ideas presented later in the text.

Criteria for Evaluating Theories

Theories arise typically from the perceptive observations and imaginative speculations of a creative scientist. This innovator is usually quite aware of the limits and deficiences of his "invention" and is disposed in the early stages of his speculation to modify it as he develops new observations and insights. Unfortunately, after its utility has been proven in a modest and limited way, the theory frequently acquires a specious stature. Having clarified certain ambiguities and survived initial criticisms, it begins to accumulate a coterie of disciples. These less creative thinkers tend to accept the theory wholeheartedly and espouse its superior explanatory powers and terminology throughout the scientific marketplace. They hold to its propositions tenaciously and defend it blindly and unequivocally against opposition. In time, it becomes a rigid and sacred dogma and, as a result, authority replaces the test of utility and empirical validity. Intelligent men become religious disciples; their theory is a doctrine of "truth," not a guide to the unknown.

Should we avoid theories knowing their frequent fate? The answer, of course, is no! Man will interpret his experience through either implicit or formal theories, regardless of the dangers and assumptions involved. Rather than dismissing theories as inevitable "religious doctrines," we should formulate criteria by which we can evaluate their genuine utility. There are several grounds upon which theories may be evaluated.

Simplicity and Parsimony. Many theories are shrouded in a dense cloak of words and concepts. Their structure

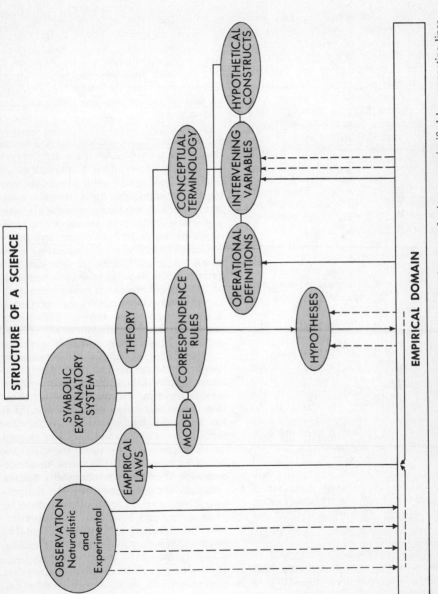

Figure 1. Structure of a science. Relationships among the elements of science are signified by connecting lines and arrows. Dotted lines denote a less formal or more imprecise relationship; straight lines indicate greater precision or formality.

is so opaque that assumptions may be concealed, principles may be difficult to extract, and consistent connections to the empirical world may be impossible to establish. In short, the structure of the theory is formulated more complexly than necessary.

The criteria of simplicity and parsimony require that a theory depend on a minimum number of assumptions and a minimum number of concepts. Alone, these criteria neither eliminate theoretical opaqueness nor verify the utility of a theory's propositions; they merely suggest that excess baggage be eliminated so that the central features of the theory can be seen more clearly. Theorists who prefer to formulate their ideas in a complex network of concepts and assumptions must carry the burden of proving the necessity of these components. Excess baggage invites only trouble and confusion.

Generality. Ideally, the number and extent of facts and data to which a theory may be generalized should not be limited. So comprehensive a system is, of course, neither feasible nor possible. However, many theories are constructed in their early stages to cover only the limited data from which they were generated; this first formulation often restricts its long-range or potential applicability. It is preferable, therefore, that the format and concepts of a theory be broad enough in scope to be extended to new data, should an elaboration be justified. Implicit in the criterion of generality, therefore, is the suggestion that the value of a theory may be gauged by its ability to generate new observations *after* its initial formulation. Despite the importance of this feature, it is wise to recognize that a disparity will exist between the *potential* range of a theory's applicability and its *actual* range of empirical support. Failure to keep this disparity in mind can lead only to erroneous generalizations.

Empirical Precision. The need to coordinate the concepts of a theory with observable data leads us to the criterion of empirical precision. The empirical criterion refers to the extent to which concepts can be anchored to assigned properties in the observable world; precision refers to the number of empirical phenomena to which each of these theoretical terms is connected. A problem arises when one attempts to balance the criterion of generality, already mentioned, with the criterion of empirical precision. How does one maintain empirical specificity, and thereby minimize ambiguity in language, while simultaneously freeing concepts to include a wide range of phenomena?

The frequent use of *intervening variables* in psychological theory results from the fact that each of these variables may be anchored to a variety of different empirical phenomena. By allowing a number of empirical events to be included in one concept, theorists may approach an ideal compromise between the criterion of generality, on the one hand, and explicitness, on the other.

Hypothetical constructs do not fulfill the empirical criterion; nevertheless, they often are necessary in the early stages of theory construction. Explanations of complex and unobservable processes may be either impossible or extremely cumbersome without them. Ultimately, hypothetical constructs should be coordinated to the empirical domain and transformed gradually into intervening variables. In general, then, theoretical concepts should be as precise and empirical as the current state of a field permits.

Derivable Consequences. Propositions or hypotheses may be derived by the systematic manipulation of several concepts in accordance with a series of correspondences rules. Unfortunately, these rules are either nonexistent or formulated imprecisely in most psychopathological theories. Because of this limitation, hypotheses derived from these theories must be evaluated carefully. After-the-fact "hypotheses" or "predictions" stated so imprecisely as to allow for different or even contradictory results must be avoided. When interrelationships among concepts are left ambiguous, the temptation arises to make "predictions" after the facts have been observed. The "prediction" is dressed up into an acceptable propositional form and then presented as a verification of the theory when, in fact, contradictory results could have also been "predicted" by the theory. The need for caution is clear: confidence in a theory's "predictions" must be restrained until the empirical hypotheses of a theory are unequivocal and genuinely predictive.

Orientation of Theories

Theories are designed as a guide to the discovery of empirical laws. Theories have a bias or *orientation* as to what kinds of laws should be sought, what empirical phenomenon should be observed, and what procedure should be used to observe these phenomena. This orientation consists, either implicitly or explicitly, of decisions made on such issues as whether to: (1) seek laws about the "unique" pattern of each individual's functioning *or* about commonalities among characteristics found in all individuals; (2) obtain data under rigorously controlled experimental procedures *or* in the settings within which events naturally occur; and (3) observe biophysical *or* intrapsychic *or* phenomenological *or* behavioral phenomena.

The data and laws produced by a theory will reflect decisions on each of these issues. Although each of the alternatives noted is a potentially fruitful approach in search of empirical laws, theorists engage in intense debates as to which of these approaches is best; the poor student wastes needless hours in trying to decide which "side" is correct. It is important to recognize at the outset that different theories ask different questions, use different procedures, and focus on different types of data. There is no "correct" choice; no rules exist in nature to tell us which methods are best or which laws are most important.

Unfortunately, the orientations of most theories are not explicit. As a result, the student is presented with a fantastic array of overlapping data and concepts which appear disconnected and contradictory and leave him dazzled and confused. Without differences in orientation clearly in mind, the student is like the young Talmudic scholar who, after immersing himself for weeks in ancient manuscripts, rose suddenly one morning, danced joyously in the streets, and shouted, "I have found the most wonderful answer; somebody please tell me the question!"

To make sense and give order to the data of his science, the student must know what kinds of laws each theory seeks to find. Only then can he construct meaning and coherence in his studies. With the goals of each theory clearly before him, he may separate them according to the laws they wish to find and compare them intelligently as to their success in answering the questions they pose in common. It should be obvious that theories seeking biochemical laws cannot be compared to theories seeking behavioral laws. And theories seeking causal sequences between past and present events should not be compared to theories seeking correlations among present events, and so on.

The student might ask at this point why different kinds of theories are needed. Cannot one theory encompass all that need be known in psychopathology? For the time being, at least, the answer must be no! At this stage of our knowledge, theories must serve as instruments to answer particular rather than universal questions. The clinician in the consulting room needs a different kind of theory to facilitate his understanding of verbal therapeutic interaction from that needed by the psychopharmacologist, who seeks to discover the effects of biochemical properties.

Recapitulating then, theories differ not only in their models, concepts, and derivation rules, but also in their orientation. This orientation is composed essentially of decisions made on three basic issues: the idiographic *or* the nomothetic approach; the experimental *or* the naturalistic approach; and different approaches in the level of data observed and conceptualized. We shall discuss next each of these three sets of alternatives.

Idiographic and Nomothetic Approaches. Some theorists seek generalizations which will hold for many individuals, whereas others are interested in the pattern with which characteristics combine within single individuals.

Typically, scientists study a specific class of phenomena until some regularity or uniformity is found which characterizes all phenomena of that class. This method, known as the *nomothetic* orientation, overlooks minor or individual variations in its search for laws common to a specific class of phenomena. Many kinds of *nomothetic* laws will be found, however, to characterize a complex organism such as man. These laws may themselves be combined in many ways; the number of combinations possible may, in fact, be infinite. The pattern with which nomothetic laws combine in particular individuals has been referred to as the *idiographic* orientation. In contrast to the nomothetic theorist, who searches for laws common to people in general, the idiographic theorist attempts to combine these laws into distinctive patterns which reflect the "uniqueness" of individuality. Both approaches ultimately are needed for scientific progress.

Nevertheless, a vigorous debate has arisen in the literature as to which approach will be "most fruitful" to the study of psychopathology (Beck, 1953; Eysenck, 1954).

The issue of "fruitfulness" depends, of course, on one's personal predilections and the immediate goals one has in mind. In this regard, the nomothetic theorist usually is a basic laboratory scientist divorced from the pressing problems which the idiographic theorist faces in his typical activity of treating disturbed individuals. Away from the complexity of the whole person, the nomothetic theorist can pursue the search for basic general laws in a rigorous and systematic fashion. In contrast, the clinician, faced with the practical problems of distressed individuals, must find ways to "piece together" the unique set of experiences which have combined to create their problems. He cannot wait for the slow accumulation of group laws by nomothetic theorists because of his immediate needs and concerns. He must now discover laws which will enable him to make sense out of the pattern of experience of a particular individual.

Given the paucity of empirical laws in psychopathology, there need be no argument as to which approach is "most fruitful"; both are fully justified. What is unjustified are contentions that one approach alone is sufficient.

Experimental and Naturalistic Approaches. Scientists accept the principle of multiple determination, that is, that events do not result from random and isolated causes, but from an orderly and lawful sequence of complex influences. A problem facing the theorist concerns the settings and methods by which he will be able to trace the sequence and strands of these multiple determinants. Two solutions have been developed: (1) the classical experimental approach which stresses the manipulation and control of variables and seeks to establish the precise sequence of cause-effect relationships and (2) the naturalistic approach by which several variables are observed in their natural or real settings and then correlated in accord with the patterns of interaction.

In the experimental method, as borrowed from classical physics, the scientist selects certain variables which he considers basic and then manipulates them in a specially arranged setting that is less complex than the one in which they naturally function. This allows him to observe the precise consequences of one set of variables upon another. Its virtue is that the contaminating or obscuring effects of irrelevant variables are removed or under tight control. Hopefully, unequivocal conclusions may be drawn about causal effects or functional relationships.

Two objections have been raised against the experimental approach: controlled settings often are artificial, and the number and nature of variables which can be studied in this fashion are limited. These objections do not apply to the naturalistic approach. In this method the scientist analyzes a complex of naturally interacting variables without intervening controls or manipulations. Cronbach describes this approach in the following (1957):

> The method, for its part, can study what man has not learned to control or can never hope to control. Nature has been experimenting since the beginning of time, with a boldness and complexity far beyond the resources of science. The . . . mission is to observe and organize the data from Nature's experiments.

Proponents of the naturalistic approach point out that experimentally oriented scientists often control or eliminate factors which should not be excluded or ignored. What does one do, they ask, when crucial variables which must be explored cannot be manipulated experimentally? To abandon an investigation because variables cannot be controlled in a classical experiment design seems foolish and may not be necessary if these variables operate in real life settings. The distinguished psychologist, Raymond Cattell, commented on this problem in this statement (1965):

> The . . . laboratory method, with its isolation of the single process, has worked well in the older sciences, but where total organisms have to be studied, the theoretical possibility must be faced that one can sometimes hope to find a law only if the total organism is included in the observations and experiences—not just a bit of its behavior.
> The fact that he can study behavior in its natural setting means that he can deal with emotionally important matters and real personality learning. Neither our ethics, nor the self-protectiveness of people themselves, will stand for psychologists giving subjects major emotional shocks or altering their whole personalities for a laboratory thesis.
> An experimenter exactly following the classical experimental design, but who happened to be a moral imbecile, might with cold logic and force of habit set out to find the effect

upon the personality of a mother of losing a child. Furthermore, he would need to "out-Herod Herod" by removing the child in half the cases, and continuing with the child in the other half of his 'controlled experiment.' Since life itself inevitably makes these tragic 'experiments,' a researcher . . . will simply compare mothers who have and have not suffered such bereavement and make his analysis of the result 'balancing' for things he cannot manipulate.

There are two methods which utilize the naturalistic approach: one is essentially intuitive and qualitative; the other is objective and quantitative. The first approach uses the data of case histories, clinical observations, and interviews; data obtained with these methods are subject to the pitfalls of memory and to the observational and inferential skills of the clinician. Although brilliant insights often have been derived in this fashion, they tend to be loosely formulated and invariably nonquantitative. More systematic and quantitative are methods which apply the technique of correlational statistics. These procedures have been referred to as multivariate methods by Cattell, who wrote (1965):

. . .the multivariate method is actually the same as in the clinical method, but it is quantitative and follows explicit calculations of laws and general conclusions. For the clinician appraises the total pattern by eye and tries to make generalizations from a good memory, whereas the multivariate experimenter actually measures all the variables and may then set an electronic computer to abstract the regularities which exist, instead of depending on human powers of memory and generalization.

In conclusion then, we may note that the experimental approach seeks to control contaminating influences and to establish precise causal connections between a limited number of variables. When complex interactions exist, or when crucial variables cannot be manipulated or controlled, the naturalistic approach may be fruitfully utilized. Both can contribute to the search for empirical laws in psychopathology.

Levels of Observation and Conceptualization. A major source of confusion for students stems from their difficulty in recognizing the existence of different levels of scientific observation and conceptualization.

As indicated earlier, the basic scientist approaches his subject somewhat differently than the practitioner. No conflict need rise. Psychopathology can be studied from many vantage points; it can be observed and conceptualized in legitimately different ways by behaviorists, phenomenologists, psychodynamicists, and biochemists. No point of observation or conceptualization alone is sufficient to encompass all of the complex and multidimensional features of psychopathology. Processes may be described in terms of conditioned habits, reaction formations, cognitive expectancies, or neurochemical dysfunctions. These levels of conceptualization cannot be arranged in a hierarchy, with one level viewed as reducible to another. Nor can they be compared in terms of some "objective truth value." These alternative levels of approach merely are different; they make possible the observation and conceptualization of different types of data and lead, therefore, to different theories and different empirical laws.

Theories are best differentiated according to the kinds of data they elect to conceptualize. These choices are purely pragmatic, and questions of comparative utility should be asked only of theories which deal with the same kinds of data. Data are the basic ingredients for concepts and for the theories which coordinate these concepts. Irrelevant controversies and confusions are avoided if the conceptual level or the kinds of data to which they refer are specified clearly. When this is done properly, the student and researcher can determine whether two concepts are comparable, whether the same conceptual label refers to different data, whether different theories apply to the same data, and so on.

There are many ways in which the subject matter of psychopathology can be differentiated according to "data levels." L'Abate (1964) has proposed levels of integration, interpretation, functioning, and development, whereas Ford and Urban (1963) have organized them in terms of degree of accessibility, order of abstraction, and hierarchical structure.

What classification scheme of levels will serve our purposes best?

The major historical traditions in psychopathology suggest a particularly useful basis for us to follow, and one which corresponds closely to the major orientations in psychopathology today. These contemporary orientations not only reflect relatively distinct historical traditions, but, perhaps more importantly, also differ in the kinds of data they conceptualize. For example, followers in the tradition of psychiatric medicine focus upon the *biophysical* substrate of pathology; those within the psychodynamic tradition of psychiatry deal with unconscious *intrapsychic* processes; theorists within the clinical-personology tradition often are concerned with conscious *phenomenological* experience; those in the academic-experimental tradition attend primarily to overt *behavioral* data; and those in the sociological-anthropological tradition are oriented to *sociocultural* data. These levels—biophysical, intrapsychic, phenomenological, behavioral and sociocultural—reflect, therefore, both different sources of data and the major theoretical orientations in psychopathology.

Scientists who are preoccupied with only a small segment of the field often have little knowledge of the work of others. Intent on a narrow approach to the subject, they lose sight of perspective, and their respective contributions are scattered and disconnected. What is needed today is a syntheses in which divergent elements of knowledge are brought together to be seen as parts of an integrated whole. Until a psychological Newton or Einstein comes along, however, the student must do the next best thing: develop an attitude by which the various branches and levels of psychopathology are viewed as an interrelated, if not an integrated, unit. He must learn the language and orientation of each of the major approaches as if they were all parts of an indivisible piece. Until such time as a bridge is created to coordinate each theory and level of approach to the others, no one theory or approach should be viewed as all-embracing, or accepted to the exclusion of others. A multiplicity of viewpoints must prevail.

Any discussion of psychopathological theory should bring us to the question of defining psychopathology. It should be obvious from the foregoing that no single definition is possible. Psychopathology will be defined in terms of the theory one employs. An idiographically oriented theorist who emphasizes the importance of phenomenological experience will include uniqueness and self-discomfort in his definition of psychopathology; a biochemical theorist will formulate his definition in terms of biochemical dysfunctions, and so on. In brief, once a particular

level and theory has been adopted, the definition of psychopathology follows logically and inevitably. Clearly, no single definition conveys the wide range of observations and orientations with which psychopathology may be explored.

Unfortunately, the observations, concepts, and propositions of the various theoretical approaches to psychopathology have not been collected within one cover. At present, no single journal covers all aspects of psychopathology either, nor is there a permanent professional organization which cuts across disciplinary lines on a regular basis. To fill this void is a monumental task and far beyond the scope of this book. At best, we hope to provide a brief panoramic view of these approaches and, hopefully, convey certain essential features.

In the following sections we will specify the major levels of theoretical analysis in greater detail. This will provide us with a picture of which data a theory has judged significant to its purposes and which it has de-emphasized. By arranging contemporary theories according to level of data observation and conceptualism, we shall be able to understand better the variety of definitions of psychopathology which have been developed. From this basis also, we should have a sound foundation for comparing the varied concepts and explanatory propositions which have been formulated regarding the development and modification of psychopathology.

References

Beck, S. J. The science of personality: nomothetic or idiographic? *Psychol. Rev.,* 1953, *60,* 353–359.

Cattell, R. B. *The Scientific Analysis of Personality,* Baltimore: Penguin Books, 1965.

Cronbach, L. J. The two disciplines of scientific psychology, *Amer. Psychol.,* 1957, *12,* 671–684.

Eysenck, H. J. The science of personality: nomothetic, *Psychol. Rev.,* 1954, *61,* 339–342.

Ford, D., and Urban, H. *Systems of Psychotherapy,* New York: Wiley, 1963.

Hebb, D. O. Alice in Wonderland, or psychology among the biological sciences. In Harlow, H., and Woolsey, C. (editors). *Biological and Biochemical Basis of Behavior,* Wisconsin: University of Wisconsin Press, 1958.

L'Abate, L. *Principles of Clinical Psychology,* New York: Grune and Stratton, 1964.

Part I

Biophysical
Theories

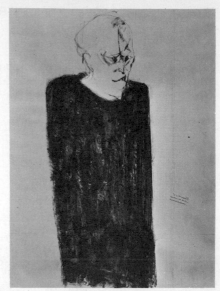

Jose Luis Cuevas—*Madman* (1954). (The Museum of Modern Art, New York, Inter-American Fund.)

INTRODUCTION

Theories at this level assume that biophysical defects and deficiencies in anatomy, physiology, and biochemistry are the primary determinants of psychopathology. According to this view, biophysical data should serve as the basis for the conceptualization of psychopathology, and biophysical methods should be the primary instruments for therapy.

Ample evidence from medical science exists to justify this biophysical "disease" model. It may be illustrated in physical medicine by infections, genetic errors, obstructions, inflammations, or other insults to normal functioning which manifest themselves overtly as fevers, fatigue, headaches, and so on. Certainly, significant progress was made in physical medicine when it shifted its focus from surface symptomatology to the biophysical disruptions which underlie them. Extending this model to psychopathology, one sees that these theorists believe that biophysical defects or deficiencies ultimately will be found for such "surface" symptoms as bizarre behavior, feelings of anguish, or maladaptive interpersonal relations. The major difference they see between psychological and biophysical disorders is that the former, affecting the central nervous system, manifests itself primarily in behavioral and social symptoms, whereas the latter, affecting other organ systems, manifests itself in physical symptoms.

Biophysical Theories:
ORIENTATION

Although the history of the disease model may be traced first to the speculations of Hippocrates and later to the formulations of William Greisinger in mid-nineteenth century Germany, it is the writings of Emil Kraepelin and Eugen Bleuler at the turn of this century which provided the modern foundations of the medical orientation. Kraepelin, designer of a major nosological system of diagnosis still in vogue today despite vigorous and justified criticisms, contended that all psychotic states stemmed from neurological or metabolic diseases. He briefly outlines the rationale of his position in the paper presented here and then turns to what he may be best remembered for, his ability to describe with clarity the overt clinical characteristics of his patients. Bleuler, despite his flirtation with psychological interpretations, holds fast to his belief, in the paper presented, that overt behavioral features of schizophrenia are merely surface expressions of physiological defects.

1. Clinical Psychiatry[*]

EMIL KRAEPELIN

The subject of the following course of lectures will be the Science of Psychiatry, which, as its name implies, is that of the treatment of mental disease. It is true that, in the strictest terms, we cannot speak of the mind as becoming diseased, whether we regard it as a separate entity or as the sum total of our subjective experience. And, indeed, from the medical point of view, it is disturbances in the *physical foundations* of mental life which should occupy most of our attention. But the incidents of such diseases are generally seen in the sphere of psychical events, a department with which the art of medicine has dealt very little as yet. Here we are not so much concerned with physical changes in size, shape, firmness, and chemical composition, as with disturbances of comprehension, memory and judgment, illusions, hallucinations, depression, and morbid changes in the activity of the will. With the help of the ideas you have derived from general pathology, you will usually be able to find your way in a new department of medicine without any serious difficulty. But here you will be utterly perplexed at first by the essentially peculiar phenomena of disease with which you will meet, until you have gradually learned to a certain extent to master the special symptomatology of mental disturbances. Of course, you will sometimes have met with isolated conditions of mental disease in everyday life, or in other hospitals—intoxication, fever delirium, and delirium tremens, or even imbecility and idiocy—but they may have impressed you more as strange and incomprehensible curiosities than as adding to your stock of medical ideas.

Insanity works a change in the mental personality, that sum of characteristics which, to our minds, represents a man's real being in a far higher degree than his physical peculiarities. Hence, our patient's whole relation to the out-

*Excerpted from lectures given at Heidelberg University, 1902.

14

side world is affected in the most comprehensive way. The knowledge of all these disturbances is a fruitful field for the investigation of mental life, not only revealing many of its universal laws, but also giving a deep insight into the history of the development of the human mind, both in the individual and in the race. It also provides us with the proper scale for comprehending the numerous intellectual, moral, religious, and artistic currents and phenomena of our social life.

But it is not these variously branching scientific relations to so many of the most important questions of human existence which make a knowledge of psychical disturbances indispensable to the physician; it is rather their extraordinary *practical importance*. Insanity, even in its mildest forms, involves the greatest suffering that physicians have to meet. Only a comparatively small percentage of mental cases are permanently and completely cured in the strictest sense of the word. And the number of the insane, which will hardly be exaggerated if we estimate it as amounting at the present moment to 200,000 in Germany alone, is apparently increasing with the most unfortunate rapidity. This increase may depend, to a great extent, on our fuller knowledge of insanity, on the more highly-developed care of the insane, and on the increasing difficulty of treating them at home, and so may be only apparent. But, considering that from one-quarter to one-third of the cases admitted to our asylums are due to the abuse of alcohol or to syphilitic infection, and that these causes of which the extension is certainly not diminishing, we cannot but suppose that the number of the insane is increasing, not only in itself, but also in its proportion to the population. The growing degeneration of our race in the future may therefore still be left an open question, but certainly it might be very greatly promoted by both these causes.

All the insane are dangerous, in some degree, to their neighbours, and even more so to themselves. Mental derangement is the cause of at least a third of the total number of suicides, while sexual crimes and arson, and, to a less extent, dangerous assaults, thefts, and impostures are often committed by those whose minds are diseased. Numberless families are ruined by their afflicted members, either by the senseless squandering of their means, or because long illness and inability to work have gradually sapped the power of caring for a household. Only a certain number of those who do not recover succumb at once. The greater part live on for dozens of years, imbecile and helpless, imposing a heavy and yearly increasing burden on their families and communities, of which the effects strike deeply into our national life.

For all these reasons, it is one of the physician's most important duties to make himself, as far as possible, acquainted with the nature and phenomena of insanity. Even though the limits of his power against this mighty adversary are very narrow, opportunity enough is afforded to every practical physician to contribute his share to the prevention and alleviation of the endless misery annually engendered by mental disease. Alcoholism and syphilis undoubtedly offer the most profitable points of attack, together with the abuse of morphia and cocaine, which so clearly owes its fatal significance to the action of medical men. Family physicians, again, can often help to prevent the marriage of the insane, or of those who are seriously threatened with insanity, and to secure a proper education and choice of occupation for children predisposed to disease. But it will be their special province to recognize dangerous symptoms in time, and, by their prompt action, to prevent suicides and accidents, and obviate the short-sighted procrastination which only too often keeps patients from coming under the care of an expert alienist until the time for practically useful treatment has long been past. Even in those numerous cases which never become insane in the narrower sense, the physician who has been trained in alienism will have such an understanding of the recognition and treatment of psychical disturbances as will amply repay him for the trouble of his years of study. Even in my own experience it has happened very often that older physicians have regretted their defective knowledge of alienism, and complained that it was only in practical life that they learned how great a part is played, in the daily round of ordinary medical practice, by the correct diagnosis of more or less morbid mental incidents. I need hardly mention that, for various reasons, such a diagnosis is in constant demand by public authorities, courts of law, and trade societies.

Of course, an intimate knowledge of Psychiatry, as of every other separate branch of medicine, can only be acquired by long and thorough occupation with the subject. Yet, even in a short time, it is possible to cast at least a general and superficial glance over the commonest forms of mental disturbance. Personal investigation and continuous observation of the greatest possible number of different cases are indispensable to this, and it is only too true that, even after one or two terms of zealous clinical study, there will still be many cases which the beginner is unable to interpret correctly by means of the knowledge with which he has been furnished or which he has acquired for himself. But one important advantage to be gained comparatively quickly is a recognition of the great *difficulties* of the subject and the correction of that simpleminded ignorance, still so widely spread, which assumes that even a non-expert may give an opinion on mental cases without any more ado.

Dementia Praecox

The presentation of clinical details in the large domain of dementia praecox meets with considerable difficulties, because a delimitation of the different clinical pictures can only be accomplished artificially. There is certainly a whole series of phases which frequently return, but between them there are such numerous transitions that in spite of all efforts it appears impossible at present to delimit them sharply and to assign each case without objection to a definite form. We shall be obliged therefore, as in paralysis, to content ourselves at first for the sake of a more lucid presentation with describing the course of certain more frequent forms of the malady without attributing special clinical value to this grouping.

As such forms I have hitherto separated from each other a *hebephrenic,* a *catatonic,* and a *paranoid* group of cases. This classification has been frequently accepted with many modifications, specially concerned with the clinical position of the paranoid diseases, as also by Bleuler in his monograph on schizophrenia; he adds, however, to it the insidious 'dementia simplex' as a special form. Räcke has made other attempts at classification; he separates out 'depressive', 'confused ex-

cited', 'stuporous', 'subacute paranoid' forms and a 'catatonia in attacks'. Wieg-Wickenthal differentiates 'dementia simplex', 'hebephrenia' with pseudomanic behaviour, 'depressive paranoid forms' and catatonia.

The undoubted inadequacy of my former classification has led me once more to undertake the attempt to make a more natural grouping, as I have in hand a larger number of possibly more reliable cases. For this purpose there were at my disposal about 500 cases in Heidelberg which had been investigated by myself, in which according to their clinical features, as well as according to the length of the time that had passed, the ultimate issue of the morbid process could be accepted with considerable probability. 'Recovered' cases were not taken into account because of the uncertainty of their significance which still exists, but only such cases as had led to profound dementia or to distinctly marked and permanent phenomena of decreased function. On grounds which will be discussed later, it is, as I believe, not to be assumed that by this choice definite clinical types have quite fallen out of the scope of our consideration; at most a certain displacement in the frequency of the individual forms would be conceivable.

The result of this attempt at a classification agrees in many points with the statements of the above-mentioned investigators. First I also think that I should delimit simple insidious dementia as a special clinical form. Next in the series comes hebephrenia in the narrower sense of silly dementia which was first described by Hecker. A third group is composed of the simple depressive or stuporous forms, a fourth of states of depression with delusions. In a fifth form I have brought together the majority of the clinical cases which go along with conditions of greater excitement; one could speak of an agitated dementia praecox. To it is nearly related the sixth form, which includes essentially the catatonia of Kahlbaum, in which peculiar states of excitement are connected with stupor. A more divergent picture is seen in the seventh and eighth groups, in which the cases are placed which run a paranoid course, according to whether they end in the usual terminal states of dementia praecox or in paranoid, relatively hallucinatory, weak-mindedness. We shall then subject to special consideration the small number of observations which present the remarkable phenomenon of confusion of speech along with perfect sense and fairly reasonable activity.

Dementia Simplex

Simple insidious dementia as it was described by Diem under the name dementia simplex consists in an *impoverishment and devastation of the whole psychic life which is accomplished quite imperceptibly*. The disease begins usually in the years of sexual development, but often the first slight beginnings can be traced back into childhood. On the other hand Pick has also described a 'primary progressive dementia of adults', but it is certainly very doubtful whether it may be grouped with dementia praecox. In our patients a deterioration of mental activity becomes very gradually noticeable. The former good, perhaps distinguished scholar, fails always more conspicuously in tasks which till then he could carry out quite easily, and he is more and more outstripped by his companions. He appears absentminded, thoughtless, makes incomprehensible mistakes, cannot any longer follow the teaching rightly, does not reach the standard of the class. While pure exercises of memory are perhaps still satisfactory, a certain poverty of thought, weakness of judgement and incoherence in the train of ideas appear always more distinctly. Many patients try by redoubled efforts to compensate for the results of their mental falling off, which is at first attributed by parents and teachers to laziness and want of good will. They sit the whole day over their work, learn by heart with all their might, sit up late at night, without being able to make their work any better. Others become idle and indifferent, stare for hours at their books without reading, give themselves no trouble with their tasks, and are not incited either by kindness or severity.

Hand in hand with this decline of mental activity there is a change of temperament, which often forms the first conspicuous sign of the developing malady. The patients become depressed, timid, lachrymose, or impertinent, irritable, malicious; sometimes a certain obstinate stubbornness is developed. The circle of their interests becomes narrower; their relations to their companions become cold; they show neither attachment nor sympathy. Not infrequently a growing estrangement towards parents and brothers and sisters becomes noticeable. The patients remain indifferent to whatever happens in the family circle, shut themselves up, limit the contact with their relatives to the least possible. Bleuler brings forward here as a frequent explanation the 'Œdipus complex', the concealed sexual inclination to one of the parents and the jealous emotions which arise from it. I consider that the generalization of that kind of case, which is certainly very rare, as belonging to the system of Freud, is wholly without foundation. It seems much more natural to me to explain the antagonism to relatives by the gloomy feeling of inferiority and the defiant resistance to it, but above all by the common experience that for a long time it has been the habit of the relatives to trace the morbid phenomena back to a moral offence, and to meet them with painful reprimands and measures. Similar antagonism is also seen quite commonly to develop in the relations with degenerate, wayward children.

Ambition and pleasure in the usual games and occasional occupations become extinct; wishes and plans for the future are silent; inclination and ability for useful occupation disappear. The patient has neither endurance nor understanding, works confusedly, begins everything the wrong way about, tries as far as possible to withdraw himself from claims on him. He remains lying in bed for days, sits about anywhere, trifles away his time in occupations of no value, devours perhaps without choice and without understanding chance and unsuitable literature, lives one day at a time without a plan. A few patients have indeed at times a certain feeling of the change, which takes place in them, often in hypochondriacal colouring; but the majority sink into dullness without being in any way sensible of it. Sometimes a certain restlessness is shown which causes the patient to take extended walks, to run away without any plan, to undertake aimless journeys. Alcohol is for him a special danger, he gives way to its temptations without resistance, and then very rapidly comes down in the world, and comes into conflict with public order and criminal law. That happens the more easily as many patients are very sensitive to intoxicating drinks.

Manic-Depressive Disease

Manic-depressive insanity, as it is to be described in this section, includes on the one hand the whole domain of so-called *periodic and circular insanity,* on the other hand *simple mania*, the greater part of the morbid states termed *melancholia* and also a not inconsiderable number of cases of *amentia* (confusional or delirious insanity). Lastly, we include here certain slight and slightest colourings of *mood*, some of them periodic, some of them continuously morbid, which on the one hand are to be regarded as the rudiment of more severe disorders, on the other hand pass over without sharp boundary into the domain of *personal predisposition.* In the course of the years I have become more and more convinced that all the above-mentioned states only represent manifestations of a *single morbid process*. It is certainly possible that later a series of subordinate forms may be described, or even individual small groups again entirely separated off. But if this happens, then according to my view those symptoms will most certainly not be authoritative, which hitherto have usually been placed in the foreground.

What has brought me to this position is first the experience that notwithstanding manifold external differences certain *common fundamental features* yet recur in all the morbid states mentioned. Along with changing symptoms, which may appear temporarily or may be completely absent, we meet in all forms of manic-depressive insanity a quite definite, narrow group of disorders, though certainly of very varied character and composition. Without any one of them being absolutely characteristic of the malady, still in association they impress a uniform stamp on all the multiform clinical states. If one is conversant with them, one will in the great majority of cases be able to conclude in regard to any one of them that it belongs to the large group of forms of manic-depressive insanity by the peculiarity of the condition, and thus to gain a series of fixed points for the special clinical and prognostic significance of the case. Even a small part of the course of the disease usually enables us to arrive at this decision, just as in paralysis or dementia praecox the general psychic change often enough makes possible the diagnosis of the fundamental malady in its most differnet phases.

Of perhaps still greater significance

than the classification of states by definite fundamental disorders is the experience that all the morbid forms brought together here as a clinical entity, *not only pass over the one into the other without recognizable boundaries, but that they may even replace each other in one and the same case*. On the one side, as will be later discussed in more detail, it is fundamentally and practically quite impossible to keep apart in any consistent way simple, periodic and circular cases; everywhere there are gradual transitions. But on the other side we see in the same patient not only mania and melancholia, but also states of the most profound confusion and perplexity, also well developed delusions, and lastly, the slightest fluctuations of mood alternating with each other. Moreover, permanent, one-sided colourings of mood very commonly form the background on which fully developed circumscribed attacks of manic-depressive insanity develop.

A further common bond which embraces all the morbid types brought together here and makes the keeping of them apart practically almost meaningless, is their *uniform prognosis*. There are indeed slight and severe attacks which may be of long or short duration, but they alternate irregularly in the same case. This difference is therefore of no use for the delimitation of different diseases. A grouping according to the frequency of the attacks might much rather be considered, which naturally would be extremely welcome to the physician. It appears, however, that here also we have not to do with fundamental differences, since in spite of certain general rules it has not been possible to separate out definite types from this point of view. On the contrary the universal experience is striking, that the attacks of manic-depressive insanity within the delimitation attempted here never lead to profound dementia, not even when they continue throughout life almost without interruption. Usually all morbid manifestations completely disappear; but where that is exceptionally not the case, only a rather slight, peculiar psychic weakness develops, which is just as common to the types here taken together as it is different from dementias in diseases of other kinds.

As a last support for the view here represented of the unity of manic-depressive insanity the circumstance may be adduced, that the various forms which it comprehends may also apparently mutually replace one another in *heredity*. In members of the same family we frequently enough find side by side pronounced periodic or circular cases, occasionally isolated states of ill temper or confusion, lastly very slight, regular fluctuations of mood or permanent conspicuous coloration of disposition. From whatever point of view accordingly the manic-depressive morbid forms may be regarded, from that of aetiology or of clinical phenomena, the course or the issue—it is evident everywhere that here points of agreement exist, which make it possible to regard our domain as a unity and to delimit it from all the other morbid types hitherto discussed. Further experience must show whether and in what directions in this extensive domain smaller sub-groups can be separated from one another.

In the first place the difference of the states which usually make up the disease, presents itself as the most favourable ground of classification. As a rule the disease runs its course in isolated attacks more or less sharply defined from each other or from health, which are either like or unlike, or even very frequently are perfect antitheses. Accordingly we distinguish first of all manic states with the essential morbid symptoms of flight of ideas, exalted mood, and pressure of activity, and *melancholia or depressive states* with sad or anxious moodiness and also sluggishness of thought and action. These two opposed phases of the clinical state have given the disease its name. But besides them we observe also clinical '*mixed forms*', in which the phenomena of mania and melancholia are combined with each other, so that states arise, which indeed are composed of the same morbid symptoms as these, but cannot without coercion be classified either with one or with the other.

2. The Physiogenic and Psychogenic in Schizophrenia

EUGEN P. BLEULER

Since Jung and myself following in Freud's footsteps pointed out, that a great part of the symptomatology of schizophrenia is to be regarded as psychic reaction, and Adolf Meyer at the same time based his well-known theory of the disease on psychic causes, some of us are often inclined to overlook that these psychic mechanisms, as they are known at the present time, do not explain the whole disease. They are only possible, if there is a certain predisposition of the brain and this disposition in schizophrenia seems to be a processive disease.

According to our conception, we can distinguish in schizophrenia, primary and secondary signs. Most of the symptoms described by Kraepelin, such as autism, delusions, illusions of memory, a part of the hallucinations, negativism, stereotypies, mannerisms and most of the catatonic signs, are secondary signs. For the explanation of all these phenomena we have to utilize the mechanisms which are also true for the normal psychology, working on the basis of the primary trouble. We consider as the main primary signs, both certain disorders in affectivity and in associations, which we have described upon other occasions. The disorder in the affectivity is the tendency of the feelings to work independently of each other, instead of working together, which becomes evident, for instance, in the ambivalence, in inadequate affective reactions, simultaneous crying and laughing, and many other observations which occur very frequently in schizophrenics. The associations, on the other hand, are no longer connected by a final aim and frequently deviate from the direction which is given in a normal person by the topic and by the aim of the central thoughts.

The purpose of this paper is to discuss for some forms and some signs in schizophrenia, what and how much can be explained by mere psychological considerations and, on the other hand, to show for what phenomena the psychological explanations are insufficient. There are even symptoms which seem to indicate that there must be physiological lesions.

The psychic mechanism is seen most clearly in paranoid forms. A working man, for instance, would like to earn more, and to be more than he actually is, but he does not get on. Even for a healthy person it is by no means pleasant to think that he himself is to blame for his failures. Everybody first looks elsewhere for the causes of his lack of success. The workman who makes impossible demands, must necessarily come into opposition or into actual conflict with his foreman and fellow-workers. This suggests to him, that these persons grudge him promotion or have given a post to one of their friends, which should have been given to him. Such a suspicion, it is true, can arise in the mind of a healthy person; but when there are primary lesions, when the affects exercise a greater influence on the process of thought than usual, the counter-concepts are suppressed and suspicion becomes more easily conviction. Hence, delusions of persecution occur in many cases. The sick person finds direct fulfillment of his wishes in his delusions. According to the popular saying, even a healthy person believes in what he wishes; but the sick person knows it and actually *is* the founder of a religion.

Some delusions of grandeur ensue, when the thinking process has become so distintegrated or, in general, so illogical that the patient no longer notices the grossest contradictions to reality. This frequently occurs after long years of delusions of persecution. Then he is emperor, Pope, Christ, or even God himself; not only is he going to make inventions, but he actually *has* made them. Here, we can distinctly see how the psychic development of the delusions depends on the progress of the primary lesion.

Perhaps a patient will come to you and first complain of all sorts of paresthesias (neurasthenic state). After a year, possibly he may come again with the same sensations, but now, in spite of all the physician's proofs to the contrary, he draws the conclusion that he is suffering from some grave bodily disease, possibly syphilis, although he has never been infected (hypochondriacal stage). Again, after a long interval, the patient is seen to be in an excited state, inimically disposed towards his surroundings; he knows now that he has enemies who are causing him unpleasurable sensations, by all sorts of machinations; the paresthesias have become proprioceptive hallucinations. He is now in the paranoid stage and decidedly psychotic. The more seriously disturbed thinking-process has drawn quite impossible inferences from the unpleasurable sensations.

In a somewhat different way, the disturbances in thinking are manifested in the case of a woman disappointed in love, who suddenly eliminates the bitter reality, and, in her hallucinations *is* engaged, married, and not infrequently a child is born. Such dream states, in contrast with mere hysterical (mere psychogenic) ones, may last for months at a time. In principle, therefore, they would be a purely psychogenic syndrome. Its schizophrenic basis, however, is clearly shown in several peculiarities; on the basis of them, as a rule, diagnosis can be made rapidly. (Lack of connection and sequence in the patient's stream of talk and in his behavior, etc.)

Psychic reactions on the basis of a morbid disposition, which are at once comprehensible, are the exalted or anxious *excitations to unpleasant events,* and also autism, the withdrawal from the unsatisfying real world into an imaginary one, which offers more to the patient. The mechanism is, therefore, similar to that in neuroses but nearly all of these signify a direct "flight into illness," and this is rare in schizophrenic reactions; such reactions stray from the right path and their schizophrenic coloring is possible only if a morbid predisposition is present; and in schizophrenia this predisposition is very clearly seen in disturbances in thought and in feeling. It is not his "complexes" as such which *cause* schizophrenia, but they *shape* the morbid picture. The fundamental disturbances, those of the thinking process and those of affectivity, develop quite independently of disagreeable experiences, from which not one of us is spared. Thus all the difficulties of the European War did not cause any increase in the number of cases of schizophrenia.

For us the alteration of the thinking-process, or, elementarily expressed, of the association, is of special importance, and, as a matter of fact, nearly all the psychogenic symptoms can be derived from it. As far as we can recognize this alteration, it is a dynamic one. Thus, we also see something similar even in those cases in which the power of the train of thought is normally weakened, as in dreams and lack of attention, and in so called mind-wandering. In schizophrenia, it is the highest control which fails where it would be necessary to act, and this again must be referred to a disturbance of the connections of all the individual functions; *for this highest control (Oberleitung) is not a special function of our soul, but the outcome, the integrated summarizing of all the individual functions.*

With this dismemberment of the connections, it is comprehensible that the logical function of thinking is disturbed by affective needs, as it is clearly evident in the example of manic forms.

Although similar association disturbances may also occur under normal circumstances, the schizophrenic thinking seems to be of direct physical origin: It shows itself in no way dependent on psychic influences, but solely on the seriousness of a fundamental process. When the disturbance is particularly severe, in acute mental aberration, catatonia and dyskinesis, it is accompanied as a rule by other symptoms, which we are rightly accustomed to regard as bodily: Raised or lowered temperature, albumen in urine, metabolic disturbances, gnashing of teeth, "Flockenlesen," fainting fits or cramps, not infrequently followed by temporary paresis of the limbs or the language, pupillary disturbances, greatly increased idiomuscular reactions, vasomotor disturbances, edema, somnolence, disturbances of the chemistry of the body, especially of the liver-functions, abnormal protein content in the spinal fluid. In many cases, too, the brain-trouble is demonstrated from the psychic side by the fact, that the confusions and delirium have absolutely the character of the "exogene" as Bonhoeffer designates it. Many cases of stupor, with their general prostration of the elementary psychic functions, conception and train of thought, often point clearly to brain-pressure, and, on autopsy, tense edema of the pia or brain-swelling is found. In the various forms of such deliria, the fundamental similarity of certain symptoms or of the whole picture to other physiogenic conditions, intoxication, fever psychoses, epileptic absences, meningitis, encephalitis cannot be denied, and in all such cases, we also find in the autopsy histological alterations of the brain tissue, which show some uniformity. But in all

chronic cases, too, decreases in the amount of ganglion cells and certain changes in the glia, furnish a proof that we are in presence of a brain lesion, of course not in the sense that the histological finding is the direct foundation of the primary psychic symptoms; it is merely an *indicator* of the existence of brain lesions, which, on the one hand, express themselves as psychic, and on the other hand as anatomical. Chronic histological findings always correspond with the clinical chronic picture, and acute changes, with acute ones. Organic symptoms are also the hyperkinesis and akinesis, which are likewise found in various diseases of the basal ganglia.

In contrast to encephalitis, affectivity in schizophrenia is not destroyed, but is, in some way, hampered in expression. Affective impulses which are in no way psychically perceptible, can be demonstrated in the psychogalvanic experiment, and the affects can again appear if a catatonic patient becomes senile, or if he is analyzed according to Freud's methods. Yet, we always obtain the impression that the affectivity is also primarily altered, but by no means in the sense of a simple destruction of all feelings as it was formerly believed.

In the case of hallucinations, we have already mentioned the excitatory states of the proprioceptive apparatus; but there are still other hallucinations which are to be attributed to a physiologic excitation of the nervous system; viz., the various kinds of a photopsia, the sensations of threads, the majority of animal visions, musical hallucinations. With respect to the latter category, it must be added that also purely psychogenic animal visions appear, but in every case, these are animals with sexual significance which are evolved from erotic complexes. Music is also heard in states of ecstasy which can be wholly, or in part, psychogenic and hysteriform.

Although we may register theoretically the majority of symptoms with great certitude, as physical or psychic, conditions in the clinical picture are often very complicated. There are catatonic spells of a purely physical, and others of a purely psychogenic nature, but when a certain psychogenic dulling of the consciousness is present, the spell may be brought about by something in connection with this disposition, which spell must then, naturally, have the commingled signs of both origins. Or a physiogenic spell increases the disintegration of the association so that the complex-tendencies, which are constantly present, can now manifest themselves by means of symptoms. The cause of the spell is physical, but the psychic symptomatology reveals the hidden complexes. Thus, it is the whole disease, and most distinctly with its acute exacerbations.

A girl is disappointed in love and has a catatonic episode. It is supposed that the disappointment is the cause of the episode, but it is only *one* of the causes; perhaps the girl has formerly experienced other equally great disappointments and has overcome them without any ill results. That the present disappointment has such results arises from the fact, that a physical process was already on the way, and when we are able to look more closely, we may find that the so-called falling in love was already a symptom and not the cause of the episode. We consequently see in these cases, too, a complete recovery, and in others, at least a disappearance of delirium, catalepsy or dyskinesis, *without any improvement in the situation*. The more serious the predisposing physical change, the less easily can the psychic causes produce an episode, or, better said, can make it manifest and vice versa. Hence, the physical and psychic symptoms and shades can mingle in all sorts of circumstances.

In *hallucinations*, we see yet other kinds of co-operation of both factors. The lack of control by the dissociation of the individual functions certainly causes the tendency to hear voices; the content, however, is determined by the complexes. Thus, in all states, the voices are the expression and confirmation of the delusions, whilst in acute delirium, it is true, they often follow in their own laws. We have seen above, how the paresthesias are transformed by the disturbance to logic and the need of justifying oneself, into bodily hallucinations, as a consequence of inimical machinations, but a fairly large portion of these same bodily hallucinations are psychogenic in later states.

In this way, the whole illness with its alterations, becomes intelligible. On the whole, schizophrenia seems to be a physical disease with a lingering *course,* which, however, can exacerbate irregularly from some reason unknown to us, into sudden episodes and then get better

again. We then see the physiogenic catatonia and delirium of exogenous character. In principle, they are capable of involution, and, so to speak, all of them really do involute, but some almost to their previous state, whilst others leave behind a more or less pronounced schizophrenic condition, the "secondary dementia" of the older school of psychiatrists. The episodes, with their changing issue, can repeat themselves, and then their psychic residues are often summarized in time into the same grave picture as, in other cases, the first episode has caused, but the same picture can develop quite imperceptibly without an acute attack. Actual chronic states seldom improve to a recovery; chronic catatonic states never.

Theoretically, reactions have to be sharply separated from the episodes, although both forms of exacerbation are in practice not always easily distinguishable from each other, and are prone to mix, but if they are really only psychogenic, they can heal to the earlier state; real deterioration is in connection with the physiogenic process. The prognosis of the psychogenic-physiogenic mixing is dependent on it, however important each of the two components may be in the picture, and then on the unfortunately incalculable capacity for involution of the physiogenic part.

Other not infrequent exacerbations are caused by the manic and the melancholic affective states, which may have quite different significances: a considerable part of these, is a symptom of a manic-depressive psychosis, which mixes with the schizophrenia. Another, belongs to schizophrenia itself, and in addition, there must be other mood-swings whose genesis is not yet exactly known. The affective states, as such, heal. The prognosis, however, becomes less favorable if the physical process exacerbates with the manic or depressive state.

The manifest disease can remain at a standstill in every phase and everything that we can perhaps bring into relation with the acute cell-modifications can involute. I believe, however, that in most cases the standstill of the brain-process permits a considerable psychic recovery, because it is less a deficiency than an intoxication, or the continuance of the process which gives the symptoms their gravity. Such standstills and involutions are often practically identical to a recovery, and many formerly pronounced sick people, are considered to be well, although in such cases the psychiatrist, as a rule, can still discover traces of the illness on closer inspection. *Improvements up to what is practically a recovery do not, therefore, contradict the diagnosis of a schizophrenia.* More for doctrinaire than for real reasons an attempt has been made to include in schizophrenia merely incurable forms. This, however, is contrary to experience. All attempts to separate deteriorating forms from non-deteriorating ones have failed. With its symptoms, as at present known, it cannot be subdivided, although I myself expect that this will be done some day. Out of three apparently like cases, one can deteriorate in a few months; the second only after several years by a new episode; the third not at all.

In acute stages, as already hinted, the purely psychogenic ones pass away without causing any injury. The acute physiogenic episodes are indeed capable of involution, and all of them involute to a certain degree, but in the majority of cases, leave slight, or serious chronic defects behind them. On these, some are purely psychic residues: a patient, for instance, who has a suicidal tendency motivated by schizophrenic depression, although he is no longer depressed, and could easily come to terms with life, now continues to try to commit suicide with the same persistence, but for no reason. Or, if in an acutely delirious state, he tore and soiled his clothing, and cannot refrain from doing so afterwards, nobody knows why. A girl who mixed up various languages and ideas in an incomprehensible confusion, keeps up the tendency by mere force of habit, and for other reasons; e.g., because she is unconsciously afraid to take up life's task again. Other "secondary" states are more closely connected with the expired, but not quite involuted, physical process.

Although a certain number of patients become deteriorated with every treatment, and others improve even in apparently severe cases, the treatment will decide in more than one-third of schizophrenic cases whether they can become social men again or not. Hence, one hospital has many, another, only few cases of improvement. Proper treatment, however, is possible only if it is known, who is accessible to our measures and at what period. Hitherto, we have not been able to

influence the physical process, however many alkaloids and gland extracts we give the patients. In acute cases, we shall, therefore, confine ourselves to expectant treatment, but we shall not trouble the patient with proceedings till the physical process takes a turn for the better; only then, shall we try to bring him back to reality. If he is left to himself, there is great danger that he will withdraw autistically into himself and lose touch with the world. Whether, in the course of a serious illness, an exacerbation occurs, is quite independent of our treatment, but the fact, that a certain patient breaks windows, soils and tears his clothes, cries, fights, *is not determined directly by the process of the disease; it belongs to the psychogenic superstructure, and it is a reaction of his complexes to inner, and particularly to outer experiences.* It is, therefore, possible to influence the patient in his symptoms. He should be made interested in some occupation, or, in grave cases, be so trained that, without his illness being improved, he gives up his bad manners and behaves better. A great deal can be accomplished with skill and patience. With many schizophrenics, not only negativistic ones, however, it is often impossible to get the necessary touch in the ordinary way; a semi-narcosis of 8 or 12 days, with somnifene or another narcotic, may bring about a complete change.

If, however, we do not wish to have all our trouble for nothing, and make the patient rebel against our measures, the right moment must be chosen for these. We must know, above all, when an acute process has so far improved that a good result is possible. Then it may happen that a patient who seemed to be quite deteriorated and was violent and noisy, can be given back to his parents, and behaves himself like a normal person from one minute to the other. We must notice when the patients have really needs to return home. Many patients have a secret animosity towards one or another members of the family; if, at this time, they are sent home, matters will go badly. Hence, we must wait till this attitude has been changed or dismiss them to another place. As the patients themselves are frequently unaware of such conditions, it is a great advantage for the physician to know all the signs that Freud has taught us to observe, which betray the concealed feelings of the patient with greater certainty than their words.

Ladies and gentlemen, no doubt a great many of the facts about which I have just spoken will be known to you: the more, therefore, may I hope for an understanding of those about which I was able only to hint. I hope, however, I have shown you how the exact knowledge of the connections of the symptoms can give us the proper directions for treating our patients and how theoretical science has also a practical utility in this matter.

Biophysical Theories:

ETIOLOGY AND DEVELOPMENT

Few theorists would deny that heredity plays a role in psychopathology, but most would insist that genetic factors can be modified substantially by learning and experience. This moderate view states that heredity operates not as a fixed constant, but as a disposition subject to the circumstances of an individual's upbringing. Franz Kallmann, the most productive genetic researcher and theorist of contemporary psychiatry, takes a more inflexible position in his paper. He refers to a body of impressive data which implicates heredity in a variety of psychopathologies. Although he admits that variations in these disorders may be produced by environmental conditions, he is convinced that these are "superficial" influences which will not prevent the individual from succumbing to his hereditary defect. The distinguished biochemist Roger Williams persuasively argues the role played by each individual's biological makeup in shaping the course of his development. To Williams, the distinctive character of a man's morphology and chemistry is the most relevant factor in understanding his experience and behavior.

3. The Genetics of Human Behavior

FRANZ J. KALLMANN

Experimental biologists are safely entrenched in the age-old esteem for progress through science and can well afford to withhold comments on the cultural and behavioral aspects of morphologic inequalities among people. It is only when such an investigator invades that particular province of psychiatry where belief in heredity in relation to personality development is equated with lack of empathy or a depraved social conscience that a sinister tinge accrues to him and his work (11, 19, 24).

In the face of such a 2-valued system of conceptualization and terminology,

Abridged from *Amer. J. Psychiat. 113*:496–501, 1956, by permission of the American Psychiatric Association.

connoting either trust or distrust in man's perfectibility, even a truly liberal psychiatrist with genetic learnings finds it difficult to cast off the onus of being an unempathetic metascientist. To be sure, were he to feel called upon to express codified value judgments regarding the original goodness or sinfulness of mankind (22), he would be out of bounds. However, it is not his fault if his investigative data arouse so much disquietude that they need a de-emotionalized climate in which to be assimilated. Meanwhile, to balance the scales, there are zealous research workers everywhere who are ardent in their views, despite the fact that they have not had the benefit of genetic training.

In the search for the roots of human behavior, it would be well to stay clear of dichotomous absolutes. In particular, the interaction of heredity and environment is formulated as a meaningless antithesis as long as vague abstractions are used in describing the properties of an organism that is most certainly both active and re-active.

Man, to be sure, mirrors his culture and the social configuration of his parental home. Yet he also forms an autonomous functional unit that perpetuates itself as the matrix of his hierarchically organized traits and self-assertive acts. The human infant, if normally endowed, is certain to possess those structural, functional, and behavioral potentialities that distinguish individuals of the human species from those of any other (15, 17). While the emergence of his individuality will depend in part on the nutritive capacities of his family group, the constructs of his mind are at no stage like a hollow shell or a *tabula rasa*, as Locke would have it (4).

In a more eclectic scheme of human personality development, the importance of genic elements in the organization of behavior patterns rests on the interdependence of organic structure and psychologic function throughout the life of the individual. There is no behavior without an organism, no organism without a genotype, and no physiologic adaptedness without continuous and integrated gene activity.

Environmental influences are vital, and after conception they gain coequality with those arising from heredity. However, only within the limits set by the genic constitution of the organism can external factors have an effect on the dynamics of physiologic functions and interactions. Beyond these limits, no power plant exists for generating behavioral potentials. Such basic phenomena as growth and maturation, homeostasis and adaptation, reflexive behavior and constitution remain chameleonic allegories without the solid foundations of genetic principles.

Man, in order to be able to maintain his present evolutionary level, must be both conditionable by culture and impressible by education. The ability to learn from others and to profit from experience is determined by the genotype, while cultural values and opportunities have to be acquired by each individual through communication with his group. Variations in basic traits are inherited to the extent that they are end-products of a chain reaction set in motion by genes.

The effect of a gene expresses itself through the control of a specific enzyme which spurs on the production of a unit difference in development or function. The outcome of this action is subject either to reinforcement or interference by nonallelic genes, that is, other genes which are not located at the same point of a chromosome.

Conversely, the occurrence of different mutants of the same gene at any one locus makes it possible for the given point to control various normal and abnormal versions of a trait. In fact the demonstration of specific pathologic changes producible by a mutant gene provides adequate proof of the existence of a normal allele. The action of the normal gene can be assumed to play an indispensable part in maintaining health and normal behavior, even if its biochemical equivalents have yet to be identified. Therefore, it is just as unfair to blame heredity for only the unpleasant events in life, as it is to hold the genes responsible for every unusual mode of behavior whose origin is still in the dark.

Broadly formulated, then, a person's phenotype may be defined as the visible expression of his moldability by environmental influences, while it is his genotype that determines his norm of reaction to the total range of possible environments during his lifetime. The implication here is that every gene-controlled mode of activity requires an operational area in which to unfold (9, 18, 23, 28, 31).

Since no part of this environmental area of operation is inert, in the sense of being ineffectual where the behavioral responses of the individual are concerned, appreciation of environmentally produced variations in the expression of gene-specific behavior components is clearly as essential to an understanding of heredity as is the knowledge of geometry to that of mathematics. Except for real instincts, which need not be learned, it is axiomatic that no type of behavior is controlled entirely by genic elements, nor is it ever the result of a single cause, genetic or nongenetic (5, 7, 33). Estimates of individual contributions are meaningful only when viewed against the backdrop of the total genetic and environmental variation observed in a population.

It has already been mentioned in this symposium that some traits occur more often in one population than in another, depending on the relative frequency of a gene in different populations. Also, non-instinctive responsiveness to conditioning influences varies in different stages of development, and from person to person at a comparable stage of development (7, 13). The aggregate of gene-specific personality constituents is so vast, and the number of interactive variables in the shaping of a behavior pattern so infinite, that every individual can count on being unique — identical twins excepted.

The gene-specific uniqueness of man's individuality is now recognized in all branches of the behavioral sciences, even if the parliamentary Bill of Acceptance has yet to be ratified by some. What differs most are the descriptive labels affixed to this uniqueness. For instance, the differentiation of early behavior patterns has been described as an "ordered sequence" that begins with the establishment of reflexive responses and gradually leads through progressive stages of maturing to the development of coordinated motor, perceptual, and intellectual functions (6); or as "hierarchical organization of traits," in the course of which the infant will in time develop a conscience and a sense of self (4); or as a process of "biosocial integration with the total family configuration" (1). Other genetic phenomena have been referred to as the result of an innate equipment "with specific power plants and tools" (25) and as a biologically determined trend toward security and homeostatic stability, identified with a striving for "survival with a minimum amount of expenditure" (2).

Despite these differences in terms used to describe the interaction of genetic and non-genetic components of behavior, there is interdisciplinary agreement on at least one general premise; namely, that those aspects of the environment which are potent in affecting the organism depend not only on the degree of maturity the organism has attained, but also on its ability to cope with extrinsic hazards. Another point of unanimity is the belief that many children are capable of working out fairly adequate ways of dealing with difficulties in their home milieu and interpersonal relationships. By the same token, the established interdependence of social aspirations and biologic needs would seem to impose certain limits on the diversity and reach of human motives and the sublimating endeavors taken up by self-determination.

Genetically, a chaotic lack of uniformity in human societies is prevented by various principles of selection, and by the fact that the cultural forces which mold, as well as the formative elements which secure moldability on the human level, are actually end-products of the same evolutionary process. Viewed in this light, they are like the 2 sides of a coin, defying analysis as independent variables (10, 12, 26). Hence, the inability to separate the 2 sets of determining factors can only in part be ascribed to the parental practice of rearing one's own children. It is more than likely, too, that this virtual inseparability will last as long as our knowledge of the constituents of the coin remains as limited as it is at present. A reflection of this state of affairs is seen in the fact that most test devices for measuring meaningful personality differences have proven refractory to standardization (8, 18, 21).

Apart from unavoidable limitations on the assessment of gene-specific personality components, the twin study method represents an excellent comparative procedure for demonstrating the significance of heredity in many behavior variations, both normal and abnormal. The effectiveness of the method is matched by its economy and versatility as a sampling procedure for investigating traits, which require vertical and longitudinal comparisons under controlled conditions, and personal contact with families from various population groups, including some whose private affairs might otherwise not be open to research. Procedurally, it is no real disadvantage that twins cannot be separated before they are born, or that they cannot be provided with 2 mothers of different age, personality, or health status.

The popular notion that the behavior patterns of 1-egg twins are alike chiefly because of unusual similarity in their early environments has yet to be substantiated. If confirmed, the argument would only strengthen, rather than weaken, any correctly formulated genetic theory. Psychodynamic concepts, too, are built on the premise that man is selective in respect to important aspects of his life experiences and so can be thought of as "creating his own environment" (2). Utilization of our "own potential formula of adjustment" evidently depends on what Sanford (27) calls the body's ability "to function at its own built-in best." Plainly, each of these elegant allegories conveys a genetic idea.

In the area of normal personality variations, gene-specific derivations have been shown by comparative twin data to range from physical, coordinative, physiognomic, and temperamental characteristics to intellectual abilities, affective regulations, and special talents (6, 14, 16, 29, 32, 34). In between are sex maturation patterns, variations in antibody production and neurohormonal alarm reactions, the capacity for longevity, and the ingredients for sustained tolerance of physiologic or psychologic stress, a highly essential prerequisite for a well-balanced personality (17, 20, 30). It is well known that each individual has his own threshold of adaptability to different types of stress, and his own pattern of stress symptom formation.

Consistent similarity in the composition of these personality components is not found in the absence of genotypic similarity. Two-egg twins of the same sex tend to differ as much in their personalities as do any siblings reared together or apart. In 1-egg twins, even pronounced differences in life experiences, however adverse, are rarely potent enough to erase basic similarities in appearance and general personality traits.

As to behavior disorders that are not sufficiently explained on a situational or experiential basis, the list of conditions for which complete twin sibship data are now available is headed by the schizophrenic and manic-depressive types of psychosis. Since these 2 disorders do not occur interchangeably in the same twin pairs, they are assumed to be genotypically specific. The potentialities for a cyclic psychosis are probably associated with a subtle disturbance in a neurohormonal control mechanism which ordinarily protects a person from having harmful extremes of emotional responses.

While the tendency to exceed the normal range of mood alterations apparently requires the mutative effect of a single dominant gene with incomplete penetrance, the metabolic deficiency in a potentially schizophrenic person is most likely the result of a recessive gene. The disordered behavior pattern produced by this specific vulnerability factor is not correlated with inadequacy of the parental home in a simple manner, but is subject to modification by mesodermal defense reactions. Psychodynamically, the pattern has been described as an integrative pleasure deficiency leading to adaptive incompetence (25).

Involutional melancholia and other non-periodic forms of depressive behavior in the involutional and senile periods have been shown by twin family data to be unrelated to the manic-depressive group of disorders. There is an indirect link with the schizophrenic genotype through certain forms of emotional instability characteristic of schizoid personality traits. Other symptoms of maladjustment in the senescent period may arise either from gene-specific metabolic dysfunctions peculiar to the senium, or from graded differences in general health and survival values.

Homosexual behavior in the adult male continues to yield a higher 1-egg concordance rate than any of the other conditions investigated. This finding points to a disarrangement in the balance between male and female maturation patterns, resulting in a shift toward an alternative minus variant in the integrative process of psychosexual maturation.

Another condition with a well-established monozygotic concordance rate of close to 100% is an entirely different defect of more obvious organicity, namely, mongolism (3). Since the corresponding rate for 2-egg co-twins does not exceed that of their later-born siblings (approximately 4%), the search for the etiologic factor in mongolism is narrowed down by twin data to a more or less permanent change in the mother's endocrine or reproductive system. Evidently, the noxious influence during a mongoloid pregnancy cannot be transient, but acts on a genetically predisposed embryo, or upon the ovum, or upon the embryo prior to the earliest stage when twinning occurs by division.

In regard to all these disorders, twin family studies are helping materially to focus attention on persisting obscurities in their etiology. Generally, the objective of genetic investigations in man is not only to demonstrate that gene-controlled phenomena play a role in the differentiation of normal and abnormal behavior patterns, but to determine how this action takes place.

In conclusion, it may be said with some measure of satisfaction that recent progress in genetics has been encouraging. Although exact studies of the subject only began at the turn of this century, advances in the cellular, structural and metabolic areas of personality organization have been remarkable. An immediate result has been the improvement of our knowledge regarding the interacting bipolarity of human life. Growing insight into this interaction will gradually unfold a better understanding of human behavior. Somewhere along this line it will be possible to explain variable behavior patterns in terms of physiochemical processes powered by genic elements.

Once this goal has been reached, psychiatrists and other workers in the behavioral sciences will no longer hesitate to welcome geneticists as allies in interdisciplinary studies of human frailties and capacities. Only then may modern man begin to recognize his potential ability to plan his own future, as well as that of the world around him. In consequence, he may learn to exercise his obligation of self-determination in this direction.

References

1. Ackerman, N. W., and Behrens, M. L. In Hoch, P. H., and Zubin, J., Eds. Psychopathology of Childhood. New York: Grune & Stratton, 1955.
2. Alexander, F. Am. J. Psychiat., 112: 692, 1956.
3. Allen, G., and Baroff, G. S. In Testimonial Volume for Prof. Tage Kemp. Acta Genetica et Statistica Medica. Basel: S. Karger, 1956.
4. Allport, G. W. Becoming: Basic Considerations for a Psychology of Personality. New Haven: Yale University Press, 1955.
5. Anastasi, A. In Hooker, D., Ed. Genetics and The Inheritance of Integrated Neurological and Psychiatric Patterns, Vol. 33. Baltimore: Williams & Wilkins, 1954.
6. Bayley, N. In Hoch, P. H., and Zubin, J., Eds. Psychopathology of Childhood. New York: Grune & Stratton, 1955.
7. Beach, F. A. In Blake, R. R., and Ramsey, G. V. Perception, An Approach to Personality. New York: Ronald Press, 1951. Also: in Wilson, J., et al. Current Trends in Psychology and The Behavioral Sciences. Pittsburgh: University of Pittsburgh Press, 1954.
8. Cronbach, L. J. In Farnsworth, P. R., Ed. Annual Review of Psychology, Vol. 7. Stanford: Annual Reviews, 1956.
9. David, P. R., and Snyder, L. H. In Rohrer, J. H., and Sherif, M., Eds. Social Psychology at The Crossroads, New York: Harper, 1951.
10. Dobzhansky, T. Evolution, Genetics, and Man. New York: J. Wiley & Sons, 1955.
11. Dreikurs, R. Internat. J. Soc. Psychiat., 1: 23, 1955.
12. Fuller, J. L. Nature and Nuture: A Modern Synthesis. New York: Doubleday, 1954.
13. Garn, S. M. Ann. N. Y. Acad. Sci., 63:537, 1955.
14. Glass, B. In Hooker, D., Ed. Genetics and The Inheritance of Integrated Neurological and Psychiatric Patterns, Vol. 33. Baltimore: Williams & Wikins, 1954. Also: J. Hopkins Mag., 6: 2, 1955.
15. Goldschmidt, R. B. Theoretical Genetics. Berkeley: University of California Press, 1955.
16. Grebe, H. A. Ge. Me. Ge., 4: 275, 1955.
17. Kallmann, F. J. Heredity in Health and Mental Disorder. New York: W. W. Norton, 1953. Also: Am. J. Human Genet., 6: 157, 1954.
18. Kallmann, F. J., and Baroff, G. S. Annual Review of Psychology, 6: 297, 1955.
19. Karpman, B., Ed. Multiple Murders (Anon. Editorial). Arch. Crim. Psychodynamics, 1: 713, 1955.
20. Lacey, J. I., and Van Lehn, R. Psychosomat. Med., 14: 71, 1952.
21. McClelland, D. C. In Farnsworth, P. R., Ed. Annual Review of Psychology. Stanford: Annual Reviews, 1956.
22. Montagu, M. F. A. Am. J. Psychiat., 112: 401, 1955.
23. Nissen, H. W. In Jones, M. R., Ed. Nebraska Symposium on Motivation. Lincoln: University Nebraska Press, 1954.
24. Pastore, N. The Nature-Nuture Controversy. New York: King's Crown Press, 1949.
25. Rado, S. Am. J. Psychiat., 110: 406, 1953; J. Nerv. Ment. Dis., 121: 389, 1955.
26. Riddle, O. The Unleashing of Evolutionary Thought. New York: Vantage Press, 1954.
27. Sanford, F. H. Am. Psychol., 10: 829, 1955.
28. Schaffner, B., Ed. Group Processes. Madison: Madison, 1955.
29. Strandskov, H. H. Eugen. Quart., 2: 152, 1955.
30. Sutton, H. E., and Vandenberg, S. G. Human Biol., 25: 318, 1953.
31. Tanner, J. M., Ed. Prospects in Psychiatric Research. Oxford: Blackwell, 1953.
32. Thurstone, L. I., Thurstone, G. T., and Strandskov, H. H. A Psychological Study of Twins. I. Distribution of Absolute Twin Differences for Identical and Fraternal Twins. Report No. 4. The Psychometric Laboratory: University of North Carolina, 1953.
33. Tinbergen, N. The Study of Instinct. Oxford: Clarendon Press, 1951.
34. Vandenberg, S. G. A comparison of identical and fraternal twins on a battery of psychological tests: A preliminary report on the University of Michigan twin study. Paper presented at A.I.B.S. Meeting, East Lansing, Michigan, Sept. 5–9, 1955.

4.   The Biological Approach to the Study of Personality

ROGER J. WILLIAMS

The study of personality logically involves trying to answer three questions: First, of what is personality composed; e.g., if two people have differing personalities, in what specific ways do they or may they differ? Second, how do distinctive personalities arise? Third, how can improvement or modification of personality be brought about?

The first question, of what is personality composed, is a difficult and complicated one, and the answers to the second and third questions hinge upon the answer to it. Our discussion in this paper will be a contribution toward the answering of all these questions. Our approach is in a sense not new but it is largely unexplored and, we believe, rich in potentialities. It has the advantage that it can be used to supplement all other approaches; it does not require the rejection of older insights regardless of their origin or how time-honored they may be.

Certainly one of the earliest attempts to account for personality differences was made by the astrologers who recognized that people differed one from another and sought to explain these differences on the basis of the influence of the heavenly bodies. The hypothesis of the astrologers has not stood up well in scientific circles, but there are numerous citizens who still believe in horoscopes and many magazines and newspapers that publish them. The tenacious belief rests, I believe, on a fundamental failure of real scientists to come up with other reasons and explanations which satisfy.

In the beginning of the nineteenth century, Gall and Spurzheim developed phrenology which was destined to be in public vogue for a number of decades. This purported to be a science essentially concerned with the relation between personality traits and the contours of people's heads. Partly because it lacked scientific validity and partly because its implications were fatalistic and deterministic, the fundamental idea has largely been discarded.

In the middle portion of the nineteenth century the possible importance of heredity as a factor in the production of personality differences was brought to the fore by the investigations and writings of Darwin and his nephew Galton. Galton, the founder of eugenics, had none of our modern information as to how complicated heredity is; his emphasis on "good" and "bad" heredity (his own, of course, was "good") was misleading and his ideas of improving the race not only flew in the face of religious teachings but were so over-simplified that they came to be regarded as unsound scientifically. The eugenic view also had the disadvantage from the standpoint of public acceptance of being impregnated with determinism.

Before the end of the nineteenth century, Freudianism came into being and has subsequently received such wide acceptance that it has dominated decades. Fundamentally, Freudianism is a system of surmises of such a nature that they have not and cannot be tested by controlled experiments. These surmises appear to some minds to be plausible to such a high degree that they demand acceptance. On the other hand, to some minds, some of the surmises appear so implausible as to demand rejection. Controlled experiments are quite outside the routine thoughts and discussions of adherents of the Freudian school.

The surmises which form the basis of the Freudian doctrine include the essential idea that personalities are built during the lifetime of the individual and that the prime factors which enter are the environmental happenings beginning on the day of birth—possibly even before —and the thoughts that are developed as a result of these happenings. Therapeutic psychoanalysis is based upon the idea that if an individual can come to understand how the events of his earlier life have developed his present unfortunate attitudes, his personality difficulties tend to evaporate. Inherent in this approach is the idea that minds are much more complex than they superficially appear to be; they are like icebergs in that there is much more "out of sight" than there is in open view.

That the Freudian approach to per-

From a paper presented at the Berkeley Conference on "Personality Development in Childhood," University of California, May 5, 1960, by permission of the author.

sonality has elements of strength is so obvious as not to require argument. It leaves room for the unknown and unexpected in human behavior (which is needed), it emphasizes the dynamic aspects of personality, and strongly encourages the belief that human beings are not powerless to change and modify their personalities and that parents have tremendous potentialities in developing the lives of their children. The wide acceptance of Freudian ideas bears out the thought that the public, including the physicians, are first people and second, if at all, scientists. Certainly a cold-blooded scientific approach would never have developed and fostered the Freudian concepts.

Freudian doctrine tacitly assumes that at the beginning of their lives individuals are substantially duplicates of one another. This doctrine is almost, if not wholly, universalized; that is, its pronouncements apply to everyone alike. Freud himself wrote, "I always find it uncanny when I can't understand someone in terms of myself."

To be sure, people develop later in life very diverse personalities, but the observed differences are, according to the Freudian school, essentially environmentally induced and the laws of development are the same for all. Freud and his followers sometimes make references to tendencies which are inherited by the human race as a whole but it is the consistent practice to disregard or minimize individual differences in heredity as a potential source of personality differences. Certainly Freudians as such have not fostered research in this area.

The neglect of hereditary factors among those who are concerned with personality disorders is so pronounced that the veteran physician, Walter C. Alvarez, has recently complained "in most of the present day books on psychiatry, there is not even a short section on heredity. The book resembles a text on paleontology written for a fundamentalist college, with not one word on evolution!"[1] Of course, the dilemma of developing an environmentalist doctrine while paying some attention to heredity is a real one. If one begins to allow heredity to make inroads and demand attention, there is no telling where the process will end; the whole structure of environmentalistic Freudianism might come tumbling down.

On hard-nosed scientific ground one does not escape from determinism by adopting an environmentalist point of view, though many seem to think so. They resist considering the importance of heredity for this reason. Rigorous scientific thinking leads us to conclude that environmentalism is just as deterministic in its implications as its hereditarianism. People say, "If we don't like one environment we can move to another," but scientific reasoning if followed implicitly leads to the conclusion that we cannot move to a new environment unless there is some stimulus in the old or the new environment which *makes us* move.

This subject is much too large to discuss in detail in this paper, but as a prelude to further discussions I will briefly state my position. In the first place I have not the slightest doubt that heredity has a great deal to do with personality development. I do not resist this idea. I do not believe this recognition leads inevitably to determinism. I do not know how or why intelligence originated on earth; I do not understand how or why free will originated or just how it works. But there are many other questions to which scientific reasoning gives me no answer. I do not even know why positive electricity attracts negative or why every particle of matter in the physical universe exerts an attractive force on every other particle. I do accept the idea of free choice, with limitations imposed by laws, as a fundamental premise. With the acceptance, as a background for my thinking, of the exercise of intelligence and free choice as prime factors in life, I do not resist the recognition of hereditary influences. Their recognition does not pin me down to determinism.

Behavioristic psychology which at its inception was *completely* environmentalistic has bolstered the environmental approach of Freudianism. This school of psychology has as a fundamental basis the facts discovered by Pavlov using dogs and commonly designated as conditioned reflexes. The development of personality thus becomes a pyramiding conditioning process whereby the developing infant is continuously modified in his responses by the stimuli he or she received.

What was not quoted by the behavioristic school were correlative findings by Pavlov which are highly pertinent. Pavlov found as a result of extensive study of many dogs that they often exhibited innate tendencies to react very differently to the same stimulus. He recognized in his dogs four basic types: (1) excitable, (2) inhibitory, (3) equilibrated, and (4) active, as well as intermediate, types.[2] He recognized enormous differences in dogs with respect to their conditionability and was by no means inclined to focus his attention solely upon the behavior of "*the* dog." Scott and others have in more recent times found ample justification for Pavlov's concern over the fundamental differences between dogs of different breeds and between individual dogs within each breed. These differences, which can be studied under controlled conditions in dogs vastly easier than in human beings, are *not* the result of training.

It is beyond dispute, of course, that dogs, cats, rats, and monkeys, for example, show species differences with respect to their patterns of conditionability. Stimuli which are highly effective for one species may be of negligible importance for another. If hereditary factors make for interspecies differences, it is entirely reasonable to suppose that intra-species differences would exist for the same reason.

Before we proceed to the principal part of our discussion it should be pointed out that the pronouncements of men whose memories we may revere must be taken in their historical context. Freud, for example, developed most of his fundamental ideas before there was any knowledge of hormones, indeed before the term "hormone" was coined. He had at this time no knowledge of present day biochemistry; the chemical factors involved in nutrition were almost wholly unknown; and he certainly had no knowledge of the close ties which exist between biochemistry and genetics. It can safely be assumed that if the youthful Sigmund Freud were reincarnated today, he would include these vast developments in endocrinology, biochemistry, and genetics in his purview, and that his thinking would follow quite different paths from those which it followed about the turn of the century.

A parallel case has existed in the field of medicine with respect to the monumental work of Louis Pasteur. Pasteur's thrilling contribution may be summarized in a single sentence: "Disease is caused by micro-organisms." To convince his contemporaries of this fact Pasteur had to overcome terrific resistance. Once established, however, the next generation not only accepted the idea but was strongly inclined to go even further and assert that disease is caused *exclusively* by micro-organisms. After Pasteur's death substantial evidence began to accumulate that disease could be caused by malnutrition. This idea in turn met with terrific resistance, possibly because this was considered a slur on Pasteur's memory. Actually, however, if the youthful Pasteur could have been reincarnated about 1900 he probably would have been one of the first to recognize the importance of malnutrition—an importance which many physicians even today do not fully recognize or welcome with open arms.

The parallel between the two cases may be discerned if we summarize Freud's contribution thus: "Personality disorders result from infantile conditioning." It appears that many followers of Freud tend to insert the word exclusively and to say "Personality disorders resort exclusively from infantile conditioning." It seems an extremely doubtful compliment to Freud's memory to follow slavishly doctrines which he—if he were alive and in possession of present day knowledge—would repudiate or radically modify.

A biological approach to personality should seek to bring from biology *everything* that can help to explain what personality is, how it originates and how it can be modified and improved. Biology has much to contribute, particularly in an area of biology which has received relatively little attention; namely, that involving anatomical, physiological, biochemical (and psychological) individuality.

It seems indefensible to assume that people are built in separate compartments, one anatomical, one physiological, one biochemical, one psychological, and that these compartments are unrelated or only distantly related to each other. Each human being possesses and exhibits unity. Certainly anatomy is basic to physiology and biochemistry, and it may logically be presumed that it is also basic to psychology.

Let us look therefore in the field of anatomy for facts which are pertinent to our problem.

Anatomists, partly for reasons of simplicity, have been prone in centuries past to concentrate on a single picture of the human body. Obvious concessions are made, when necessary, in considering the male and the female of the species, and always anatomists have been aware that within these two groups there are variations and anomalies. Only within the past decade,[3] however, has comprehensive information been published which indicates how great these inter-individual variations are and how widespread they are in the general population.

It makes no difference where we look, whether at the skeletal system, the digestive tract, the muscular system, the circulatory system, the respiratory system, the endocrine system, the nervous system, or even at the microscopic anatomy of the blood, we find tremendous morphological variations within the so-called normal range.

For example, normal stomachs vary greatly in shape and about six-fold in size. Transverse colons vary widely in the positions at which they cross over in the abdomen and pelvic colon patterns vary widely. Arising from the aortic arch are two, three, four, and sometimes five and six branch arteries; the aorta itself varies greatly in size and hearts differ morphologically and physiologically so that their pumping capacities in healthy young men vary widely. The size of arteries and the branching patterns are such that in each individual the various tissues and organs are supplied with blood unequally well, resulting in a distinctive pattern of blood supply for each.

Morphological differences in the respiratory systems of normal people are basic to the fact that each person exhibits a distinctive breathing pattern as shown in the spirograms of different individuals made under comparable conditions.

Each endocrine gland is subject to wide variation among "normal" individuals. Thyroid glands vary in weight about six-fold,[4] and the protein-bound iodine of the blood which measures the hormonal output varies to about the same degree.[5] Parathyroid glands also vary about six-fold in total weight in so-called "normal" individuals, and the number of lobes varies from 2–12.[4] The most prevalent number of lobes is 4, but some anatomists estimate that not over fifty per cent of the population have this number. The number of islets of Langerhans, which are responsible for insulin production, vary over a ten-fold range in diabetes-free individuals.[6] The thickness of the adrenal cortex, where the critical adrenal hormones arise, is said to vary from 0.5 mm to 5 mm (ten-fold).[7]

The morphology of the pituitary glands which produce about eight different hormones is so variable, when different healthy individuals are compared, as to allow for several-fold differences in the production of the individual hormones.[8,9,10] The male sex glands vary in weight from 10 to 45 grams[4c] in so-called "normal" males and much more than this if those with "sub-normal" sex development are included. The female sex glands vary in weight over a five-fold range and the number of primordial ova present at the birth of "normal" female infants varies over a thirteen-fold range.[4d] It is evident that all individuals possess distinctive endocrine systems and that the individual hormonal activities may vary over a several-fold range in individuals who have no recognized hormonal difficulty.

The nervous system is, of course, particularly interesting in connection with the personality problem, and the question arises whether substantial variations exist. The classification of the various kinds of sensory nerve endings, for example, is by no means complete nor satisfactory, and the precise functioning of many of the recognized types is unknown. Investigations involving "cold spots," "warm spots," and "pain spots" on the skin indicate that each individual exhibits a distinctive pattern of each. In a relatively recent study of pain spots in twenty-one healthy young adults, a high degree of variation was observed.[11] When subjected to carefully controlled test conditions the right hand of one young man "A" showed seven per cent of the area tested to be "highly sensitive," while in another, "B" the right hand showed one hundred per cent "highly sensitive" areas. On A's hand, forty-nine per cent of the area registered "no pain" under standard pain producing test conditions. On B's hand, however, there was no area which registered "no pain."

It is evident that there is room for wide variations with respect to the numbers and distributions of sensory nerve endings in different individuals. That such differences exist is indicated by the extreme diversity in the reactions of individuals to many stimuli such as those involving seeing, hearing, and tasting. An entire lecture could be devoted to this subject alone.

The branching of the trunk nerves is as distinctive as that of the blood vessels.[3] Anson, for example, shows eight patterns of the branching of the facial nerve, each type representing, on the basis of examination of one hundred facial halves, from 5 to 22 per cent of the specimens. About 15 per cent of people do not have a direct pyramidal nerve tract in the spinal column; an unknown percentage have three splanchnic nerves as compared with the usual two; recurrent laryngeal nerves may be wholly unbranched or may have as many as six branches;[12] the termination of the spinal cord varies in different individuals over a range of three full vertebrae.[3]

Variations in brain anatomy have received little attention. Thirteen years ago, however, Lashley in a review wrote:[13] "The brain is extremely variable in every character that has been subjected to measurement. Its diversities of structure within the species are of the same general character as are the differences between related species or even between orders of animals. . . . Even the limited evidence at hand, however, shows that individuals start life with brain differing enormously in structure; unlike in number, size, and arrangement of neurons as well as in grosser features."

Unfortunately, partly due to the complexity of the problem, there is no information whatever available as to how these enormous anatomical differences are related to the equally striking personality differences which are commonplace. Recently there has been published, primarily for the use of surgeons, an extensive study of differences in brain anatomy.[14]

Up to the present in our discussion we have paid attention only to certain facts of biology—those in the field of anatomy. Before we consider other areas—physiology, biochemistry, and psychology—it seems appropriate to note whether we have made any progress in uncovering facts that have important implications for personality development.

Consider the fact (I do regard it a fact and not a theory) that every individual person is endowed with a distinctive gastrointestinal tract, a distinctive circulatory system, a distinctive endocrine system, a distinctive nervous system, and a morphologically distinctive brain; furthermore that the differences involved in this distinctiveness are never trifling and often are enormous. Can it be that this fact is inconsequential in relation the problem of personality differences?

I am willing to take the position that this fact is of the *utmost* importance. The material in the area of anatomy alone is sufficient to convince anyone who comes upon the problem with an open mind that here is an obvious frontier which should yield many insights. Those who have accepted the Freudian idea that personality disorders arise from infantile conditioning will surely be led to see that, *in addition*, the distinctive bodily equipment of each individual infant is potentially important.

The failure of psychologists—and of biologists, too—to deal seriously with innate individual differences in connection with many problems probably has deep roots.

McGill has said, "Experimental psychologists . . . ignore individual differences almost as an item of faith."[15] The same statement holds, in the main, for physiological psychologists, physiologists, and biochemists. Anatomists have adopted in the past (and some do even at present) the same attitude. Generally speaking, individual differences are flies in the ointment which need to be removed and disregarded. Every subject becomes vastly simpler and more "scientific" when this is done.

If one is pursuing knowledge about personality, however, neglect of innate individual differences is fatal. All of biology and all of psychology have suffered, in my opinion, from at least a mild case of "universalitis," an overruling desire to generalize immediately—oftentimes long before sufficient facts are gathered to give the generalization validity. This desire to generalize is of itself laudable, but the willingness to do so without an adequate background of information is unscientific and has devastating effects in the area of personality study.

The most treacherous type of premature generalization is the one that is not stated, but is merely accepted as obvious or axiomatic. Such a generalization is hidden, for example, in the famous line of Alexander Pope "The proper study of mankind is man.'' This common saying *assumes* the existence of a meaningful prototype, *man*, a universalized human being —an object of our primary concern. From the standpoint of the serious realistic study of personality, I object to this implied generalization. If we were to alter Pope's line to read "The proper study of mankind is men," we would have detracted from its poetic excellence but we would have added immeasurably to its validity in the area of personality study.

"Universalitis" is probably born of fundamental egotism. If one can make sweeping generalizations, they are self-gratifying, they can be readily passed on to disciples, the atmosphere seems to clear, life becomes simple, and we approach being gods. It is more pleasant often to retain one's conceit than it is to be realistically humble and admit ignorance. "Universalitis" is thus a sign of immaturity. When personality study has grown up it will recognize realistically the tremendous diversity in personalities, the classification of which is extremely difficult and must be based upon far more data than we now have.

With these ideas as additional background for our thinking let us consider some of the other aspects of biology. Physiologically and biochemically, distinctiveness in gastrointestinal tracts is just as marked as is the distinctiveness in anatomy. The gastric juices of 5,000 individuals free from gastric disease were found to contain from 0–4300 units of pepsin.[16] The range of hydrochloric acid in a smaller study of normal individuals was from 0.0 to 66.0 milliequivalents per liter.[17] No one can deny the probability that large variations also exist in the digestive juices which cannot be so readily investigated. Some "normal" hearts beat more than twice as fast as others,[18] some have pumping capacities at least three times as large as others,[19] and the blood of each individual is distinctive. The discovery of the existence of "blood groups" was just the beginning of our knowledge of the individuality of the blood. Enzyme levels in the blood, which are a reflection of fundamental biochemical differences, vary from one well individual to another over substantial ranges, sometimes ten-fold or even thirty-fold or more.[20]

Our neuromuscular systems are far from assembly line products as can easily be demonstrated by a study of motor skills and by a large number of physiological tests. Our senses are by no means identical, as has been made clear by taste tests for PTC and many other substances,[21] by tests involving sense of smell (verbenas,[22] hydrocyanic acid[23]), sense of sight (peripheral vision, foveal size, flicker fusion, and related phenomena, eighteen types of color "blindness"), sense of balance, pitch discriminations and hearing acuities at different frequencies, etc.', etc. From the tremendous variation in the action of specific drugs and chemicals on different individuals, we gain further evidence of fundamental differences in physiology and biochemistry.[24]

Thurston's pioneering work on primary mental abilities called attention to the fact that human minds have different facets, and that some individuals may be relatively well endowed with respect to arithmetical facility, for example, while being relatively deficient in word familiarity or spatial imagery. Others may be strong in the area of word familiarity but weak in rote memory or arithmetic. Guilford has more recently suggested that there are at least forty facets to human minds, involving a group of memory factors, four groups of thinking factors, the latter involving abilities relating to discovering, evaluating, and generating ideas.[25] All of this leaves room for a multitude of mental patterns (patterns of conditionability) which it seems reasonable to suppose must be related to the enormous variation in the anatomy of human brains. People even when confronted with the same facts, do not think alike, and this appears to have a sound anatomical as well as psychological basis.

Those social anthropologists and other social scientists, who regard culture as the one factor which determines what an individual will be like, often say, or imply, that adult members of a society bear a very great resemblance to each other because of the similarities of their upbringing. In view of this common implication it may be well to ask whether inborn differentness and distinctiveness fades out as a result of the adjustment of the individuals to the culture to which they are exposed.

That this is not the case is indicated by the results of a game played anonymously with a group of 140 adults. They were given the following list of twenty desirable items, each of which was to be rated 0, 1, 2, 3, 4, or 5 depending on its satisfaction-giving value for the individual making the anonymous rating.

1. Animals, pets of all kinds
2. Babies, enjoyment of
3. Bargaining, buying and selling
4. Beauty, as seen through the eyes
5. Conversation, all kinds
6. Creative work
7. Exploring, travel
8. Food, eating of all kinds
9. Gardening
10. Medical care
11. Music, all kinds
12. Nature, enjoyment of
13. Odors, perfumes, etc.
14. Ownership of property
15. Reading, all kinds
16. Religious worship
17. Routine activities
18. Self adornment
19. Sex
20. Shows, all kinds

The results showed clearly that every individual was distinct and different from every other individual. No two patterns were alike even with respect to a half dozen items; no pattern had a faint resemblance to the average for the group. Furthermore, the distinctiveness of each was not based upon minor differences in ratings; every item on the list was rated 0 by some individuals; every item was rated 5 by some individuals. In fact every item received, by members of this group, every possible rating from 0 to 5!

At the risk of being naive, it appears that the whole story we have been unfolding hangs together. Individual infants are endowed with far-reaching anatomical distinctiveness; each has a distinctive endocrine system, a highly distinctive nervous system, a highly distinctive brain. The same distinctiveness carries over into the sensory and biochemical realms, and into their individual psychologies. It is not surprising therefore that each individual upon reaching adulthood exhibits a distinctive pattern of likes and dislikes not only with respect to trivialities but also with respect to what may be regarded the most important things in life.

That culture has a profound influence on our lives no one should deny. The serious question arises, however, as to the relative position that different factors occupy in producing distinctive personalities. To me it seems probable that one's dis-

tinctive endocrine system and one's distinctive brain morphology are more important factors than the toilet training one receives as an infant.

We cannot state as a demonstrated fact that differences in brain morphology or in endocrine systems have much to do with personality differences. On the other hand we have no rigorous scientific proof that toilet training has any substantial effect on personality development. We can only surmise. In one sense, personality study is in its very early infancy.

Another pertinent question—simple but important—awaits a clear answer: Are patterns of brain morphology inherited? On the basis of what is known about the inheritance of other morphological features including fingerprints and the branching of blood vessels in the chest, etc., it may be *inferred* that specific morphological features in the brain are handed down by inheritance, but we do not have definite proof.

A fact which makes the study of the inheritance of such morphological features difficult is that expressed by geneticists David and Snyder.[26] "It has become more and more widely recognized that single-gene differences which produce readily distinguishable discontinuities in phenotype variation are completely non-representative of the bulk of genetic variability in any species." Multiple gene effects are extremely common and in many cases, because of the complexity of the inheritance process, it is impossible to trace them in families or to know when and where such effects may be expected to arise. This complication is not the only one which exists; there is also the possibility (and certainty in some species) of maternal influence (cytoplasmic) which does not follow the rules of gene-centered genetics, and can thus throw one's calculations off.[27]

The complications of broad genetic study are so great that closely inbred animals, which, according to the simpler concepts of genetics, should be nearly identical in body make-up, are often relatively far from it. Even within relatively closely inbred groups of animals each has a distinctive pattern of organ weights, a distinctive excretion pattern, and at the same time a distinctive pattern of behavioral responses.

The technique of twin studies also has its pitfalls. Monozygotic twins have, according to the simpler concepts of Mendelian genetics, identical inheritance. Actually, however, because of cytoplasmic factors or other unknowns, they appear not to have. It is a common observation that so-called "identical" twins vary markedly in their resemblance to each other. Sometimes they have almost indistinguishable facial features and very similar temperaments. In other cases, however, they are readily distinguished one from another by facial features and/or by temperaments. Our study of excretion patterns suggests that these show in monozygotic twins a high degree of similarity but not an identity. Kallman states, "Discordance between them [monozygotic twins] is not, as is commonly assumed, a measure merely of postnatal or even prenatal development; it may also have a genetic component."[28]

Consideration of the available facts leads me to suppose, in the absence of completely definitive information, that differences in brain morphology, in endocrine patterns, in digestive, circulatory, muscular, and nervous systems, etc., have important roots in heredity. It is difficult to see how such differences as exist could arise independent of heredity. The exact mechanisms whereby all these differences are inherited will probably be obscure many decades hence.

The recognition of hereditary factors does not, by any means, exclude from consideration the dynamic aspects of personality development. Potentialities and conditionabilities are inherited, not fixed, characteristics. The widespread idea that personalities are developed from early childhood is fully in accord with an appreciation of the hereditary factors. Conditioning still takes place but the recognition of innate biological differences calls attention to distinct make-up that each newborn baby possesses. Conditioning does not take place starting with assembly-line babies, each one, according to Watson, possessing exactly the same potentialities to develop into a "doctor, lawyer, artist, merchant, chief, and yes, even beggarman and thief."

We have two choices in personality study: one is to neglect hereditary factors as we have done in the past decades, in which case progress will come to a full stop; the other is to recognize the numerous individual differences to be observed in the various areas of biology and study them intensively and ascertain their pertinence.

If we adopt the latter course this means

the cultivation of spontaneity in research and perhaps a de-emphasis on theory until some valuable data are collected. Hebb has recently called attention to the weakness of the "design of experiment" approach.[29] "It assumes that the thinking is done in advance of experimentation, since it demands that the whole program be laid out in advance; it tends also, in its own Procrustean way, to confirm or deny the ideas with which one began the experiment, but its elaborate mathematical machinery is virtually certain to exclude the kind of unexpected result that gives one new ideas. . . . We must not let our epistemological preconceptions stand in the way of getting research done. We had much better be naive and productive than sophisticated, hypercritical and sterile."

To tackle in one giant undertaking the problem of understanding, characterizing, and cataloguing all personalities from the biological or any other point of view seems hopeless. A strategy which seems far from hopeless, however, involves studying *one at a time* various personality characteristics to ascertain what biological roots they may have. The personality characteristics to be chosen for investigation should, obviously, be as definite as possible. They might include not only matters of temperament or emotion but also the ability to perform specified types of mental processes, or they might include personality problems of numerous types.

Studying even one particular personality characteristic to ascertain its biological roots is a large undertaking and might involve making scores, possibly hundreds, of measurements on every individual subjected to study. If one has some rational basis for selecting wisely the measurements to be made, the number of desirable measurements might be reduced. This fact would constitute an argument for selecting as the "personality problem" to be investigated, one for which the type of biological roots *might be* successfully guessed in advance. Such might include hyper- or hyposexuality, homosexuality, obesity, depressions, alcoholism, insomnia, accident proneness, etc. When one after another of personality disorders have been studied from this standpoint, it seems very likely that the whole picture will begin to clear and that the study of specific personality characteristics and problems will become successively easier the farther it progresses. What I am considering is obviously a relatively long range proposal.

Such a type of study as I am suggesting is not in line with the vast amount of experimentation which is currently fashionable. It is very common, for example, to develop a measurement and then apply it to large numbers of people. It is almost or totally unheard of to apply a large series of measurements to a relatively few individuals to determine their individual distinctive patterns. This must be done if we are to find the biological roots of personality characteristics, and psychologists should be warned that the major part of the work must be done in the area of biology, and the biological scientists concerned cannot be looked upon as minor contributors.

Digressing for a moment, it has been with this thought in mind that I have objected strenuously to the current widespread implication that "behavioral sciences" constitute a distinct group including psychology, sociology, and social anthropology and excluding the biological sciences. Hidden in this classification is the *assumption* that biological factors are of no importance in behavior and that conditioning is the whole story. It actually may well be, however, that anatomy, physiology, and biochemistry are, from the standpoint of the practical potentialities, the most important behavioral sciences at our disposal.

In connection with tracing the biological roots of personality characteristics or problems, a highly important part of the strategy is to recognize what I have elsewhere called "disconformities" in the various measurements that are made.[30] High or low values within the so-called "normal range," for example, are disconformities. Such values are abundant and may be highly meaningful, and more important (because of their wider occurrence) than "abnormalities," especially when, as is often the case, the adopted "norms" are selected arbitrarily and without any rational basis whatever.

One of the most encouraging aspects of this type of study is the potential application of high-speed computers to study biological disconformity patterns, and their pertinence to particular personality characteristics or personality problems. Techniques for studying patterns are in their infancy, but the possibilities are most alluring. It may spur our interest in these possibilities to know that, according to recent reports from the Soviet Medical Academy, an electronic diagnosing machine has been constructed. This utilizes, no doubt, some of the mathematical principles and techniques that would be useful in personality study.

Parenthetically, but very briefly, it may be stated that a study of disconformity patterns such as we have suggested is also urgent for reasons other than those involving personality study. These patterns constitute the basis for the complex patterns of innate susceptibilities which all individuals have for all types of diseases.

Space will not permit a discussion of the numerous ways in which my own discipline, biochemistry, impinges on personality problems.[31] The effects of various chemicals on personality behavior, the correlations between brain metabolism and behavior, the effects of various hormones on personality characteristics are all well recognized. What is not so well recognized is that each individual's body chemistry is distinctive and different, and that complex biochemical roots of personality characteristics are likely to be found when we look for them with due care and thoroughness.

Before I close this discussion, I want to stress a most important environmental factor which is capable of contributing enormously to healthy personality development.

The monumental work of Beadle and Tatum[32] demonstrated for the first time the vital connection between genes and enzymes, and, in effect, between heredity and biochemistry. Their work made clear the inevitable basis for individual body chemistry. As a direct consequence of this finding, it becomes inevitable that the nutritional needs of genetically distinctive individuals are quantitatively not the same. Carrying the idea still further it becomes inescapable that the brain cells of individual people do not have quantitatively identical nutritional needs.

It has been amply demonstrated that malnutrition of various kinds can induce personality disorders. This was observed in the starvation studies of Keys and associates,[33] in thiamin deficiency studies,[34] in amino acid deficiency studies,[35] and perhaps most notably in pellagra where unequivocal insanity may result from niacin deficiency and can be abolished promptly by administration of the missing vitamin. It has also been repeatedly that inadequacy of prenatal nutrition can cause all sorts of development difficulties and abnormalities in the growing fetus.

One of the most obvious environmental measures that can be taken to insure favorable personality development is to see, for example, that the nervous system of each distinctive individual, with his distinctive needs, receives prenatally and postnatally the best possible nourishment. Nourishment of brain cells like the nourishment of the other cells throughout the body can be maintained at many levels of excellence, and of course achieving the best is no small order.

Serious attention to nutrition which must involve the utilization of substantial manpower and a great deal of human ingenuity and persistence can, I believe, make tremendous contributions to our knowledge of personality states and personality disorders, and to the alleviation and prevention of personality difficulties.

In conclusion I would emphasize that the biological approach to personality, outstandingly important as I believe it to be, is not a substitute for all other valid approaches. Whatever we may know or may be able to accomplish by other approaches, if valid, is not lost. Consideration of the biological approach expands our horizon and gives us a much broader view. In my opinion the insight we may gain from this approach will be most valuable and productive. I should reiterate also what I have said before, that personality study is in its early infancy.

References

1. Alvarez, Walter C., *Practical Leads to Puzzling Diagnoses*, J. B. Lippincott, Philadelphia, Pa., 1958, p. 181.
2. Maiorov, F. P., *History of Study on Conditioned Reflexes*, 2nd Rev. and Completed ed., U.S.S.R. Academy of Sciences, Moscow and Leningrad, 1954, p. 190. (In Russian.)
3. Anson, Barry J., *Atlas of Human Anatomy*, W. B. Saunders Co., Philadelphia, Pa. and London, England, 1951.
4(a). Grollman, Arthur, *Essentials of Endocrinology*, J. B. Lippincott Co., Philadelphia, Pa., 2nd ed., 1947, p. 155.
4(b). *Ibid.*, p. 247.
4(c). *Ibid.*, p. 460.
4(d). *Ibid.*, p. 497.
5. Williams, Roger J., *Biochemical Individuality*, John Wiley & Sons, New York, N.Y., 1956, p. 53.
6. Pincus, Gregory, and Thimann, Kenneth V., eds., *The Hormones*, Academic Press, Inc., New York, N. Y., 1948, Vol. 1, p. 303.
7. Goldzieher, Max A., *The Endocrine Glands*, D. Appleton-Century Co., New York, N.Y. and London, England, 1939, p. 589.
8. Rasmussen, A. T., *Am. J. Anat.*, 42, 1–27 (1928).
9. Rasmussen, A. T., *Endocrinology*, 12, 129–524 (1924).
10. Rasmussen, A. T., *Endocrinology*, 12, 129–150 (1928).
11. Tindall, George T., and Kunkle, E. Charles, *A.M.A. Archives of Neurology and Psychiatry*, 77, 605–610 (1957).
12. Rustad, William H., *Clin. Endocrinol. Metabolism*, 14, 87–96 (1954).
13. Lashley, K. S., *Psychological Reviews*, 54, 333–334 (1947).
14. Schattenbrand, Georges, and Bailey, Percival, *Introduction to Stereotaxis, with an Atlas of the Human Brain* (3 Vols.), Georg Thieme, Verlag, Stuttgart; Grune and Stratton, New York, N. Y., 1959.
15. McGill, W. J., *Amer. Psych. Ass'n. Symposium: Behavior Genetics and Differential Psychology*, New York, Sept. 4, 1957.
16. Osterberg, Arnold E., Vanzant, Frances R., Alvarez, Walter C., and Rivers, Andrew B., *Am. J. Digestive Diseases*, 3, 35–41 (1936).
17. Bernstein, Ralph E., *J. Lab. Clin. Med.*, 40, 707–717 (1952).
18. Heath, Clark W., et al., *What People Are*, Harvard University Press, Cambridge, Mass., 1945, p. 126.
19. King, C. C., et al., *J. Applied Physiol.*, 5, 99–110 (1952).
20. Williams, Roger J., *Biochemical Individuality*, John Wiley & Sons, New York, N. Y., 1956, pp. 69–79.
21. *Ibid.*, pp. 127–130.
22. Blakeslee, A. F., *Proc. Natl. Acad. Sci.*, 48, 298–299 (1918); *J. of Heredity*, 23, 106 (1932).
23. Kirk, R. L., and Stenhouse, N. S., *Nature*, 171, 698–699 (1953).
24. Williams, Roger J., *Biochemical Individuality*, John Wiley & Sons, New York, 1956, pp. 106–118.
25. Guilford, J. P., *Science*, 122, 875 (1955).
26. David, P. R., and Snyder, L. H., *Social Psychology at the Crossroads*, Harper and Bros., New York, N. Y., 1951, pp. 61–62.
27. Williams, Roger J., *J. of Heredity*, 51, 91–98 (1960).
28. Kallmann, F. J., *Am. J. Human Genetics*, 6, 157–162 (1954).
29. Harlow, Harry F., and Woolsey, Clinton N., eds., *Biological and Biochemical Bases of Behavior*, The University of Wisconsin Press, Madison, Wisconsin, 1958, p. 464.
30. Williams, Roger J., *Texas Reports Biol. and Med.*, 18, 168–185 (1960).
31. Williams, Roger J., *Biochemical Individuality*, John Wiley & Sons, New York, N. Y., 1956, pp. 197–209.
32. Beadle, G. W., and Tatum, E. L., *Proc. Natl. Acad. Sci.*, 27, 499–506 (1941).
33. Keys, Ancel, "Experimental Induction of Neuropsychoses by Starvation," in *Biology of Mental Health and Disease*, Paul B. Hoeber, Inc., New York, N. Y., 1952, pp. 515–525.
34. Wilder, Russell M., "Experimental Induction of Psychoneuroses through Restriction of Intake of Thiamine," in *Biology of Mental Health and Disease*, Paul B. Hoeber, Inc., New York, N. Y., 1952, pp. 531–538.
35. Rose, W. C., personal communication.

Biophysical Theories:

PATHOLOGICAL PATTERNS

How can the various forms of psychopathology best be classified? To the biophysical theorist, the answer lies in terms of those
features of biological make-up which dispose individuals to pathology. Pathological behavior patterns that are correlated consistently with measurable morphological characteristics offer a
beginning toward a quantitative and stable psychiatric classification, according to William Sheldon. In his paper, Sheldon formulates an "operational" classification of psychiatric disorders
based on his exhaustive studies of body build and temperament.
In contrast to his forerunner, Ernst Kretschmer, Sheldon's theoretical speculations are founded on years of quantitative research.
Kurt Goldstein, eminent neurological theorist, has argued vigorously for the view that brain diseases are significant in that they
precipitate a complex sequence of psychological changes in the
patient. In the paper published here, he spells out the classical
signs associated with neurological damage, differentiating clearly
those features which stem primarily from the disease and those
which reflect the patient's psychological efforts to cope with them.

5.   Constitutional Psychiatry

WILLIAM H. SHELDON

A.   STRUCTURAL CONCEPTS

Constitution.   The organizational or
underlying pattern. Literally, the way a
thing *stands together.* The whole aggregate of the relatively fixed and deep-seated
structural and behavioral characteristics
that collectively differentiate a personality.
Perhaps the most satisfactory way to start
an examination of the constitutional pattern of a human being is photographically,
although this is only a beginning and
offers but an anchorage or frame of reference for constitutional description. Behind the objective and overt aspects of
morphology lie individual differences
first in those aspects of morphology
which are not outwardly revealed, such
as the structure, dysplasias, and *t* component of internal organs, of the nervous system, of the endocrine glands,
and so on; and further, individual differences in physiology and chemistry. All
of these differences contribute to and make
up what is referred to as personality. The
term *constitution* implies only a certain
relatedness and orderliness or patterning
with respect to the underlying aspects of
personality. In so far as the student of constitution addresses his energies to the
study of external morphology he is but
trying to anchor (to something taxonom-
ically describable) an approach to personality as a whole, in its physiological and
immunological and psychological as well
as morphological aspects.

The Somatotype.   A quantification
of the primary components determining
the morphological structure of an individual. In practice the somatotype is a series
of three numerals, each expressing the

Abridged from *Varieties of Delinquent Youth,*
pages 14–62, 1949, by William H. Sheldon, E. M.
Hartl, and Eugene McDermott. By permission of
Professor Sheldon, copyright holder.

approximate strength of one of the primary components in a physique. The first numeral always refers to *endomorphy,* the second to *mesomorphy,* the third to *ectomorphy.* When a 7-point scale is used the somatotype 7–1–1 is the most extreme endomorph, the 1–7–1 is the most extreme mesomorph, and the 1–1–7 is the most extreme ectomorph. The somatotype 4–4–4 falls at the midpoint of the scale with respect to all three primary components.

Endomorphy, or the first component: Relative predominance in the bodily economy of structure associated with digestion and assimilation. Relatively great development of the digestive *viscera.* In embryonic life the endoderm, or inner embryonic layer, grows into what becomes the functional element in a long tube, stretched or coiled from mouth to anus with a number of appendages. This is the digestive tube. Together with its appendages it is sometimes called the vegetative system. Its organs make up the bulk of the viscera. Endomorphy means relative predominance of the vegetative system, with a consequent tendency to put on fat easily. Endomorphs have low specific gravity. They float easily in the water. When well nourished they tend toward softness and roundness throughout the body, but it should be remembered that in learning to gauge one of the components it is necessary to learn to gauge the other two at the same time.

Mesomorphy, or the second component: Relative predominance of the mesodermally derived tissues, which are chiefly bone, muscle, and connective tissue. These are the somatic structures, or the motor organ-systems. Mesomorphs tend toward massive strength and muscular development. When their endomorphy is low, so that they remain lean, they retain a hard rectangularity of outline. If endomorphy is not low, mesomorphs tend to "fill out" heavily and to grow fat in middle life. However, because of the heavy underlying skeletal and muscular structure, they remain solid. When fat they are "hard-round," in contrast with the "soft-roundness" of endomorphy, and they continue in the general mold and in the proportions of athletic shapeliness. Endomorphs get roly-poly, globular, and pendulous. Mesomorphs just swell up in their generally athletic mold. Mesomorphs are of higher specific gravity than endomorphs. They

are less buoyant in water but because of superior muscular power are nevertheless often good swimmers. The mesomorphic heart and blood vessels are large, and the skin seems relatively thick because of heavy reinforcement with underlying connective tissue.

Ectomorphy, or the third component: Relative predominance of the skin and its appendages, which include the nervous system. All of these tissues are derived from the ectodermal embryonic layer. In the ectomorph there is relatively little bodily mass and relatively great surface area—therefore greater sensory exposure to the outside world. Endomorphs and mesomorphs appear to be biological conservatives, the former investing faith in superior assimilative power or digestive ability, the latter in superior resistive substance and striking power. Ectomorphs seem to have departed from *both* of these essential biological insurances and to have embarked on an exteroceptive adventure. They have given up mass for surface, in a sense suppressing the primacy of both the digestive organ-system and the motor organ-system in favor of the sensory organ-system. The Italian School of Clinical Anthropology (DiGiovanni, Viola, Pende; *see* VHP, Chapter 2) calls them hyperevolutes, suggesting that in departing from the secure advantages of the coarser and heavier bodies of the endomorphs and mesomorphs (in favor of extending the sensorium externally), they tend to move out toward the end of an evolutionary limb whence it may be difficult to return. Morphologically, ectomorphy means flatness and fragility throughout the body, with a comparatively high height/weight index.

Mesomorphic endomorphs; endomorphic mesomorphs; ectomorphic mesomorphs; mesomorphic ectomorphs; endomorphic ectomorphs; ectomorphic endomorphs: These terms refer to physiques in which all three of the primary morphological components are of different strength. Figure 1 is a schematic two-dimensional presentation of the somatotypes in which these six various "families" are spatially delineated. An endomorphic mesomorph is an individual in whom mesomorphy predominates, with endomorphy second in order to strength, and ectomorphy third. Example: the somatotype 3–5–2.

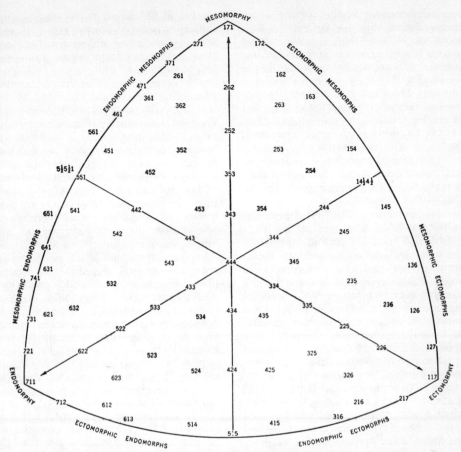

A SCHEMATIC TWO-DIMENSIONAL PROJECTION OF THE THEORETICAL SPATIAL RELATIONSHIPS AMONG THE KNOWN SOMATOTYPES

Figure 1

B. BEHAVIORAL CONCEPTS

Temperament. According to Webster: (1) A mixing in due proportion; (2) The internal constitution with respect to balance or mixture of qualities or components; (3) The peculiar physical and mental character of an individual; (4) Frame of mind or type of mental reactions characteristic of an individual.

The original meaning of the Greek verb is to mix. As I use the term, temperament is simply some quantification of the mixture of components that a person presents. In this literal sense temperament at the morphological level is the somatotype. At a slightly more dynamic or behavioral level it is the pattern of the mixture of the three primary components *vis-*

cerotonia, somatotonia, and *cerebrontonia.* At more complex and more culturally conditioned levels, temperament may be defined more elaborately and may embrace any schema for quantification of the manifest components of a personality that a psychologist can devise. In the academic exercise published in the second volume of this series (VT) it was shown that temperament can be measured at a level sufficiently basic to correlate about +.80 with the primary morphological components. It of course does not necessarily follow that the measurement of temperament at such a comparatively basic level is the most useful thing a psychologist can do with his time, especially if he should choose to stop at that level.

Temperament is the pattern at *all* levels. But as I use the term it is a little more specific than that. It is *the pattern quantitatively expressed, in terms of some schema of components which offers a frame of reference for an operational psychology.* The most difficult and most important task of the psychologist is that of making his choice of primary variables, or of getting down to primary components; that is to say, components which offer a basis for general quantitative comparison, and cannot be further factored. For elaboration of this exceedingly important point, see VHP, Chapter 5.

VISCEROTONIA. The first component of temperament, measured at the least-conditioned level of dynamic expression. Endomorphy is the same component measured at a purely structural or morphological level. Endomorphy is expressed by the morphological consequences of a predominance of the first component. Viscerotonia constitutes the primary or most general behavioral expression of the same predominance; that is to say, predominance of the digestive-assimilative function—the gut function. A detailed ostensive definition of viscerotonia is presented in VT, pages 31–48. Twenty defining traits which when quantitatively scaled can be used to measure the first component at this level are those in the first column of Table 1.

In briefest summary viscerotonia is manifested by relaxation, conviviality, and gluttony for food, for company, and for affection or social support. When this component is predominant the primary motive in life seems to be assimilation and conservation of energy.

SOMATOTONIA. The second component of temperament, measured at the least-conditioned level of dynamic expression. Mesomorphy is the same component measured at the morphological level. Somatotonia expresses the function of movement and predation—the somatic function. A detailed ostensive definition of somatotonia is presented in VT, pages 49–68. Twenty defining traits which can be used to measure this component at the "lowest dynamic level" are those in the second column of Table 1.

In briefest summary somatotonia is manifested by bodily assertiveness and by desire for muscular activity. When this component is predominant the primary

motive of life seems to be the vigorous utilization or expenditure of energy. Somatotonics love action and power. Their motivational organization seems dominated by the soma.

CEREBROTONIA. The third component of temperament, measured at the least-conditioned level of dynamic expression. Ectomorphy is the same component at the morphological level. Cerebrotonia appears to express the function of exteroception, which necessitates or involves cerebrally mediated inhibition of both of the other two primary functions. It also involves or leads to conscious attentionality and thereby to substitution of symbolic ideation for immediate overt response to stimulation. Attendant upon this latter phenomenon are the "cerebral tragedies" of hesitation, disorientation, and confusion. These appear to be by-products of overstimulation, which is doubtless one consequence of an overbalanced investment in exteroception. A detailed ostensive definition of cerebrotonia is presented in VT, pages 69–94. Twenty defining traits which can be used to measure cerebrotonia are those in the third column of Table 1.

In briefest summary cerebrotonia is manifested by (1) inhibition of both viscerotonic and somatotonic expression, (2) hyperattentionality or overconsciousness. When this component is predominant one of the principal desires of life seems to be avoidance of overstimulation—hence love of concealment and avoidance of attracting attention. While cerebrotonia seems to result from an evolutionary development in the direction of purchasing increased exteroception at the cost of *both* vegetative mass and motor strength, the *manifest traits* of cerebrotonia (in a crowded society) are associated largely with escaping the painful consequences of the increased exteroception thus attained. Yet cerebrotonia is probably in itself far from painful. There is a certain elemental ecstasy in the heightened attentionality just as there is a somatotonic ecstasy in vigorous muscular action and a viscerotonic ecstasy in first-rate digestive action.

The Suffix-otic. As in *viscerotic, somatorotic, cerebrotic;* also *viscerosis, somatorosis, cerebrosis.* This suffix signifies an abnormal or pathological overmanifes-

TABLE 1. THE SCALE FOR TEMPERAMENT

Name   Date   Photo No.   Scored by

I VISCEROTONIA. . . .	II SOMATOTONIA. . . .	III CEREBROTONIA. . . .
( ) 1. Relaxation in Posture and Movement	( ) 1. Assertiveness of Posture and Movement	( ) 1. Restraint in Posture and Movement, Tightness
( ) 2. Love of Physical Comfort	( ) 2. Love of Physical Adventure	— 2. Physiological Over-response
( ) 3. Slow Reaction	( ) 3. The Energetic Characteristic	( ) 3. Overly Fast Reactions
— 4. Love of Eating	( ) 4. Need and Enjoyment of Exercise	( ) 4. Love of Privacy
— 5. Socialization of Eating	— 5. Love of Dominating, Lust for Power	( ) 5. Mental Overintensity, Hyperattentionality, Apprehensiveness
— 6. Pleasure in Digestion	( ) 6. Love of Risk and Chance	( ) 6. Secretiveness of Feeling, Emotional Restraint
( ) 7. Love of Polite Ceremony	( ) 7. Bold Directness of Manner	( ) 7. Self-conscious Motility of the Eyes and Face
( ) 8. Sociophilia	( ) 8. Physical Courage for Combat	( ) 8. Sociophobia
— 9. Indiscriminate Amiability	( ) 9. Competitive Aggressiveness	( ) 9. Inhibited Social Address
— 10. Greed for Affection and Approval	— 10. Psychological Callousness	— 10. Resistance to Habit, and Poor Routinizing
— 11. Orientation to People	— 11. Claustrophobia	— 11. Agoraphobia
( ) 12. Evenness of Emotional Flow	— 12. Ruthlessness, Freedom from Squeamishness	— 12. Unpredictability of Attitude
( ) 13. Tolerance	( ) 13. The Unrestrained Voice	( ) 13. Vocal Restraint, and General Restraint of Noise
( ) 14. Complacency	— 14. Spartan Indifference to Pain	— 14. Hypersensitivity to Pain
— 15. Deep Sleep	— 15. General Noisiness	— 15. Poor Sleep Habits, Chronic Fatigue
( ) 16. The Untempered Characteristic	( ) 16. Overmaturity of Appearance	( ) 16. Youthful Intentness of Manner and Appearance
( ) 17. Smooth, Easy Communication of Feeling, Extraversion of Viscerotonia	— 17. Horizontal Mental Cleavage, Extraversion of Somatotonia	— 17. Vertical Mental Cleavage, Introversion
— 18. Relaxation and Sociophilia under Alcohol	— 18. Assertiveness and Aggression under Alcohol	— 18. Resistance to Alcohol, and to other Depressant Drugs
— 19. Need of People when Troubled	— 19. Need of Action when Troubled	— 19. Need of Solitude when Troubled
— 20. Orientation toward Childhood and Family Relationships	— 20. Orientation toward Goals and Activities of Youth	— 20. Orientation toward the Later Periods of Life

Note: The thirty traits with brackets constitute collectively the short form of the scale.

tation of the primary component named. The extra syllable—*or*—is put in *somatorotic* for euphony and to maintain the syllabic parallel with *somatotonic*. Since the term *neurotic* is prepsychological in the sense that it came into use during an era before primary components had been defined, and when it was the custom to blame psychopathology vaguely on "nerves" or "glands," this term is not definitive. To call a person "neurotic" is about as meaningful as calling him "glandotic." If an individual is neurotic he is either viscerotic, somatorotic, cerebrotic, or a combination of any two or all three.

The Suffix-penic. As in *viscero-penic, somatopenic, cerebropenic;* also *visceropenia, somatopenia, cerebropenia.* The suffix signifies *lack of*, or an abnormally low degree of the component named. Cf. *leukopenia,* lack of white corpuscles.

C. BABEL IN PSYCHIATRY

For anyone who has had firsthand contact with problems of delinquency the point will require no urging that the criminologist and the psychiatrist are fishing in the same pond. Both are dealing with temperamental pathology in its various manifestations, and in the last analysis a psychiatry or a criminology can be only about as good, or as true and useful, as the conception of temperament which it uses for its frame of reference.

One of the major hypotheses in Constitutional Psychology is that structure and function, or somatotype and temperament, are best viewed as a continuum. We are therefore not in this study primarily concerned with correlation between somatotype and temperament, for by hypothesis such a correlation is no source of new light but only a measure of the accuracy with which quantification has been accomplished at different levels of objectivity in the measurement of the same thing. In the second volume of the series, *Varieties of Temperament,* a crucial exercise on this correlational topic was presented. As the primary components of temperament were operationally defined and scaled in that study, the correlation between them and the primary components of the somatotype turned out to be

of the order +.80. Here we are not concerned with a repetition of such an exercise but are after more elusive game than statistical correlation between structure and function. That correlation is taken for granted. The problem now is to describe temperamental pathology, and if possible thereby to reflect a little light on the vast turmoil of verbality that psychiatric thinking and writing have created.

One of the things the human clan needs urgently is an operational psychiatry. It might turn out to be a keystone for the often prayed-for science of humanics. But to get an operational psychiatry it will first be necessary to establish the habit of systematically describing psychiatric behavior. Read cases 86 through 89 and I think it will be apparent enough, even if you have been exposed to some kind of psychiatric instruction, that what you have studied is confusion. Neither the Kraepelinian typology, which is still in almost universal use, nor the currently popular psychoanalytic slang* really brings order to the vagaries of human temperament any more than the crude morphological typologies of the Christian era, which could be called a biological age of shame, brought order to the study of human structure.

Observation of our series of 200 boys was not begun as a psychiatric exercise. The descriptions and notations on manifest temperament were routine to constitutional study. But they soon brought us squarely against the problem of psychiatric classification. Four-fifths of the youngsters had been "seen" by one or another kind of psychiatrist, and many were under constant psychiatric observation while at the

---

*The term *psychoanalytic slang* is used not in disparagement of Freud or of his work, for I hold both in high regard. It is used as about the most descriptive way of referring to the garbled and careless use of Freudian concepts which during the past two decades has become popular in American psychiatry and social work. On reading the biographies it will be apparent that smatterings of Freudian "language" have seeped through to half or more of the youths of the series. These boys, and many of the social workers who have coached or have ridden herd on them, "talk Freud" with about as much insight and understanding as the average city urchin has of Christianity when he "talks Jesus." In this country psychoanalytic jargon has become a superficial and a vulgar fad—a form of slang. Priests of the Freudian church are partly responsible, for they have commercialized and prostituted Freud's teaching as possibly no religious preachment was ever prostituted before.

Inn. As psychiatric diagnoses and recommendations piled up, the necessity for integrating two kinds of language—our operational structure-function language and the eclectic typologizing of the psychiatric fraternity—became increasingly urgent.

It was not uncommon to find that as many as a dozen different psychiatric diagnoses and interpretations had been made on a youngster, and *sometimes the dozen would embrace the entire repertory of the Kraepelinian typology*. That is to say, the youth would at various times have been given diagnoses not only mutually contradictory and pointing in opposite directions therapeutically, but he would be taken entirely around the clock and would have *all* the possible diagnoses.

It grew clearer every day that a vocabulary problem of the most serious nature existed in the psychiatric field, that in fact the vocabulary the psychiatrists were trying to use was nonoperational. It didn't work. We held a series of seminars on the question, and invited several of our consulting psychiatrists to come and help thrash it out. One in particular, Dr. Bryant Moulton, spent many hours with us over this difficult and fascinating question.

For many years, in my attempts to correlate constitutional characteristics with psychiatric findings, I had been baffled by the lack of any quantifiable (operational) variables by which the psychiatric findings could be expressed. Patients were diagnosed as suffering from manic-depressive psychosis, *or* paranoid schizophrenia *or* hebephrenic schizophrenia, and so on. It was always a matter of either-or. Psychiatry had developed as a branch of clinical practice, where a patient either "had something" or didn't have it. If he had it, it was either measles *or* scarlet fever *or* perhaps a heat rash in Latin. In clinical medicine the either-or approach possesses a certain cogency, for there *are* disease entities which you can have or not have. But in psychology there is little use for such an approach. The constitutional psychologist tries to describe the behavior of a personality; that is to say, of an organic structure in action. His first job (I believe) is to describe the structure, in terms of the most primary or universal components of structure that he can measure. That done, the job is to describe the

behavior in terms of similarly basic behavioral components. Then the constitutional psychologist proceeds, or should proceed, to a consideration of the details of behavior in the light of the details of structure. In any event he deals mainly with components of structure and behavior, not with either-or phenomena.

We were confronted with the fact that psychiatry offered no handles that a psychologist could take hold of. It postulated no hierarchy of variables that were amenable to quantification or, therefore, to correlation. In short, psychiatry, with its either-or criteria, did not appear to present a psychologically true-to-life discipline. It seemed clear that if a psychologist were to hope to make progress in the interpretation and correlation of psychiatric phenomena, he must first translate these into a system of variables with which he could operate. Moreover this was something we had to do before the general subject of delinquency could be expected to make sense. It was clear enough that delinquent and psychopathic behavior overlapped like the shingles of a house, that to get at one was impossible without at the same time getting at the other.

In short, we found it necessary to formulate a new approach to psychiatric classification before we could integrate constitutional morphology and temperament with the vast wealth of specific information that was being accumulated through psychiatric study and referral.

D. FROM DISEASE ENTITIES TO COMPONENTS

Where, then, in terms of operational concepts or in terms of structure-function language could a beginning be made toward psychiatric classification? This was a problem on which much of the potential usefulness of a study of delinquency seemed to hinge.

It was evident that in psychiatric circles there had long been a tendency to rely on some variation of a three-pole typology for a diagnostic frame of reference. At the "psychotic" level, for example, it was common to hear that, in general, three kinds of psychotic personality (together with mixtures) were to be encountered: cases showing *affective exaggeration;* those showing *paranoid pro-*

jection; and those showing *hebephrenic regression.* Also at the "psychoneurotic" level a similar tripolar typology was usually assumed to exist, and was embraced within the concepts *hysterical, psychasthenic,* and *neurasthenic* psychoneurosis.

In the closing decade of the last century Kraepelin, by including both mania and melancholia under the general heading of *manic-depressive psychosis,* and by setting this new entity off against *dementia praecox,* had postulated a fundamental dichotomy in the field of the functional psychoses. But Bleuler's conception of *schizophrenia* as a group or pattern of psychotic *reactions* soon largely supplanted the disease-entity conception of dementia praecox and led to renewed activity in the direction of classifying or "naming kinds" of schizophrenia.

Among most present-day practicing psychiatrists quite a sharp distinction is made between schizophrenic patterns in which a hostile or harsh reaction *against* seems to be the predominant temperamental "set" of the patient, and patterns characterized by reaction *away from* (i.e., by apathy, withdrawal from social contact, refusal or failure to participate or to take an interest). The reaction against is often buttressed by more or less extensive and systematized delusions in support of the central fixed idea—delusions usually of persecution and of the subject's own importance. The subject distorts his world of actual experience to fit his primary attitude. Hence the term *paranoid.* The paranoid patient, even when psychotic (which is only to say, *seriously* deranged), is "in there fighting" against something. He has not given up, has not jettisoned his cargo. There is still a somatotonic drive and it is aimed against something.

The reaction away from is of an entirely different nature, and the essential difference lies in the fact that the somatotonic drive is absent. It is as if the subject had lost, or had never had somatotonia. The drive to do things, to achieve, to dominate and triumph over others, to exercise and perfect the muscles, to compete and to fight—in short, somatotonia—is conspicuously absent. If any of this component ever was present it has been jettisoned, thrown overboard. The jettisoning may have been necessary to save the subject from further disastrous consequences of his ill-sustained and poorly executed efforts at normal or culturally

expected somatotonic aggression. This is probably as plausible a "mechanism" as any to explain the pathological somatopenia; but the essential fact is the somatopenia, whatever its origin.

One conspicuous corollary of the jettisoned pattern of personality is what psychiatrists call regressive behavior. The subject seems to regress or fall back to what is in some respects an infantile level of behavior. He may lose all ability to take care of himself, even sphincter control. There is marked lack of energy and of motivation. He may fail to respond at all to social stimulation and to conversational contact. He may have to be fed, bathed, and dressed, and in general cared for as an infant. He is then said to have regressed to a *hebephrenic* (infant mind) state.

Objections can be well taken to the use of the term hebephrenic in this sense. It is only in some respects that the subject has become like an infant; that is to say, in his helplessness. Infants, on the other hand, are normally of vigorous motivation, are alertly somatotonic and within the limits of their repertory of muscular skills are inclined to be aggressively somatotonic and to "go after" what they want. Infants—normally vigorous ones—have not jettisoned anything. It is merely that their executive department has not yet caught up with their desires. To use the idea of infant-mind or infant-like as a description of the most extreme and helpless form of mental pathology, even if it is said in Greek, is not very good semantics. These patients have not "regressed"; you can't really go back in this life. They have reacted away from the problems and competitions of life. They have jettisoned their second component and they show a pathological somatopenia. A better term than hebephrenic might be *oneirophrenic* (dream mind). However, we need not further labor the terminological aspect of the problem at this point in the development of the theme.

The distinction between mental aberration in which the *against* reaction is predominant and that in which the *away from* reaction predominates is as sharp a distinction as is to be found in psychiatry. The psychiatrically conventional single-word symbols for the two reaction patterns are, respectively, *paranoid* and *hebephrenic.*

Thus one end point of the original

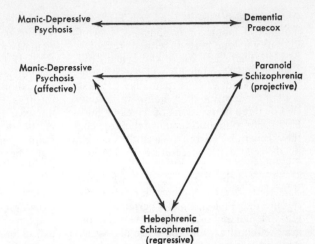

Figure 2. Illustrating the Kraepelinian Typology.

Kraepelinian psychotic dichotomy has as it were grown apart into two end points. Figure 2 A has grown into Figure 2 B, and a tripolar orientation has replaced a bipolar one. One of the poles, that called hebephrenic, seems to make a degree of operational sense in terms of pathological somatopenia, a concept with biological meaning. What about the other two poles? Can any sense be made of these from a biological point of view?

The reaction patterns that psychiatrists conventionally label *manic-depressive* psychosis all have one essential characteristic in common. The subject always has a low threshold of reaction. There is also a low threshold of emotional expression. He is feebly inhibited. In the "manic" state, which may be chronic or intermittent, he expresses elation and euphoria on slight provocation or without any apparent provocation. In the "depressed" state, which also may be chronic or intermittent, he similarly expresses emotional sorrow, dejection, or self-deprecation without externally apparent justification. The emotion itself may range from extreme elation to extreme dejection; indeed, it may be any emotion. It is the uninhibitedly free expression of the emotion that is constant. Similarly with respect to action of all kinds, here too it is the lack of inhibition, the lack of the cerebrotonic function, that is constant.

During the phase called manic expansiveness, that is to say, when the subject is active, the constant feature is lack of normal constraint in both emotional and somatic expression. He is maladaptively hyperactive; he is responsive, like the proverbial dog in a forest of telephone poles. There may be euphorial emotionalism, motor overactivity, flight of ideas, press of speech, poor attentional focus, hypersuggestibility, uninhibited eroticism, bizarre exhibitionism; and with it all a forceful keyed-up vigor of physical expression far beyond that for which the situation seems to call. All this is simply a description of somatotonia gone wild; pathological somatotonia, or somatorosis.

But in the phase called depression, or depressive melancholy, the dominant feature is not somatorosis but viscerosis —pathologically uncontrolled expression of viscerotonia, or lack of inhibition of affectivity. The subject is physically and mentally slowed up; overrelaxed, overly dependent, overly expressive of his now melancholy feelings. He has become untempered. In the viscerotic phase he is as uninhibitedly viscerotic as he is uninhibitedly somatorotic in the somatorotic phase.

The term manic-depressive psychosis does not then describe a disease entity, but a pattern of reaction in which the constant feature is pathological absence of inhibition. That is to say, the subject is cerebropenic. The result of the cerebropenia depends of course on the underlying temperamental endowment of the individual; that is what will determine his manner of expression. If he is mesomorphic and vigorous, strong and healthy, capable of sustained, violent exertion and of standing up well under it—if he is all this *and* cerebropenic—he will probably maintain a manic or hypomanic level of activity for long periods without recourse to rest. There are some who remain hypomanic all through life. These are athletes of a kind. One of them may exhaust a whole generation of contemporaries and two or three generations of wives or husbands, not to mention minor relatives; but they generally go out pleasantly enough in the end with a cerebral or cardiac "accident."

Such is the "pure manic," who is a comparative rarity. Similarly rare are cases of pure depression, or of "permanent aggressive melancholy." Far more common are the mixtures, and there are almost as many varieties of these as there are individuals. Typically there is some alternation between the somatorotic and the viscerotic cerebropenia, and there are cases where the individual seems to be caught in a regular rhythm or cycle of the two phases, as if he had to suspend the manic activity every so often to rest and recharge his battery. But I think that clear-cut examples of such a rhythmic cycle are less common than the term *cycloid psychosis*, which is often used instead of manic-depressive psychosis, would imply. What we find is not a disease entity but a more or less maladaptive reaction pattern characterized constantly by two things: (1) overly vigorous response, either visceral-emotional or somatic, or both; (2) feeble inhibition or lack of cerebrotonia.

We may then perhaps say that another of the poles in the tripolar schema of Figure 2 B seems to make some degree of operational sense. There may possibly be psychiatric meaning in the biological phenomenon of pathological cerebropenia. What about the third pole, which in the figure is labelled *paranoid?*

The reaction patterns that psychiatrists call paranoid, or paranoid projection—the reactions against—have as a constant characteristic a singular *lack of compassion*. The subject is without the bowels of mercy. According to his temperament and his strength he may look upon his world and his contemporaries as his persecutors or as legitimate objects of his own destructive fury. In either case his bond with his kind is one of hate, scorn, resentment, defiance; and all of this he "projects" against his environment. If he is weak the reaction pattern is more covert

that overt. It then takes the form of involved delusional ideation centered particularly around the main idea of persecution. If he is strong—physically strong —overt aggression and an arrogant manner combine with opinionated superciliousness to produce quite a remarkably unpleasant personality. The strong paranoids are ugly customers, especially in a pulpit or a state legislature.

There are as many different kinds of the maladaptive paranoid-projection reaction as there are of the maladaptive affective or of the jettisoning reactions. Common to all paranoia is the lack of participant compassion. The affective psychotic on the other hand is one vast bowel of compassion. He tends to enfold his world in a cosmic Dionysian embrace, and he is so participant in *everything* that the focus of his energy is lost in ubiquity. He is at one with it all. The paranoid is unable to be at one with any of it. He cannot relax and accept; cannot accept comfort; cannot deliberately enjoy food, company, or the glories of digestion; he finds no joy in the social amenities, no "fulfillment" in knowing people and in knowing about them; he cannot express emotion smoothly; has neither tolerance nor complacency; cannot achieve mutual dependency with other people and so cannot invest hope outside himself, except abstractly. Alcohol has no good effect— it makes him not more viscerotonic but more paranoid. These are all traits of visceropenia. But this personality cannot jettison. Cut off from the main channels of viscerotonic expression (the reaction toward), yet constrained to carry on, there is only one direction that the reaction can take. The reaction is against. It may be against at a very high and idealistic level, as in the case of Prometheus against Zeus, and this may in the long run be a "good" reaction—good for both man and Zeus. It may somehow even be good for Prometheus, and may contribute to the working out of his destiny, but Prometheus remains blood brother to Paranoius.

Biologically, the paranoid reaction seems to stem from lack of, or from interference with, the normal expression of viscerotonia. The reaction against is a visceropenic reaction. This appears to be the constant in the formula, and if the appearance is not a misleading one, it would seem possible that all three of the poles

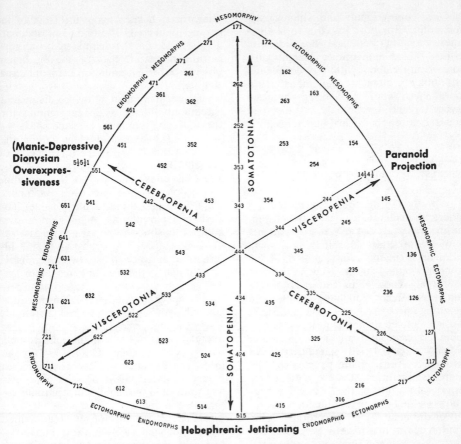

Figure 3. A Tripolar Psychiatric Orientation.

in the tripolar schema of Figure 2 B may make biological sense. Figure 2 B might then be drawn a little differently to take the form of Figure 3. Up to the present point all this is of course speculative. We are following some of the steps in the formulation of what may be called a speculative hypothesis. Hypothetically the three conventional poles for classification of the functional psychoses fall respectively *opposite* the three established poles for morphological and temperamental classification. The Dionysian-affective psychoses, in this hypothetical construct, are manifestations of something gone wrong either in the constitutional endowment or in the temperamental manifestations of the third component. Similarly for the paranoid-projective psychoses with respect to the first component; and for the hebephrenic-jettisoning psychoses with respect to the second component.

In the study of morphology and temperament we had made no progress beyond the types of Hippocrates until we emerged from the idea of typologies, or of dichotomies and trichotomies, and substituted for all that the conception of components capable of multidimensional distribution and therefore leading to a morphological and a temperamental taxonomy which the familiar biological distribution curves would fit—multidimensionally. The first two volumes of the Constitution series describe the steps leading to those two respective taxonomies. The question that now intruded itself was this: Could we taken the same step in psychiatry, at last emerging from the Laocoön-like struggle to describe the mentally aberrant in terms of biologically unreal disease entities or types of reaction? Could we emerge from this and substitute for it a taxonomy psychologically operational and biologically true to life? In short, could mental aberrancy be described and diagnosed in terms of demonstrable, quantifiable components falling within a continuum with other biological phenomena? If it could, there would be a bridge between psychiatry and psychology, and the road might open to a biological humanics.

E. A HYPOTHETICAL PSYCHIATRIC INDEX

During the decade following 1935 I undertook exploratory constitutional studies on two groups of psychiatric patients at Worcester State Hospital, on a small group of 50 in the Army, and on 3,800 psychotic patients in the New York State mental hospitals. This latter group included all of the available male cases in the state who were under 30 and were at the time labeled dementia praecox (schizophrenia); also all available males under 45 who were labeled manic-depressive psychosis. Study of the psychiatric and diagnostic histories of these patients together with study of the physical constitution yielded a remarkable demonstration of the need for an operational frame of reference in diagnosis.

It is a common thing, not only in the New York mental hospitals but in every other mental hospital with which I am familiar, to find that the diagnosis of a psychotic case has been changed half a dozen or more times—usually about as many times as there have been changes of diagnosing officer. Yet even in this madness there is method. One observation first struck me forcibly at Worcester and later was borne out in the New York State study and in the Army. *It is the patients who fall in a particular range of somatotypes whose diagnoses get changed the most.* These are of two groups: (1) the the midrange somatotypes; and (2) those falling near the morphological poles. *There is a clearly discernible tendency toward greater diagnostic agreement when the somatotype falls near any one of the three hypothetical psychiatric poles.*

A morphological 5-5-1, 4-5-1, or 5-4-1 who is psychotic has an excellent chance to be labeled manic or manic-depressive and to keep the label. A 1-4-5 or 1-5-4 is almost equally likely to continue through his diagnostic history as a paranoid; and a 4-1-5 or 5-1-4, or even a 4-2-5 or 5-2-4 seems to be almost certain to get and to keep the tag hebephrenic schizophrenia (or schizophrenia simplex).

That this tendency toward diagnostic agreement should disappear among the the midrange somatotypes, such as the 4-4-3's and 3-4-4's, or even among the 3-5-3's and 4-5-3's might well be expected. But it also disappears, and just about as conspicuously, at the morphological poles. 7-2-1's and 6-2-1's, for example, are just about as likely to get labeled hebephrenic as manic-depressive, and in this somatotype area there is a remarkable tendency for hesitation and alternation between these two diagnoses.

Similarly the extreme mesomorphs, 2-7-1's, 1-7-1's, 1-6-2's, and so on perplex the psychiatrists. These mesomorphs get labeled both manic and paranoid, rarely hebephrenic (although not infrequently "catatonic," which seems to be a wastbasket category). One 2-7-1 in the first series I studied at Worcester had been diagnosed as a manic-depressive psychotic five times and paranoid schizophrenic six times—ten changes of diagnosis alternating between two diagnoses. He seemed to be balanced right in the middle, between those two diagnostic typologies, and I think that in fact he was so balanced. His biological position was almost perfectly centered between the two psychiatric poles.

The extreme ectomorphs, 1-1-7's, 1-2-7's, and even the far commoner 2-2-6's appear to defy diagnosis by the conventional Kraepelinian typology in about the same way. Many a dreary hour of psychiatric case conference drains off into the weighty business of deciding whether such a patient is *a* hebephrenic or *a* paranoid schizophrene; and then next month in deciding it back the other way again. The criteria on which such diagnostic decisions rest are more often derived from verbalistic hairsplitting than from inquiry into the biological nature of the patient.

For patients at all three morphological poles psychiatric diagnosis seems to run into conflict and tends to hesitate between *two* alternatives. In dealing with the midrange somatotypes the typological psychiatrist is confronted with a still more difficult diagnostic problem. The midrange people, with all three of the primary biological components more or less equally represented, tend naturally enough under varying circumstances to manifest more or less of all three of the primary psychiatric components. At times a psychotic with the somatotype 4–5–3 is very likely to behave like a manic-depressive, at times he will be singularly paranoid, at times he may be "hebephrenic as hell." Often he may be simply stuporous. His most common diagnosis is catatonic schizophrenia.

Now *catatonic* is one diagnostic term in common psychiatric use which has been defined in almost every way psychiatrically imaginable. Henderson and Gillespie* defined catatonia as "an alternating state characterized by a stage of depression, a stage of excitement and a stage of stupor." Many psychiatrists, particularly those of European training, follow Kraepelin in applying the term catatonic dementia praecox (schizophrenia) to virtually all cases of functional psychosis that show a mixture or alternation of *all three* primary psychiatric components.

In the original Kraepelinian typology there was first the primary dichotomy of manic-depressive psychosis and dementia praecox; second, a division of dementia praecox into the three types, paranoid, hebephrenic, and catatonic. The catatonic type, which Kraepelin considered the most common, has always been diagnosed in practice mainly by the fact of shifts between manic-like excitement, stuporous depressions, and both paranoid-like and hebephrenic-like reaction patterns—all or any of these mixed in various proportions, according to the temperament of the patient. Some of the patients with this mixed picture spend much of their time in a cataleptic state, or state of sustained immobility. Many psychiatrists have adopted that characteristic as the critical or definitive one for the diagnosis of catatonic. Others, finding that catalepsy is by no means a constant feature, have considered it incidental. Still others, especially those not trained under the Kraepelinian tradition, have looked on "catatonic" as a mere wastebasket adjective more or less synonymous with "mixed"

and so have not used the term diagnostically at all. In the mental hospitals of some states today as many as 70 per cent of the schizophrenic patients are labeled catatonic; in those of some other states the term catatonic rarely appears. The consequence of all this has been rather general confusion over the term catatonic and an increasing tendency to avoid use of it, except as a synonym for mixed.

Kraepelin later added a fourth "type" of dementia praecox—the *simplex* or simple type. The identifying characteristic is absence of any definite trend; simply a general falling away of interest and a general falling back or lack of effective adaptivity. Kraepelin described this as consisting of an "impoverishment . . . of the whole psychic life, which is accomplished quite imperceptibly." No particular manic tendency, excitement or depression, or paranoid reaction. There is general apathy or emotional dulling, and a sinking away from life. The individual is born and remains a weak nonentity. A more descriptive term than schizophrenia simplex might be, simply, mental asthenia. In short, schizophrenia simplex is a term commonly applied to a psychotic personality that seems to stay in the middle with respect to all three of the primary psychiatric components, and so never shows a pronounced tendency toward any of them. The catatonic also in the long run falls in the middle, but this is because, in the course of time, he reveals all the primary psychiatric components in some strength, and all this divergent psychiatric "strength" cancels itself out.

We have now considered all the main conventional categories in the Kraepelinian diagnostic schema, which remains in almost universal psychiatric use wherever the European languages predominate. We can see that Kraepelin covered the ground remarkably well, that he included in his typology just about all of the possible main directions of variation of pattern. His is a first-rate typology. First, there is a "type of reaction pattern" extending out into each of the primary dimensions of possible extension. These are the manic-depressive, the paranoid, and the hebephrenic reaction patterns. Second, there is a name for those personalities which, upon showing tendencies along all of these dimensions, nevertheless average out somewhere near the ori-

*A Textbook of Psychiatry (6th ed., New York, 1946), p. 316.

gin or center point. These are the catatonics. Finally, there is a name for those personalities that go nowhere at all, but *simply* stay at nothingness. These are the simplexes.

But typologies do not offer an operational frame of reference for social science. Even the best of typologies can offer no more than a preliminary scaffolding which may mark out the main lines along which an operational science is to develop. The question we now have to consider is that of whether or not the whole field of psychiatric description— and therefore perhaps of psychological description in general—is ready for translation from the current typological to an operational frame of reference.

The picture as we have reviewed it can be diagrammatically summarized as in Figure 4. Here all the Kraepelin psychotic types are written into a hypothetical three-dimensional structure. But along with these typological designations there is also the suggestion of a quantitative frame of reference. At what may be called the apex or pole of the region of manic-depressive psychosis is the symbol $\psi 7-1-1$.* A personality plotted at this point on the diagram would be visualized as overwhelmingly Dionysian (a 7 in that component), and as altogether lacking in any signs of either of the other two primary psychiatric components. Similarly the symbol $\psi 1-7-1$ marks the pole for the territory of paranoid psychosis, and $\psi 1-1-7$ marks the hebephrenic pole.

One other point of great psychiatric interest will perhaps have already oc-

---

*The Greek ψ here stands for psychiatric, and this symbol placed in front of the three familiar numerals commonly used to define the somatotype indicates that we are now considering a *psychiatric*, not a morphological index.

The psychiatric index is expressed in the same way as the morphological index, or somatotype, but the poles for the psychiatric components fall opposite those used for the morphological components. This means that the three coordinates of the psychiatric system are rotated with respect to the coordinates of the morphological system. The rotation is about the center axis determined by the points 4–4–4, 3–3–3, 2–2–2, etc. Also in this center axis are the points 7–7–7 and 1–1–1.

What has actually happened in the change over from the somatotype designations to the psychiatric designations is simply a clockwise rotation of the poles through one-sixth of a complete turn, or through 60 degrees. The psychiatric 7–1–1 is just 60 degrees ahead of the somatotype 7–1—1, and the same is true of other corresponding numerals except those in the center axis, which remain fixed.

curred to anyone who in his thinking has begun to substitute the idea of a psychiatric index for the Kraepelinian typology. Psychotic personalities falling in the northwest sector of the distribution (see Figure 1, p. 41) are frequently referred to as "cycloid," or manic-depressive. At times they show manic euphorial aggression, at other times overt melancholic depression. Some individuals appear to present a rhythmic alternation between the two moods. For the northwest psychiatric territory the term cycloid has long been in common use and is almost interchangeable with manic-depressive.

But anyone who will take the trouble to observe a group of psychiatric patients, while keeping in mind the structural frame of reference of Figure 1, will soon become aware of the same cycloid phenomenon in the northeast and south that is seen in the northwest. Among paranoid schizophrenes who present about the same strength in mesomorphy as in ectomorphy there is very much the same alternation between somatic aggression and ideational substitutive hostility as there is between euphorial and melancholic expression among the patients who are well balanced in mesomorphy and endomorphy. And the same cycloid phenomenon is seen at the south, among the hebephrenic patients who show about the same strength in endomorphy and ectomorphy. These patients often alternate between bizarre, irrelevant affect and bizarre, irrelevant ideation.

When psychiatric behavior is described against an operational frame of reference the alternational or cycloid phenomenon is seen to be general—not specific to the manic-depressive pattern. Moreover the alternation is not limited to a swinging back and forth across what I have called the psychiatric poles; that is to say, across the poles of cerebropenia, visceropenia, and somatopenia. The cycloid alternation is just about as conspicuous across the poles of the primary components as across the psychiatric poles. That is to say, the swing is also seen across the poles of viscerosis, somatorosis, and cerebrosis. Endomorphs frequently show a cycloid alternation between overt melancholic depression and bizarre, irrelevant affect. Mesomorphs are likely to swing between manic-euphorial aggression and somatic aggression, and ectomorphs be-

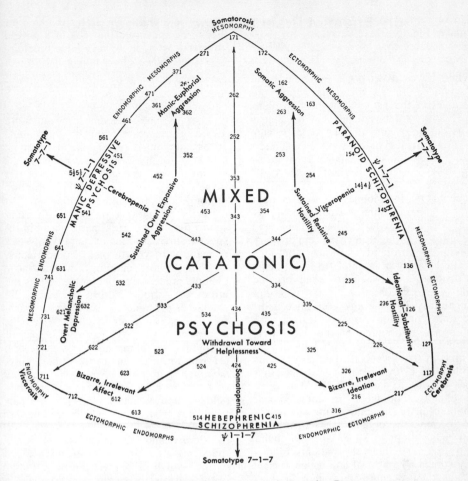

Figure 4. Diagram for the Psychotic Reaction Patterns.

tween ideational-substitutive hostility and bizarre, irrelevant ideation.

Among psychiatric patients of mid-range somatotype the alternations of mood and of behavior tend to become complex and some of these patients show, at different times, the definitive criteria for *all* of the Kraepelinian typological diagnoses. These are the people who get labeled catatonic. We cannot say whether or not there is usually some logical sequence, some "rhyme and reason," in their variations. There may be and somebody may find a good doctoral dissertation in the problem of working out relationships between overt constitutional factors and catatonic patterns.

In fairness to the psychiatric practitioners who have fallen into the conventional habit of applying the term cycloid only to the northwest sector, it should be pointed out that the alternation phenomenon is in fact more dramatic in that quarter than elsewhere. This is because all expressiveness reaches its maximal volume at the pole of the first psychiatric component. That is the area of pathological cerebropenia, where inhibition of expressiveness is at its physiological minimum and all reaction is therefore maximal. It was doubtless to be expected that the phenomenon of swinging back and forth between two partially incompatible kinds of reaction would first be noticed in the sector where behavior is most overtly accentuated. To point out that the cycloid pattern is seen elsewhere as well as in the northwest does not detract from the usefulness of the concept or from the brilliance of Kretschmer's classic description of the cycloid—meaning manic-depressive—temperament.

6. Effect of Brain Damage on Personality

KURT GOLDSTEIN

When I was asked to speak before the Psychoanalytic Association about the changes of the personality in brain damage, I was somewhat hesitant because I was not quite sure that I would be able to make myself understood by an audience which thinks mainly in such different categories and speaks in such a different terminology from my own. I finally accepted the invitation, because I thought that members of the Association apparently wanted to hear what I think and because it brought me the opportunity to express an old idea of mine—the idea that it is faulty in principle to try to make a distinction between so-called organic and functional diseases, as far as symptomatology and therapy are concerned.[1] In both conditions, one is dealing with abnormal functioning of the same psychophysical apparatus and with the attempts of the organism to come to terms with that. If the disturbances—whether they are due to damage to the brain or to psychological conflicts—do not disappear spontaneously or cannot be eliminated by therapy, the organism has to make a new adjustment to life in spite of them. Our task is to help the patients in this adjustment by physical and psychological means; the procedure and goal of the therapy in both conditions is, in principle, the same.

This was the basic idea which induced a group of neurologists, psychiatrists, and psychotherapists—including myself—many years ago, in 1927, to organize the Internationale Gesellschaft für Psychotherapei in Germany and to invite all physicians interested in psychotherapy to meet at the First Congress of the Society. Psychotherapists of all different schools responded to our invitation, and the result of the discussions was surprisingly fruitful. At the second meeting in 1927, I spoke about the relation between psychoanalysis and biology.[2] During the last twenty years, in which I have occupied myself intensively with psychotherapy, I have become more and more aware of the similarity of the phenomena of organic and psychogenic conditions.

It is not my intention to consider the similarities in this paper. I want to restrict myself to the description of the symptomatology and the interpretation of the behavior changes in patients with damage to the brain cortex, particularly in respect to their personality, and would like to leave it to you to make comparisons.

The symptomatology which these patients present is very complex.[3] It is the effect of various factors of which the change of personality is only one. Therefore, when we want to characterize the change of personality, we have to separate it from the symptoms due to other factors: (1) from those which are the effect of *disturbance of inborn or learned patterns* of performances in special performance fields—such as motor and sensory patterns; (2) from those which are the *expression of the so-called catastrophic conditions;* and (3) from those which are the *expression of the protective mechanisms* which originate from the attempt of the organism to avoid catastrophies.

In order to avoid terminological misunderstandings, I want to state what I mean by personality: Personality shows itself in behavior. Personality is the mode of behavior of a person in terms of the capacities of human beings in general and in the specific appearance of these capacities in a particular person. Behavior is always an entity and concerns the whole personality. Only abstractively can we separate behavior into parts—as for instance, bodily processes, conscious phenomena, states of feelings, attitudes, and so on.[4]

According to my observation, all the

From *Psychiatry, 15*: 245–260, 1952. Reprinted by special permission of The William Alanson White Psychiatric Foundation, Inc. Copyright 1952 by The Foundation.

[1]See K. Goldstein, "Ueber die gleichartige functionelle Bedingtheit der Symptome in organischen und psychischen Krankheiten," *Monatsschrift fur Psychiatrie und Neurologie,* 1924, *57,* 191.

[2]K. Goldstein, "Die Beziehungen der Psychoanalyse zur Biologie"; in *Verhandlungen d. Congresses fur Psychotherapie in Nauheim* (Leipzig: Hirzel, 1927).

[3]See K. Goldstein, *Aftereffects of Brain Injuries in War* (New York: Grune & Stratton, 1942).

[4]See K. Goldstein, *The Organism; A Holistic Approach to Biology* (New York: American Book Co., 1939), pp. 310 ff.

phenomena of behavior become understandable if one assumes that all the behavior of the organism is determined by one trend,[5] the *trend to actualize itself* —that is, its nature and all its capacities. This takes place normally in such harmony that the realization of all capacities in the best way possible in the particular environment is permitted. The capacities are experienced by a person as various *needs* which he is driven to fulfill with the cooperation of some parts of the environment and in spite of the hindrance by other parts of it.

Each stimulation brings about some disorder in the organism. But after a certain time—which is determined by the particular performance—the organism comes back, by a process of *equalization,* to its normal condition. This process guarantees the constancy of the organism. A person's specific personality corresponds to this constancy. Because realization has to take place in terms of different needs and different tasks, the behavior of the organism is soon directed more by one than by another need. This does not mean that organismic behavior is determined by separate needs or drives. All such concepts need the assumption of a controlling agency. I have tried to show in my book, *The Organism,* that the different agencies which have been assumed for this purpose have only made for new difficulties in the attempt to understand organismic behavior; they are not necessary if one gives up the concept of separate drives, as my theory of the organism does. All of a person's capacities are always in action in each of his activities. The capacity that is particularly important for the task is in the foreground; the others are in the background. All of these capacities are organized in a way which facilitates the self-realization of the total organism in the particular situation. For each performance there is a definite figure ground organization of capacities; the change in the behavior of a patient corresponds to the change in the total organism in the form of an alteration of the normal pattern of figure-ground organization.[6]

Among patients with brain damage we can distinguish between alterations which occur when an area belonging to a special performance field—such as a motor or sensory area—is damaged somewhat isolatedly, and alterations which occur when the personality organization itself is altered. In lesions of these areas —according to a dedifferentiation of the function of the brain cortex[7]—qualities and patterns of behavior (both those developing as a result of maturation and those acquired by learning) are disturbed. Indeed, these patterns never occur isolatedly. They are always embedded in that kind of behavior which we call personality. The personality structure is disturbed particularly by lesions of the frontal lobes, the parietal lobes, and the insula Reili; but it is also disturbed by diffuse damage to the cortex—for instance, in paralysis, alcoholism, and trauma, and in metabolic disturbances such as hypoglycemia. The effect of diffuse damage is understandable when we consider that what we call personality structure apparently is not related to a definite locality of the cortex[8] but to a particular complex function of the brain which is the same for all its parts. This function can be damaged especially by lesions in any of the areas I have mentioned. The damage of the patterns certainly modifies the personality too. Although for full understanding of the personality changes, we should discuss the organization of the patterns and their destruction in damaged patients, that would carry us too far and is not absolutely necessary for our discussion. I shall therefore restrict my presentation to consideration of the symptoms due to damage of the personality structure itself.[9]

There would be no better way of getting to the heart of the problem than by demonstrating a patient. Unfortunately I have to substitute for this a description of the behavior of patients with severe damage of the brain cortex. Let us consider a man with an extensive lesion of the frontal lobes.[10] His customary way of living does not seem to be very much disturbed. He is a little slow; his face

[5]See K. Goldstein, *Human Nature in the Light of Psychopathology* (Cambridge: Harvard University Press, 1940), p. 194.

[6]Goldstein, *The Organism, op. cit.,* p. 109.

[7]*Ibid.,* p. 131.

[8]*Ibid.,* pp. 249 ff.

[9]See K. Goldstein, *Handbuch der normalen und pathalogischen Physiologie* (Berlin: J. S. Springer, 1927), Vol. 10, pp. 600 ff. and 813.

[10]K. Goldstein, "The Significance of the Frontal Lobes for Mental Performances," *Journal of Neurology and Psychopathology,* 1936, *17,* 27–40; and "The Modifications of Behavior Consequent to Cerebral Lesions," *Psychiatric Quarterly,* 1936, *10,* 586.

is rather immobile, rather rigid; his attention is directed very strictly to what he is doing at the moment—say, writing a letter, or speaking to someone. Confronted with tasks in various fields, he gives seemingly normal responses under certain conditions; but under other conditions he fails completely in tasks that seem to be very similar to those he has performed quite well.

This change of behavior becomes apparent particularly in the following simple test: We place before him a small wooden stick in a definite position, pointing, for example, diagonally from left to right. He is asked to note the position of the stick carefully. After a half minute's exposure, the stick is removed; then it is handed to the patient, and he is asked to put it back in the position in which it was before. He grasps the stick and tries to replace it, but he fumbles; he is all confusion; he looks at the examiner, shakes his head, tries this way and that, plainly uncertain. The upshot is that he cannot place the stick in the required position. He is likewise unable to imitate other simple figures built of sticks. Next we show the patient a little house made of many sticks—a house with a roof, a door, a window, and a chimney. After we remove it, we ask the patient to reproduce the model. He succeeds very well.

IMPAIRMENT OF ABSTRACT CAPACITY

If we ask ourselves what is the cause of the difference in his behavior in the two tasks, we can at once exclude defects in the field of perception, action, and memory. For there is no doubt that copying the house with many details demands a much greater capacity in all these faculties, especially in memory, than putting a single stick into a position which the patient has been shown shortly before. A further experiment clarifies the situation. We put before the patient two sticks placed together so as to form an angle with the opening pointing upward (V). The patient is unable to reproduce this model. Then we confront him with the same angle, the opening downward this time (Λ), and now he reproduces the figure very well on the first trial. When we ask the patient how it is that he can reproduce the second figure but not the

first one, he says, "This one has nothing to do with the other one." Pointing to the second one, he says, "That is a roof"; pointing to the first, "That is nothing."

These two replies lead us to an understanding of the patient's behavior. His first reply makes it clear that, to him, the two objects with which he has to deal are totally different from one another. The second answer shows that he apprehends the angle with the opening downward as a concrete object out of his own experience, and he constructs a concrete thing with the two sticks. The two sticks that formed an angle with the opening upward apparently did not arouse an impression of a concrete thing. He had to regard the sticks as representations indicating directions in abstract space. Furthermore, he had to keep these directions in mind and rearrange the sticks from memory as representatives of these abstract directions. To solve the problem he must give an account to himself of relations in space and must act on the basis of abstract ideas. Thus we may conclude that the failure of the patient in the first test lies in the fact that he is unable to perform a task which can be executed only by means of a grasp of the abstract. The test in which the opening of the angle is downwards does not demand this, since the patient is able to grasp it as a concrete object and therefore to execute it perfectly. It is for the same reason that he is able to copy the little house, which seems to us to be so much more complicated. From the result of his behavior in this and similar tasks we come to the assumption that these *patients are impaired in their abstract capacity.*

The term "abstract attitude," which I shall use in describing this capacity, will be more comprehensible in the light of the following explanation.[11] We can distinguish two different kinds of attitudes, the concrete and the abstract. In the concrete attitude we are given over passively and bound to the immediate experience of unique objects or situations. Our thinking and acting are determined by the immediate claims made by the particular aspect of the object or situation. For instance, we act concretely when

---

[11]See K. Goldstein and M. Scheerer, *Abstract and Concrete Behavior,* Psychological Monographs. No. 239, 1941.

we enter a room in darkness and push the button for light. If, however, we reflect that by pushing the button we might awaken someone asleep in the room, and desist from pushing the button, then we are acting abstractively. We transcend the immediately given specific aspect of sense impressions; we detach ourselves from these impressions, consider the situation from a conceptual point of view, and react accordingly. Our actions are determined not so much by the objects before us as by the way we think about them: the individual thing becomes a mere accidental representative of a category to which it belongs.

The impairment of the attitude toward the abstract shows in every performance of the brain-damaged patient who is impaired in this capacity. He always fails when the solution of a task presupposes this attitude; he performs well when the appropriate activity is determined directly by the stimuli and when the task can be fulfilled by concrete behavior. He may have no difficulty in using known objects in a situation that requires them; but he is totally at a loss if he is asked to demonstrate the use of such an object outside the concrete situation, and still more so if he is asked to do it without the real object. A few examples will illustrate this.

The patient is asked to blow away a slip of paper. He does this very well. If the paper is taken away and he is asked to think that there is a slip of paper and to blow it away, he is unable to do do so. Here the situation is not realistically complete. In order to perform the task the patient would have to imagine the piece of paper there. He is not capable of this.

The patient is asked to throw a ball into open boxes situated respectively at distances of three, nine, and fifteen feet. He does that correctly. When he is asked how far the several boxes are from him, he is not only unable to answer this question but unable even to say which box is nearest to him and which is farthest.

In the first action, the patient has only to deal with objects in a behavioral fashion. It is unnecessary for him to be conscious of this behavior and of objects in a world separated from himself. In the second, however, he must separate himself from objects in the outer world and give himself an account of his actions and of the space relations in the world facing him. Since he is unable to do this, he fails. We could describe this failure also by saying that the patient is unable to deal with a situation which is only possible.

A simple story is read to a patient. He may repeat some single words, but he does not understand their meaning and is unable to grasp the essential point. Now we read him another story, which would seem to a normal person to be more difficult to understand. This time he understands the meaning very well and recounts the chief points. The first story deals with a simple situation, but a situation which has no connection with the actual situation of the patient. The second story recounts a situation he is familiar with. Hence one could say the patient is able to grasp and handle only something which is related to himself.

Such a patient almost always recognizes pictures of single objects, even if the picture contains many details. In pictures which represent a composition of a number of things and persons, he may pick out some details; but he is unable to understand the picture as a whole and is unable to respond to the whole. The patient's real understanding does not depend on the greater or smaller number of components in a picture but on whether the components, whatever their number, hang together concretely and are familiar to him, or whether an understanding of their connection requires a more abstract synthesis on his part. He may lack understanding of a picture even if there are only a few details. If the picture does not reveal its essence directly, by bringing the patient into the situation which it represents, he is not able to understand it. Thus one may characterize the deficiency as an inability to discover the essence of a situation which is not related to his own personality.

CATASTROPHIC CONDITIONS

Impairment of abstraction is not the only factor which produces deviations in the behavior of patients, as I have stated before. Another very important factor is the occurrence of a catastrophic condition.[12] When a patient is not able to ful-

---

[12]Goldstein, *The Organism, op. cit.*, pp. 35 ff.

fill a task set before him, this condition is a frequent occurrence. A patient may look animated, calm, in a good mood, well-poised, collected, and cooperative when he is confronted with tasks he can fulfill; the same patient may appear dazed, become agitated, change color, start to fumble, become unfriendly, evasive, and even aggressive when he is not able to fulfill the task. His overt behavior appears very much the same as a person in a state of anxiety. I have called the state of the patient in the situation of success, *ordered condition;* the state in the situation of failure, *disordered or catastrophic condition.*

In the catastrophic condition the patient not only is incapable of performing a task which exceeds his impaired capacity, but he also fails, for a longer or shorter period, in performances which he is able to carry out in the ordered state. For a varying period of time, the organism's reactions are in great disorder or are impeded altogether. We are able to study this condition particularly well in these patients, since we can produce it experimentally by demanding from the patient something which we know he will not be able to do, because of his defect. Now, as we have said, impairment of abstraction makes it impossible for a patient to account to himself for his acts. He is quite unable to realize his failure and why he fails. Thus we can assume that catastrophic condition is not a reaction of the patient to failure, but rather belongs intrinsically to the situation of the organism in failing. For the normal person, failure in the performance of a non-important task would be merely something disagreeable; for the brain-injured person, however, as observation shows, any failure means the impossibility of self-realization and of existence. The occurrence of catastrophic condition is not limited therefore to special tasks; any task can place the patient in this situation, since the patient's self-realization is endangered so easily. Thus the same task produces anxiety at one time, and not at another.

Anxiety

The conditions under which anxiety occurs in brain-injured patients correspond to the conditions for its occurrence in normal people in that what produces anxiety is not the failure itself, but the resultant danger to the person's existence. I would like to add that the danger need not always be real; it is sufficient if the person images that the condition is such that he will not be able to realize himself. For instance, a person may be in distress because he is not able to answer questions in an examination. If the outcome of the examination is not particularly important, then the normal person will take it calmly even though he may feel somewhat upset; because it is not a dangerous situation for him, he will face the situation and try to come to terms with it as well as he can by using his wits, and in this way he will bring it to a more or less successful solution. The situation becomes totally different, however, if passing the examination is of great consequence in the person's life; not passing the examination may, for instance, endanger his professional career or the possibility of marrying the person he loves. When self-realization is seriously in danger, catastrophe may occur together with severe anxiety; when this occurs, it is impossible for the person to answer even those questions which, under other circumstances, he could solve without difficulty.

I would like to clarify one point here —namely, that anxiety represents an emotional state which does not refer to any object. Certainly the occurrence of anxiety is connected with an outer or inner event. The organism, shaken by a catastrophic shock, exists in relation to a definite reality; and the basic phenomenon of anxiety, which is the occurrence of disordered behavior, is understandable only in terms of this relationship to reality. But anxiety does not originate from the experiencing of this relationship. The brain-injured patient could not experience anxiety, if it were necessary for him to experience this relationship to reality. He is certainly not aware of this objective reality; he experiences only the shock, only anxiety. And this, of course holds true for anxiety in general. Observations of many patients confirm the interpretation of anxiety by philosophers, such as Pascal and Kierkegaard, and by psychologists who have dealt with anxiety—namely, that the source of anxiety is the inner experience of not being confronted with anything or of being confronted with nothingness.

In making such a statement, one must distinguish sharply between *anxiety* and *fear*—another emotional state which is very often confused with anxiety.[13] Superficially, fear may have many of the characteristics of anxiety, but intrinsically it is different. In the state of fear we have an object before us, we can meet that object, we can attempt to remove it, or we can flee from it. We are conscious of ourselves, as well as of the object; we can deliberate as to how we shall behave toward it, and we can look at the cause of the fear, which actually lies before us. Anxiety, on the other hand, gets at us from the back, so to speak. The only thing we can do is to attempt to flee from it, but without knowing what direction to take, since we experience it as coming from no particular place. We are dealing, as I have shown explicitly elsewhere, with qualitative differences, with different attitudes toward the world. Fear is related, in our experience, to an object; anxiety is not—it is only an inner state.

What is characteristic of the object of fear? It is something inherent in the object itself, at all times? Of course not. At one time an object may arouse only interest, or be met with indifference; but at another time it may evoke the greatest fear. In other words, fear must be the result of a specific relationship between organism and object. What leads to fear is nothing but the experience of the possibility of the onset of anxiety. What we fear is the impending anxiety, which we experience in relation to some objects. Since a person in a state of fear is not yet in a state of anxiety but only envisions it—that is, he only fears that anxiety may befall him—he is not so disturbed in his judgment of the outer world as the person in a state of anxiety. Rather, driven as he is by the tendency to avoid the onset of anxiety, he attempts to establish special contact with the outer world. He tries to recognize the situation as clearly as possible and to react to it in an appropriate manner. Fear is conditioned by, and directed against, very definite aspects of the environment. These have to be recognized and, if possible, removed. Fear sharpens the senses, whereas anxiety renders them unusable. Fear drives to action; anxiety paralyzes.

From these explanations it is obvious that in order to feel anxiety it is not necessary to be able to give oneself an account of one's acts; to feel fear, however, presupposes that capacity. From this it becomes clear that our patients do not behave like people in a state of fear—that is, they do not intentionally try to avoid situations from which anxiety may arise. They cannot do that because of the defect of abstraction. Also from our observation of the patients we can assume that they do not experience fear and that they only have the experience of anxiety.

Anxiety, a catastrophic condition in which self-realization is not possible, may be produced by a variety of events, all of which have in common the following: There is a discrepancy between the individual's capacities and the demands made on him, and this discrepancy makes self-realization impossible. This may be due to external or internal conditions, physical or psychological. It is this discrepancy to which we are referring when we speak of "conflicts." Thus we can observe anxiety in infants, in whom such a discrepancy must occur frequently, particularly since their abstract attitude is not yet developed or not fully. We also see anxiety in brain-injured people, in whom impairment of abstraction produces the same discrepancy. In normal people, anxiety appears when the demands of the world are too much above the capacity of the individual, when social and economic situations are too stressful, or when religious conflicts arise. Finally we see anxiety in people with neuroses and psychoses which are based on unsolvable and unbearable inner conflicts.

THE PROTECTIVE MECHANISMS

The last group of symptoms to be observed in brain-injured patients are the behavior changes which make it possible for the patient to get rid of the catastrophic condition—of anxiety.[14] The

[13]See K. Goldstein, "Zum Problem der Angst," *Allg. ärztl. Ztschr. f. Psychotherap, u. psych. Hygiene,* 1929, *2,* 409–437. Also, Goldstein, *The Organism, op. cit.,* p. 293.

[14]Goldstein, *The Organism, op. cit.,* p. 40 ff.

observation of this phenomenon in these patients is of special interest since it can teach us how an organism can get rid of anxiety without being aware of its origin and without being able to avoid the anxiety voluntarily. After a certain time these patients show a diminution of disorder and of catastrophic eactions (anxiety) even though the defect caused by the damage to the brain still exists. This, of course, can occur only if the patient is no longer exposed to tasks he cannot cope with. This diminution is achieved by definite changes in the behavior of the patients: They are withdrawn, so that a number of stimuli, including dangerous ones, do not reach them. They usually stay alone; either they do not like company or they want to be only with people whom they know well. They like to be in a familiar room in which everything is organized in a definite way. They show extreme orderliness in every respect; everything has to be done exactly at an appointed time—whether it is breakfast, dinner, or a walk. They show excessive and fanatical orderliness in arranging their belongings; each item of their wardrobe must be in a definite place—that is, in a place where it can be gotten hold of quickly, without the necessity of a choice, which they are unable to make. Although it is a very primitive order indeed, they stick fanatically to it; it is the only way to exist. Any change results in a state of very great excitement. They themselves cannot voluntarily arrange things in a definite way. The orderliness is maintained simply because the patients try to stick to those arrangements which they can handle. This sticking to that which they can cope with is characteristic for their behavior; thus any behavior change can be understood only in terms of this characteristic behavior.

An illustration of this characteristic behavior is the fact that they always try to keep themselves busy with things that they are able to do as a protection against things that they cannot cope with. The activities which engross them need not be of great value in themselves. Their usefulness consists apparently in the fact that they protect the patient. Thus a patient does not like to be interrupted in an activity. For instance, although a patient may behave well in a conversation with someone he knows and likes, he does not like to be suddenly addressed by someone else.

We very often observe that a patient is totally unaware of his defect—such as hemiplegia or hemianopsia—and of the difference between his state prior to the development of the symptoms and his present state. This is strikingly illustrated by the fact that the disturbances of these patients play a very small part in their complaints. We are not dealing simply with a subjective lack of awareness, for the defects are effectively excluded from awareness, one might say. This is shown by the fact that they produce very little disturbance—apparently as the result of compensation. This exclusion from awareness seems to occur particularly when the degree of functional defect in performance is extreme. We can say that defects are shut out from the life of the organism when they would seriously impair any of its essential functions and when a defect can be compensated for by other activities at least to the extent that self-realization is not essentially disturbed.

One can easily get the impression that a patient tries to deny the experience of the functional disturbance because he is afraid that he will get into a catastrophic condition if he becomes aware of his defect. As a matter of fact, a patient may get into a catastrophic condition when we make him aware of his defect, or when the particular situation does not make possible an adequate compensation. Sometimes this happens—and this is especially interesting—when the underlying pathological condition improves and with that the function.

A patient of mine who became totally blind by a suicidal gunshot through the chiasma opticum behaved as if he were not aware of his blindness; the defect was compensated for very well by his use of his other senses, his motor skill, and his knowledge and intelligence. He was usually in a good mood; he never spoke of his defect, and he resisted all attempts to draw his attention to it. After a certain time, the condition improved; but at the same time he realized that he could not recognize objects through his vision. He was shocked and became deeply depressed. When he was asked why he was depressed, he said, "I cannot see." We might assume that in the beginning the patient denied the defect intentionally because he could not bear it. But why then did he not deny it when he began to see? Or we might assume that in the beginning he did not deny his blindness, but that in total blindness an adjustment occurred in terms of a change of behavior for which vision was not necessary; and because of this it was not necessary for him to realize his blindness. The moment he was able to see, he became aware of his defect and was no longer able to eliminate it. The exclusion of the blindness defect from awareness could thus be considered a secondary effect of the adjustment. But in this patient who was mentally undisturbed a more voluntary denial cannot be overlooked. A voluntary denial is not possible in patients with impairment of abstraction as in brain-injured patients. Here the unawareness of the defect can only be a secondary effect—an effect of the same behavior, which we have described before, by which the brain-injured person is protected against catastrophes which may occur because of his defect. As we have said, the patient, driven by the trend to realize himself as well as possible, sticks to what he is able to do; this shows in his whole behavior. From this point of view, the patient's lack of awareness of his defect, as well as his peculiarities in general, becomes understandable. For instance, in these terms, it is understandable why an aphasic patient utters a word which is only on the normal fringe of the word that he needs; for the word that he needs to use is a word that he cannot say at all or can say only in such a way that he could not be understood and would as a result be in distress.[15] Thus a patient may repeat "church" instead of "God," "father" instead of "mother," and so on; he considers his reaction correct, at least as long as no one makes him aware of the fact that his reaction is wrong. This same kind of reaction occurs in disturbances of recognition, of feelings, and so on.

One is inclined to consider the use of wrong words or disturbances of recognition, actions, and feelings as due to a special pathology; but that is not their origin. Since these disturbances are reactions which represent all that the individual is able to execute, he recognizes them as fulfillment of the task; in this way, these reactions fulfill this need to such a degree that no catastrophe occurs. Thus the protection appears as a passive effect of an active "correct" procedure and could not be correctly termed denial, which refers to a more intentional activity, "conscious" or "unconscious."

This theory on the origin of the protective behavior in organic patients deserves consideration, particularly because the phenomena observed in organic patients shows such a similarity to that observed in neurotics. One could even use psychoanalytic terms for the different forms of behavior in organic patients. For instance, one might use the same terms that Anna Freud[16] uses to characterize various defense mechanisms against anxiety. Both neurotic and organic patients show a definite similarity in behavior structure and in the purpose served by that structure. In organic patients, however, I prefer to speak of protective mechanisms instead of defense mechanisms; the latter refers to a more voluntary act, which organic patients certainly cannot perform, as we have discussed earlier. In neurotics, the development of defense mechanisms generally does not occur so passively through organismic adjustment, as does the development of protective mechanisms in the organic patients; this is in general the distinction between the two. It seems to me that this distinction is not true in the case of neurotic children, however; some of these children seem to develop protective mechanisms in a passive way, similar to organic patients. Such mechanisms can perhaps be found in other neurotics. Thus, in interpreting these mechanisms, one should take into account the possibility of confusing the neurotic patient with the organic patient.

I would like to add a last word with regard to the restrictions of the personality and of the world of these patients which is brought about by this protective behavior. The restrictions are not as disturbing in the brain-injured patients as is the effect of defense mechanisms in neuroses. In a neurotic, defense mechanisms represent a characteristic part of

---

[15]Goldstein, *Language and Language Disturbances, op. cit.,* p. 226.

[16]A. Freud, *The Ego and the Mechanisms of Defense* (New York: International University Press, 1946).

the disturbances he is suffering from; but the organic patient does not become aware of the restriction since his protective mechanisms allow for some ordered form of behavior and for the experience of some kind of self-realization—which is true, of course, only as long as the environment is so organized by the people around him that no tasks arise that he cannot fulfill and as long as the protecting behavior changes are not hindered. This is the only way the brain-damaged person can exist. The patient cannot bear conflict—that is, anxiety, restriction, or suffering. In this respect he differs essentially from the neurotic who is more or less able to bear conflict. This is the main difference which demands a different procedure in treatment; in many respects, however, treatment can be set up in much the same way for both.[17] In treating these patients, it is more important to deal with the possible occurrence of catastrophe rather than with the impairment of abstraction, for my observations of a great many patients for over ten years indicate that the impairment of abstraction cannot be alleviated unless the brain damage from which it originated

is eliminated. There is no functional restitution of this capacity by compensation through other parts of the brain. Improvement of performances can be achieved only by the building up of substitute performances by the use of the part of concrete behavior which is preserved; but this is only possible by a definite arrangement of the environment.

I am well aware that my description of the personality change in brain damage is somewhat sketchy. The immense material and the problems involved, so manifold and complex, make a more satisfactory presentation in such a brief time impossible. I hope that I have been successful in outlining, to the best of my ability, the essential phenomena and problems of these patients. In addition, I trust that I have shown how much we can learn from these observations for our concept of the structure of the personality, both normal and pathological, and for the treatment of brain-damaged patients and also, I hope, of patients with so-called psychogenic disorders.

---

[17]See K. Goldstein, "The Idea of Disease and Therapy," *Review of Religion*, 1949, *14*, 229–240.

THERAPY

It should not be surprising that biophysical theorists prefer biophysical methods for treating psychopathology. According to them, the primary source of the difficulty exists in the biophysical make-up of the patient. It follows logically then that efforts should be made to remedy the defect directly. The fact that few of these "defects" have been specified or even localized has not deterred the development of biophysical therapies. The chapter by Lothar Kalinowsky and Paul Hoch summarizes the rather checkered history of theories of biophysical therapy, and offers incisive commentaries on their respective merits as theories and as therapies. In a different vein, Harold Himwich presents a detailed review of the biophysical substrate underlying the action of the new psychopharmacologic agents. Here he demonstrates the complex steps required to track down the varied and intricate neurophysiological reactions to these drugs.

7. Theories of Somatic Treatment

LOTHAR KALINOWSKY and PAUL HOCH

Psychiatry differs from other fields of medicine in a deplorable lack of facts on which all psychiatrists can agree. There is no generally accepted etiology of most mental diseases, and the entire foundation of the specialty of psychiatry is based on theories believed by some, and opposed by others. It is, therefore, not surprising that attempts to explain treatment procedures vary with the theoretical approach of the observer. This in itself leads to differences in explaining the mode of action of treatments. The matter is complicated by the fact that all psychiatric treatments were found empirically, and only later theories were developed to explain their action. Many theories were offered for one individual method, and efforts to find a common denominator for several treatments with similar effects have also been made. None of these attempts was satisfactory. The following chapter tries to list the theories presented in the literature, and to scrutinize their validity.

PHARMACOTHERAPY

While in the field of the later discussed shock treatments, theories were primarily based on the individual belief of those who developed them, pharmacotherapy offered a more scientific basis of theoretical considerations. It must not be overlooked, however, that no theoretical concepts led to the introduction of any of the new drugs into psychiatry. Even the hope that they would contribute to a better understanding of the pathophysiological manifestations underlying psychiatric disorders, was not fulfilled. The same hope had been expressed, when the shock treatments were introduced. Thus far, all forms of therapy were equally disappointing in this respect. In pharmacotherapy the interest of the basic sciences was greater than in previous somatic treatments, and it was justified to expect that this chemical approach would

From *Somatic Treatments in Psychiatry*, Chapter 7, Grune and Stratton, 1961, by Lothar B. Kalinowsky and Paul B. Hoch. By permission of the publisher and Dr. Kalinowsky.

lead to better knowledge of the biochemical basis of psychopathological manifestations and their changes under the influence of known chemicals. Actually, the various theories presented for the action of the empirically found neuroleptics are still quite speculative. Some clearly defined theories on certain antidepressant drugs turned out to be inapplicable to other drugs with the same clinical effect. The following theoretical considerations are presented mainly as a starting point for further efforts.

The main basis for theory formation in pharmacotherapy is animal experimentation and observations in humans. Most pharmacological properties have already been described in the chapters on the various drugs or groups of drugs. Here, only some studies concentrating on theoretical implications will be added.

There is essential agreement on the regions of the brain on which the phenothiazines act. The regions of the brain that are affected are the thalamus, the hypothalamus, the reticular formation and the remainder of the extra-pyramidal system. Clinically one of the most prominent side-effects of this group of drugs are the extrapyramidal manifestations (parkinsonism, dystonia, and akathisia). Many of these symptoms have been compared to those occurring in encephalitis lethargica which affects similar areas of the brain. The potency of a phenothiazine appears to increase in association with the incidence of extrapyramidal effects. Stimulation of the reticular formation formation alerting system produces characteristic low amplitude rapid waves in the EEG associated with arousal of the organism. In small doses chlorpromazine blocks this arousal pattern, but in large doses its action is reversed and the alerting system may be stimulated. Wase el al. have demonstrated the specificity of chlorpromazine for the reticular formation radiochemically.

The phenothiazines also have antiadrenergic activity. Dell and his group have shown experimentally that, after blockage of adrenergic intra-reticular mechanisms by chlorpromazine, the spontaneous activity of the reticular formation is diminished. There is no longer a reaction to adrenaline liberated through nociceptive stimulation, and the reticular formation becomes more sensitive to inhibiting influences. The animal receiving

chlorpromazine has a reduced spontaneous activity, fall asleep readily, and, if it is awakened, the waking state is not maintained. Dell suggests that certain neurones of the reticular formation are adrenergic in nature and that consequently adrenaline or a related substance can have a central reticular action.

Phenothiazines have been found to block the central actions of norepinephrine analogs such as mescaline and amphetamine and of parenterally administered catechol amines. The substance used for the latter purpose is DOPA—dihydroxyphenylalanine—the amino acid precursor of the catechol amines which, when given intravenously to rabbits, produces typical sympathetic effects. Its breakdown product has a marked resemblance to norepinephrine. The excitement and increased psychomotor activity consequent upon the sympathetic stimulation are blocked by chlorpromazine. It has been suggested that chlorpromazine blocks the sympathetic activities by interfering with the action of norepinephrine in the brain. However, this does not account for all the action of these drugs in psychiatric illness, such as on delusions and hallucinations, which are also alleviated together with the diminution of increased psychomotor activity.

Saunders has suggested the following hypothesis for the action of the phenothiazines, Raufwolfia alkaloids and iproniazid. He suggests that in schizophrenia transamination is excessive in the brain, while in depression it is oxidative deamination which is excessive. The transamination reaction is catalysed by ionic copper, with pyridoxine as the co-enzyme. Chlorpromazine and reserpine are able to form complexes and/or chelates with copper and to modify the action of copper—catalysed enzymes. They both increase copper plasma levels. Chlorpromazine and reserpine may, therefore, provide copper in the necessary physico-chemical state to control transaminase reactions at the proper rate.

Charatan has put forward the theory that chlorpromazine, as a tertiary ammonium compound, gives rise to free base in the central nervous system which has the property of entering nerve cells. It will achieve its maximum effects according to the density of the cell population. Thus selective concentration in the basal ganglia including the thalamus would lead to interference with corticothalamic circuits and a reduction in the pathologically increased psychomotor activity.

Gliedman and Horsley Gantt considered the greatest value of the tranquilizing drugs to be their ability to insulate organisms from stimuli to which they are subjected, but to which they do not have learned meanings. In acute excitement states, due to overwhelming stress, there might be a breakdown of learned reactions with a residue of heightened unlearned reactivity and consequent hyper-motor and hyper-autonomic activity. There might also be overactivity consequent upon a failure to have learned appropriate responses to stressful situations.

Pavlovian techniques, applied by Soviet psychiatrists, lead, according to J. Wortis, to the conclusion that chlorpromazine (aminazine) has a dual therapeutic role: The general inhibition of an animal exposed to overwhelming stimulation is relieved by the drug because of its dampening effect on overstimulation. At the same time, the drug promotes a reorganization of the disordered conditioned responses.

Interesting attempts at distinguishing between the effects of phenothiazine on the cells and on the regulating centers of the two opposing parts of the vegetative nervous system were made by C. and H. Selbach. Few studies were made to investigate the effect of the neuroleptics on metabolism. An exception is the work by Consbrough and Faust who tried to correlate the treatment effect of phenothiazine and reserpine in various endogenous psychoses with changes of serum protein levels. They observed a characteristic lowering of serum albumen and rise of serum alpha-globulin in patients who responded to therapy. The changes of serum protein levels were only minimal, when therapeutic results were poor.

Himwich paid particular attention to the manner in which specific "tranquilizers" affect specific areas of the brain. Some of his conclusions are that the phenothiazines and also the barbiturates suppress the midbrain reticular formation, and that the rauwolfia derivatives stimulate it, and that meprobamate has no particular effect on this activating system. Serotonin is influenced by phenothiazines and rauwolfia derivatives but not by barbiturates and meprobamate. These last two drugs are also clinically very similar, but they differ in the depressive effect of barbiturates on the hypothalamus which meprobamate does not have. Aside from the midbrain reticular formation the activating system consists of diffused thalamo-cortical projections which may be influenced by the drugs in different ways. The second great system involved in emotion is the limbic system (rhinencephalon) or Papez circuit which is stimulated by the neuroleptic drugs but depressed by meprobamate and barbiturates. Similar attempts at stimulation of drug action on various parts of the brain were made by Kraines whose studies also include the psychoanaleptics.

The more clinically and psychopathologically oriented theories are mentioned in the clinical chapters. Freyhan's concept that the effect of neuroleptic drugs is dependent on hypomotility can be found under "central nervous system side-effects of chlorpromazine," where the question of the relationship between extrapyramidal manifestations and therapeutic effect will also be discussed.

The action of the various new drugs have also been explained in psychoanalytical terms. At the time this book goes to press Sarwer-Foner edited a volume with numerous contributions on "The Dynamics of Psychiatric Drug Therapy." We can only refer to this book which is not yet available to us with the exception of a contribution by Ostow. He infers that neuroleptics and antidepressants primarily affect a function which Freud hypothesized "psychic energy," which is ultimately derived at from instinctual impetus. Ostow stipulates that the phenothiazines decrease the amount of psychic energy available to the ego, while iproniazid increases it.

There are many psychoanalysts who reject pharmacotherapeutic support to patients on psychotherapy for theoretical reasons. It is difficult to see why, for instance, a patient should not be given relief by means of drugs because it has been claimed that this may diminish his efforts to work out his problems with the psychotherapist. A more valid objection to the use of the new drugs is that such symptoms as feelings of depersonalization might be produced by certain drugs, and, like other side-effects, interfere with the patient's cooperation in the analytical session. The question to what extent the new drugs really aid in psychotherapy is still open, and we agree with Sargant that in some cases older sedatives such as phenobarbital may be more helpful than the neuroleptics.

Concepts regarding the group of antidepressant drugs which found the greatest theoretical interest, were discussed in the section on monoamine oxidase inhibitors. Strangely enough, this rather hypothetical effect of iproniazid and similar drugs gave the name to this entire group of analeptics, and the term had to be explained together with their pharmacological properties prior to the discussion of the individual drugs.

INSULIN AND CONVULSIVE TREATMENTS

In the area of shock treatments, many theories have been presented, many of them without actual foundation in facts. Some overlap, and some express the same idea in different terms. This made it possible for Gordon to collect the surprising number of fifty different theories. We still agree with Nolan D. C. Lewis that "at the present time there is no theory as to the nature of the shock treatments sufficiently comprehensible to be taken very seriously."

The therapeutic action is explained by some authors on an organic basis, others believe that shock treatments effect essentially a psychogenic cure. The so-called somatic theories will be discussed first. The first explanation was advanced by Sakel concerning insulin treatment. The theory of insulin action was obviously evolved during or after the introduction of the treatment as an afterthought. Sakel himself realized that his theory was not too convincingly elaborated. He once wrote: "The mistakes in theory should not be counted against the treatment itself, which seems to be accomplishing more than the theory behind it."

Sakel believed that the nerve cell develops an exaggerated activity, becomes oversensitive to the normal stimuli of the outside world and elaborates these stimuli excessively. "To restore normal conditions again," he writes, "one has to either limit the supply of excitant material, or else diminish combustion in the cell by muffling it." He conceives the action of insulin as being due to neutralization of the excitant, which he believes to be a hormone, and to the vagotonic muffling of the cell. He further assumes that in schizophrenics, the phylogenetically youngest intracellular connections are injured, and the more ancient nerve pathways are activated. As the disease progresses, these normally obliterated pathways dominate the scene. The stronger the harmful influence of the disease, more and more deeply seated pathways are involved successively until phylogenetically ancient pathway patterns are reached which prove to be resistant to the toxic influences. Sakel also assumes a short-circuiting of the pathways between the nerve cells. Insulin shock treatment, according to him, reverses all these processes by blockading the cell through influence on the vegetative centers so that the injured or confused pathways are not exposed to further stimuli. By means of this artificial rest, the normal pathways recuperate and attain their former prominence. In schizophrenia, vegetative subcortical centers are assumed to be the site of the primary disturbance, of which the abnormal psychotic symptoms are secondary manifestations.

It is apparent that this hypothesis of Sakel's is far too vague and speculative to offer convincing evidence on the action of insulin shock. It leaves completely unresolved the questions as to how and where this overaction of the nervous system originates in schizophrenia, and, furthermore, what kind of physical-chemical process is responsible for the "blockade" of the cell or the short-circuiting of the pathways. Nor does this theory elucidate the etiology of schizophrenia which is a necessary shortcoming of all theories on treatments of this disease.

A similar theory centering on cell destruction was evolved more recently by Arnold. He assumes that insulin leads to an acute disorganization of carbohydrate metabolism of the ganglion cell which first interferes with cell function and ends in cell destruction. This effect of insulin is limited to those ganglion cells which for genetic reasons are predisposed to a disturbance in carbo-hydrate metabolism.

Meduna's introduction of the met-razol treatment was based on premises which proved to be incorrect, but, as so often happens in science, an errone-ous working hypothesis yielded an ef-fective therapeutic weapon. We owe to it not only the pharmacological con-vulsive therapy but also the electric con-vulsive therapy for which no new theories have been developed by their inventors. Meduna's theoretical basis for the introduction of the convulsive treatment was the assumption that epilepsy and schizophrenia are antago-nistic to each other. He found, in his clinical studies, that these two dis-orders very rarely occurred together. Moreover, his biochemical investiga-tions supported this theory as deter-minations of uric acid, creatinine, ni-trogen content, and blood sugar sug-gested that schizophrenics and epilep-tics had a different biochemistry. In ad-dition, he made clinical observations which emphasized the beneficial effects of spontaneously occurring epileptic con-vulsions in schizophrenic patients.

Meduna's assumption that schizo-phrenia and epilepsy are antagonistic to each other has been refuted by a num-ber of authors. The biochemistry of both disorders is so complicated and still so obscure, that no theory of similarity or antagonism regarding these two diseases can be formulated at the present time. Recently, in strong contrast to von Meduna's original concept of a biolog-ical antagonism between the two dis-eases, attempts have been made to es-tablish a positive relationship between schizophrenia and epilepsy on the basis of electroencephalographic findings. This, however, was disproved by Hoch, who demonstrated in a genetic, electroenceph-alographic, and clinical study that the two disorders are neither related nor opposed to each other. The observation by Meduna that spontaneous epileptic attacks in schizophrenia influence favorably the clinical symptomatology is probably more valid. However, contrary to clinical evi-dence brought forward by other workers, Esser, on the basis of 10,000 patients surveyed in the literature, arrives at the conclusion that epileptic convulsions are not infrequent in catatonia and in many cases are not followed by improvement.

But the main argument against von Meduna's theory is the fact that con-vulsive treatment is most effective in the manic-depressive psychoses. The great therapeutic value of convulsive therapy in the affective disorders was recognized, but not until several years after the theo-retical foundation for the treatment of schizophrenia with convulsions had been developed. A theory of a biological an-tagonism, therefore, would have to be extended to cover the affective psycho-ses as well.

After Sakel and Meduna had given the first theoretical explanations for the treatments devised by them, other au-thors advanced theories which were partly elaborations of previous ones; again, others suggested some new mech-anisms that might be responsible for the improvement, with more and more em-phasis on the common denominators in view of the great similarity in the effec-tiveness of insulin and convulsive ther-apies. Georgi believes that alteration of the nerve cell membrane is responsible for the success of these therapies. Evi-dence of this membrane alteration is found in a reduction in the amount of sugar in the cell, which is produced slowly in the hypoglycemic coma and quickly with metrazol and electric shock. Demole and Freudenberg expressed simi-lar ideas. Von Angyal believes that hy-poglycemia affects the metabolism in the brain cells due to reduction of the sugar content followed by compensa-tion and an increased metabolism stim-ulating the cells that are in a state of malfunction or degeneration. Similarly. Küppers thinks that metabolic exhaus-tion in the nerve cells due to insulin provokes a counteraction and finally re-stores the cells to normal functioning. An unknown toxic substance is assumed by Danziger to accumulate in the body. This substance might depress the rate of heat production by inhibiting one of the respiratory enzymes. Shock therapy is assumed to remove the postulated toxic material. This idea is similar to the as-sumption that in epilepsy the convulsion eliminates toxic substances, and insulin, by way of sweating, does the same. Cerletti formulated the theory that con-vulsions bring the organism to a state which is close to death, thereby arousing a reaction of extreme biologic defense in producing a substance he calls ago-nine, which exerts the therapeutic effect. Pappalardo explains the effect of shock as well as of fever therapies as means of modifying the defense mechanism of the organism via the reticuloendothelial system. Ewald believes that all shock treatments have a marked influence on the diencephalon whose regulatory mechanisms are intensely stimulated under any kind of shock treatment. He speaks of a "massage of the diencephalic centers" and states that changes in the vegetative regulation, expressing themselves, among other symptoms, by increased weight, are the important therapeutic factors. His theory follows logically his ideas on the origin of schizophrenia which he localized essentially in the diencephalon. In a paper on electric shock therapy, Ewald and Haddenbrock list various observations to support this theory.

A similar concept is Delay's and Mallet's, that the shock treatments exert a sedative effect on hyperthymias (manic states) and a stimulating effect on hypothymias (depressive states). The action of the treatment is explained as excitation of the diencephalon in the hyperthymias and as depression of the diencephalon in the hypothymias. Thus, it is postulated that the vegetative centers in the brain are influenced. Delmas-Marsalet's theory of dissolution and reconstruction of the mechanism of ECT is in many respects related. Delay and also Delmas-Marsalet expounded their theories in monographs on the subject.

Attempts were made to determine whether cerebral oxidation was the common denominator for the action of all shock treatments. High insulin doses prevent the utilization of carbohydrates by the central nervous system and indirectly reduce the oxidation of the brain, as demonstrated in human beings by Damashek and Myerson, and in animals by Himwich et al. Oxygen consumption of the brain drops during insulin treatment and the basal metabolism of the nervous system is reduced by about 60 per cent. The reduction in the metabolism of the brain is actually even greater if we consider that during hypoglycemia the circulation time of the blood in the brain is reduced by about 25 per cent. Serejski is of the opinion that it is not so much the reduction of oxygen as the inability to utilize oxygen that is important in this metabolic alteration. He finds relatively high oxygen content in the veins of the brain during insulin treatment. Convulsive treatments do not produce anoxemia for as long a period as does insulin, but anoxemia is present temporarily, during and shortly after the convulsion, due to the vasoconstriction which the convulsion produces. In electrically induced convulsions, Wortis et al. found interference with oxygen uptake. Due to the anoxia, a reduction in brain metabolism ensues, to be supplanted by a compensatory hyperactivity after the convulsion. In the light of experience with ECT under anesthesia during which the patient is not anoxic but rather oversaturated with oxygen, it is difficult to maintain the theory of anoxia as an important factor in this treatment.

Gellhorn believes that the sympathetic adrenal system dominates the vagoinsulin system in the normal person. In schizophrenia, however, clinical evidence exists pointing to a deficient sympathetic reactivity. The therapeutic effect of shock treatments in schizophrenia is due to the stimulation of the sympathetic adrenal system. This leads to a shift in the balance existing between the centers of the sympathetic adrenal and vagoinsulin systems. Prolonged excitation of the sympathetic centers by the shock treatments restores the disturbed autonomic balance and exerts far reaching effects on the cortex itself. According to Gellhorn, the fact that inhibited conditioned reflexes can be restored by subjecting the animal to insulin coma or to convulsions supports this interpretation. In insulin coma treatment and prolonged narcosis, the hypothalamic stimulation is a release phenomenon, the cortical control being abolished; in convulsive treatment, direct excitation of the hypothalamus takes place. Ivanov-Smolenskii also believes that the common therapeutic factor in shock treatments is the production of cortical decompression or inhibition coupled with subcortical release and vegetative mobilization. Abely et al. hold that the effect of ECT is determined by a short sympathetic stimulation followed by prolonged para-sympathetic excitation with stimulation of the anterior hypothalamus and the acidophile cells of the hypophysis. We repeatedly expressed the view that ECT exerts its influence on the diencephalon. This view based on clinical observations regarding sleep, weight, and menstrual changes, was supported by M. Roth in electroencephalographical studies which also suggested the primary effect of ECT on the diencephalon.

There is no doubt that changes in the vegetative nervous system can be demonstrated experimentally and clinically during and following shock treatment. It is also apparent that vegetative regulations are changed, as evidenced by improvement in sleep, appetite, weight, digestion, and circulation. It is still uncertain, however, whether or not these changes are concomitant manifestations occurring with mental improvement rather than the basis of mental improvement. It has not been demonstrated conclusively that an alteration in vegetative regulations is the actual cause of schizophrenia; therefore, biochemical changes during successful treatment are not necessarily the cause of mental improvement. Moreover, these theories do not take into consideration the differences which exist between manic-depressive psychoses and schizophrenia and some other mental conditions in which shock treatments are generally effective in varying degrees. At present the most important point to recognize is that, as different forms of treatments may achieve the same results, none of them can be considered specific for a particular mental disease.

Of particular interest is the response to treatment of organic psychoses. The removal of psychotic syndromes in general paresis, of post-infectious psychoses and even psychotic syndromes in cases of pernicious anemia, led Fernandes and Polonio to the conclusion that the shock therapies and leucotomy have no bearing on the etiological causes of the psychoses. According to their concepts, psychotic symptoms arise from deviations of biopsychological functions caused by the noxious factors which, once in existence, may persist for a longer or shorter time. It seems doubtful, however, whether this must necessarily lead to the conclusion that we treat only symptoms or groups of symptoms, if we do not want to extend Bonhoeffer's concept of symptomatic psychoses to the symptoms of schizophrenia or manic-depressive psychosis, assuming that schizophrenia is a toxic disease acting secondarily on the brain.

On the basis of histopathological examinations, Stief formulated the theory that hypoglycemic coma and convulsive therapy produce spasms in the brain capillaries which eliminate diseased nerve cells, thereby bringing about the desired therapeutic results. That the vascular origin of cellular changes is disputed was discussed in the chapters on neuropathology. A more important objection to this theory is that there is no conclusive histopathological evidence that in schizophrenia diseased cortical cells are present in sufficient quantity to be responsible for the mental pathology. Stief's theory fits with the theories of the efficacy of frontal lobotomy. In the light of these concepts, shock treatment is considered a milder form of surgical procedure. While shock treatments may temporarily impair the function of cortical cells, in frontal lobotomy pathways are permanently cut between the cortical and subcortical centers. Both procedures supposedly lead to a reduction in cortical stimulation. LaValette assumes that the organic reaction in convulsive therapy produces a personality change on which the patient can reconstruct his personality.

Coma has also been credited as being the common therapeutic factor, whether caused by hypoglycemia or by convulsive therapy. Not only is coma brought about in hypoglycemia but the patient is in an equally comatose condition during and shortly after a convulsion as indicated by the term "electrocoma treatment" (Fettermann). Coma as the common denominator was suggested not only by those who consider therapeutically effective the pathophysiologic changes occurring in the brain during coma, but also by some who incline to psychologic explanations.

Quite recently, one of the few available experimental studies on clarifications of some of the main problems in ECT were published in a monograph by Ottosson. His questions concern the assumption of most clinicians that the convulsion rather than the electric current is responsible for a therapeutic effect, and, secondly, whether the memory impairment is a consequence of the seizure or a direct effect of the current as had been assumed by those who claimed diminished memory impairment with certain modifications of current. Ottosson uses the anticonvulsive effect of "lidocaine," a local anesthetic which abolishes electrically induced seizures and grand mal attacks in epileptics. He applied ECT to three groups, all of them receiving barbiturate and succinyl choline. The first two groups were given supraliminal and liminal electric stimuli, and it is shown that the electroencephalographic pattern is the same, characterized by an electric silence followed by delta waves. The lidocaine-modified seizures of the third group had hardly any electric silence and no delta activity. The clinical improvement is impaired, when lidocaine is given, and the conclusion can be drawn that the depression-relieving effect must be due to seizure activity and not to the current as such. The memory impairment, however, is only slightly less in ECT with lidocaine which permits the conclusion that a great part of the memory disturbance is accounted for by effects of the current other than the seizure. This most informative study on the action of ECT should be an important basis for any future research on the theory of ECT.

Soon after the first organic theories of the action of insulin coma and convulsive therapy appeared, other psychiatrists expressed a psychogenic point of view. These workers believe that the somatic part of the treatment is only incidental and that prolonged sleep, insulin, or convulsive therapies only prepare the soil for intensive psychotherapy. Meier was one of the first to advance the idea that the more intimate contact with physician and nurses produced by shock treatments exerts a marked psychotherapeutic effect on the patient. Somewhat similar views have been expressed by Schatner and O'Neill, who reason that with the patient helpless and dependent, the physician becomes a mother surrogate, the patient establishes a better transference and therefore becomes more psychotherapeutically approachable. This is true of insulin treatment, which requires a great deal of attention, but is less applicable to electric shock treatment, where the patient is returned to the general ward soon after the treatment or returns home soon after an office treatment. Furthermore, in many

private institutions with large medical staffs, considerable attention was paid to the individual patient before the shock era; yet the results were not comparable to those with shock treatment. If rendering the patient helpless or unconscious were sufficient to produce recovery, many other forms of treatment, such as fever treatment, anesthesias, continuous sleep would be as effective as the shock treatments but such is not the case.

Another group of authors, emphasize the psychotherapeutic value of the psychic "shock." They assume that the treatments actually produce a shock in the patient. It is difficult to prove or disprove this idea. However, it is quite evident that the so-called shock treatments usually do not produce any mental shock. Also on the physical level, physiologists and pathologists object to the designation of these treatments as "shock" treatments because there are no phenomena observed similar to surgical shock which is a different and fairly well defined pathological condition. Some of these theories were evolved only because the patient was actually visualized as undergoing some form of mental shock. The patient is usually amnesic during insulin or convulsive treatment and is unable to report on his experiences or impressions during the state of unconsciousness. This naturally does not mean that there are no experiences in that condition, but since it is impossible to obtain any facts on these perceptions, it is pure assumption to say that the experience is that of mental shock. Jelliffe, and others believe that the patients undergo the experience of impending death followed by the feeling of rebirth, and the impetus of these sensations is so great that it breaks the autism of the patient and eliminates the regression and narcissism. We mentioned previously that these experiences of impending death are rather uncommon in insulin-treated patients and in those treated with electric convulsive therapy. Furthermore, there is the question of why it is that all the medieval tortures inflicted on the insane failed to produce impressive therapeutic results, especially when they were inflicted on a conscious person in whom the so-called emotional shock or death threat must have been much more intense. Millett and Moses found that in patients treated by electric shock the treatment is desired because it is felt to be a fitting punishment acceptable from the hands of a trusted and kind doctor-father who really wishes to do no injury but to temper retribution with mercy. Ideas of battering down the patient's defense mechanism, are based more on the impressions of the person who sees the treatment than on those of the patient himself. Some patients are concerned about the convulsion even before they receive the first treatment. This anticipatory fear produces associations of punishment, annihilation. But the fear *of* the treatment should always be differentiated from the fear *produced by* the treatment. Furthermore, many patients who display fear in connection with shock treatments do not improve, while many who display no fear do improve. In electric shock treatment it is a common experience that psychoneurotics express more fear of the treatment than any other group of patients and yet they show the poorest results.

Schilder tried to combine psychogenic and organic theories, stating that the victory over the death threat expressed in the epileptic fit and lingering in the perceptual and aphasic difficulty enables the individual to start life and normal relations with human beings all over again. The hypomanic elation which often follows the epileptic fit is the joy of rebirth; the previous fixations of libido lying in a more personal layer of experience are removed by recovery from a catacylsmic catastrophe in the depth of the organism. "But," Schilder emphasizes, although "the results of the treatment are psychologically understood, it does not mean that metrazol treatment acts as a psychologic agent in the common sense. Its effects are deeper than the effects of what is called psychic influence. This is an organic treatment reflected in psychologic attitudes. Just as in insulin treatment, the organic processes of regeneration are put in action, metrazol convulsions seem to bring with themselves a reconstruction which also serves the more labile organic structures which serve emotions and which are damaged by the process of schizophrenia. The forces liberated by metrazol and insulin treatment come from layers which are generally not accessible to the processes which are usually called psychic."

Flescher feels that the therapeutic process of ECT implies a specific and dynamic pathogenous element which cannot be referred to a higher psychic level such as fear or need of help. He himself tries to understand ECT through the function of epileptic attacks, in which, according to him, considerable amounts of destructive energies are discharged.

Psychoanalytic theories of shock treatment have been formulated by Jelliffe, Glueck, Bychowski, and others. Glueck believes that the shock treatment facilitates emotional catharsis and is a highly condensed recapitulation of the process by means of which the fate of the egodystonic impulses is determined—the process which takes place normally in cases of ontogentic development and artificially in the course of psychoanalytic therapy. Bychowski believes that in the psychoses the pathologic ego dominates the healthy one which experiences a rebirth and fortification through insulin; between these two a battle rages until the shock reduces the pathologic ego. The cathartic abreaction then permits psychoanalytic approach and influence. Frosch and Impastato maintain that the various clinical changes seen during and following shock therapy reflect the degree to which the ego defenses succeed in controlling the emergence of previously repressed libidinous and aggressive impulses consequent to the drastic physical assault of the convulsion and the attendant disorders of memory defect and altered body image.

There have been some who assert that the amnesia produced in convulsive shock treatment is a therapeutic factor. For instance, the theory of Brain and Strauss postulates the presence of faulty electrical patterns in the brain, which are altered by the treatment, the resulting amnesia allowing time for the brain to become accustomed to simplified patterns. It should be pointed out, however, that amnesia does not occur regularly in shock treated patients. It is not often present in the insulin-treated patients, and it is usually temporary. The loss of familiarity which plays a certain role in the psychological literature on ECT (Zubin, Janis) has the same weak point as the amnesia theory, namely, that often the organic symptoms are either not present or clear up in a short time after the treatment, and yet, in many cases the recovery persists. The temporary blotting out of symptoms of all kinds does not affect the ultimate outcome of therapy.

A neurophysiologic-adaptive theory was presented by Fink et al. who stated that in ECT an induced change in brain function precedes the milieu in which behavioral changes can occur depending on the characterologic disposition of the subject. As indices of cerebral function they measured the degree of induced delta activity in the EEG, and changes in orientation and awareness of illness after intravenous injection of amobarbital sodium. In the amobarbital test the patient is asked a standard set of questions, and changes in orientation, denial of illness, confabulation and reduplication are considered as indicative of altered brain function. It was found that patients with high denial scores are those who improve best under ECT. These findings were considered to support the hypothesis advanced by Weinstein and Kahn that the mechanism of therapeutic action of electrically induced convulsions lies in the creation of altered brain function in which the patient might express his problems in a new symbolic fashion, particularly in the form of denial. Other theories also tend to combine physiological and psychological mechanisms. In analogy to similar insulin theories, Benda using Selye's general adaptation syndrome, considers the convulsion as a severe stress to which the body adapts and thereby mobilizes general defences. Ploog applies ideas about psychic counter regulation to ECT. L. Alexander tried to come to a better understanding of the mode of action by means of a study of the distinctive operations of the ego.

In connection with psychogenic theories of shock treatment, it is necessary to discuss again the question of psychotherapy in conjunction with these treatments. The theoretical implication of this question is whether the somatic treatments are treatments in their own right, or whether they are only part of the over-all psychological treatment of the patient, or, as is still claimed by many, an adjunct to psychotherapy. Sakel, in his first publications, designated insulin shock treatment as an or-

ganic treatment. He mentioned the fact that probings or psychotherapeutic attempts with respect to hallucinations and delusions, especially in paranoid patients, were unwarranted for they upset the patient and might provoke a relapse. Most workers agree that intensive analytical psychotherapy should not be carried out simultaneously with insulin treatment as the patient is in no condition to digest such material; that is especially true as regards sexual and particularly homosexual conflicts. If psychotherapy is given during insulin treatment, it is best to give reassurance in order to assist the patient in solving some of his superficial conflicts and to discuss with him some of his most disturbing psychotic experiences. The best time to do this is after he wakens, when he is in a state of relaxation and maximum approachability. In patients whose improvement is more stabilized, psychotherapeutic sessions can be held in the afternoons of insulin treatment days. The special aspects of this question in electric shock patients have been discussed in the section on this treatment.

Practically no study is available that proves the necessity of psychotherapy by comparing the results in patients who received psychotherapy with those who did not. Furthermore, psychotherapy covers a wide range of activity from simple reassurance to psychoanalysis, and in many instances it is not stated what type of psychotherapy was applied. In some of those institutions where the best results with shock treatments were obtained and where the largest number of cases was treated, only very superficial psychotherapy was and is applied. Their results were apparently not worse and indeed sometimes even better than those indicated by statistics from hospitals where it was possible to apply intensive psychotherapy in conjunction with or after shock therapy. This question is of great importance and more research should be concentrated on it.

An attempt was made by Knight to designate the organic forms of treatment and especially shock therapy as "strong arm method" in contrast to the "gentle" form of treatment, meaning psychotherapy or psychoanalysis. Hoch took exception to this differentiation of therapy. Shock treatments, lobotomy, and other procedures were not devised to intimidate patients, to purge patients, or to force them to desist from expressing symptoms. The treatments were introduced as the basis of certain theoretical conceptions and, more important, of empirical observations. Some of the theoretical concepts which were offered as a basis of these treatments turned out to be invalid. The same, however, can be said for many psychoanalytic concepts.

Empirically, the organic treatments produced results. The evaluation of these results is naturally open to discussion, and no final determination of their value has as yet been made. Even so, we know approximately what they are able to accomplish. The organic treatments rapidly accumulated considerable statistical material which could be analyzed and criticized. By comparison, the psychotherapeutic approaches have practically no statistics or the number of patients evaluated and reported is very small. Therefore, it is more difficult to appraise the efficacy of these treatments; this is especially true for psychoanalytical treatment in the psychoses. The indiscriminate use of the somatic treatments, particularly of electric shock therapy, must be deplored. However, indiscriminate use of psychotherapy also occurs. For instance, we do not think that treatment with analysis or other psychotherapy is justified in a markedly depressed patient who is not able to establish a good transference with the therapist, and becomes agitated due to a procedure that he is unable to follow and which brings up traumatic material which, in his state of agitation and agony he is unable to digest. These patients often become worse under such treatment but usually very quickly recover with electroshock treatments.

In all theoretical considerations of shock therapy there is a great tendency to single out certain observational factors, such as memory impairment or confusion, unconsciousness, and so on, and to try to explain all the actions of the treatment by one or the other of these changes seen. We are in full agreement with Von Baeyer that the shock treatments are not etiological treatments because the basic personality organization, the matrix on which the psychosis grows, is not touched. The recurrence of manic-depressive psychosis or the frequent relapses in shock-treated schizophrenics indicates that even though symptoms of the disorder can sometimes be fully removed, some of the underlying basic factors are not eliminated. With such special drugs as mescaline, pervitin, etc., it is possible to reactivate the psychosis, which also would indicate that a complete elimination of the etiological mechanisms is not achieved. However, lack of etiological basis should not be assumed as an argument against any form of treatment. Many valuable methods in other fields of medicine are proof that it would be entirely unjustified to reject methods because they are purely symptomatic in nature. It may be said here that this objection has been raised against the psychosurgical procedures, whose theoretical implications will now be discussed.

PSYCHOSURGERY

Theories which try to explain *frontal lobotomy and other psychosurgical procedures* are fewer in number than those brought forward for the shock treatments, and have a better foundation in clinical observation, although it must be repeated that none is entirely satisfactory. The hypothesis of Egaz Moniz, who introduced frontal lobotomy, has been mentioned already. It is in certain ways too general to be useful, and some of his specific statements concerning mental illness as being caused by faulty fiber connections are not generally accepted.

Freeman and Watts demonstrated that the therapeutic results were obtained by section of the thalamofrontal radiation followed by a degeneration of the dorsal medial nucleus of the thalamus which, in turn, produces a bleaching of the affect. They assume that the dorsal medial nucleus of the thalamus is the physical substrata of emotion. Their explanation that the so-called functional psychoses are produced by worry, which is reduced by the operation because the self-involvement of the patient is reduced, is too simple an explanation on the origin of the functional psychoses, even though a nucleus of truth may be in it. Their belief that without the frontal lobes, which have a tendency to overelaborate on anxiety and worry, no functional psychoses could develop, is open to question: elimination of the frontal lobe functions in many patients does not improve the psychosis, and relapses after frontal lobotomy may occur which would not be the case if existence of frontal lobe function were the sole prerequisite for a functional psychosis. It is probable that the origin of the functional psychoses goes beyond the function of the frontal lobe and involves other than the cortical areas of the brain as well.

Partridge, in his monograph on prefrontal leucotomy, clearly states that the modus operandi of leucotomy is not solved. He believes that the most important change after lobotomy is in the thalamus. He considers the thalamus an organ which integrates perceptions, emotions, and patterns of behavior, and believes it is also linked with the hypothalamus, through which autonomic influences are exerted. Partridge feels the schizophrenic disturbances are due to an impairment of this integrating function, which is seemingly favorably altered after operation. This actually does not solve the complicated question of improvements and personality damage seen after psychosurgery but does focus attention on a part of the brain which is probably implicated in mental sickness. Halstead, Hebb, and lately Landis have offered hypotheses based on their psychological investigations. Their description of the alterations which take place after frontal lobe surgery illuminates some aspects of the impairment of function in the frontal lobes without, however, offering a comprehensive understanding of all the alterations of function which are seen. They do not illuminate the etiology of the disorders involved, and do not actually explain the modus operandi of the surgical procedures.

Studies made on different brain-operated patients indicate that a very intimate relationship exists between the cerebral cortex and thalamus, and that a two-way circuit exists between the cortical gray matter and the subcortical gray matter, which mutually influence each other. Therefore, personality alterations can be achieved by ablating cortex, operating on the thalamus, or by cutting connections between thalamus and cortex. Today the connections between frontal lobe and thalamus are especially emphasized. However, it is necessary to recall that the long association fibers connecting the cortical areas of different lobes are also of great importance. We believe that these twofold connections within the cortical areas, and between cortex and thalamus explain why after frontal lobotomy the alterations of psychic functioning are not more severe. The basic intellectual and emotional functioning of the individual remains intact after frontal lobotomy even though the more subtle cognitive and connative performances are altered. If the basic functions of the person were concentrated in the frontal lobes alone, we could expect personality function after frontal lobotomy to show very serious alterations which actually are not even seen after frontal lobectomy. The changes are much less marked than prior theories of the function of the frontal lobe have indicated. Most likely, when parts of the frontal lobe are separated from other parts of the brain, the other cortical areas are able to take over. We believe that the basic intellectual and emotional life of the individual which is necessary for his personality functioning is not localized in the frontal lobe alone, but is distributed over the whole cortex, with the thalamus also having some function in it. This, of course, does not contradict the observation that the highest symbolic functions, such as creativeness, planning and the fusion of emotional and intellectual performances, depend on normal functioning by the frontal lobes. We do not believe that psychosurgery alters the basic structure of the neurosis or psychosis. Most patients who have undergone psychosurgery show in general unchanged dynamics. The retention of the basic psychodynamic structure is clearly seen in schizophrenic patients, and it is possible with drugs like mescaline to reactivate the original psychosis even some time after the operation. The symptoms which reappear are usually not as intense but are the same in quality. Therefore, we believe that psychosurgery points to an important problem in psychiatric therapy. Most of our treatments, especially the psychotherapeutic ones, mainly consider the qualitative approach to the different disorders. By analyzing the psychodynamic factors in a case we try to find out what conflicts in what constellations produce the emotional disorder. Thus we may overlook the fact that many of these conflicts can be present in a person without emotional disease becoming apparent until the symptoms become so marked that he is obsessed by his fears or dominated by his hallucinations and delusions. Only these dominating symptoms are eliminated or reduced by psychosurgery. An analogy exists in patients who suffer from intractable pain, where the pain is not eliminated but the patient's response to the perception of the pain experience is altered by the operation. We think that in psychosurgery we are dealing with a quantitative treatment which leaves many of the underlying disease processes unimpaired; the patient, however, does not perceive his difficulties any more, is no longer disorganized by them, and is thereby enabled to function. The same quantitative approach is applicable to the therapeutic effect of the neu-

roleptic drugs which may not always remove certain symptoms completely but reduce them sufficiently to allow the patient to live with them.

FINAL REMARKS

The discussion of the theoretical aspects of the various somatic treatments has shown that most of them are poorly understood, or even entirely obscure in their mode of action. The expectation that the newer somatic treatments would throw some light on the etiology of the mental disorders for which they are applied, has not yet been fulfilled. A great deal of research will still be necessary to explain the mode of action of the treatments hitherto available, and thus help us at some future day to arrive at better understood means of treating psychotic disorders. At present, we can say only that we are treating empirically disorders whose etiology is unknown, with methods whose action is also shrouded in mystery.

8. Psychopharmacologic Drugs

HAROLD E. HIMWICH

The last few years have seen the increasing use of a new group of drugs effective for overactive psychotic patients and presenting interesting and important differences from procedures and drugs previously employed in the management of individuals with such behavioral disorders. In fact, in order to give an appropriate name to these drugs, it was necessary to invent a nomenclature. Many terms, all emphasizing one or another aspect of the actions of these drugs, have been devised. The one most frequently used is *tranquilizer,* indicating a sedative or calming effect without enforcement of sleep. Others are *ataraxic (1),* denoting peace of mind, and *neuroleptic*

and *neuroplegic,* indicating diminutions in the intensity of nerve function. This group of drugs, however, may be regarded as an advance guard of a long-awaited pharmacologic attack not limited only to hyperactive disturbed patients, but also to be directed against other types of behavioral disorders. To this division of drugs the term *psychotropic (2),* or action on the mind, has been applied. *Neuropharmacologic* refers to the branch of pharmacology to which these drugs belong. The title *psychopharmacologic drugs (3, 4),* possesses certain advantages, for it indicates a medicine which influences the mind by affecting its morphologic substrate, the brain.

The chief usefulness of the new drugs, which at present lies in the field of psychiatry, is being extended into the

Abridged from *Science 127*:59–72, Jan. 10, 1958, by permission of the American Association for the Advancement of Science and the author.

many medical and surgical specialties. It is true that a drug not only changes favorably the malfunction of the organ for which it is intended but also acts, perhaps to a lesser extent, on the entire body. Either indirectly, by their influence on the brain, or by their influence on the peripheral nerves, the new drugs exert potent effects on the viscera of the body, including the gastrointestinal tract and the cardiorespiratory system and the endocrine glands.

But the impact of these new drugs has extended far beyond their immediate practical use in the management of disease. They are also employed by the clinical investigator who is seeking to unravel the tangled skein of abnormal behavior as well as by the psychologist who delves into intricacies of accepted normal patterns. Neurochemists and neurophysiologists have taken advantage of the tranquilizers to use them as tools in their investigations and meanwhile are uncovering their physiological actions in the brain and elsewhere in the body. These studies, made on man and lower animals, permit an analysis of the structure and function of the central nervous system, impossible before. Not that the methods are new, but the tranquilization resulting from the application of these drugs has not been previously observed. Perhaps most important, the new drugs may aid in the production of a desirable change in our culture and remove mental disease from the field of mysticism and superstition. They may convince the public that mental disease is not a thing to be ashamed of and that it should be placed in the same category as any other disease which can be treated by medical means.

CLINICAL ASPECTS

At this time it is hardly necessary to emphasize the magnitude of the problem of mental disease. The title of Gorman's recent book, *Every Other Bed (5),* is suggested by the fact that half of the sickbeds in our country are occupied by mental patients. The financial requirements for the maintenance of these hospitals are correspondingly great. The money comes chiefly out of the taxpayers' pockets. Only comparatively wealthy families can bear the cost of maintaining one of their members in a private institution.

The growing population of our mental hospitals indicates that advances prior to the advent of new drugs were not adequate to cope with the problem of mental disease. Much was left to be desired, therefore, from the therapeutic viewpoint. Psychoanalysis is a better weapon in the management of the neuroses than of the psychoses. Electroshock is a comparatively severe procedure, for electrodes are applied to the temples of the patient and a brief, measured current is passed through his brain. The patient becomes momentarily unconscious and undergoes a convulsion. Electroshock greatly benefits patients with depression and is of value in the management of excessively hyperactive patients to maintain the uneasy status quo which characterizes hospitals not using tranquilizing drugs. Insulin hypoglycemia appears to be more effective than electroshock for certain types of schizophrenia but requires highly trained physicians and is costly. In insulin hypoglycemia, the patients receive doses of insulin large enough to reduce the level of sugar in the blood. The brain is thus deprived of its chief foodstuff, and the patient sinks into coma. Another method for treating the distraught patient is to stupefy or anesthetize him with an adequate dose of one of the barbiturate drugs.

Though the immediate situation can thus be met, it is not necessarily followed by improvement in behavior. With the tranquilizing drugs, however, the patient is improved without significant interruption of consciousness—a highly desirable goal in the successful therapeutic process. Even if his manic excitement is extreme and if he must be given a correspondingly large dose, which renders him sleepy, he can be easily awakened and in general can go on with his prescribed hospital activities. With the new drugs, more patients have been returned to society from the state hospitals than with any previous therapeutic regime. We therefore seem to be entering a new era in the treatment of mental disease, and it remains to be seen how far this advance will take us.

SCHIZOPHRENIA

What are the mental disorders to which these new drugs are applied? The field of mental disease is complex. It is not a case of a single mental disease. On the contrary, there are many categories, and each one includes several varieties. Schizophrenia is the chief disorder met with in our psychotic population. We do not know the cause of schizophrenia, and this makes it necessary to limit our attack on it to empirical methods. But this is not unusual in the history of medicine, for the majority of therapeutic successes were produced on an empirical basis; witness the use of quinine long before the plasmodium of malaria was discovered.

Because the origin of schizophrenia is not known, that disease must be characterized chiefly by its symptoms. These are many and varied and, in general, may be divided into four types, which may change and merge into each other. The clinical picture is therefore not constant, and at different times the signs of one or another of these four types predominate. One of the characteristics of schizophrenia is emotional blunting, and this is a prominent change in the *simple* type. The psychiatrist is quick to observe the diagnostic paucity of facial expression and regards it as an outward lack of emotional expression or affect. Some individuals with inadequate personalities, who lose one job after another, belong to this group of patients. Sometimes the patient wears a silly and inappropriate grin. If such a patient, like Mr. M. on one of our wards, exhibits restless hyperactivity, at least that aspect of his disorder can be corrected by a tranquilizing drug.

An abnormality of the thought process is another characteristic of schizophrenia and is developed most highly in the *hebephrenic* type. Sentences spoken may have meaning for the patient but to others are neither coherent nor logical. In the most serious distortion of the thought process, the spoken word ceases to assume sentence form and is called "word salad." Mrs. H. replies to all questions with the unintelligible statement "16-21 telephone pole." That phrase includes her usual conversational limits. After receiving a new experimental tranquilizer, she informed us, in well constructed sentences, that she was born in a small village, consisting of six homes, and that her home was situated near a telephone pole numbered 16-21.

Delusions or false ideas and hallucinations, or false sensory impressions, are characteristic of the *paranoid* type.

Unlike the utterances of the hebephrenic, which cannot be comprehended by the physician, those of the paranoid patient are readily understood but reveal lack of relation to reality. Mrs. G., one of the patients in our hospital, has suffered intensely for a long time from well-developed delusions of a gigantic "crime-ring" which is out to get her, even penetrating into the confines of the Galesburg State Research Hospital. Recently, when she was receiving a test drug, a new serenity was observed in her demeanor. When asked about the "crime ring," she smiled, made a deprecating gesture with her hand, and said it did not bother her any more. In fact, she doubted whether it existed. This is an evident amelioration and was maintained as long as the patient remained on this medication.

In general, hallucinations, which also occur in mental disease other than schizophrenia, yield more readily to these drugs than do delusions. Mrs. S. has placed cotton plugs in her ears for many years to shut out the voices that were so hostile and were giving her such a bad time. During a period in which she was receiving one of the test drugs, she came in for an interview without the cotton plugs in her ears. The voices no longer tormented her, or at least not to the same extent as previously.

In the *catatonic* type of schizophrenia there are marked distortions of motor activity. Stupor is one aspect, and whether with or without stupor, posturing and the assumption and maintenance of bizarre positions and mannerisms are observed. After one has raised the arm of such a patient, the patient may keep his arm up for a long time. When he walks he may change his direction by turning at right angles only. A catatonic may also go into a furor, a period of wild overactivity, and become highly destructive.

Here we come to a very important use of tranquilizing drugs—namely, a calming action which is being applied to various kinds of destructive patients and not only to combative schizophrenics. Taking chlorpromazine and reserpine as examples, we find two different kinds of pharmacologic actions characteristic of this group of drugs. The first, which counteracts such symptoms of schizophrenia as dissociated thought, hallucinations, and delusions, has just been described. The second drug effect is of a different type and causes a general toning down of emotional reactions and physical activity. If the ability to correct the thought processes of the hebephrenic and the paranoid patients is regarded as a specific antipsychotic power of chlorpromazine and reserpine, then the use of these drugs to combat excessive activity may be considered a nonspecific result. As has been pointed out by Barsa, these two results do not necessarily occur together; either may be observed without the other (6). The calming action of the drug cuts across the diagnostic categories of mental disease, for it is employed in all types of overactive patients, irrespective of the diagnosis. It can even be given to an individual who has no behavioral abnormalities, and in such a normal person a reduction of activity and a diminution in the response to environmental stimuli will be noted.

USE WITH HYPERACTIVE PATIENTS

It must be remembered that patients with psychoses are sent to psychiatric hospitals most often because they display behavior which is not socially compatible. Psychotics who can carry on outside the hospital gates are not necessarily sent to such institutions. When a patient presents behavioral disorders that menace the life and limb of other individuals as well as his own, it is essential that he enter a hospital where he can be properly treated.

Types of hyperactive patients who secure benefits from this sedative influence include the manic, whose disorder is chiefly that of mood or affect, which is greatly elevated; the schizo-affective, in whom abnormal elation is associated with deterioration of mental abilities; and the patient with a toxic psychosis, as in delirium tremens. These patients have their hyperactivity and abnormally increased initiative reduced to more reasonable levels so that they cease to wear themselves out and are no longer a trial to the ward attendants and their fellow-patients. This is a tremendous advantage for hospitals with highly disturbed patients. Isolation rooms, where a dangerous patient was formerly incarcerated, are no longer required. Mechanical restraints, sedative wet packs, electroshock, and deep barbiturate medication are prescribed only infrequently. As a result, many of these patients can now be liberated from physical restraints as well as from the psychological constraints of a locked ward. The ward doors have been opened, and privileges have been given to many patients, permitting them to traverse hospital halls and attend various therapeutic activities—recreational, occupational, and industrial. Thus, treatments have not only been made more humane, with greater benefit to the patient, but have also effected improvement in the staff morale of the mental institutions. A hospital atmosphere is being established in state institutions to an extent that was not previously possible. One now feels that a mental hospital is not a place for the expedient management of an intolerable situation but rather a treatment center for the amelioration of disease, like hospitals devoted to other kinds of disorders.

One patient will receive most benefit from a certain tranquilizing agent, and a second from another. This is not the place to compare the therapeutic efficacy of the various tranquilizers, especially in such an early state of their development, but it is obvious that some produce a deeper sedative action than others. Each of the accepted tranquilizing drugs, when given in adequate dosage, is of aid to disturbed patients, but our experience (7) with hyperactive patients has been widest with chlorpromazine (8) and reserpine (9), drugs which have profound sedative or calming actions. But there is no way to foretell which drug will be most effective for a given patient, and therefore the psychiatrist should be prepared to employ any one in an emergency. Some, like azacyclonol (7, 10), can bring about better social adjustment, so that the atmosphere on the ward becomes friendlier, especially among patients who are only moderately disturbed. The choice of a tranquilizing drug must be decided empirically; the best one for a given patient can be found only by the process of elimination.

The most dramatic improvements are observed in the first acute attack or in the chronic patient who has developed an acute exacerbation of his disorder. At our hospital, however, tranquilizing drugs have also been found to exert marked benefit in patients with schizophrenia of long duration—that is, chronic schizophrenia, as documented in the case histories presented above. But the improvements were mainly seen in patients with obvious active schizophrenic processes— those who had hallucinations and delusions or who were hyperactive, agitated, and tense. Blocked, retarded, and apathetic schizophrenics are more difficult to help. This greater intractability of the so-called "burned-out" patients, who have survived a more active phase of their disorder and who seem free of schizophrenic symptoms and excessive physical activity, is also observed with previous methods of treating deteriorated, passive schizophrenics.

Similarly, senile patients who are irritable, quarrelsome, and apprehensive show greater improvements than patients who exhibit negativism, apathy, and withdrawal. It would appear that tranquilizing drugs are less valuable for the senile patient who does not display signs of agitation. For the same reason, depressions not accompanied by anxiety and tension are less apt to be ameliorated by a psychopharmacologic agent. The treatment of the passive patient is therefore more difficult. In individuals with hypertension, apparently free from behavioral abnormalities, the use of these drugs may lead to a worsening of the mental condition if the profound sadness of a depression is induced.

PSYCHONEUROSES

Mental diseases milder than the psychoses are the psychoneuroses or neuroses, and in some forms of these disorders tranquilizing drugs are of value. In contradistinction to the psychotic patient, the neurotic acts, by and large, as if reality has the same meaning for him as for most people. He is not subjected to persecution by a "crime ring" and does not have other bizarre experiences. He suffers, however, from great anxiety, which may not be readily identified with any particular object. Yet this anxiety is expressed in bodily symptoms: palpita-

tion, breathlessness, weakness of limbs, tremors and pains that plague him. For that reason, in some patients, the anxiety is associated with a particular organ: the heart, the lungs, or the stomach. Neurotics who must be active in order to escape their disturbing fears are usually not helped by tranquilizers. In contrast, those with internal tensions, who cannot sleep despite use of such sedative drugs as the barbiturates, often gain relief from a psychopharmacologic agent.

FOR THE "NORMAL" POPULATION

These drugs also exhibit decided usefulness for the members of our so-called normal population who are subjected to intolerable stress. A businessman with a demanding and unreasonable supervisor or a woman with insufficient funds to run her home according to her ideal standard can gradually build up an emotional impasse so that perspective is lost, as the darker side of the situation is increasingly magnified, until a state of panic may develop. Restoration to a more objective evaluation of the situation may be secured by psychotherapeutic discussions with a physician, and an important action of tranquilizing drugs is to render the patient more receptive to other kinds of therapy. In fact, at times a psychopharmacologic drug may be essential for a successful psychiatric interview. Ephemeral disturbances—for example, the anxiety and tension aroused by an impending surgical operation—can be pleasantly dissipated by a small dose of a tranquilizing agent.

SIDE REACTIONS

I have not mentioned the matter of occasional undesirable side reactions of the new drugs (11). In the first place, the drugs cause much less inconvenience than the mental disorder of the psychotic patient. Some patients can be managed by a temporary reduction of dosage—for example, a patient who exhibits an excessive fall of blood pressure. Others can be treated by a drug which counteracts the undesirable changes; a tremor of the hands resembling that of Parkinsonism can be relieved by an anti-Parkinson drug. Patients with brain injury are more likely to exhibit a convulsion than those with an intact organ (*12*). The production of lactation and menstrual changes by chlorpromazine and reserpine and the power of the latter to impair libido in the male are subjects for research. Fortunately, serious complications occur only rarely. A small number of patients develop jaundice, a sign of liver involvement. In some instances there may be a reduction of white blood cells. A failure in the formation of these cells is dangerous because it diminishes the resistance of the body to disease. But, on the whole, the treatment of thousands of psychotic patients with the new drugs has been relatively safe, because most are resistant to these side effects. This resistance, however, does not apply to neurotic patients, who seem more sensitive to side reactions and even on comparatively low dosage complain of fatigue, prostration, dizziness, and nausea.

It is apparent, then, that state hospitals have been placed on a much better basis by the use of the tranquilizing drugs, especially in the management of highly disturbed patients. The same, however, can not be said of psychiatrists whose private practice is concerned chiefly with neurotic patients. But it is also true that many patients who were formerly sent to a mental institution can now be treated outside the hospital gates. Some psychotic individuals can continue to lead productive lives and need not go to a psychiatric hospital at all. During the acute phase, they may be controlled by tranquilizing drugs in a general hospital and later may be maintained outside the hospital on appropriate doses of these medicines. On the other hand, apathetic psychotics who are not in conflict socially but who are rather withdrawn, inactive, and without signs of agitation, usually cannot be raised to a higher adaptive level. They are still the despair of the psychiatrist. In evaluating the present clinical position of the psychopharmacologic drugs, it must be understood that the production of tranquilization, though a desirable end in itself, also aids other forms of therapy. A potent factor in the successful treatment of a patient with disorganized or disturbed behavior is a satisfactory relationship with a psychiatrist, and an important result of tranquilization is the facilitation of such a beneficial relationship.

THEORY FOR THERAPEUTIC EFFECTS

To bridge the gap between our information of the pharmacologic actions of reserpine and chlorpromazine and their therapeutic results is a goal greatly to be desired. Unfortunately, we do not have sufficient data or even the basic neurophysiologic facts to do this. It is realized that such speculations on the mode of action of tranquilizers in man are largely based on observations of animals—a doubtful procedure. Moreover, there is a genuine logical difficulty, for it has not been proved that the behavioral improvements noted with use of these drugs are due to the pharmacologic effects. The two diverse groups of phenomena may be related to each other only by a common causative factor —namely, the drug. But it is useful to make the assumption that the medicines are causes of the clinical changes as a device to clarify our thinking in seeking indications for the direction of future research in the field of psychopharmacology.

In our analyses of the therapeutic results of reserpine and chlorpromazine, we found that they are of two different kinds: one is a calming of the individual and other is directed against schizophrenic manifestations. Can each of these two different clinical improvements be related to specific actions of the drugs? The decreased reactivity of tranquilized patients may be ascribed in part to the depletion of the catechol amines, the depletion depriving the organism of part of the mechanism of reactivity. Obviously, tension and anxiety, whether evoked by real or imaginary emergencies, will nevertheless mobilize the autonomic nervous system. Not only adrenaline and noradrenaline but also other hormones, including serotonin and acetylcholine, are probably released during threatening emergencies. Thus, in general, a pharmacologic action of these drugs is to remove part of the mobilization mechanism, and the beneficial results include tranquilization and decreases of anxiety and tension. Turning to the electrophysiological portion of this analysis, we find ourselves examining the parts of the brain which help to regulate the activity of the neurohormones. A neuronal depression of the reticular formation and of the hypothalamus diminishes the actions of these portions of the brain. This depression can only render more profound the decrease in reactivity due to the emptying of the neurohormonal storehouses.

Animal experiments indicate a close relationship between rhinencephalic structure and the emotions, while drug studies have disclosed the sensitivity of the amygdala to chlorpromazine and reserpine. But here we see that a similar final effect of tranquilization is associated with an action which is quite the reverse of that seen in the hypothalamus. Inhibition of nerve function is not observed. On the contrary, the affected areas reveal abnormal hyperactivity. Does the drug induced aberrant operation of the amygdala interfere with the functions of the rhinencephalon, and, if so, does such an interference afford a basis for the second action of these drugs against schizophrenic symptoms? It would seem that the normal contribution of the amygdala to the economy of the brain cannot continue when that structure is being subjected to seizures (13). Perhaps the rhinencephalic chain ceases to act physiologically because of the functional failure of the amygdaloid link—a failure which makes for a loss in a connection between the most primitive brain area (concerned with emotion), the midbrain reticular formation, and the later developed rhinencephalon.

The diminution in reactivity of the organism probably influences the quantity or intensity of the emotional impact on the cortex. But it is difficult see how such an amelioration can change the quality of thought so that the dissociated "word salad" of the hebephrenic patient can become less incoherent, more logical and comprehensible. One can appreciate that a decrease in emotional intensity might mitigate the violence in the expression of hallucinatory and delusional material, but again it is more difficult to understand how such a mitigation can cause the correction of schizophrenic mentation. For that change, thinking must be altered in quality.

Though the various parts of the brain work together as a unit in a coordinated manner, we have seen that certain structures, both cortical and subcortical, are more involved than others in our emotional life. Similarly, as is pointed out by Bailey (14), some subcortical regions add a crude awareness, but for the discriminative contribution to that complex function, the cortex must be included in a prominent position. The cingulate gyrus, which is a part not only of the rhinencephalon but also of the cortex, may be the area where the abnormal elements concerned with awareness and thinking enter into discriminative conscious activity. It is not said that rhinencephalic structures do not affect emotional reactions, but it is suggested, as a working hypothesis, that the cessation of rhinencephalic function is a possible factor in the prevention of the morbid thinking of schizophrenia. This would indicate that the disease process of schizophrenia is tied up with the malfunction of certain brain areas and that the rhinencephalic circle carries impulses which are sources of the pathologic psychophysiology of schizophrenia. It is realized that a change of behavior produced by a loss of the contribution from a specific brain area, whether due to to a physical extirpation or to functional incapacitation, does not prove that pathology in that area is the source of the disease. The removal of a part of the brain may interfere with the function of another region more directly concerned with the disease process. For example, an origin of the pathologic course may lie within the septal region, as is indicated by the work of Heath and his colleagues (15), or the warped emotional reactions may find their earlier expression in the midbrain reticular formation. But at least it can be said that the anatomic site sensitive to drug action bears a relationship to schizophrenia, because the functional diversion of that area may correct the symptomatology of the disorder.

PATHS OF RESEARCH

A review of the present pharmacologic data can serve to throw light on paths for future exploration. One series of observations has emphasized quantitative changes causing shifts in the neurohormonal balance, involving excesses or deficits of acetylcholine, adrenaline, noradrenaline, serotonin, or serotoninlike substances. Concentrations of serotonin in the brain can be increased by the administration of its precursor, 5-hydroxytryptophan, which provokes disturbances in the electroencephalogram and in the behavior of the rabbit (16) (Fig. 1). Apparently, 5-hydroxytryptophan enters the brain rapidly and, presumably, is transformed into serotonin. But that does not demonstrate that serotonin is excessive in hyperactive psychotic patients (17) or that their improvement is necessarily due to the decrease of serotonin in the brain. On the other hand, there is a recent suggestion that Marsilid, which increases the serotonin content of the brain, benefits depressed patients (18). Again, that does not prove that patients are depressed because of abnormally low levels of serotonin in the brain. But it must be admitted that this circumstantial evidence is of such interest that it calls for further investigation of these possibilities.

An experiment to throw light on this subject would be to determine the cerebral serotonin contents in the brains of psychotic patients and compare them with those of nonpsychotics. A start has been made. Costa and Aprison have demonstrated that serotonin is a normal constituent of the human brain just as it is of the brain of lower animals (12). However, it can be said conservatively that the suggestion of Woolley and Shaw (18) on the role of serotonin is an attractive one and that it has been useful in turning up new material (19). For example, Shaw and Woolley (20) have synthesized compounds which block serotonin, including BAB, the benzyl analog of bufotenin, and BAS, the benzyl analog of serotonin (Fig. 1). We have employed BAS in the treatment of schizophrenics on the possibility that it may exert a reserpinelike action (19). The salutary results on these psychotic patients were very encouraging, but the side reactions contraindicate the clinical use of BAS.

It is not justifiable, however, to separate the role of serotonin from that of the catechol amines, for both are affected simultaneously by reserpine and probably by other tranquilizing drugs. A strong point in favor of the catechol amines is that one of them, deoxyephedrine, is able to substitute for depleted catechol amines in the brain (21). Mice and monkeys, under the influence of reserpine and showing the depression, reduced mobility, and the hunched posture typically produced by that drug, are dramatically restored to apparently normal activity by deoxyephedrine. Another line of investigation is concerned more with qualitative changes in the neurohormones than with quantitative ones, and it implicates a metabolic factor in schizophrenia. This work cannot be reviewed here, but it involves the more rapid oxidation of adrenaline (22) or the production of abnormal oxidation products of that neurohormone (23). As a result of an abnormal enzyme system, the metabolism of adrenaline is perverted, and an aberrant metabolic product, which may be a pathogenic factor in schizophrenia, is formed (24).

At this time, when theories of schizophrenia are actively multiplying, it would seem that the two different aspects of quantitative and qualitative changes in the hormones are not mutually exclusive. One example is afforded by Hoffer, who suggests that there are two basic conditions for the production of schizophrenia—an increase in the concentration and activity of acetylcholine within the brain and an abnormal metabolic diversion of adrenaline to some aberrant indole compound (25).

The inclusion of electrical changes of brain areas in our field of research diversifies the problem still more. At the present state of development of psychopharmacology it is difficult to apply William of Occam's razor, for each successful drug seems to differ from the others. Perhaps when we know more, the attack will be simplified by a unitary hypothesis on the pharmacologic actions of these drugs. We are therefore left with a number of tempting speculations, and the judgment of the investigator will largely determine which one will be emphasized in his researches.

The fact that we have effective drugs will not stop the production of better ones. In that process, a guiding principle is concerned with a characteristic of the brain—the fact that it, more than any other organ, is sensitive to changes in the chemical structure of a drug *(26)*. Illustrations may be drawn from the phenothiazine derivatives. Profound differences in the intensity of the therapeutic effects and the distribution of the side reactions *(27)* may be produced either by the replacement of the chlorine (Cl) atom of the nucleus with another chemical or by an alteration in the number of carbon atoms between the two nitrogen atoms (N) of the side chain. We are looking forward to the discovery of compounds of new chemical structures, to be used for types of patients who require not tranquilization but other kinds of therapeutic aid—for example, for the blocked and retarded individual who must be stimulated without an increase of hostility or an activation of hallucinations and delusions.

We have seen, however, that thus far in the field of psychopharmacology, practice has outstripped theory. Though we recognize that tranquilizers correct certain schizophrenic symptoms, there is less agreement on the mechanism by which the improvements are achieved. Whether or not drugs effect cures is a problem for the future. But the practical value of the advance should not be underestimated. It may be compared with the advent of insulin, which counteracts symptoms of diabetes without removing their cause.

References

1. Fabing, H. D. "The dimensions of neurology," presidential address, Am. Acad. of Neurology (1955).
2. Gerard, R. W. *Science 125,* 201 (1957).
3. Himwich, H. E. *J. Nervous Mental Disease 122,* 413 (1955).
4. ——, "Discussion of Papers on Basic Observations of New Psychopharmacological Agents." *Psychiat. Research Rept. No. 4* (1956), pp. 24–31. Examples include (i) *Rauwolfia* alkaloids: reserpine (Serpasil, Ciba Pharmaceutical Co.); deserpidine (Harmonyl, Abbott Laboratories); rescinnamine (Moderil, Chas. Pfizer & Co.). (ii) Phenothiazine derivatives: chlorpromazine (Thorazine, Smith, Kline & French Laboratories); promazine (Sparine, Wyeth Laboratories); mepazine (Pacatal, Warner-Chilcott Laboratories); perphenazine (Trilafon, Schering Corp.); proclorperazine (Compazine, Smith, Kline & French Laboratories); thiopropazate (Dartal, G. D. Searle & Co.); triflupromazine (Vesprin, E. R. Squibb & Son; Adazine, Upjohn Co.). (iii) Diphenylmethane derivatives: azacyclonol (Frenquel, William S. Merrell Co.); hydroxyzine (Atarax, R. J. Roerig &

Co.); benactyzine (Suavitil, Merck, Sharp & Dohme); phenyltoloxamine (PRN, Bristol Laboratories). (iv) Substituted propanediols: meprobamate (Miltown, Wallace Laboratories; Equanil, Wyeth Laboratories).
5. Gorman, M. *Every Other Bed* (World, New York, 1956).
6. Barsa, J. A. *Am. J. Psychiat. 114,* 74 (1957.)
7. Rinaldi, F., Rudy, L. H., Himwich, H. E., *ibid. 112,* 678 (1956).
8. Kinross-Wright, V., *ibid. 111,* 907 (1955); Goldman, D. *J. Am. Med. Assoc. 157,* 1274 (1955); Lehman, H. A. *Arch. Neurol. Psychiat. 71,* 227 (1954).
9. Kline, N., Barsa, J., Gosline, E. *Am. J. Psychiat. 17,* 352 (1956).
10. Brown, N. L. *J. Nervous Mental Disease 123,* 130 (1956); Rinaldi, F., Rudy, L. H., Himwich, H. E. *Am. J. Psychiat. 112,* 343 (1955); Rinaldi, F. *et. al.,* in *Tranquilizing Drugs,* Himwich, H. E., Ed. (Am. Assoc. Advance. Sci., Washington, D.C., 1957); Proctor, R. C., in *Alcoholism, Basic Aspects and Treatment,* Himwich, H. E., Ed. (Am. Assoc. Advance. Sci., Washington, D.C., 1957), pp. 133–139.
11. Kline, N. S., Barsa, J., Gosline, E. in *Tranquilizing Drugs,* Himwich, H. E., Ed. (Am. Assoc. Advance. Sci., Washington, D.C., 1957), pp. 149–161; Ferguson, J. T. "The relative values of drugs in the various psychiatric syndromes," *Psychiat. Research Rept. No. 4* (1956), pp. 35–43; Tuteur, W. and Lepson, D. in *Tranquilizing Drugs,* Himwich, H. E., Ed. (Am. Assoc. Advance. Sci., Washington, D.C., 1957), pp. 163–172.
12. Rudy, L. H., Himwhich, H. E., Rinaldi, F. "A clinical evaluation of psychopharmacological agents in the management of disturbed mentally defective patients," in *Trans. Soc. Biol. Psychiat. 11,* (1957).
13. Buscaino, M. *Scientia Med. Ital. 5,* 44 (1956).
14. Bailey, P. "Neurosurgical data on states of consciousness," Congr. Neurol. Sci. Brussels, Belgium (1957).
15. Heath, R. B. *et al.,* "Pharmacological and biological psychotherapy," presented at the annual meeting of the American Psychiatric Assoc., Chicago, Ill. (May 1957).
16. Udenfriend, S., Weissbach, H., Bogdanski, D. F. *J. Biol. Chem. 224,* 803 (1956); Shore, P. A., and Brodie, B. B. *Proc. Soc. Explt. Biol. Med. 94,* 433 (1957).
17. Costa, E., Rinaldi, F., Himwich, H. E. "Some relationships between tranquilization indolalkylamines and brain structure," presented at the Intern. Symposium on Psychotropic Drugs, Milan, Italy (May 1957).
18. Saunders, J. C., Radinger, N., Kline, N. S. "A theoretical and clinical approach to treating depressed and regressed patients with iproniazid," paper read at 12th annual meeting, Society of Biological Psychiatry (1957).
19. Rudy, L. H. *et al.* "Clinical evaluation of benzyl analog of serotonin (BAS): a tranquilizing drug," presented before the Society of Biological Psychiatry, Atlantic City, N.J. (June 1957).
20. Shaw, E. N., and Woolley, D. W. *J. Pharmacol, Exptl. Therap. 116,* 164 (1955).

21. Everett, G. M., Toman, J. E. P., Smith, A. H., Jr. *Federation Proc. 16,* 295 (1957).
22. Akerfeldt, S. "Serological reaction of psychiatric patients to n, n-dimethy-p-phenylene diamine," presented at annual meeting of American Psychiatric Assoc. (May 1957).
23. Leach, B. E. *et al., Arch. Neurol. Psychiat. 76,* 635 (1956); Hoffer, A., and Kenyon, M. *ibid. 77,* 437 (1957); Rinkel, M., Hyde, R. W., Solomon H. C. *Diseases of Nervous System 15,* 3 (1954).
24. Heath, R. G. *et al.,* in preparation.
25. Hoffer, A. *J. Clin. Explt. Psychopathol. 18,* 27 (1957).
26. Abood, L. G., and Romanchek, L. *Ann. N.Y. Acad. Sci. 66,* 812 (1957); Grenell, R. G. *ibid. 66,* 826 (1957); Ayd, F. J., Jr. *J. Am. Geriatric Soc. 5,* 1 (1957); Fazekas, J. F. *et al.,* in Alcoholism, Himwich, H. E., Ed. (Am. Assoc. Advance. Sci., Washington, D.C., 1957), pp. 125–132; Gallagher, W. J. *et al.* in *Tranquilizing Drugs,* H. E. Himwich, Ed. (Am. Assoc. Advance. Sci., Washington, D.C., 1957), pp. 133–147; Rudy, L. H., Himwich, H. E., Tasher, D. C. *Am. J. Psychiat. 113,* 979 (1957).
27. Himwich, H. E., Rinaldi, F., Willis, D. J. *Nervous Mental Disease 124,* 53 (1956).

Biophysical Theories

CRITICAL EVALUATION

The belief that tangible biophysical defects or deficiencies are the cause of mental disorders has not gone unchallenged. Evidence in support of this notion has not been demonstrated convincingly and has spurred adherents of other viewpoints to question the wisdom of pursuing the search for these defects. Thomas Szasz's article, for example, contends that the concept of mental disease itself is merely a myth, a false verbal analogy founded on the erroneous application of a medical model to psychopathology. In contrast, Seymour Kety does not question the legitimacy of the biophysical approach, but merely examines a number of biochemical hypotheses in detail, and finds them either ill-conceived or lacking in empirical support.

9. The Myth of Mental Illness

THOMAS S. SZASZ

My aim in this essay is to raise the question "Is there such a thing as mental illness?" and to argue that there is not. Since the notion of mental illness is extremely widely used nowadays, inquiry into the ways in which this term is employed would seem to be especially indicated. Mental illness, of course, is not literally a "thing"—or physical object—and hence it can "exist" only in the same sort of way in which other theoretical concepts exist. Yet, familiar theories are in the habit of posing, sooner or later—at least to those who come to believe in them—as "objective truths" (or "facts"). During certain historical periods, explanatory conceptions such as deities, witches, and microorganisms appeared not only as theories but as self-evident *causes* of a vast number of events. I submit that today mental illness is widely regarded in a somewhat similar fashion, that is, as the cause of innumerable diverse happenings. As an antidote to the complacent

use of the notion of mental illness—whether as a self-evident phenomenon, theory, or cause—let us ask this question: What is meant when it is asserted that someone is mentally ill?

In what follows I shall describe briefly the main uses to which the concept of mental illness has been put. I shall argue that this notion has outlived whatever usefulness it might have had and that it now functions merely as a convenient myth.

MENTAL ILLNESS AS A SIGN OF BRAIN DAMAGE

The notion of mental illness derives its main support from such phenomena as syphilis of the brain or delirious conditions—intoxications, for instance—in which persons are known to manifest various peculiarities or disorders of thinking and behavior. Correctly speaking, however, these are diseases of the brain, not of the mind. According to one school of thought, *all* so-called mental illness is of this type. The assumption is made that some neurological defect, perhaps

From *Amer. Psychol.* 15:113–118, 1960, by permission of the American Psychological Association and the author.

a very subtle one, will ultimately be found for all the disorders of thinking and behavior. Many contemporary psychiatrists, physicians, and other scientists hold this view. This position implies that people *cannot* have troubles —expressed in what are *now called* "mental illnesses"—because of differences in personal needs, opinions, social aspirations, values, and so on. *All problems in living* are attributed to physicochemical processes which in due time will be discovered by medical research.

"Mental illnesses" are thus regarded as basically no different than all other diseases (that is, of the body). The only difference, in this view, between mental and bodily diseases is that the former, affecting the brain, manifest themselves by means of mental symptoms; whereas the latter, affecting other organ systems (for example, the skin, liver, etc.), manifest themselves by means of symptoms referable to those parts of the body. This view rests on and expresses what are, in my opinion, two fundamental errors.

In the first place, what central nervous system symptoms would correspond to a skin eruption or a fracture? It would *not* be some emotion or complex bit of behavior. Rather, it would be blindness or a paralysis of some part of the body. The crux of the matter is that a disease of the brain, analogous to a disease of the skin or bone, is a neurological defect, and not a problem in living. For example, a *defect* in a person's visual field may be satisfactorily explained by correlating it with certain definite lesions in the nervous system. On the other hand, a person's *belief*—whether this be a belief in Christianity, in Communism, or in the idea that his internal organs are "rotting" and that his body is, in fact, already "dead"—cannot be explained by a defect or disease of the nervous system. Explanations of this sort of occurrence—assuming that one is interested in the belief itself and does not regard it simply as a "symptom" or expression of something else that is *more interesting*—must be sought along different lines.

The second error in regarding complex psychosocial behavior, consisting of communications about ourselves and the world about us, as mere symptoms of neurological functioning is *epistemo-logical*. In other words, it is an error pertaining not to any mistakes in observation or reasoning, as such, but rather to the way in which we organize and express our knowledge. In the present case, the error lies in making a symmetrical dualism between mental and physical (or bodily) symptoms, a dualism which is merely a habit of speech and to which no known observations can be found to correspond. Let us see if this is so. In medical practice, when we speak of physical disturbances, we mean either signs (for example, a fever) or symptoms (for example, pain). We speak of mental symptoms, on the other hand, when we refer to a patient's *communications about himself, others, and the world about him.* He might state that he is Napoleon or that he is being persecuted by the Communists. These would be considered mental symptoms *only* if the observer believed that the patient was *not* Napoleon or that he was *not* being persecuted by the Communists. This makes it apparent that the statement that "*X* is a mental symptom" involves rendering a judgment. The judgment entials, moreover, a covert comparison or matching of the patient's ideas, concepts, or beliefs with those of the observer and the society in which they live. The notion of mental symptom is therefore inextricably tied to the *social* (including *ethical*) *context* in which it is made in much the same way as the notion of bodily symptom is tied to an *anatomical* and *genetic context* (Szasz, 1957a, 1957b).

To sum up what has been said thus far: I have tried to show that for those who regard mental symptoms as signs of brain disease, the concept of mental illness is unnecessary and misleading. For what they mean is that people so labeled suffer from diseases of the brain; and, if that is what they mean, it would seem better for the sake of clarity to say that and not somthing else.

MENTAL ILLNESS AS A NAME FOR PROBLEMS IN LIVING

The term "mental illness" is widely used to describe something which is very different than a disease of the brain. Many people today take it for granted that living is an arduous process. Its hardship for modern man, moreover, derives not so much from a struggle for biological survival as from the stresses and strains inherent in the social intercourse of complex human personalities. In this context, the notion of mental illness is used to identify or describe some feature of an individual's so-called personality. Mental illness—as a deformity of the personality, so to speak—is then regarded as the *cause* of the human disharmony. It is implicit in this view that social intercourse between people is regarded as something *inherently harmonious,* its disturbance being due solely to the presence of "mental illness" in many people. This is obviously fallacious reasoning, for it makes the abstraction "mental illness" into a *cause*, even though this abstraction was created in the first place to serve only as a shorthand expression for certain types of human behavior. It now becomes necessary to ask: "What kinds of behavior are regarded as indicative of mental illness, and by whom?"

The concept of illness, whether bodily or mental, implies *deviation from some clearly defined norm*. In the case of physical illness, the norm is the structural and functional integrity of the human body. Thus, although the desirability of physical health, as such, is an ethical value, what health *is* can be stated in anatomical and physiological terms. What is the norm deviation from which is regarded as mental illness? This question cannot be easily answered. But whatever this norm might be, we can be certain of only one thing: namely, that it is a norm that must be stated in terms of *psychosocial, ethical,* and *legal* concepts. For example, notions such as "excessive repression" or "acting out an unconscious impulse" illustrate the use of psychological concepts for judging (so-called) mental health and illness. The idea that chronic hostility, vengefulness, or divorce are indicative of mental illness would be illustrations of the use of ethical norms (that is, the desirability of love, kindness, and a stable marriage relationship). Finally, the widespread psychiatric opinion that only a mentally ill person would commit homicide illustrates the use of a legal concept as a norm of mental health. The norm from which deviation is measured whenever one speaks of a mental illness is a *psychosocial and*

ethical one. Yet, the remedy is sought in terms of *medical* measures which—it is hoped and assumed—are free from wide differences of ethical value. The definition of the disorder and the terms in which its remedy are sought are therefore at serious odds with one another. The practical significance of this covert conflict between the alleged nature of the defect and the remedy can hardly be exaggerated.

Having identified the norms used to measure deviations in cases of mental illness, we will now turn to the question: "Who defines the norms and hence the deviation?" Two basic answers may be offered: *(a)* It may be the person himself (that is, the patient) who decides that he deviates from a norm. For example, an artist may believe that he suffers from a work inhibition; and he may implement this conclusion by seeking help *for* himself from a psychotherapist. *(b)* It may be someone other than the patient who decides that the latter is deviant (for example, relatives, physicians, legal authorities, society generally, etc.). In such a case a psychiatrist may be hired by others to do something *to* the patient in order to correct the deviation.

These considerations underscore the importance of asking the question "Whose agent is the psychiatrist?" and of giving a candid answer to it (Szasz, 1956, 1958). The psychiatrist (psychologist or nonmedical psychotherapist), it now develops, may be the agent of the patient, of the relatives, of the school, of the military services, of a business organization, of a court of law, and so forth. In speaking of the psychiatrist as the agent of these persons or organizations, it is not implied that his values concerning norms, or his ideas and aims concerning the proper nature of remedial action, need to coincide exactly with those of his employer. For example, a patient in individual psychotherapy may believe that his salvation lies in a new marriage; his psychotherapist need not share this hypothesis. As the patient's agent, however, he must abstain from bringing social or legal force to bear on the patient which would prevent him from putting his beliefs into action. If his *contract* is with the patient, the psychiatrist (psychotherapist) may disagree with him or stop his treatment; but he cannot engage others to obstruct the patient's aspirations.

Similarly, if a psychiatrist is engaged by a court to determine the sanity of a criminal, he need not fully share the legal authorities' values and intentions in regard to the criminal and the means available for dealing with him. But the psychiatrist is expressly barred from stating, for example, that it is not the criminal who is "insane" but the men who wrote the law on the basis of which the very actions that are being judged are regarded as "criminal." Such an opinion could be voiced, of course, but not in a courtroom, and not by a psychiatrist who makes it his practice to assist the court in performing its daily work.

To recapitulate: In actual contemporary social usage, the finding of a mental illness is made by establishing a deviance in behavior from certain psychosocial, ethical, or legal norms. The judgment may be made, as in medicine, by the patient, the physician (psychiatrist), or others. Remedial action, finally, tends to be sought in a therapeutic—or covertly medical—framework, thus creating a situation in which *psychosocial, ethical,* and/or *legal deviations* are claimed to be correctible by (so-called) *medical action.* Since medical action is designed to correct only medical deviations, it seems logically absurd to expect that it will help solve problems whose very existence had been defined and established on nonmedical grounds. I think that these considerations may be fruitfully applied to the present use of tranquilizers and, more generally, to what might be expected of drugs of whatever type in regard to the amelioration or solution of problems in human living.

THE ROLE OF ETHICS IN PSYCHIATRY

Anything that people *do*—in contrast to things that *happen* to them (Peters, 1958)—takes place in a context of value. In this broad sense, no human activity is devoid of ethical implications. When the values underlying certain activities are widely shared, those who participate in their pursuit may lose sight of them altogether. The discipline of medicine, both as a pure science (for example, research) and as a technology (for example, therapy), contains many ethical considerations and judgments. Unfortunately, these are often denied,

minimized, or merely kept out of focus; for the ideal of the medical profession as well as of the people whom it serves seems to be having a system of medicine (allegedly) free of ethical value. This sentimental notion is expressed by such things as the doctor's willingness to treat and help patients irrespective of their religious or political beliefs, whether they are rich or poor, etc. While there may be some grounds for this belief—albeit it is a view that is not impressively true even in these regards—the fact remains that ethical considerations encompass a vast range of human affairs. By making the practice of medicine neutral in regard to some specific issues of value need not, and cannot, mean that it can be kept free from all such values. The practice of medicine is intimately tied to ethics; and the first thing that we must do, it seems to me, is to try to make this clear and explicit. I shall let this matter rest here, for it does not concern us specifically in this essay. Lest there be any vagueness, however, about how or where ethics and medicine meet, let me remind the reader of such issues as birth control, abortion, suicide, and euthanasia as only a few of the major areas of current ethicomedical controversy.

Psychiatry, I submit, is very much more intimately tied to problems of ethics than is medicine. I use the word "psychiatry" here to refer to that contemporary discipline which is concerned with *problems in living* (and not with diseases of the brain, which are problems for neurology). Problems in human relations can be analyzed, interpreted, and given meaning only within given social and ethical contexts. Accordingly, it *does* make a difference—arguments to the contrary notwithstanding—what the psychiatrist's socioethical orientations happen to be; for these will influence his ideas on what is wrong with the patient, what deserves comment or interpretation, in what possible directions change might be desirable, and so forth. Even in medicine proper, these factors play a role, as for instance, in the divergent orientations which physicians, depending on their religious affiliations, have toward such things as birth control and therapeutic abortion. Can anyone really believe that a psychotherapist's ideas concerning religious belief, slavery, or other similar issues play no role in his practical work? If they do make a difference, what are we to infer from it? Does it not seem reasonable that we ought to have different psychiatric therapies—each expressly recognized for the ethical positions which they embody—for, say, Catholics and Jews, religious persons and agnostics, democrats and communists, white supremacists and Negroes, and so on? Indeed, if we look at how psychiatry is actually practiced today (especially in the United States), we find that people do seek psychiatric help in accordance with their social status and ethical beliefs (Hollingshead & Redlich, 1958). This should really not surprise us more than being told that practicing Catholics rarely frequent birth control clinics.

The foregoing position which holds that contemporary psychotherapists deal with problems in living, rather than with mental illness and their cures, stands in opposition to a currently prevalent claim, according to which mental illness is just as "real" and "objective" as bodily illness. This is a confusing claim since it is never known exactly what is meant by such words as "real" and "objective." I suspect, however, that what is intended by the proponents of this view is to create the idea in the popular mind that mental illness is some sort of disease entity, like an infection or a malignancy. If this were true, one could *catch* or *get* a "mental illness," one might *have* or *harbor* it, one might *transmit* it to others, and finally one could get *rid* of it. In my opinion, there is not a shred of evidence to support this idea. To the contrary, all the evidence is the other way and supports the view that what people now call mental illnesses are for the most part *communications* expressing unacceptable ideas, often framed, moreover, in an unusual idiom. The scope of this essay allows me to do no more than mention this alternatively theoretical approach to this problem (Szasz, 1957c).

This is not the place to consider in detail the similarities and differences between bodily and mental illnesses. It shall suffice for us here to emphasize only one important difference between them: namely, that whereas bodily disease refers to public, physicochemical occurrences, the notion of mental illness is used to codify relatively more private, sociopsychological happenings of which the observer (diagnostician) forms a part. In other words, the psychiatrist does not stand *apart* from what he observes, but is, in Harry Stack Sullivan's apt words, a "participant observer." This means that he is *committed* to some picture of what he considers reality—and to what he thinks society considers reality—and he observes and judges the patient's behavior in the light of these considerations. This touches on our earlier observation that the notion of mental symptom itself implies a comparison between observer and observed, psychiatrist and patient. This is so obvious that I may be charged with belaboring trivialities. Let me therefore say once more that my aim in presenting this argument was expressly to criticize and counter a prevailing contemporary tendency to deny the moral aspects of psychiatry (and psychotherapy) and to substitute for them allegedly value-free medical considerations. Psychotherapy, for example, is being widely practiced as though it entailed nothing other than restoring the patient from a state of mental sickness to one of mental health. While it is generally accepted that mental illness has something to do with man's social (or inter-personal) relations, it is paradoxically maintained that problems of values (that is, of ethics) do not arise in this process.* Yet, in one sense, much of psychotherapy may revolve around nothing other than the elucidation and weighing of goals and values—many of which may be mutually contradictory—and the means whereby they might best be harmonized realized, or relinquished.

The diversity of human values and the methods by means of which they may be realized is so vast, and many

---

*Freud went so far as to say that: "I consider ethics to be taken for granted. Actually I have never done a mean thing" (Jones, 1957, p. 247). This surely is a strange thing to say for someone who has studied man as a social being as closely as did Freud. I mention it here to show how the notion of "illness" (in the case of psychoanalysis, "psychopathology," or "mental illness") was used by Freud—and by most of his followers—as a means for classifying certain forms of human behavior as falling within the scope of medicine, and hence (by *fiat*) outside that of ethics!

of them remain so unacknowledged, that they cannot fail but lead to conflicts in human relations. Indeed, to say that human relations at all levels—from mother to child, through husband and wife, to nation and nation—are fraught with stress, strain, and disharmony is, once again, making the obvious explicit. Yet, what may be obvious may be also poorly understood. This I think is the case here. For it seems to me that—at least in our scientific theories of behavior—we have failed to *accept* the simple fact that human relations are inherently fraught with difficulties and that to make them even relatively harmonious requires much patience and hard work. I submit that the idea of mental illness is now being put to work to obscure certain difficulties which at present may be inherent—not that they need be unmodifiable—in the social intercourse of persons. If this is true, the concept functions as a disguise; for instead of calling attention to conflicting human needs, aspirations, and values, the notion of mental illness provides an amoral and impersonal "thing" (an "illness") as an explanation for *problems in living* (Szasz, 1959). We may recall in this connection that not so long ago it was devils and witches who were held responsible for men's problems in social living. The belief in mental illness, as something other than man's trouble in getting along with his fellow man, is the proper heir to the belief in demonology and witchcraft. Mental illness exists or is "real" in exactly the same sense in which witches existed or were "real."

CHOICE, RESPONSIBILITY, AND PSYCHIATRY

While I have argued that mental illnesses do not exist, I obviously did not imply that the social and psychological occurrences to which this label is currently being attached also do not exist. Like the personal and social troubles which people had in the Middle Ages, they are real enough. It is the labels we give them that concerns us and, having labelled them, what we do about them. While I cannot go into the ramified implications of this

problem here, it is worth noting that a demonologic conception of problems in living gave rise to therapy along theological lines. Today, a belief in mental illness implies—nay, requires—therapy along medical or psychotherapeutic lines.

What is implied in the line of thought set forth here is something quite different. I do not intend to offer a new conception of "psychiatric illness" nor a new form of "therapy." My aim is more modest and yet also more ambitious. It is to suggest that the phenomena now called mental illnesses be looked at afresh and more simply, that they be removed from the category of illnesses, and that they be regarded as the expressions of man's struggle with the problem of *how* he should live. The last mentioned problem is obviously a vast one, its enormity reflecting not only man's inability to cope with his environment, but even more his increasing self-reflectiveness.

By problems in living, then, I refer to that truly explosive chain reaction which began with man's fall from divine grace by partaking of the fruit of the tree of knowledge. Man's awareness of himself and of the world about him seems to be a steadily expanding one, bringing in its wake an ever larger *burden of understanding* (an expression borrowed from Susanne Langer, 1953). *This burden, then, is to be expected and must not be misinterpreted.* Our only *rational* means for lightening it is *more understanding,* and appropriate *action* based on such understanding. The main alternative lies in acting as though the burden were not what in fact we perceive it to be and taking refuge in an outmoded theological view of man. In the latter view, man does not fashion his life and much of his world about him, but merely lives out his fate in a world created by superior beings. This may logically lead to pleading nonresponsibility in the face of seemingly unfathomable problems and difficulties. Yet, if man fails to take increasing responsibility for his actions, individually as well as collectively, it seems unlikely that some higher power or being would assume this task and carry this burden for him. Moreover, this seems hardly the proper time in human history for obscuring the issue of man's responsibility for his actions by hiding it behind the skirt of an all-explaining conception of mental illness.

CONCLUSIONS

I have tried to show that the notion of mental illness has outlived whatever usefulness it might have had and that it now functions merely as a convenient myth. As such, it is a true heir to religious myths in general, and to the belief in witchcraft in particular; the role of all these belief-systems was to act as *social tranquilizers,* thus encouraging the hope that mastery of certain specific problems may be achieved by means of substitutive (symbolic-magical) operations. The notion of mental illness thus serves mainly to obscure the everyday fact that life for most people is a continuous struggle, not for biological survival, but for a "place in the sun," "peace of mind," or some other human value. For man aware of himself and of the world about him, once the needs for preserving the body (and perhaps the race) are more or less satisfied, the problem arises as to what he should do with himself. Sustained adherence to the myth of mental illness allows people to avoid facing this problem, believing that mental health, conceived as the absence of mental illness, automatically insures the making of right and safe choices in one's conduct of life. But the facts are all the other way. It is the making of good choices in life that others regard, retrospectively, as good mental health!

The myth of mental illness encourages us, moreover, to believe in its logical corollary: that social intercourse would be harmonious, satisfying, and the secure basis of a "good life" were it not for the disrupting influences of mental illness or "psychopathology." The potentiality for universal human happiness, in this form at least, seems to me but another example of the I-wish-it-were-true type of fantasy. I do believe that human happiness or well-being on a hitherto unimaginably large scale,

and not just for a select few, is possible. This goal could be achieved, however, only at the cost of many men, and not just a few being willing and able to tackle their personal, social, and ethical conflicts. This means having the courage and integrity to forego waging battles on false fronts, finding solutions for substitute problems—for instance, fighting the battle of stomach acid and chronic fatigue instead of facing up to a marital conflict.

Our adversaries are not demons, witches, fate, or mental illness. We have no enemy whom we can fight, exorcise, or dispel by "cure." What we do have are *problems in living*—whether these be biologic, economic, political, or sociopsychological. In this essay I was concerned only with problems belonging in the last mentioned category, and within this group mainly with those pertaining to moral values. The field to which modern psychiatry addresses itself is vast, and I made no effort to encompass it all. My argument was limited to the proposition that mental illness is a myth, whose function it is to disguise and thus render more palatable the bitter pill of moral conflicts in human relations.

References

Hollingshead, A. B., and Redlich, F. C. *Social class and mental illness.* New York: Wiley, 1958.

Jones, E. *The life and work of Sigmund Freud.* Vol. III. New York: Basic Books, 1957.

Langer, S. K. *Philosophy in a new key.* New York: Mentor Books, 1953.

Peters, R. S. *The concept of motivation.* London: Routledge & Kegan Paul, 1958.

Szasz, T. S. Malingering: "Diagnosis" or social condemnation? *AMA Arch Neurol. Psychiat.,* 1956, *76,* 432–443.

Szasz, T. S. *Pain and pleasure; A study of bodily feelings.* New York: Basic Books, 1957. (a)

Szasz, T. S. The problem of psychiatric nosology: A contribution to a situational analysis of psychiatric operations. *Amer. J. Psychiat.,* 1957, *114,* 405–413. (b)

Szasz, T. S. On the theory of psychoanalytic treatment. *Int. J. Psycho-Anal.,* 1957, *38,* 166–182. (c)

Szasz, T. S. Psychiatry, ethics and the criminal law. *Columbia Law Rev.,* 1958, *58,* 183–198.

Szasz, T. S. Moral conflict and psychiatry, *Yale Rev.,* 1959, in press.

10.   Biochemical Hypotheses of Schizophrenia

SEYMOUR S. KETY

Biochemistry, which has had notable success in elucidating etiologic factors in many areas of medicine, has also been brought to bear on the problem of schizophrenia. Although these efforts have not to date been successful in demonstrating a biochemical "lesion," a number of arguments can be made to support the viewpoint that chemical factors operate significantly and specifically in schizophrenia.

Perhaps the strongest of these arguments is the good evidence for the operation of genetic factors in the transmission of schizophrenia,[92] consisting of a higher concordance rate for the disorder in the monozygotic twins of afflicted individuals[43,57,59,67,99] and in the biologic families of schizophrenics where early adoption or removal from their natural parents has served to disentagle the operation of genetic and environmental factors in its transmission.[50,64,93]

Another argument which has been used is the ability of a number of exogenous chemical substances (iodides, mescaline, LSD, amphetamine, iproniazid, psilocybin) or some endogenous biochemical disturbances (porphyria, thyroid disorders) to produce psychoses resembling schizophrenia in some or many of its features.

Biochemical hypotheses and findings related to schizophrenia have been the subject of several exhaustive and critical reviews of which only a few are cited for further reference.[22,61,63,109] In spite of the large number of abnormal chemical findings which have been reported in schizophrenia, few have been independently confirmed and on none is there general agreement with regard to its significance. This may be attributed to the operation of an inordinate number of variables, difficult to control, which are associated with the clinical studies of schizophrenia.

Despite the phenomenologic similarities which permitted the concept of schizophrenia to emerge, there is little evidence that all of its forms have a common etiology of pathogenesis. Errors involved in the study of relatively small samples from heterogeneous populations may help to explain the frequency with which findings of one group fail to be confirmed by another.

Most biochemical research in schizophrenia has been carried out in patients with a long history of hospitalization in institutions where overcrowding is difficult to avoid and hygienic standards cannot always be maintained. It is easy to imagine the spread of chronic infections such as infectious hepatitis among such patients, and one wonders how often this may account for findings attributable to disturbed hepatic function or elevated plasma titres of antibody globulins. Even in the absence of previous or current infection, the development of a characteristic pattern of intestinal flora in a group of patients living together for long periods of time may occasionally contribute to the finding of what appear to be deviant metabolic pathways.

The variety and quality of the diet of the institutionalized schizophrenic is rarely comparable to that of the non-hospitalized normal control. In the case of the acute schizophrenic, the weeks of continual turmoil which precede recognition of the disorder are hardly conducive to a normal dietary intake. It is not surprising that a dietary vitamin deficiency has been found to account for at least one biochemical abnormality which had been attributed to schizophrenia.[77] Horwitt[55] found signs of liver dysfunction during long periods of borderline protein ingestion.

Emotional stress is known to cause profound changes in man, in adrenocortical and thyroid function, in excretion of water, electrolytes, creatinine, epinephrine and norepinephrine, to mention only a few recently reported findings. On the other hand, physical inactivity would be expected to produce changes in a number of body functions. Schizophrenic illness is often characterized by indolence and lack of exercise or by marked emotional dis-

From Leopold Bellak and Laurence Loeb (Eds.), *The Schizophrenic Syndrome*. New York: Grune & Stratton, 1969. pp. 155–171. Reprinted by permission of Grune & Stratton, Inc. and the author.

turbance in the basal state and frequently exaggerated anxiety in response to routine and research procedures. The disturbances in behavior and activity which mark the schizophrenic process would also be expected to cause deviations from the normal in many biochemical and metabolic measures: in urinary volume and concentration, in energy and nitrogen metabolism, in the state and activity of numerous organ systems and metabolic pathways. The biochemical changes which are secondary to the psychologic and behavioral state of the patient are often of interest in themselves; it is important, however, not to attribute to them etiologic roles.

Another incidental feature of the schizophrenic patient which differentiates him from the normal control and from many other types of patient is the long list of therapies to which he may have been exposed. The ataractic drugs which are often used over extended periods of time are particularly prone to produce metabolites which appear in the urine and interfere with a number of chemical determinations long after the drug has been withdrawn.

With this combination of many variables and the subjective judgments necessary for diagnosis and the evaluation of clinical course, it is not unexpected that subjective bias would from time to time affect the results of research in schizophrenia and make even more necessary in that field than in many others the employment of rigorous research design.

ENERGY METABOLISM

A decrease in basal metabolism was found in schizophrenia by earlier workers, although more recent work has not confirmed this,[89] and hypotheses attributing the disease to disturbances in the fundamental mechanisms of energy supply or conversion in the brain have been formulated but on the basis of rather inadequate evidence. Kelsey and co-workers[60] found a decreased B.M.R. in their series of schizophrenics to be associated with an increased uptake of ^{131}I by the thyroid, correctible by the addition of iodine to the diet, and attributed it to a lack of that element in the institutional diet. Periodic catatonia and some other schizophreniform psychoses seem to be associated with disturbances in thyroxine or thyrotropic hormone regulation,[21,41] but little evidence exists to suggest that such disturbances are characteristic of schizophrenia generally.

The oxygen consumption and blood flow of the brain as a whole have been found to lie within the normal range in a variety of forms of schizophrenia,[65] and although localized changes in these functions have sometimes been postulated, there is no evidence to support this supposition. The clear consciousness usually present in schizophrenia does not suggest the manifestation of cerebral anoxia.

Richter[89] has pointed out the uncontrolled factors in earlier work which implicated a defect in carbohydrate metabolism as a characteristic of the schizophrenic process. The finding in schizophrenia of an abnormal glucose tolerance in conjunction with other evidence of hepatic dysfunction, or evidence of a retarded metabolism of lactate by the schizophrenic,[2] does not completely exclude hepatic disease, nutritional deficiencies or the psychophysiologic influences on carbohydrate metabolism as possible sources of error. Horwitt and associates[56] were able to demonstrate and correct similar abnormalities by altering the dietary intake of the B group of vitamins.

A deficiency of glucose-6-phosphate dehydrogenase, known to occur in 10-20 per cent of American Negroes, has been found to show an incidence significantly different from normal in Negro catatonic and paranoid schizophrenics,[19] an observation which has received partial confirmation by an independent group.[29] Findings that schizophrenia is associated with cellular changes in oxidative phosphorylation or in the uptake[44] or metabolism of glucose[35] require further confirmation.[17]

It is difficult to believe that a generalized defect in energy metabolism, a process fundamental to every cell in the body, could be responsible for the highly specialized features of schizophrenia. For this reason, perhaps, interest has developed in other aspects of metabolism, the substrates or products of which appear to have some special role in the brain.

PROTEIN

Although Gjessing[41] found definite alterations in bodily nitrogen balance correlated with and sometimes preceding the changes in mental state of periodic catatonics, there has been no evidence to indicate a major change in protein metabolism for schizophrenia generally. On the other hand, some interest has been focused recently on more specific protein constituents or the metabolism of particular amino acids or their amines.

Interest in the possible presence of an abnormal protein constituent of blood of schizophrenics was stimulated by a report, in 1958, that a serum fraction obtained from schizophrenic patients was capable of causing some of the symptoms of that disorder when injected into nonschizophrenic volunteers.[49] This material, which was given the name "taraxein," appeared to have some relationship to ceruloplasmin, the copper-containing globulin of normal plasma which the same group had found to be elevated in schizophrenia[71] and, upon its intravenous injection, to produce rapid clinical improvement.[48] Very recently, Martens, in a thorough examination of the relationships between ceruloplasmin and schizophrenia,[76] has reported an equivalent elevation of serum copper in that disorder and in delirium tremens. In a controlled, double blind series he was unable to confirm the earlier report of clinical improvement following intravenous injections of ceruloplasmin. One attempt to replicate the production of psychotic symptoms in volunteers by means of taraxein was not successful,[91] and to date the original findings have not been confirmed in a significant and well controlled series.

A number of groups, however, have reported evidence compatible with the thesis that an abnormal protein is present to a greater extent in the blood of some schizophrenics than in normals and that this substance is capable of producing certain behavioral, metabolic, or cellular changes in lower animals. Haddad and Rabe,[45] replicating and extending an earlier report by Malis,[73] found some evidence for an antigenic abnormality in the pooled serum of chronically ill schizophrenic patients. More recent studies by this group using different immunologic methods have yielded negative results which they do not regard as conclusive. Faurbye, Lundberg and Jensen[23] were unable to confirm Malis' results. Using another approach, Vartanyan[108] has found evidence for an immunologic abnormality in schizophrenia. Heath and co-workers[47] have advanced an autoimmune concept as the biologic basis of schizophrenia. The studies with fluorescent antibodies, electrophysiologic, immunologic and behavioral observations, on which the concept is based, await independent confirmation. Precipitin reactions have yielded positive[79] and negative[58,84,90] results with respect to the occurrence of specific proteins in the serum of schizophrenics.

Fessel and co-workers[26,28] have reported increases in 4S and 19S macroglobulins in a considerable proportion of schizophrenic patients and the ability to differentiate schizophrenic from manic depressive patients on this basis. Mental stress in nonpsychotic individuals was found to elevate the same macroglobulins.[27] Certain of these findings have been confirmed by two independent groups.[66,97] Gammack and Hector,[37] while failing to confirm Fessel's findings, observed a highly significant increase in the α-globulin fraction and the haptoglobin component in the serum of schizophrenics. They also questioned the specificity of such findings which occur frequently in many types of chronic disease. Others have not confirmed this increase in haptoglobins.[72] It seems fair to conclude that to the present time no abnormal protein characteristic of schizophrenia has been characterized by physicochemical technics.

Some special properties of the plasma of schizophrenics have been reported by workers using various biologic assays. Bishop[11] has reported evidence for the effect of plasma from schizophrenic patients upon learning and retention of learning in the rat. Other investigators[8,112] found a slowing of rope climbing activity in rats injected with whole serum or certain fractions from schizophrenic patients as compared with normal fractions. The specificity of this response for schizophrenia has not been demonstrated and later findings were not confirmatory.[96] German[38] reported an effect of serum of schizophrenics on cortical evoked responses in rats which in later more rigorously controlled studies he and his associates were unable to confirm.[39] In well controlled studies of the effects of plasma from psychotic patients on behavior, Ferguson and Fisher[25] have reported observations using a precision timing task in cebus monkeys in which a highly significant delay in responsiveness was produced by the injection of plasma from some newly admitted catatonic patients. It is of interest that in their studies plasma from normal individuals under preoperative stress produced a similar but not as marked slowing of response.

Frohman and his associates[34] have reported increases in the ratio of lactate-to-pyruvate in the medium after chicken erythrocytes are incubated with plasma or plasma fractions of some schizophrenic patients as compared to normal controls. Mangoni and associates[74] have been unable to confirm this. In a subsequent paper, Frohman and associates[36] were able to demonstrate this difference in the lactate:pyruvate ratio only when the subjects had engaged in moderate exercise before the blood samples were drawn; no appreciable difference was found when the subjects were at complete rest, in normal activity, or exercising vigorously. This, plus the fact that exercise affected the lactate:pyruvate ratio in the incubation mixture more than did the presence or absence of schizophrenia, suggests the need for better definition of what may be a large number of variables involved in this reaction.

Recently, Ryan, Brown and Durell[94] have succeeded in clarifying some of the fundamental processes involved in the ability of human plasma to affect the lactate production of chicken erythrocytes, which appears to be the determining variable of the lactate:pyruvate ratio. In their test system, lactate production by aerobic glycolysis did not occur in completely intact erythrocytes but was contingent upon and correlated with hemolysis. This, in turn, was caused by a complement-requiring antibody present in variable titre in all human plasma tested. The plasma of schizophrenics could not be reliably distinguished from that of

nonschizophrenic patients from the same hospital.[95] Turner and Chipps[107] found a higher heterophile hemolysin titre in the blood of schizophrenics than of nonschizophrenics. Chronic alcoholics, however, also showed a higher titre of the hemolysin. Although Frohman and his associates have consistently found this phenomenon with higher frequency among schizophrenics, a possibility which remains to be ruled out is that the titre of this antibody is more closely related to a history of chronic hospitalization and greater exposure to a variety of antigens than to the presence of schizophrenia. An interesting further possibility is the significantly greater antibody responsiveness of schizophrenic patients than normal or depressed individuals to a standard antigen challenge.[33a]

The evidence with regard to the biologic or behavioral effects of the plasma of schizophrenics is far from conclusive at the present time. Most of the effects reported have failed of confirmation and none have been shown to be properties of plasma which are characteristic of schizophrenia.

Further work is necessary to determine to what extent the abnormalities in plasma found by physico-chemical analysis, when they are confirmed, are characteristic of schizophrenia or a reflection of the stress, exposure to chronic endemic infections, dietary or other adventitious factors which accompany the disorder and are associated with chronic institutionalization.[61]

AMINO ACIDS AND AMINES

Although an earlier report indicated abnormalities in amino acid excretion in schizophrenia,[114] this has not been confirmed. Much interest, on the other hand, has been attached to the possibility that abnormal metabolism of one or another amine could be of etiologic importance in schizophrenia.[51] The great sensitivity and relative nonspecificity of chromatographic methods and the ease with which findings may be affected by exogenous factors such as diet or drugs increase the likelihood of false positives in this area, and great caution must be exercised in identifying the particular metabolite which appears to be involved or interpreting the significance which should be attached to it.[42,75]

The significance of an unidentified Ehrlich positive substance ("the mauve spot") attributed to a new form of schizophrenia by Hoffer and Osmond[52] has been brought into question by O'Reilly and his associates[80,81] who found it with high frequency in the urines of patients with affective psychosis, alcoholism, psychoneurosis, personality disorders and cancer.

TRANSMETHYLATION

In 1952, Osmond and Smythies[82] pointed out some similarities between mescaline psychosis and schizophrenia and between that drug and epinephrine. They included a biochemical note by Harley-mason which stated, in part:

It is extremely probable that the final stage in the biogenesis of adrenaline is a transmethylation of noradrenaline, the methyl group arising from methionine or choline. It is just possible that a pathological disordering of its transmethylation mechanism might lead to methylation of one or both of its phenolic hydroxyl groups instead of its amino group. . . . Methylation of phenolic hydroxyl groups in the animal body is of rare occurrence but a significant case has been reported recently. . . . It is particularly interesting to note that out of a series of phenylethylamine derivations tested by Noteboom, 3,4-dimethoxyphenylethylamine was the most potent in producing catatonia in animals.

Since that time the transmethylation of norepinephrine to epinephrine has been established,[12] while Axelrod, Senoh and Witkop[5] have demonstrated the O-methylation of both catecholamines as an important step in their normal metabolism.

The suggestion that pathologic transmethylation may occur in schizophrenia was further strengthened by the recognition that a number of psychotomimetic agents, in addition to mescaline, were methylated congeners of normal body metabolites. On this basis, Hoffer and associates[53] used niacin and niacinamide, methyl accepters, in an effort to inhibit competitively the possible abnormal process. They reported beneficial results which have not been independently confirmed. In 1961,

Pollin, Cardon and Kety[86] tested this hypothesis by administering large doses of L-methionine to chronic schizophrenic patients in conjunction with a monoamine oxidase inhibitor to permit the accumulation of any monoamines formed. This substance is an essential precursor of S-adenosylmethionine, the active substance which was shown by Cantoni[18] to transfer its methyl group to accepter compounds in the process of transmethylation. In some of the patients during the administration of the L-methionine there was a brief intensification of psychosis which involved an exacerbation of some of the schizophrenic symptoms. No other amino acids tested (glycine, tyrosine, phenylalanine, tryptophan, histidine, glutamine) were associated with this phenomenon. The intensification of psychosis in schizophrenics with methionine has since, in essence, been confirmed by four other groups[1,15,46,83] and in addition, Brune and Himwich[16] found that betaine, another methyl donor, was equally effective in accentuating psychotic symptoms in schizophrenics. Baldessarini and Kopin[6] found that feeding L-methionine to rats produced a significant increase in S-adenosylmethionine concentration in the liver and brain. Axelrod[4] demonstrated the presence in normal mammalian tissue of an enzyme capable of methylating normal metabolites, i.e., tryptamine and serotonin to their dimethyl derivatives for which psychotomimetic properties have been reported.

DIMETHOXYPHENYLETHYLAMINE

In 1962, Friedhoff and Van Winkle[32] examined the urine of patients with early schizophrenia and reported the occurrence of 3,4-dimethoxyphenylethylamine (DMPEA), to which Harley-Mason had alluded as a possible abnormally methylated metabolite. This compound is a dimethylated derivative of dopamine and closely related to mescaline, which represents a trimethylated congener of this biogenic amine.

Since 1962 a number of groups have attempted to confirm the excretion of DMPEA in schizophrenia and further to define the variables which affect it.

Friedhoff and Van Winkle[32] had found it in the urine of 15 of 19 schizophrenics and in none of 14 normal urines. Kuehl and associates[68] confirmed its presence in 7 of 22 schizophrenics and in none of 10 normals. Takesada and associates[105] found it in 70 of 78 (90 per cent) schizophrenics but also in 35 of 67, or 52 per cent, of normals. Faurbye and Pind,[24] who modified the method to increase its sensitivity and to avoid interference by phenothiazine metabolites, were unable to detect DMPEA in the urine of 15 schizophrenics and 10 normals. Perry, Hansen and Macintyre[85] were unable to find the compound in 10 schizophrenics on a diet free of fruits and vegetables. After finding DMPEA in the urine of 4 out of 6 schizophrenics and 2 of 3 controls, Studnitz and Nyman[104] demonstrated its disappearance when the same individuals were placed on a pure carbohydrate regimen.

In an extensive series in which biochemical determinations and psychiatric diagnoses were made independently, Bourdillon and his associates[14] reported the presence of a "pink spot" having some of the characteristics of DMPEA in the urines of 46 of 84 (55 per cent) schizophrenics, while it was absent in all of 17 nonschizophrenic patients and 149 normal controls. A second experiment with less striking results showed a low incidence (3 per cent) of the spot in the urine of paranoid patients and a 29 per cent incidence in nonparanoid schizophrenics. Drug administration which was not controlled could have been different in type of drug or dosage for different diagnostic categories. Drugs or their metabolites are known to interfere with DMPEA determinations, and at least one group[24] has observed a phenothiazine metabolite with Rf value and color reactions similar to DMPEA which persisted in the urine for as long as 25 days after withdrawal of the drug. Williams[110] has examined the technic used by Bourdillon and found it relatively insensitive to DMPEA. Further studies by his group[111] and by others using more specific technics[7,13] have indicated that Bourdillon's "pink spot" was not, in fact, DMPEA and that DMPEA is not excreted in abnormal amounts by schizophrenics. Friedhoff,[33] on the other hand, on the basis of its behavior in six solvent sys-

tems, a number of color reactions, thin layer and gas chromatography and melting point determinations, has concluded that the material he has found in the urine of schizophrenics is identical to DMPEA. Although this substance, when administered to schizophrenics is rapidly converted to 3,4-dimethoxy-phenyl-acetic acid,[31] Kuehl and associates[69] could not detect a significant difference in the excretion of that acid between normal subjects and schizophrenics.

These findings—the intensification of psychosis in schizophrenics by methionine or betaine, the increase in S-adenosylmethionine in the brain and liver of rats by methionine feeding, the existence of at least one enzyme capable of transmethylating normal metabolites to psychoto-mimetic compounds, the evidence obtained by some workers for the excretion of DMPEA in a substantial number of schizophrenics —are compatible with the hypothesis that the process of biologic transmethylation is somehow disturbed in schizophrenia with the production or persistence of excessive amounts of methylated derivatives of normal metabolites capable of inducing some of the symptoms of schizophrenia. That hypothesis, however, is far from having been validated. Although methionine and betaine are the only ones of a large number of amino acids which have been shown capable of briefly exacerbating psychosis in some schizophrenics, it has not been established that the clinical changes resulted from any specific methylated derivatives, and the possibility that this was a nonspecific toxic psychosis or a peculiarly schizophrenic response to nonspecific toxic changes has not been ruled out. Haydu, et al.,[46] who confirm the ability of methionine to exacerbate schizophrenic symptomatology, found an ameliorating effect from hydroxychloroquine and suggest that the clinical effects of these agents result from their activation or suppression of thiol groups. A special sensitivity of schizophrenics to methionine has not been established although a similar regimen of methionine without iproniazid in a small number of normal volunteers produced no hint of a psychotic reaction.[62] The accumulated evidence for the excretion of dimethoxyphenylethylamine in association with some forms of schizophrenia is as yet inconclusive. Several groups have been unable to confirm it and the possibility that it is an artifact of drug therapy has not been completely ruled out. There is evidence that some dietary factors are necessary for its appearance although the same is true for phenylketonuria and does not argue against its significance or relevance to schizophrenia. On parenteral administration to man, DMPEA has not been shown to produce perceptible mental effects,[31] but this does not preclude an effect from higher concentrations locally within the brain. The transmethylation hypothesis appears to require and merit further examination and development.

INDOLEAMINES

Although Woolley[113] was impressed with indirect evidence for the possibility of a disorder in serotonin metabolism in schizophrenia, significant differences between schizophrenic and normal populations with respect to this amine or its metabolites have not been established.[61] Earlier findings of indolic compounds (indole acetamide and 6-hydroxyskatole) with abnormal frequency in the urine of schizophrenics[78,101] have more recently been found to a similar extent in the urine of other types of mental patient and are probably to be attributed to exogenous or non-disease-related factors.[20,100,115]

Tryptamine excretion may have some significance in schizophrenia since an increase has been found to occur in such patients before a period of exacerbation.[9] An increase in urinary tryptophan metabolites has also been observed following the administration of methionine,[10,102,103] and it has been suggested that the conversion of tryptamine to its hallucinogenic methylated derivative may occur. Aside from one positive report,[30] the search for dimethyltryptamine or dimethylserotonin in the urine of schizophrenics has yielded negative results.[98,102,106]

EPINEPHRINE

The hypothesis that adrenochrome or other abnormal metabolites of circulating epinephrine were formed in schizophrenia and accounted for many of the symptoms[54] has received careful scrutiny made possible by the recently acquired knowledge of the normal metabolism of this hormone.[3] No evidence was found for the abnormal metabolism of labeled epinephrine infused into schizophrenic patients,[88] and in one study which accounted almost entirely for the excreted label in terms of unchanged epinephrine and four metabolites (3-methoxy-4-hydroxymandelic acid, metanephrine, 3,4-dihydroxymandelic acid, and 3-methoxy-4-dihydroxyphenylglycol), no qualitative or quantitative differences were found in this pattern between chronic schizophrenics and normal volunteers.[70] The infusion of epinephrine into schizophrenics was not found to intensify the psychosis[87] which would have been expected if the psychosis were associated with abnormal metabolites of circulating epinephrine.

SUMMARY AND CONCLUSIONS

Although it would be difficult to demonstrate that a definitive increase in our knowledge of biochemical mechanisms in the schizophrenic psychoses has occurred in the past decade, substantial progress has nonetheless been made. There is an increasing awareness of the complexity of the problem and of the sophistication of research design necessary to cope with it. Most important, there has been a burgeoning of fundamental knowledge in biochemistry and neurochemistry and their interaction with behavior on which depend meaningful hypotheses relating to schizophrenia and from which may eventually come an understanding of whatever biochemical mechanisms operate significantly in its etiology, pathogenesis, or therapy.

Before the etiology of any syndrome has been established, it is idle to regard it as a single disease, and, in the case of schizophrenia, the striking resemblance which certain temporal lobe epilepsies or chronic intoxications (bromidism, iodism, amphetamine psychosis, porphyria) bear to it makes tenable the possibility that the syndrome may emerge from different etiologic pathways. Recognition of such a possibility aids in the interpretation of genetic and biologic findings and would facilitate the characterization of more specific subgroups.

Those interested in exploring the biologic aspects of schizophrenic disorders cannot with impunity ignore the psychologic, social, and other environmental factors which operate significantly at various stages of their development. Leaving aside etiologic considerations, it is clear that exogenous factors may precipitate, intensify, or ameliorate the symptoms and confound the biologic picture. To what extent the classical psychologic features of chronic schizophrenia are created by prolonged isolation and hospitalization will become apparent with the increasing adoption of community-oriented treatment. Examples are readily found in which uncontrolled nutritional, infectious, or pharmacologic variables may have accounted for specific biochemical abnormalities in populations of chronic schizophrenics. These secondary variables are so manifold that it is hard to imagine a design which could anticipate and control them all, and successive studies concentrating on particularly relevant controls will probably continue to be called for. There is, in addition, much to be said for broadening the scope of the typical sample from chronic hospitalized schizophrenia to the early, more acute, remitting, episodic, or periodic forms[21,40] in which it may not only be possible to obviate some of the difficulties imposed by chronic hospitalization and drug administration but, by study of the same patient in psychotic and nonpsychotic states, to avoid the effects of interindividual variance.

An unavoidable difficulty at the present time is the fact that the crucial processes of diagnosis and evaluation of change are based almost entirely on subjective estimates. It is not insensitivity which diminishes the reliability of such measures as much as their vulnerability to bias; failure to recognize and guard against this source of error probably accounts for much of the inconsistency in the study of schizophrenia not only from biologic but also from sociologic and psychologic points of view.

The single-gene-single-enzyme concept of the biologic disorder in schizophrenia was encouraged by the very high concordance rate found in monozygotic twins in earlier studies. More recent twin studies in which selective bias in sampling has been more effectively controlled have yielded a concordance rate of 40 per cent or less. Studies with adopted schizophrenics[64,93] where environmental factors can be more successfully controlled have still reinforced the importance of genetic factors but have emphasized the genetic transmission of a vulnerability to schizophrenia or to a variety of personality or character disorders. This suggests that personality or intelligence may be more appropriate models for schizophrenia than phenylketonuria. A polygenic inadequacy interacting with particular life situations seems more compatible with all of the evidence.[92] The biologic component of the schizophreniform illnesses may lie in the mechanisms which underlie arousal, inhibition, perception, cognition, affect, or the complex relationships among them, all of which appear to be involved at one time or another. Although a single chemical substance such as mescaline or lysergic acid diethylamide may produce disturbances in all of these areas, it would be well to keep in mind the possibility that more complex neurochemical, neurophysiologic and psychologic interactions may form the biologic substrate of schizophrenia.

References

1. Alexander, F., Curtis, G. C., Sprince, H., & Crosley, A. P. L-Methionine and L-tryptophan feedings in nonpsychotic and schizophrenic patients with and without tranylcypromine. *Journal of Nervous and Mental Disease*, 1963, *137*, 135–142.
2. Altschule, M. D., Henneman, D. H., Holliday, P., & Goncz, R,-M. Carbohydrate metabolism in brain disease. VI. Lactate metabolism after infusion of sodium d-lactate in manic-depressive and schizophrenic psychoses. *AMA Archives of Internal Medicine*, 1956, *98*, 35–38.
3. Axelrod, J. Metabolism of epinephrine and other sympathomimetic amines. *Physiological Review*, 1959, *39*, 751–776.
4. Axelrod, J. Enzymatic formation of psychotomimetic metabolites from normally occurring compounds. *Science*, 1961, *134*, 343.

5. Axelrod, J., Senoh, S., & Witkop, B. O-Methylation of catecholamines *in vivo, Journal of Biological Chemistry,* 1958, *233,* 697–701.

6. Baldessarini, R. J., & Kopin, I. J. Assay of tissue levels of S-adenosylmethionine. *Anal. Biochem,* 1963, *6,* 289–292.

7. Bell, C. E., & Somerville, A. R. Identity of the "pink spot." *Nature,* 1966, *211,* 1405–1406.

8. Bergen, J. F., Pennell, R. B., Saravis, C. A., & Hoagland, H. Further experiments with plasma proteins from schizophrenics. *In* R. G. Heath, (Ed.). *Serological fractions in Schizophrenia.* New York: Harper & Row, 1963. pp. 67–76.

9. Berlet, H. H., Bull, C., Himwich, H. E., Kohl, H., Matsumoto, K., Pscheidt, G. R., Spaide, J., Tourlentes, T. T., & Valverde, J. M. Endogenous metabolic factor in schizophrenic behavior. *Science,* 1964, *144,* 311–313.

10. Berlet, H. H., Matsumoto, K., Pscheidt, G. R., Spaide, J., Bull, C., & Himwich, H. E. Biochemical correlates of behavior in schizophrenic patients. *Archives of General Psychiatry,* 1965, *13,* 521–531.

11. Bishop, M. P. Effects of plasma from schizophrenia subjects upon learning and retention in the rat. *In* R. G. Heath, (Ed.). *Serological fractions in schizophrenia.* New York: Harper & Row, 1963. pp. 77–91.

12. Blaschko, H. The development of current concepts of catecholamine formation. *Pharmacological Review,* 1959, *11,* 307–316.

13. Boulton, A. A., & Felton, C. A. The "pink spot" and schizophrenia. *Nature,* 1966, *211,* 1404–1405.

14. Bourdillon, R. E., Clarke, C. A., Ridges, A. P., Sheppard, P. M., Harper, P., & Leslie, S. A. "Pink spot" in the urine of schizophrenics. *Nature,* 1965, *208,* 453–455.

15. Brune, G. G., & Himwich, H. E. Effects of methionine loading on the behavior of schizophrenic patients. *Journal of Nervous and Mental Disease,* 1962, *134,* 447–450.

16. Brune, G. G., & Himwich, H. E. Biogenic amines and behavior in schizophrenic patients. In *Recent advances in biological psychiatry,* Vol. 5. New York: Plenum Press, 1963. pp. 144–160.

17. Buhler, D. R., & Ihler, G. S. Effect of plasma from normal and schizophrenic subjects on the oxidation of labeled glucose by chicken erythrocytes. *Journal of Laboratory and Clinical Medicine,* 1963, *62,* 306–318.

18. Cantoni, G. L. S-Adenosylmethinine: a new intermediate formed enzymatically from L-methionine and adenosine-triphosphate. *Journal of Biological Chemistry,* 1953, *204,* 403–416.

19. Dern, R. J., Glynn, M. F., & Brewer, G. J. Studies on the influence of hereditary G-6-PD deficiency in the expression of schizophrenic patterns. *Clinical Research,* 1962, *10,* 80.

20. Dohan, F. C., Ewing, J., Graff, H., & Sprince, H. Schizophrenia: 6-hydroxyskatole and environment. *Archives of General Psychiatry,* 1964, *10,* 420–422.

21. Durell, J., Lidow, L. S., Kellam, S. F., & Shader, R. I. Interrelationships between regulation of thyroid gland function and psychosis. *Research Publications: Association for Research in Nervous and Mental Disease,* 1966, *43,* 387–399.

22. Durell, J., & Schildkraut, J. J. Biochemical studies of the schizophrenic and affective disorders. *In* S. Arieti, (Ed.). *American handbook of psychiatry,* Vol. III. New York: Basic Books, 1966. pp. 423–457.

23. Faurbye, A., Lundberg, L., & Jensen, K. A. Studies on the antigen demonstrated by Malis in serum from schizophrenic patients. *Acta Pathalogica et Microbiologica Scandinavica,* 1964. *61,* 663–651.

24. Faurbye, A., & Pind, K. Investigation on the occurrence of the dopamine metabolite 3,4-dimethoxyphenylethylamine in the urine of schizophrenics. *Acta Psychiatrica Scandinavica,* 1964, *40,* 240–243.

25. Ferguson, D. C., & Fisher, A. E. Behavior disruption in cebus monkeys as a function of injected substances. *Science,* 1963, *139* 1281–1282.

26. Fessel, W. J. Macroglobulin elevations in functional mental illness. *Nature,* 1962, *193,* 1005.

27. Fessel, W. J. Mental stress, blood proteins and the hypothalamus: experimental results showing effect of mental stress upon 4S and 19S proteins. *Archives of General Psychiatry,* 1962, *7,* 427–435.

28. Fessel, W. J., & Grunbaum, B. W. Electrophoretic and analytical ultracentrifuge studies in sera of psychotic patients: elevation of gamma globulins and macroglobulins, and splitting of alpha$_2$ globulins. *Annals of Internal Medicine,* 1961, *54,* 1134–1145.

29. Fieve, R. R., Brauninger, G., Fleiss, J., & Cohen, G. Glucose-6-phosphate dehydrogenase deficiency and schizophrenic behavior. *Journal of Psychiatric Research,* 1965, *3,* 255–262.

30. Fischer, E., Fernandez-Lagravere, T. A., Vazquez, A. J., & Di Stefano, A. O. A bufotenin-like substance in the urine of schizophrenics. *Journal of Nervous and Mental Disease,* 1961, *133,* 441–444.

31. Friedhoff, A. J., & Hollister, L. E. Comparison of the metabolism of 3,4-dimethoxyphenylethylamine and mescaline in humans. *Biochemical Pharmacology,* 1966, *15,* 269–273.

32. Friedhoff, A. J., & Van Winkle, E. The characteristics of an amine found in the urine of schizophrenic patients. *Journal of Nervous and Mental Disease,* 1962, *135,* 550–555.

33. Friedhoff, A. J., & Van Winkle, E. New developments in the investigation of the relationship of 3,4-dimethoxyphenylethylamine to schizophrenia. *In* H. E. Himwich, S. S. Kety, and J. R. Smythies, (Eds.). *Amines and Schizophrenia.* Oxford: Pergamon Press, 1967. pp. 19–21.

33a. Friedman, S. B., Cohen, J., & Iker, H. Antibody response to cholera vaccine. Differences between depressed, schizophrenic, and normal subjects. *Archives of General Psychiatry,* 1967, *16,* 312–315.

34. Frohman, C. E., Czajkowski, N. P., Luby, E. D.,

Gottlieb, J. S., & Senf, R. Further evidence of a plasma factor in schizophrenia. *Archives of General Psychiatry*, 1960, 2, 263–267.

35. Frohman, C. E., Latham, L. K., Beckett, P. G. S., & Gottlieb, J. S. Evidence of a plasma factor in schizophrenia. *Archives of General Psychiatry*, 1960, 2, 255–262.

36. Frohman, C. E., Latham, L. K., Warner, K. A., Brosius, C. O., Beckett, P. G. S., & Gottlieb, J. S. Motor activity in schizophrenia; effect on plasma factor. *Archieves of General Psychiatry*, 1963, 9, 83–88.

37. Gammack, D. B., & Hector, R. I. A study of serum proteins in acute schizophrenia. *Clinical Science*, 1965, 28, 469–475.

38. German, G. A. Effects of serum from schizophrenics on evoked cortical potentials in the rat. *British Journal of Psychiatry*, 1963, 109, 616–623.

39. German, G. A., Antebi, R. N., Dear, E. M. A., & McCance, C. A further study of the effects of serum from schizophrenics on evoked cortical potentials in the rat. *British Journal of Psychiatry*, 1965, 111, 345–347.

40. Gjessing, L. R. Studies of periodic catatonia. II. The urinary excretion of phenolic amines and acids with and without loads of different drugs. *Journal of Psychiatry Research*, 1964, 2, 149–162.

41. Gjessing, R. Disturbances of somatic functions in catatonia with a periodic course, and their compensation. *Journal of Mental Science*, 1938, 84, 608–621.

42. Goldenberg, H., Fishman, V., Whittier, J., & Brinitzer, W. Urinary aromatic excretion patterns in schizophrenia. *Archives of General Psychiatry*, 1960, 2, 221–230.

43. Gottesman, I. I., & Shields, J. Schizophrenia in twins: sixteen years' consecutive admissions to a psychiatric clinic. *Diseases of the Nervous System*, 1966, 27, (Suppl.), 11–19.

44. Haavaldsen, R., Lingjaerde, O., & Walaas, O. Disturbances of carbohydrate metabolism in schizophrenics: effect of serum fractions from schizophrenics on glucose uptake of rat diaphragm *in vitro*. *Confinia Neurologica/Borderland of Neurology*, 1958, 18, 270.

45. Haddad, R. K., & Rabe, A. An antigenic abnormality in the serum of chronically ill schizophrenic patients. *In* R. G. Heath, (Ed.). *Serological fractions in schizophrenia*. New York: Harper & Row, 1963. pp. 151–157.

46. Haydu, G. G., Dhrymiotis, A., Korenyi, C., & Goldschmidt, L. Effects of methionine and hydroxychloroquine in schizophrenia. *American Journal of Psychiatry*, 1965, 122, 560–564.

47. Heath, R. G., & Krupp, I. M. The biologic basis of schizophrenia: an autoimmune concept. *In* O. Walaas, (Ed.). *Molecular basis of some aspects of mental activity*, Vol. 2. London: Academic Press, 1967. pp. 313–344.

48. Heath, R. G., Leach, B. E., Byers, L. W., Martens, S., & Feigley, C. A. Pharmacological and biological psychotherapy. *American Journal of Psychiatry*, 1958, 114, 683–689.

49. Heath, R. G., Martens, S., Leach, B. E., Cohen, M., & Feigley, C. A. Behavioral changes in nonpsychotic volunteers following the administration of taraxein, the substance obtained from serum of schizophrenic patients. *American Journal of Psychiatry*, 1958, 114, 917–920.

50. Heston, L. L. Psychiatric disorders in foster home reared children of schizophrenic mothers. *British Journal of Psychiatry*, 1966, 112, 819–825.

51. Himwich, H. E., Kety, S. S., & Smythies, J. R. (Eds.). *Amines and schizophrenia*. Oxford: Pergamon Press, 1967.

52. Hoffer, A., & Osmond, H. Malvaria: A new psychiatric disease. *Acta Psychiatrica Scandinavica*, 1963, 39, 335–366.

53. Hoffer, A., Osmond, H., Callbeck, M. J., & Kahan, I. Treatment of schizophrenia with nicotinic acid and nicotinamide. *Journal of Clinical and Experimental Psychopathology*, 1957, 18, 131–158.

54. Hoffer, A., Osmond, H., & Smythies, J. Schizophrenia: A new approach. II. Result of a year's research. *Journal of Mental Science*, 1954, 100,, 29–45.

55. Horwitt, M. K. Report of Elgin Project No. 3 with emphasis on liver dysfunction. In *Nutrition symposium*, Series No. 7. New York: National Vitamin Foundation, 1953. pp. 67–83.

56. Horwitt, M. K., Liebert, E., Kreisler, O., & Wittman, P. Investigations of human requirements for B-complex vitamins. In *National Research Council Bulletin No. 116*. Washington, D.C.: National Academy of Sciences, 1948.

57. Inouye, E. Similarity and dissimilarity of schizophrenia in twins. *In Proceedings of the Third World Congress of Psychiatry*, Vol. I, Montreal: 1961. pp. 524–530.

58. Jensen, K., Clausen, J., & Osterman, E. Serum and cerebrospinal fluid proteins in schizophrenia. *Acta Psychiatrica Scandinavica*, 1964, 40, 280–286.

59. Kallmann, F. J. The genetic theory of schizophrenia. An analysis of 691 schizophrenic twin index families. *American Journal of Psychiatry*, 1946, 103, 309–322.

60. Kelsey, F. O., Gullock, A. H., & Kelsey, F. E. Thyroid activity in hospitalized psychiatric patients. *AMA Archives of Neurological Psychiatry*, 1957, 77, 543–548.

61. Kety, S. S. Biochemical theories of schizophrenia. *Science*, 1959, 129, 1528–1532, 1590–1596.

62. Kety, S. S. Possible relation of central amines to behavior in schizophrenic patients. *Federal Proceedings*, 1961, 20, 894–896.

63. Kety, S. S. Current biochemical approaches to schizophrenia. *New England Journal of Medicine*, 1967, 276, 325–331.

64. Kety, S. S., Rosenthal, D., Wender, P. H., & Schulsinger, F. The types and prevalence of mental illness in the biological and adoptive families of adopted schizophrenics. *Journal of Psychiatric Research*, 6, (Suppl.), 1968.

65. Kety, S. S., Woodford, R. B., Harmel, M. H., Freyhan, F. A., Appel, K. E., & Schmidt, C. F. Cerebral blood flow and metabolism in schizophrenia. The effects of barbiturate seminarcosis, insulin coma and electro-

shock. *American Journal of Psychiatry,* 1948, *104,* 765–770.

66. Kopeloff, L. M., & Fischel, E. Serum levels of bactericidin and globulin in schizophrenia. *Archives of General Psychiatry,* 1968, *9,* 524–528.

67. Kringlen, E. Schizophrenia in twins: An epidemiological-clinical study. *Psychiatry,* 1966, *29,* 172–184.

68. Kuehl, F. A., Jr., Hichens, M., Ormond, R. E., Meisinger, M. A. P., Gale, P. H., Cirillo, V. J., & Brink, N. G. Para-O-methylation of dopamine in schizophrenic and normal individuals. *Nature,* 1964, *203,* 154–155.

69. Kuehl, F. A., Jr., Ormond, R. E., & Vandenheuvel, W. J. A. Occurrence of 3,4-dimethoxyphenylacetic acid in urines of normal and schizophrenic individuals. *Nature,* 1966, *211,* 606–608.

70. LaBrosse, E. H., Mann, J. D., & Kety, S. S. The physiological and psychological effects of intravenously administered epinephrine and its metabolism in normal and schizophrenic men. III. Metabolism of 7-H^3-epinephrine as determined in studies on blood and urine. *Journal of Psychiatric Research,* 1961, *1,* 68–75.

71. Leach, B. E., Cohen, M., Heath, R. G., & Martens, S. Studies of the role of ceruloplasmin and albumin in adrenaline metabolism. *AMA Archives of Neurological Psychiatry,* 1956, *76,* 635–642.

72. Lovegrove, T. D., & Nicholls, D. M. Haptoglobin subtypes in a schizophrenic and control population. *Journal of Nervous and Mental Disease,* 1965, *141,* 195–196.

73. Malis, C. Y. *K Etiologii Schizofrenii.* Moscow: Medgiz, 1959.

74. Mangoni, A., Balazs, R., & Coppen, A. J. The effect of plasma from schizophrenic patients on the chicken erythrocyte system. *British Journal of Psychiatry,* 1963, *109,* 231–234.

75. Mann, J. D., & LaBrosse, E. H. Urinary excretion of phenolic acids by normal and schizophrenic male patients. *Archives of General Psychiatry,* 1959, *1,* 547–551.

76. Martens, S. *Effects of exogenous human ceruloplasmin in the schizophrenia syndrome.* Stockholm: Tryckeri Balder AB, 1966.

77. McDonald, R. K., Weise, V. K., Evans, F. T., & Patrick, R. W. Studies on plasma ascorbic acid and ceruloplasmin levels in schizophrenia. *In* J. Folch-Pi (Ed.). *Chemical pathology of the nervous system.* Oxford: Pergamon Press, 1961. pp. 404–412.

78. Nakao, A., & Ball, M. The appearance of a skatole derivative in the urine of schizophrenics. *Journal of Nervous and Mental Disease,* 1960, *130,* 417–419.

79. Noval, J. J., & Mao, T. S. S. Abnormal immunological reaction of schizophrenic serum. *Federal Proceedings,* 1966, *25,* 560.

80. O'Reilly, P. O., Ernest, M., & Hughes, G. The incidence of malvaria. *British Journal of Psychiatry,* 1965, *111,* 741–744.

81. O'Reilly, P. O., Hughes, G., Russell, S., & Ernest, M. The mauve factor: An evalua-

tion. *Diseases of the Nervous System,* 1965, *26,* 562–568.

82. Osmond, H., & Smythies, J. Schizophrenia: A new approach. *Journal of Mental Science,* 1952, *98,* 309–315.

83. Park, L., Baldessarini, R. J., & Kety, S. S. Methionine effects on chronic schizophrenics. *Archives of General Psychiatry,* 1965, *12,* 346–351.

84. Pennell, R. B., Pawlus, C., Saravis, C. A., & Scrimshaw, G. Further characterization of a human plasma component which influences animal behavior. *Transactions of the New York Academy of Science,* 1965, *28,* 47–58.

85. Perry, T. L., Hansen, S., & Macintyre, L. Failure to detect 3,4-dimethoxyphenylamine in the urine of schizophrenics. *Nature,* 1964, *202,* 519–520.

86. Pollin, W., Cardon, P. V., & Kety, S. S. Effects of amino acid feedings in schizophrenic patients treated with iproniazid. *Science,* 1961, *133,* 104–105.

87. Pollin, W., & Goldin, S. The physiological and psychological effects of intravenously administered epinephrine and its metabolism in normal and schizophrenic men. II. Psychiatric observations. *Journal of Psychiatric Research,* 1961, *1,* 50–67.

88. Resnick, O., & Elmadjian, F. Excretion and metabolism of dl-epinephrine 7-C^{14}-d-bitartrate infused into schizophrenic patients. *American Journal of Physiology,* 1956, *187,* 626.

89. Richter, D. Biochemical aspects of schizophrenia. *In* D. Richter (Ed.). *Schizophrenia: Somatic aspects.* London: Pergamon Press, 1957, pp. 53–75.

90. Rieder, H. P., Ritzel, G., Spiegelberg, H., & Gnirss, F. Serologische Versuche zum Nachweis von "Taraxein," *Experientia,* 1960, *16,* 561–562.

91. Robins, E., Smith, K., & Lowe, I. P. Discussion of clinical studies with taraxein. *In* H. A. Abramson (Ed.). *Neuropharmacology: Transactions of the Fourth Conference.* New York: Josiah Macy Jr. Foundation, 1957. pp. 123–135.

92. Rosenthal, D., & Kety, S. S. (Eds.). The transmission of schizophrenia. *Journal of Psychiatric Research,* 1968, *6* (Suppl.).

93. Rosenthal, D., Wender, P. H., Kety, S. S., Schulsinger, F., Welner, J., & Ostergaard, L. Schizophrenics' offspring reared in adoptive homes, *Journal of Psychiatric Research,* 1968, (Suppl.).

94. Ryan, J. W., Brown, J. D., & Durell, J. Antibodies affecting metabolism of chicken erythrocytes: Examination of schizophrenic and other subjects. *Science,* 1966, *151,* 1408–1410.

95. Ryan, J. W., Steinberg, H. R., Green, R., Brown, J. D., & Durell, J. Controlled study of effects of plasma of schizophrenic and nonschizophrenic psychiatric patients on chicken erythrocytes. *Journal of Psychiatric Research,* 1968, *6,* 33–44.

96. Sanders, B. E., Small, S. M., Ayers, W. J., Oh, Y. H., & Axelrod, S. Additional studies on plasma proteins obtained from schizophrenics and controls. *Transactions of*

the New York Academy of Science, 1965, *28*, 22–39.

97. Sapira, J. D. Immunoelectrophoresis of the serum of psychotic patients. *Archives of General Psychiatry*, 1964, *10*, 196–198.

98. Siegel, M. A sensitive method for the detection of N,N-dimethylserotonin (bufotenin) in urine; failure to demonstrate its presence in the urine of schizophrenic and normal subjects. *Journal of Psychiatric Research*, 1965, *3*, 205–211.

99. Slater, E. *Psychotic and neurotic illnesses in twins*. London: H. M. Stationery Office, 1953.

100. Sohler, A., Noval, J. J., & Renz, R. H. 6-Hydroxyskatole sulfate excretion in schizophrenia. *Journal of Nervous and Mental Disease*, 1963, *137*, 591–596.

101. Sprince, H., Houser, E., Jameson, D., & Dohan, F. C. Differential extraction of indoles from the urine of schizophrenic and normal subjects. *Archives of General Psychiatry*, 1960, *2*, 268–270.

102. Sprince, H., Parker, C. M., Jameson, D., & Alexander, F. Urinary indoles in schizophrenic and psychoneurotic patients after administration of tranylcypromine (parnate) and methionine or tryptophan. *Journal of Nervous and Mental Disease*, 1963, *137*, 246–251.

103. Sprince, H., Parker, C. M., Jameson, D., & Josephs, J. A. Effect of methionine on nicotinic acid and indoleacetic acid pathways of tryptophan metabolism *in vivo*. *Proceedings of the Society for Experimental Biology and Medicine*, 1965, *119*, 942–946.

104. Studnitz, W. V., & Nyman, G. E. Excretion of 3,4-dimethoxyphenylethylamine in schizophrenia. *Acta Psychiatrica Scandinavica*, 1965, *41*, 117–121.

105. Takesada, M., Kakimoto, Y., Sano, I., & Kaneko, Z. 3,4-dimethoxyphenylethylamine and other amines in the urine of schizo-

phrenic patients. *Nature*, 1963, *199*, 203–204.

106. Takesada, M., Miyamoto, E., Kakimoto, Y., Sano, I., & Kaneko, Z. Phenolic and indole amines in the urine of schizophrenics. *Nature*, 1965, *207*, 1199–1200.

107. Turner, W. J., & Chipps, H. I. A heterophil hemolysin in human blood. I. Distribution in schizophrenics and non-schizophrenics. *Archives of General Psychiatry*, 1966, *15*, 373–377.

108. Vartanyan, M. E. Immunological investigation of schizophrenia. Zh. Nevropat. Psikhiat. Korsakov, 1963, *63*, 3–12.

109. Weil-Malherbe, H. The biochemistry of the functional psychoses. In *Advances in enzymology*, Vol. XXIX. New York: Interscience Publishers, 1967. pp. 479–553.

110. Williams, C. H. The pink spot. *Lancet*, 1966, *1*, 599–600.

111. Williams, C. H., Gibson, J. G., & McCormick, W. O. 3,4-dimethoxyphenylethylamine in schizophrenia. *Nature*, 1966, *211*, 1195.

112. Winter, C. A., Flataker, L., Boger, W. P., Smith, E. V. C., & Sanders, B. E. The effects of blood serum and of serum fractions from schizophrenic donors upon the performance of trained rats. In J. Folch-Pi, (Ed.). *Chemical pathology of the nervous system*. Oxford: Pergamon Press, 1961. pp. 641–646.

113. Woolley, D. W. *The biochemical bases of psychoses*. New York: Wiley, 1962.

114. Young, H. K., Berry, H. K., Beerstecher, E., & Berry, J. S. Metabolic patterns in schizophrenic and control groups. *In Biochemical Institute Studies IV*, University of Texas Publication No. 5109. Austin: University of Texas, 1951. pp. 189–197.

115. Yuwiler, A., & Good, M. H. Chromatographic study of "Reigelhaupt" chromogens in urine. *Journal of Psychiatric Research*, 1962, *1*, 215–227.

Part II

Intrapsychic Theories

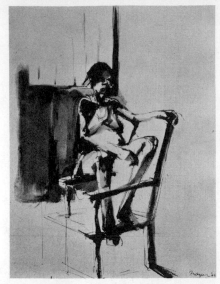

Michael Mazur—*Her Place*. (The Museum of Modern Art, Gift of Mrs. Bertram Smith.)

INTRODUCTION

The emphasis given to early childhood experience by intrapsychic theorists represents their contention that disorders of adulthood are a direct product of the continued and insidious operation of past events. To them, knowledge of the past provides information indispensable to understanding adult difficulties. To the question "What is the basis of adult disorders?" they would answer: the anxieties of childhood and the progressive sequence of defensive maneuvers which were devised to protect against a recurrence of these feelings.

Intrapsychic theorists contend that these two determinants of adult behavior, childhood anxieties and defensive maneuvers, are unconscious, that is, cannot be brought to awareness except under unusual conditions. It is the search for these unconscious processes which is the distinguishing feature of the intrapsychic approach. The obscure and elusive phenomena of the unconscious are the data which they uncover and use for their concepts. These data consist, first, of repressed childhood anxieties that persist within the individual and attach themselves insidiously to ongoing experiences, and, second, of unconscious adaptive processes which protect the individual against the resurgence of these anxieties. The *intrapsychic* label we have attached to these theorists reflects, therefore, their common focus on these two elements of the unconscious.

ORIENTATION

Our presentation of the intrapsychic approach begins with a contribution by Sigmund Freud for two reasons. First, in recognition of the fact that his monumental works are the foundation upon which all other intrapsychic theories are based and, second, to demonstrate the bridge he attempted to build between the biophysical and the intrapsychic orientations. Freud anchored many of his concepts to the biological make-up of man, a view that was rejected or overlooked by several of his followers. In the selection reprinted, drawn from one of his major publications, Freud attempted to summarize the central features of his theoretical work. Here he chose to stress two central ideas: the role and development of the biological instincts and the workings of unconscious processes.

Among the major theorists who have continued and enriched the intrapsychic tradition none has played a more significant or creative role than Heinz Hartmann. Hartmann retained Freud's notion of biological instincts, but proposed that constructive "ego" instincts exist within man which enable him to develop in a healthy and constructive fashion. In contrast to Freud, who believed that disorders arose as a function of destructive instinctual drives, Hartmann contended that pathological development occurs when constructive ego instincts fail to develop. In the article presented here, Hartmann examines the philosophical under-pinnings of intrapsychic theory. He outlines the major assumptions of this approach and offers a series of counter-arguments to those who who have criticized "psychoanalysis" as lacking scientific and theoretical rigor.

11. The Metapsychology of Instincts, Repression and the Unconscious

SIGMUND FREUD

I: INSTINCTS

The view is often defended that sciences should be built up on clear and sharply defined basal concepts. In actual fact no science, not even the most exact, begins with such definitions. The true beginning of scientific activity consists rather in describing phenomena and then in proceeding to group, classify and correlate them. Even at the stage of de-

scription it is not possible to avoid applying certain abstract ideas to the material in hand, ideas derived from various sources and certainly not the fruit of the new experience only. Still more indispensable are such ideas—which will later become the basal concepts of the science—as the material is further elaborated. They must at first necessarily possess some measure of uncertainty; there can be no question of any clear delimitation of their content. So long as they remain in this condition, we come to an understanding about their meaning by repeated references to the material of ob-

From *Collected Papers of Sigmund Freud* edited by Ernest Jones, Basic Books, Inc., 1959, by permission of the publisher.

servation, from which we seem to have deduced our abstract ideas, but which is in point of fact subject to them. Thus, strictly speaking, they are in the nature of conventions; although everything depends on their being chosen in no arbitrary manner, but determined by the important relations they have to the empirical material—relations that we seem to divine before we can clearly recognize and demonstrate them. It is only after more searching investigation of the field in question that we are able to formulate with increased clarity the scientific concepts underlying it, and progressively so to modify these concepts that they become widely applicable and at the same time consistent logically. Then, indeed, it may be time to immure them in definitions. The progress of science, however, demands a certain elasticity even in these definitions. The science of physics furnishes an excellent illustration of the way in which even those 'basal concepts' that are firmly established in the form of definitions are constantly being altered in their content.

A conventional but still rather obscure basal concept of this kind, which is nevertheless indispensable to us in psychology, is that of an *instinct*. Let us try to ascertain what is comprised in this conception by approaching it from different angles.

First, from the side of physiology. This has given us the concept of *stimuli* and the scheme of the reflex arc, according to which a stimulus applied *from the outer world* to living tissue (nervous substance) is discharged by action *towards the outer world*. The action answers the purpose of withdrawing the substance affected from the operation of the stimulus, removing it out of range of the stimulus.

Now what is the relation between 'instinct' and 'stimulus'? There is nothing to prevent our including the concept of 'instinct' under that of 'stimulus' and saying that an instinct is a stimulus to the mind. But we are immediately set on our guard against treating instinct and mental stimulus as one and the same thing. Obviously, besides those of intinctual origin, there are other stimuli to the mind which behave far more like physiological stimuli. For example, a strong light striking upon the eye is not a stimulus of instinctual origin; it is one, however, when the mucous membrane of the esophagus becomes

parched or when a gnawing makes itself felt in the stomach.[1]

We have now obtained material necessary for discriminating between stimuli of instinctual origin and the other (physiological) stimuli which operate on our minds. First, a stimulus of instinctual origin does not arise in the outside world but from within the organism itself. For this reason it has a different mental effect and different actions are necessary in order to remove it. Further, all that is essential in an external stimulus is contained in the assumption that it acts as a single impact, so that it can be discharged by a single appropriate action—a typical instance being that of motor flight from the source of stimulation. Of course these impacts may be repeated and their force may be cumulative, but that makes no difference to our notion of the process and to the conditions necessary in order that the stimulus may be dispelled. An instinct, on the other hand, never acts as a momentary impact but always as a constant force. As it makes its attack not from without but from within the organism, it follows that no flight can avail against it. A better term for a stimulus of instinctual origin is a 'need'; that which does away with this need is 'satisfaction'. This can be attained only by a suitable (adequate) alteration of the inner source of stimulation.

We thus find our first conception of the essential nature of an instinct by considering its main characteristics, its origin in sources of stimulation within the organism and its appearance as a constant force, and thence we deduce one of its further distinguishing features, namely, that no actions of flight avail against it. Now, in making these remarks, we cannot fail to be struck by a fact which compels us to a further admission. We do not merely accept as basal concepts certain conventions which we apply to the material we have acquired empirically, but we also make use of various complicated postulates to guide us in dealing with psychological phenomena. We have already cited the most important of these postulates; it remains for us expressly to lay stress upon it. It is of a biological nature, and makes use of the concept of 'purpose' (one might

---

[1]Assuming, of course, that these internal processes constitute the organic basis of the needs described as thirst and hunger.

say, of adaptation of the means to the end) and runs as follows: the nervous system is an apparatus having the function of abolishing stimuli which reach it, or of reducing excitation to the lowest possible level: an apparatus which would even, if this were feasible, maintain itself in an altogether unstimulated condition. Let us for the present not take exception to the indefiniteness of this idea and let us grant that the task of the nervous system is—broadly speaking—*to master stimuli*. We see then how greatly the simple physiological reflex scheme is complicated by the introduction of instincts. External stimuli impose upon the organism the single task of withdrawing itself from their action: this is accomplished by muscular movements, one of which reaches the goal aimed at and, being the most appropriate to the end in view, is thenceforward transmitted as an hereditary disposition. Those instinctual stimuli which emanate from within the organism cannot be dealt with by this mechanism. Consequently, they make far higher demands upon the nervous system and compel it to complicated and interdependent activities, which effect such changes in the outer world as enable it to offer satisfaction to the internal source of stimulation; above all, instinctual stimuli oblige the nervous system to renounce its ideal intention of warding off stimuli, for they maintain an incessant and unavoidable afflux of stimulation. So we may probably conclude that instincts and not external stimuli are the true motive forces in the progress that has raised the nervous system, with all its incomparable efficiency, to its present high level of development. Of course there is nothing to prevent our assuming that the instincts themselves are, at least in part, the precipitates of different forms of external stimulation, which in the course of phylogenesis have effected modifications in the organism.

If now we apply ourselves to considering mental life from a biological point of view, an 'instinct' appears to us as a borderland concept between the mental and the physical, being both the mental representative of the stimuli emanating from within the organism and penetrating to the mind, and at the same time a measure of the demand made upon the energy of the latter in consequence of its connection with the body.

We are now in a position to discuss certain terms used in reference to the concept of an instinct, for example, its impetus, its aim, its object and its source.

By the *impetus* of an instinct we understand its motor element, the amount of force or the measure of the demand upon energy which it represents. The characteristic of impulsion is common to all instincts, is in fact the very essence of them. Every instinct is a form of activity; if we speak loosely of passive instincts, we can only mean those whose aim is passive.

The *aim* of an instinct is in every instance satisfaction, which can only be obtained by abolishing the condition of stimulation in the source of the instinct. But although this remains invariably the final goal of every instinct, there may yet be different ways leading to the same goal, so that an instinct may be found to have various nearer or intermediate aims, capable of combination or interchange. Experience permits us also to speak of instincts which are *inhibited in respect of their aim,* in cases where a certain advance has been permitted in the direction of satisfaction and then an inhibition or deflection has occurred. We may suppose that even in such cases a partial satisfaction is achieved.

The *object* of an instinct is that in or through which it can achieve its aim. It is the most variable thing about an instinct and is not originally connected with it, but becomes attached to it only in consequence of being peculiarly fitted to provide satisfaction. The object is not necessarily an extraneous one: it may be part of the subject's own body. It may be changed any number of times in the course of the vicissitudes the instinct undergoes during life; a highly important part is played by this capacity for displacement in the instinct. It may happen that the same object may serve for the satisfaction of several instincts simultaneously, a phenomenon which Adler calls a 'confluence' of instincts. A particularly close attachment of the instinct to its object is distinguished by the term *fixation:* this frequently occurs in very early stages of the instinct's development and so puts an end to its mobility, through the vigorous resistance it sets up against detachment.

By the *source* of an instinct is meant that somatic process in an organ or part of the body from which there results a stimulus represented in mental life by an instinct. We do not know whether this process is regularly of a chemical nature or whether it may also correspond with the release of other, *e.g.* mechanical, forces. The study of the sources of instinct is outside the scope of psychology; although its source in the body is what gives the instinct its distinct and essential character, yet in mental life we know it merely by its aims. A more exact knowledge of the sources of instincts is not strictly necessary for purposes of psychological investigation; often the source may be with certainty inferred from the aims.

Now what instincts and how many should be postulated? There is obviously a great opportunity here for arbitrary choice. No objection can be made to anyone's employing the concept of an instinct of play or of destruction, or that of a social instinct, when the subject demands it and the limitations of psychological analysis allow of it. Nevertheless, we should not neglect to ask whether such instinctual motives, which are in one direction so highly specialized, do not admit of further analysis in respect of their sources, so that only those primal instincts which are not to be resolved further could really lay claim to the name.

I have proposed that two groups of such primal instincts should be distinguished: the *self-preservative* or *ego*-instincts and the *sexual* instincts. But this proposition has not the weight of a necessary postulate, such as, for instance, our assumption about the biological 'purpose' in the mental apparatus (*v. supra*); it is merely an auxiliary construction, to be retained only so long as it proves useful, and it will make little difference to the results of our work of description and classification if we replace it by another. The occasion for it arose in the course of the evolution of psychoanalysis, which was first employed upon the psychoneuroses, actually upon the group designated transference neuroses (hysteria and obsessional neurosis); through them it became plain that at the root of all such affections there lies a conflict between the claims of sexuality and those of the ego. It is always possible that an exhaustive study of the other neurotic affections (especially of the narcissistic psychoneuroses, the schizophrenias) may oblige us to alter this formula and therewith to make a different classification of the primal instincts. But for the present we do not know what this new formula may be, nor have we met with any argument which seems likely to be prejudicial to the contrast between sexual and ego-instincts.

An attempt to formulate the general characteristics of the sexual instincts would run as follows: they are numerous, emanate from manifold organic sources, act in the first instance independently of one another and only at a late stage achieve a more or less complete synthesis. The aim which each strives to attain is 'organ-pleasure'; only when the synthesis is complete do they enter the service of the function of reproduction, becoming thereby generally recognizable as sexual instincts. At their first appearance they support themselves upon the instincts of self-preservation, from which they only gradually detach themselves; in their choice of object also they follow paths indicated by the ego-instincts. Some of them remain throughout life associated with these latter and furnish them with libidinal components, which with normal functioning easily escape notice and are clearly recognizable only when disease is present. They have this distinctive characteristic —that they have in a high degree the capacity to act vicariously for one another and that they can readily change their objects. In consequence of the last-mentioned properties they are capable of activities widely removed from their original modes of attaining their aims (sublimation).

Our inquiry into the various vicissitudes which instincts undergo in the process of development and in the course of life must be confined to the sexual instincts, for these are the more familiar to us. Observation shows us that an instinct may undergo the following vicissitudes:

Reversal into its opposite,
Turning round upon the subject,
Repression,
Sublimation.

Since I do not intend to treat of sublimation here and since repression requires a special chapter to itself, it only remains for us to describe and discuss the two first points. Bearing in mind that there are tendencies which are opposed to the instincts pursuing a straightforward course, we may regard these vicissitudes as modes of defence against the instincts.

The *reversal* of an instinct *into its op-*

posite may on closer scrutiny be resolved into two different processes: a change from active to passive, and a reversal of the content. The two processes, being essentially distinct, must be treated separately.

Examples of the first process are met with in the two pairs of opposites: sadism-masochism and scoptophilia-exhibitionism. The reversal here concerns only the aims of the instincts. The passive aim (to be tortured, or looked at) has been substituted for the active aim (to torture, to look at). Reversal of content is found in the single instance of the change of love into hate.

The *turning round* of an instinct *upon the subject* is suggested to us by the reflection that masochism is actually sadism turned round upon the subject's own ego, and that exhibitionism includes the love of gazing at the subject's own body. Further, analytic observation leaves us in no doubt that the masochist also enjoys the *act* of torturing when this is being applied to himself, and the exhibitionist the exposing of someone in being exposed himself. So the essence of the process is the change of the object, while the aim remains unchanged.

The fact that, at that later period of development, the instinct in its primary form may be observed side by side with its (passive) opposite deserves to be distinguished by the highly appropriate name introduced by Bleuler: *ambivalence*.

These considerations regarding the developmental history of an instinct and the permanent character of the intermediate stages in it should make instinct-development more comprehensible to us. Experience shows that the degree of demonstrable ambivalence varies greatly in individuals, groups and races. Marked ambivalence of an instinct in a human being at the present day may be regarded as an archaic inheritance, for we have reason to suppose that the part played in the life of the instincts by the active impulses in their original form was greater in primitive times than it is on an average to-day.

The transformation of the 'content' of an instinct into its opposite is observed in a single instance only—the changing of *love into hate*. It is particularly common to find both these directed simultaneously towards the same object, and this phenomenon of their co-existence furnishes the most important example of ambivalence of feeling.

The case of love and hate acquires a special interest from the circumstance that it resists classification in our scheme of the instincts. It is impossible to doubt the existence of a most intimate relation between these two contrary feelings and sexual life, but one is naturally unwilling to conceive of love as being a kind of special component-instinct of sexuality in the same way as are the others just discussed. One would prefer to regard loving rather as the expression of the whole sexual current of feeling, but this idea does not clear up our difficulties and we are at a loss how to conceive of an essential opposite to this striving.

Loving admits of not merely one, but of three antitheses. First there is the antithesis of loving—hating; secondly, there is loving—being loved; and, in addition to these, loving and hating together are the opposite of the condition of neutrality or indifference. The second of these two antitheses, loving—being loved, corresponds exactly to the transformation from active to passive and may be traced to a primal situation in the same way as the scoptophilic instinct. This situation is that of *loving oneself,* which for us is the characteristic of narcissism. Then, according to whether the self as object or subject is exchanged for an extraneous one, there results the active aim of loving or the passive one of being loved, the latter remaining nearly related to narcissism.

Perhaps we shall come to a better understanding of the manifold opposites of loving if we reflect that our mental life as a whole is governed by *three polarities,* namely, the following antitheses:

Subject (ego)—Object (external world),
Pleasure—Pain,
Active—Passive.

The antithesis of ego—non-ego (outer), *i.e.* subject—object, is, as we have already said, thrust upon the individual being at an early stage, by the experience that it can abolish external stimuli by means of muscular action but is defenceless against those stimuli that originate in instinct. This antithesis remains sovereign above all in our intellectual activity and provides research with a fundamental situation which no amount of effort can alter. The polarity of pleasure—pain depends upon a feeling-series, the significance of which in determining our actions (will) is paramount and has already been emphasized. The antithesis of active and passive must not be confounded with that of ego-subject—external object. The relation of the ego to the outer world is passive in so far as it receives stimuli from it, active when it reacts to these. Its instincts compel it to a quite special degree of activity towards the outside world, so that, if we wished to emphasize the essence of the matter, we might say that the ego-subject is passive in respect of external stimuli, active in virtue of its own instincts. The antithesis of active—passive coalesces later with that of masculine—feminine, which, until this has taken place, has no psychological significance. The fusion of activity with masculinity and passivity with femininity confronts us, indeed, as a biological fact, but it is by no means so invariably complete and exclusive as we are inclined to assume.

II: REPRESSION

One of the vicissitudes an instinctual impulse may undergo is to meet with resistances the aim of which is to make the impulse inoperative. Under certain conditions, which we shall presently investigate more closely, the impulse then passes into the state of *repression*. If it were a question of the operation of an external stimulus, obviously flight would be the appropriate remedy; with an instinct, flight is of no avail, for the ego cannot escape from itself. Later on, rejection based on judgement (*condemnation*) will be found to be a good weapon against the impulse. Repression is a preliminary phase of condemnation, something between flight and condemnation; it is a concept which could not have been formulated before the time of psycho-analytic research.

It is not easy in theory to deduce the possibility of such a thing as repression. Why should an instinctual impulse suffer such a fate? For this to happen, obviously a necessary condition must be that attainment of its aim by the instinct should produce 'pain' instead of pleasure. But we cannot well imagine such a contingency. There are no such instincts; satisfaction of an instinct is always pleasurable. We should have to assume certain peculiar circumstances, some sort of process which changes the pleasure of satisfaction into 'pain'.

In order the better to define repression we may discuss some other situations in which instincts are concerned. It may happen that an external stimulus becomes internal, for example, by eating into and destroying a bodily organ, so that a new source of constant excitation and increase of tension is formed. The stimulus thereby acquires a far-reaching similarity to an instinct. We know that a case of this sort is experienced by us as *physical pain*. The aim of this pseudo-instinct, however, is simply the cessation of the change in the organ and of the pain accompanying it. There is no other direct pleasure to be attained by cessation of the pain. Further, pain is imperative; the only things which can subdue it are the effect of some toxic agent in removing it and the influence of some mental distraction.

The case of physical pain is too obscure to help us much in our purpose. Let us suppose that an instinctual stimulus such as hunger remains unsatisfied. It then becomes imperative and can be allayed by nothing but the appropriate action for satisfying it; it keeps up a constant tension of need. Anything like a repression seems in this case to be utterly out of the question.

So repression is certainly not an essential result of the tension produced by lack of satisfaction of an impulse being raised to an unbearable degree. The weapons of defence of which the organism avails itself to guard against that situation must be discussed in another connection.

Let us instead confine ourselves to the clinical experience we meet with in the practice of psychoanalysis. We then see that the satisfaction of an instinct under repression is quite possible; further, that in every instance such a satisfaction is pleasurable in itself, but is irreconcilable with other claims and purposes; it therefore causes pleasure in one part of the mind and 'pain' in another. We see then that it is a condition of repression that the element of avoiding 'pain' shall have acquired more strength than the pleasure of gratification. Psycho-analytic experience of the transference neuroses, moreover, forces us to the conclusion that repression is not a defence-mechanism present from the very beginning, and that it cannot occur until a sharp distinction has been established between what is conscious and what is unconscious: that *the essence of repression lies simply in the function of rejecting and keeping something out of consciousness*. This conception of repression would be supplemented by assuming that, before the mental organization reaches this phase, the other vicissitudes which may befall instincts, *e.g.* reversal into the opposite or turning round upon the subject, deal with the task of mastering the instinctual impulses.

It seems to us now that in view of the very great extent to which repression and the unconscious are correlated, we must defer probing more deeply into the nature of repression until we have learnt more about the structure of the various institutions in the mind—and about what differentiates consciousness from the unconscious. Till we have done this, all we can do is to put together in purely descriptive fashion some characteristics of repression noted in clinical practice, even though we run the risk of having to repeat unchanged much that has been said elsewhere.

Psycho-analysis is able to show us something else which is important for understanding the effects of repression in the psychoneuroses. It shows us, for instance, that the instinct-presentation develops in a more unchecked and luxuriant fashion if it is withdrawn by repression from conscious influence. It ramifies like a fungus, so to speak, in the dark and takes on extreme forms of expression, which when translated and revealed to the neurotic are bound not merely to seem alien to him, but to terrify him by the way in which they reflect an extraordinary and dangerous strength of instinct. This illusory strength of instinct is the result of an uninhibited development of it in phantasy and of the damming-up consequent on lack of real satisfaction. The fact that this last result is bound up with repression points the direction in which we have to look for the true significance of the latter.

In reverting to the contrary aspect, however, let us state definitely that it is not even correct to suppose that repression withholds from consciousness all the derivatives of what was primally repressed. If these derivatives are sufficiently far removed from the repressed instinct-presentation, whether owing to the process of distortion or by reason of the number of intermediate associations, they have free access to consciousness. It is as though the resistance of consciousness against them was in inverse proportion to their remoteness from what was originally repressed. During the practice of the psycho-analytic method, we continually require the patient to produce such derivatives of what has been repressed as, in consequence either of their remoteness or of distortion, can pass the censorship of consciousness. Indeed, the associations which we require him to give, while refraining from any consciously directed train of thought or any criticism, and from which we reconstruct a conscious interpretation of the repressed instinct-presentation, are precisely derivatives of this kind. We then observe that the patient can go on spinning a whole chain of such associations, till he is brought up in the midst of them against some thought-formation, the relation of which to what is repressed acts so intensely that he is compelled to repeat this attempt at repression. Neurotic symptoms, too, must have fulfilled the condition referred to, for they are derivatives of the repressed, which has finally by means of these formations wrested from consciousness the right of way previously denied it.

We can lay down no general rule concerning the degree of distortion and remoteness necessary before the resistance of consciousness is abrogated. In this matter a delicate balancing takes place, the play of which is hidden from us; its mode of operation, however, leads us to infer that it is a question of a definite degree of intensity in the cathexis of the unconscious—beyond which it would break through for satisfaction. Repression acts, therefore, in a *highly specific* manner in each instance; every single derivative of the repressed may have its peculiar fate—a little more or a little less distortion alters the whole issue. In this connection it becomes comprehensible that those objects to which men give their preference, that is, their ideals, originate in the same perceptions and experiences as those objects of which they have most abhorrence, and that the two originally differed from one another only by slight modifications. Indeed, as we found in the origin of the fetish, it is possible for the original instinct-presentation to be split into two, one part undergoing repression, while the remainder, just on account of its intimate association with the other, undergoes idealization.

The same result as ensues from an increase or a decrease in the degree of distortion may also be achieved at the other end of the apparatus, so to speak, by a modification in the conditions producing pleasure and 'pain.' Special devices have been evolved, with the object of bringing about such changes in the play of mental forces that what usually gives rise to 'pain' may on this occasion result in pleasure, and whenever such a device comes into operation the repression of an instinct-presentation that is ordinarily repudiated is abrogated. The only one of these devices which has till now been studied in any detail is that of joking. Generally the lifting of the repression is only transitory; the repression is immediately re-established.

Observations of this sort, however, suffice to draw our attention to some further characteristics of repression. Not only is it, as we have just explained, *variable* and *specific*, but it is also exceedingly *mobile*. The process of repression is not to be regarded as something which takes place once for all, the results of which are permanent, as when some living thing has been killed and from that time onward is dead; on the contrary, repression demands a constant expenditure of energy, and if this were discontinued the success of the repression would be jeopardized, so that a fresh act of repression would be necessary. We may imagine that what is repressed exercises a continuous straining in the direction of consciousness, so that the balance has to be kept by means of a steady counter-pressure. A constant expenditure of energy, therefore, is entailed in maintaining a repression, and economically its abrogation denotes a saving. The mobility of the repression, incidentally, finds expression also in the mental characteristics of the condition of sleep which alone renders dream-formation possible. With a return to waking life the repressive cathexes which have been called in are once more put forth.

Finally, we must not forget that after all we have said very little about an instinctual impulse when we state it to be repressed. Without prejudice to the repression such an impulse may find itself in widely different conditions; it may be inactive, *i.e.* cathected with only a low degree of mental energy, or its degree of cathexis (and consequently its capacity for activity) may vary. True, its activity will not result in a direct abrogation of the repression, but it will certainly set in motion all the processes which terminate in a breaking through into consciousness by circuitous routes. With unrepressed derivatives of the unconscious the fate of a particular idea is often decided by the degree of its activity or cathexis. It is an everyday occurrence that such a derivative can remain unrepressed so long as it represents only a small amount of energy, although its content is of such a nature as to give rise to a conflict with conscious control. But the quantitative factor is manifestly decisive for this conflict; as soon as an idea which is fundamentally offensive exceeds a certain degree of strength, the conflict takes on actuality, and it is precisely activation of the idea that leads to its repression. So that, where repression is concerned, an increase in energic cathexis operates in the same way as an approach to the unconscious, while a decrease in that energy operates like distance from the unconscious or like distortion. We understand that the repressing tendencies can find a substitute for repression in a weakening or lessening of whatever is distasteful to them.

We now wish to gain some insight into the mechanism of the process of repression, and especially we want to know whether it has a single mechanism only, or more than one, and whether perhaps each of the psycho-neuroses may be distinguished by a characteristic repression-mechanism peculiar to itself. At the outset of this inquiry, however, we encounter complications. The mechanism of a repression becomes accessible to us only when we deduce it from its final results. If we confine our observations to the results of its effect on the ideational part of the instinct-presentation, we discover that as a rule repression creates a *substitute-formation*. What then is the mechanism of such a substitute-formation, or must we distinguish several mechanisms here also? Further, we know that repression leaves *symptoms* in its train. May we then regard substitute-formation and symptom-formation as coincident processes, and, if this is on the whole possible, does the mechanism of substitute-formation coincide with that of repression? So far as we know at present, it seems probable that the two are widely divergent, that it is not the repression itself which produces substitute-formations and symptoms, but that these latter constitute indications of a *return of the repressed* and owe their existence to quite other processes. It would also seem advisable to examine the mechanisms of substitute and symptom-formation before those of repression.

Obviously there is no ground here for speculation to explore: on the contrary, the solution of the problem must be found by careful analysis of the results of repression observable in the individual neuroses. I must, however, suggest that we should postpone this task, too, until we have formed reliable conceptions of the relation of consciousness to the unconscious.

III: THE UNCONSCIOUS

Psycho-analysis has taught us that the essence of the process of repression lies, not in abrogating or annihilating the ideational presentation of an instinct, but in withholding it from becoming conscious. We then say of the idea that it is in a state of 'unconsciousness,' of being not apprehended by the conscious mind, and we can produce convincing proofs to show that unconsciously it can also produce effects, even of a kind that finally penetrate to consciousness. Everything that is repressed . must remain unconscious, but at the very outset let us state that the repressed does not comprise the whole unconscious. The unconscious has the greater compass: the repressed is a part of the unconscious.

How are we to arrive at a knowledge of the unconscious? It is of course only as something conscious that we know anything of it, after it has undergone transformation or translation into something conscious. The possibility of such translation is a matter of everyday experience in psycho-analytic work. In order to achieve this, it is necessary that the person analysed should overcome certain resistances, the very same as those which at some earlier time placed the material in question under repression by rejecting it from consciousness.

In many quarters our justification is disputed for assuming the existence of an unconscious system in the mind and for employing such an assumption for purposes of scientific work. To this we can reply that our assumption of the existence of the unconscious is *necessary* and *legitimate,* and that we possess manifold *proofs* of the existence of the unconscious. It is necessary because the data of consciousness are exceedingly defective; both in healthy and in sick persons mental acts are often in process which can be explained only by presupposing other acts, of which consciousness yields no evidence. These include not only the parapraxes[2] and dreams of healthy persons, and everything designated a mental symptom or an obsession in the sick; our most intimate daily experience introduces us to sudden ideas of the source of which we are ignorant, and to results of mentation arrived at we know not how. All these conscious acts remain disconnected and unintelligible if we are determined to hold fast to the claim that every single mental act performed within us must be consciously experienced; on the other hand, they fall into a demonstrable connection if we interpolate the unconscious acts that we infer. A gain in meaning and connection, however, is a perfectly justifiable motive, one which may well carry us beyond the limitations of direct experience. When, after this, it appears that the assumption of the unconscious helps us to construct a highly successful practical method, by which we are enabled to exert a useful influence upon the course of conscious processes, this success will have won us an incontrovertible proof of the existence of that which we assumed. We become obliged then to take up the position that it is both untenable and presumptuous to claim that whatever goes on in the mind must be known to consciousness.

We can go further and in support of an unconscious mental state allege that only a small content is embraced by consciousness at any given moment, so that the greater part of what we call conscious knowledge must in any case exist for very considerable periods of time in a condition of latency, that is to say, of unconsciousness, of not being apprehended by the mind. When all our latent memories are taken into consideration it becomes totally incomprehensible how the existence

---

[2] *e.g.,* slips of the tongue, mislaying of objects, etc. — TRANS.

of the unconscious can be gainsaid. We then encounter the objection that these latent recollections can no longer be described as mental processes, but that they correspond to residues of somatic processes from which something mental can once more proceed. The obvious answer to this should be that a latent memory is, on the contrary, indubitably a residuum of a mental process. But it is more important to make clear to our minds that this objection is based on the identification—not, it is true, explicitly stated but regarded as axiomatic—of conscious and mental. This identification is either a *petitio principii* and begs the question whether all that is mental is also necessarily conscious, or else it is a matter of convention, of nomenclature. In this latter case it is of course no more open to refutation than any other convention. The only question that remains is whether it proves so useful that we must needs adopt it. To this we may reply that the conventional identification of the mental with the conscious is thoroughly unpractical. It breaks up all mental continuity, plunges us into the insoluble difficulties of psychophysical parallelism, is open to the reproach that without any manifest grounds it overestimates the part played by consciousness, and finally it forces us prematurely to retire from the territory of psychological research without being able to offer us any compensation elsewhere.

At any rate it is clear that the question—whether the latent states of mental life, whose existence is undeniable, are to be conceived of as unconscious mental states or as physical ones—threatens to resolve itself into a war of words. We shall therefore be better advised to give prominence to what we know with certainty of the nature of these debatable states. Now, as far as their physical characteristics are concerned, they are totally inaccessible to us; no physiological conception nor chemical process can give us any notion of their nature. On the other hand, we know for certain that they have abundant points of contact with conscious mental processes; on being submitted to a certain method of operation they may be transformed into or replaced by conscious processes, and all the categories which we employ to describe conscious mental acts, such as ideas, purposes, resolutions and so forth, can be applied to them. Indeed, of many of these latent states we have to assert that the only point in which they differ from states which are conscious is just in the lack of consciousness of them. So we shall not hesitate to treat them as objects of psychological research, and that in the most intimate connection with conscious mental acts.

The stubborn denial of a mental quality to latent mental processes may be accounted for by the circumstance that most of the phenomena in question have not been objects of study outside psychoanalysis. Anyone who is ignorant of the facts of pathology, who regards the blunders of normal persons as accidental, and who is content with the old saw that dreams are froth[3] need only ignore a few more problems of the psychology of consciousness in order to dispense with the assumption of an unconscious mental activity. As it happens, hypnotic experiments, and especially post-hypnotic suggestion, had demonstrated tangibly even before the time of psycho-analysis the existence and mode of operation of the unconscious in the mind.

The assumption of an unconscious is, moreover, in a further respect a perfectly *legitimate* one, inasmuch as in postulating it we do not depart a single step from our customary and accepted mode of thinking. By the medium of consciousness each one of us becomes aware only of his own states of mind; that another man possesses consciousness is a conclusion drawn by analogy from the utterances and actions we perceive him to make, and it is drawn in order that this behaviour of his may become intelligible to us. (It would probably be psychologically more correct to put it thus: that without any special reflection we impute to everyone else our own constitution and therefore also our consciousness, and that this identification is a necessary condition of understanding in us.) This conclusion—or identification—was formerly extended by the ego to other human beings, to animals, plants, inanimate matter and to the world at large, and proved useful as long as the correspondence with the individual ego was overwhelmingly great; but it became more untrustworthy in proportion as the gulf between the ego and the non-ego widened. To-day, our judgment is already

---

[3][·Träume sind Schäume.·]

in doubt on the question of consciousness in animals; we refuse to admit it in plants and we relegate to mysticism the assumption of its existence in inanimate matter. But even where the original tendency to identification has withstood criticism —that is, when the non-ego is our fellowman—the assumption of a consciousness in him rests upon an inference and cannot share the direct certainty we have of our own consciousness.

Now psycho-analysis demands nothing more than that we should apply this method of inference to ourselves also—a proceeding to which, it is true, we are not constitutionally disposed. If we do this, we must say that all the acts and manifestations which I notice in myself and do not know how to link up with the rest of my mental life must be judged as if they belonged to someone else and are to be explained by the mental life ascribed to that person. Further, experience shows that we understand very well how to interpret in others (*i.e.* how to fit into their mental context) those same acts which we refuse to acknowledge as mentally conditioned in ourselves. Some special hindrance evidently deflects our investigations from ourselves and interferes with our obtaining true knowledge of ourselves.

Now this method of inference, applied to oneself in spite of inner opposition, does not lead to the discovery of an unconscious, but leads logically to the assumption of another, second consciousness which is united in myself with the consciousness I know. But at this point criticism may fairly make certain comments. In the first place, a consciousness of which its own possessor knows nothing is something very different from that of another person and it is questionable whether such a consciousness, lacking, as it does, its most important characteristic, is worthy of any further discussion at all. Those who have

contested the assumption of an unconscious system in the mind will not be content to accept in its place an unconscious consciousness. Secondly, analysis shows that the individual latent mental processes inferred by us enjoy a high degree of independence, as though each had no connection with another, and knew nothing about any other. We must be prepared, it would appear, to assume the existence not only of a second consciousness in us, but of a third and fourth also, perhaps of an infinite series of states of consciousness, each and all unknown to us and to one another. In the third place—and this is the most weighty argument of all—we have to take into account that analytic investigation reveals some of these latent processes as having characteristics and peculiarities which seem alien to us, or even incredible, and running directly counter to the well-known attributes of consciousness. This justifies us in modifying our inference about ourselves and saying that what is proved is not a second consciousness in us, but the existence of certain mental operations lacking in the quality of consciousness. We shall also, moreover, be right in rejecting the term 'subconsciousness' as incorrect and misleading. The known cases of *'double conscience'* (splitting of consciousness) prove nothing against our view. They may most accurately be described as cases of a splitting of the mental activities into two groups, whereby a single consciousness takes up its position alternately with either the one or the other of these groups.

In psycho-analysis there is no choice for us but to declare mental processes to be in themselves unconscious, and to compare the perception of them by consciousness with the perception of the outside world through the sense-organs; we even hope to extract some fresh knowledge from the comparison.

12. Psychoanalysis as a Scientific Theory

HEINZ HARTMANN

When some forty-five years ago Freud (12) wrote for the first time about the philosophical interests in analysis, his main point was that philosophy could not avoid taking fully into account what he then called "the hypothesis of unconscious mental activities." He also mentioned that philosophers may be interested in the interpretation of philosphical thought in terms of psychoanalysis —adding, though, here as elsewhere, that the fact that a theory or doctrine is determined by psychological processes of many kinds does not necessarily invalidate its scientific truth. Since then, the knowledge of human behavior and motivation we owe to analysis has greatly increased, has become much more comprehensive but also more specific; and this development has certainly influenced not only social science, anthropology, and medicine, but also philosophy in a broad sense. This does not, though, necessarily mean that analysis can "answer" what one usually calls philosophical problems; it usually means that it leads to looking at them from a new angle. Some of its potentialities in this respect have been made use of only rather scantily so far. I am thinking, for example, of its possible contribution toward a better understanding of ethical problems. The interest psychoanalysis may have for philosophers has clearly two aspects: it resides partly in the new psychological findings and theories of analysis, but also in certain questions of methodology raised by Freud's and other psychoanalysts' approach to the study of man.

In speaking of psychoanalysis one often refers to a therapeutic technique. One may also refer to a method of psychological investigation whose main aspects are free association and interpretation; or, finally, to a body of facts and theories (Freud, 13). In this last sense, we would certainly consider as psychoanalytical any knowledge gained directly by Freud's method of investigation; but many of us would today consider analysis to include related procedures such as the application of psychoanalytic insights to data of direct child observation, a field which has grown in importance in the last two decades. Of the three aspects just mentioned, it is the method of exploration that has undergone the least change; it is commonly used in a situation defined by a certain set of rules and referred to as the psychoanalytic situation or the psychoanalytic interview. The therapeutic technique has been repeatedly modified, and psychoanalytic theory has gone through a series of more or less radical modifications, by Freud and by others. I want to emphasize that the interrelations among these three aspects are, in analysis, a central topic—though in the context of this presentation I can refer to them only occasionally.

The theories of psychoanalysis follow principles of systematization, as do theories in other fields. Freud, however, did not speak of analysis as a "system," but rather accentuated its unfinished character, its flexibility, and the tentative nature of a considerable part of it. Actually, adjustments and reformulations of various aspects of theory have repeatedly become necessary. There are chapters such as the psychology of the dream, of libidinal development, of anxiety, and of symptom formation, that have been more systematically worked out than others. Psychoanalysis is obviously far from being a closed system of doctrines, though it has sometimes been represented as such. Also, though some fundamental tenets of psychoanalysis are accepted by all (Freudian) analysts, agreement on all of them is obviously lacking.

There is in analysis a hierarchy of hypotheses as to their closeness to observation, their generality, and the degree to which they have been confirmed. It appears that a neater classification as to these points and a higher degree of systematization (considering the different levels of theorizing) than exist today would not only facilitate my task in discussing psycho-analysis as a scientific theory but also clarify the standing of

Abridged from *Psychoanalysis, Scientific Method and Philosophy* edited by Sidney Hook, pages 3–35, New York University Press, 1959, by permission of the publisher and the author.

analysis as a scientific discipline. Promising efforts in this direction have been made and are being made by analysts and also by nonanalysts, but as yet no complete and systematical outline drawn from this angle is available; a recent work by David Rapaport (30), soon to be published, may come close to performing this task. This is probably the reason, or one of the reasons, that in more or less general presentations of psychoanalysis references to its history abound, and the reader will forgive me if they do in this paper too, at least in its first part. I shall mostly refer to the work of Freud, because most of the more general theories of analysis have their origin in it, and because he is in many ways more representative of psychoanalytic thinking than anybody else.

Often historical explanations are substituted for system; an attempt is made to clarify the function of propositions in their relation to others by tracing their place in the development of analysis. Also, without such historical reference it happens over and over again that analytical hypotheses are dealt with on one level, so to say, which belong to different phases of theory formation, and some of which have actually been discarded and replaced by others. Again, because of the comparatively low level of systematization, I think it is true that even today a thorough knowledge of at least some chapters of analytic theory cannot be acquired without knowledge of its history (Hartmann, 16).

From the beginning, explanations of human behavior in terms of propositions about unconscious mental processes have been an essential part and one characteristic feature of psychoanalysis. I may, then, start by introducing Freud's concepts of unconscious processes. He makes a distinction between two forms of unconscious mental activity. The one, called preconscious, functions more or less as conscious activities do. It is not conscious, in a descriptive sense, but can become conscious without having to overcome powerful counterforces. Where such overcoming of resistances is necessary, as is the case with repressed material, we speak of unconscious processes in the stricter, the dynamic, sense of the word. The dynamic impact of these latter unconscious processes on human behavior —and not only in the case of mental

disease—is one main tenet of Freud's theory of unconscious mental activities.

There is rather wide agreement that conscious data are insufficient for the explanation of a considerable part of behavior, and particularly of those aspects that were first studied in analysis. However, its critics have repeatedly claimed that the introduction of unconscious processes is superfluous. The explanation needed could be stated, or should be sought for, in terms of the more reliable data of brain physiology. The question here is not just whether, and why, explanations based on such data would be per se more reliable, nor why psychological hypotheses about mental processes ought not to be introduced in explaining human behavior. We have also to consider the fact that, given the actual state of brain physiology, many and even comparatively simple aspects of behavior of the kind we are dealing with in analysis cannot be explained. To rely on brain physiology alone would mean to renounce explanation of the greatest part of the field that psychoanalysis has set out to explain. Or, if one should insist on attempting an explanation on physiological grounds, the resultant hypotheses would of necessity be considerably more tenuous and more speculative even than psychoanalytic hypotheses are suspected to be by its critics today.

Freud, well trained in the anatomy and physiology of the brain, actually started out by attempting to devise a physiological psychology that could provide him with concepts and hypotheses to account for his clinical insights. But beyond a certain point this approach proved of no use. He was thus led to replace it by a set of psychological hypotheses and constructs; and this step represents probably the most important turning point in the history of psychoanalysis. It was the beginning in analysis of psychological theory, the heuristic value of which he found to be greatly superior—a point that, I think, has been corroborated by its subsequent development.

But it is true that even after this radical turn in his approach Freud held on to the expectation, shared by many analysts, that one day the development of brain physiology would make it possible to base psychoanalysis on its findings and theories. He did not think this would happen during his lifetime, in which he proved to be right. In the meantime certain, though limited, parallels between analytic propositions and discoveries in the physiology of the brain have become apparent. Also, the usefulness of some psychoanalytic hypotheses for their field has been recognized by a least some representatives of brain research (Adrian, 1). As to the psychology of unconscious processes, I think it can be said that Freud in developing that part of analysis was much less interested in the ultimate "nature" or "essence" of such processes—whatever this may mean—than in finding a suitable conceptual framework for the phenomena he had discovered.

While Freud, after the first years of his scientific work, relinquished the attempt to account for his findings in terms of physiology, it is nevertheless characteristic of some of his psychoanalytic theorizing that he used physiological models. He was guided by the trend in German physiology which has been designated as the physicalist school (Bernfeld, 5), whose representatives were, among others, Helmholtz and Bruecke, the latter being one of Freud's teachers. Certain aspects of the psychology of neurosis, for example, led him to introduce into psychoanalysis the concept of regression (to earlier stages of development), which had been used in the physiology of his day; this concept, though, acquired new meaning in the context in which he used it. Also, in making "function" the criterion for defining what he called the mental systems (ego, id, superego), Freud used physiology as a model. But this no longer implies any correlation to any specific physiological organization (Hartmann, Kris, Loewenstein, 21). The value of such borrowings or analogies has, of course, to be determined in every single instance by confronting their application with tested knowledge (data and hypotheses). Physiological models (also occasionally physical models, as is obvious, for instance, in Freud's concept of a "mental apparatus") have been used also by other psychoanalysts (see Kubie in a recent lecture) in order to illustrate certain characteristics of mental phenomena or to suggest a new hypothesis. The use even of metaphors need not of necessity lead into muddled thinking once their place in theory has been clearly delineated. The

danger that earlier implications of those model concepts might impair their fruitful use in the new context of psychoanalysis has on the whole been successfully avoided (Hartmann-Kris-Loewenstein).

The broadening of the scope of psychology that came about as the consequence of the inclusion of propositions about unconscious mental processes meant, first of all, that many aspects of a person's life history that had never been explained before—and that, as a matter of fact, one had not even tried to explain—could be accounted for in terms of the individual's experience and dispositions. Causation in the field of personality is traceable only at its fringes without this broadening of theory. Freud was a strict determinist and often stated that to fill that gap in earlier psychological approaches, partly because of which the study of personality had been unsatisfactory, was one of his primary aims in developing analytic theory. More recently it has been said, by the mathematician von Mises (29), that the observations correspond rather to statistical than to causal relations. I may mention at this point that this interest in the causation of mental phenomena included, quite naturally, also the interest in what we call the genetic viewpoint, since Freud's attention had been drawn to many facts of early childhood which had been unknown, and regularities in the relationships between early childhood situations and the behavior of the adult had become apparent. With Freud, the investigation of highly complex series of experience and behavior, extending over long periods of time, soon moved into the center of interest. Developmental research was to become equally important for psychoanalytic theory and practice. It is significant that the reconstructive approach in analysis led not only to the discovery of a great wealth of childhood material in every individual case, but also to the ascertainment of typical sequences of developmental phases. The genetic approach has become so pervasive, not only in psychopathology but also in psychoanalytic psychology in general, that in analysis phenomena are often grouped together, not according to their descriptive similarities but as belonging together if they have a common genetic root (oral character, anal character). It was only much later that this predominance of a genetic conceptualization was counterbalanced by a sharper distinction between genesis and function, to which I shall shortly return in speaking of the structural point of view.

Here I want to add that while I just spoke of the study of the individual's "life history," it would be misleading (though it actually has been done) to classify this aspect of analysis as an historical discipline. This misinterpretation may be traceable to its comparison with archaeology, which Freud occasionally uses. It is true that most analytical knowledge has been gained in the psychoanalytic interview and that the concern with developmental problems refers primarily to the history of individuals. But this should not obfuscate the fact that the aim of these studies is (besides its therapeutic purpose) to develop lawlike propositions which then, of course, transcend individual observations.

At this point I should like briefly to summarize the role of psychoanalysis as a psychology of motivation, bearing in mind that nowadays psychoanalysis takes into consideration the interaction of the individual with his environment, as well as his so-called "inner-psychic" processes. The study of these psychic processes constitutes what, in analysis, we call "metapsychology," a term that signifies not (as it might seem) that which is beyond psychology altogether, but simply those psychological investigations that are not limited to conscious phenomena, and that formulate the most general assumptions of analysis on the most abstract level of theory. Metapsychology is concerned with the substructures of personality, with the ego, the id, and the superego which are defined as units of functions. The id refers to the instinctual aspect, the ego to the reality principle and to the "centralization of functional control" (to borrow a term from brain physiology). The superego has its biological roots in the long dependency on the parents and in the helplessness of the human child; it develops out of identification with the parents; and it accounts for the fact that moral conflict and guilt feelings become a natural and fundamental aspect of human behavior. The theoretical and clinical advantage of the structural formulations, referring to the distinction of ego, id, superego, has several reasons. The most important is probably that the de-

marcation lines of the three systems, ego, id, superego are geared to the typical conflicts of man: conflicts with the instinctual drives, with moral conscience, and with the outside world. The paramount importance on neurotic *and* normal development of these conflicts, and of the ways to solve them, was one of the earliest discoveries of Freud and has remained central in psychoanalytic practice and theory ever since.

Critics of analysis often tend to underrate the wealth of individual data on which it is built. But on the other hand, it also happens that the theoretical nature of concepts like libido is not fully realized; for example, libido is often identified with sexual experience, or as a mere generalization of some observable connections.

In the beginnings of psychoanalysis (even after the importance of unconscious processes had been realized), Freud still adhered more or less strictly to associationism. But when he found conflict to be a primary motivating force of behavior, and specifically an important etiological agent in neurosis, he gradually developed the concept of mental tendencies and purposive ideas. Psychoanalysis became a psychology of motivation, the motives being partly, but not generally, considered in analogy with those consciously experienced. There originated the idea of wishes, in certain circumstances, warded off by defensive techniques. He discovered the role of repression and later of other defense mechanisms, like projection, isolation, undoing, and so on. The consideration of mental processes from this angle of synergistic or antagonistic motivating forces is what has been known since as the dynamic aspect of psychoanalysis. The systematic and objective study of conflict has remained one of its essential aspects and has proved a necessary and fruitful avenue to the explanation of human behavior. This was a second bold step in the development of psychoanalysis. The importance of "conflict" had, of course, been known in religious and philosophical doctrines and in literature, but scientific psychology before Freud had had no means to approach the subject.

The dynamic factors involved in both sides of a conflict were, for some time, rather poorly defined. It was, then, again primarily data of analytical observation that led to the realization of the dominance of the instinctual drives among the motivating forces. I am referring here to Freud's discovery of infantile sexuality. This discovery was, at the time, considered by many as the product of revolting imagination; today, it can easily be confirmed in every nursery.

Even at the period when instinctual motivation seemed to be pretty much ubiquitous, the basic fact of conflict was not overlooked. Self-preservative instinctual drives were, at the time, thought of as the opponents of sexuality. Besides this, the concept of overdetermination, referring to the multiple motivation of all human behavior, continued also through the phase in which motivation was, on the level of general theory, nearly always considered instinctual.

Again, to fit it to his field of observation Freud has to modify the concept of "instinct" commonly used in other fields. His term, in German, *Trieb,* in English, "instinctual drive," or "drive," is certainly not identical with what one refers to in speaking of the instincts of lower animals. His concept of drives had to prove its usefulness with respect to human psychology. Here, the sources of the drives are of much less importance than their aims and their objects. The lesser rigidity of the human drives, the comparatively easy shift of the aims, the freeing of many activities from a rigid connection with one definite instinctual tendency, the comparative independence from and variety of possible response to outer and inner stimuli have to be taken into account in considering the role of the drives in human psychology. Still, the psychoanalytic theory of instinctual drives is broad enough to show also many impressive parallels with the findings of a modern school of zoologists (ethnologists).

The concept of a continuity of this driving force allows the consideration of a great variety of mental acts from the angle of their investment with drive energy. Also in this way it is possible to understand the close relationship of many mental processes which, looked at from the surface, would appear to be entirely heterogeneous. The capacity for displacement or transformation into various kinds of human activities; also the motivational role traceable through and specific on all levels of man's growth from

birth to maturity; their central role in typical conflicts; and the fact that they involve relations to human objects—these are some of the psychologically essential aspects of the psychoanalytic concept of human drives. According to Freud, sexuality and aggression are, among all the drives one could describe, those that come closest to fulfilling the demands psychoanalysis makes on a concept of drives.

The concept of mental energy was then elaborated in the sense that it is the drives that are the main sources of energy in what Freud calls the "mental apparatus." However, a strictly speaking quantifying approach to these energic problems has so far not been developed. Or rather: while it is possible to speak of a greater or lesser degree of, let's say, a resistance (against the uncovering of some hidden material), we have no way of measuring it. To account for the difference in the unconscious and the conscious (and preconscious) processes Freud postulated two forms of energy distribution, conceptualized as, respectively, primary and secondary processes. The primary processes represent a tendency to immediate discharge, while the secondary processes are guided by the consideration of reality. This distinction is again both theoretically significant and clinically quite helpful. The thesis that behavior is to be explained also in terms of its energic cathexis is what we call, in analysis, the economic viewpoint.

The regulation of energies in the mental apparatus is assumed to follow the pleasure principle, the reality principle (derived from the pleasure principle under the influence of ego-development), and a tendency to keep the level of excitation constant or at a minimum. There are parallels to this in hypotheses formulated by others, and again the use of physical and physiological models played a role in the Freudian concepts.

The three aspects of psychoanalytic theory I have mentioned so far—the topographical (conscious-preconscious-unconscious), the dynamic, and the economic (energic)—represent Freud's first approach to what he called "metapsychology." It is postulated that a satisfactory explanation of human behavior includes its consideration in relation to all aspects of metapsychology. The "meta" in this term points to a theory going "beyond" the investigation of conscious phenomena. The word, generally accepted in psychoanalysis, has proved misleading for many outside analysis. Actually, "metapsychology" is nothing but a term for the highest level of abstraction used in analytic psychology.

A fourth aspect of metapsychology, called structural, was explicitly stated considerably later, though it was implicit in earlier theoretical thinking on mental conflicts. The forces opposing the drives in typical conflict formations, warding them off and forcing them to compromise formations (of which the neurotic symptom may serve as an example), are today conceptualized as an essential aspect of what we call the ego. At the core of this concept formation is the recognition of the relevant differences between instinctual tendencies which strive for discharge, and other tendencies that enforce postponement of discharge and are modifiable by the influence of the environment. This means, of course, that the dynamic and economic viewpoints can no longer be limited to the vicissitudes of instinctual drives. The original concept of a defensive ego had to be broadened to include in the ego those nondefensive functions of the mental apparatus that are noninstinctual in character. Many of these are not, or not necessarily, part of the conflictual set-up; we call them today "the nonconflictual sphere of the ego" (Hartmann, 15). Here belong (though they too may be involved in conflict, without, however, originating in it) perception, thinking, memory, action, and so on. It is likely that in man not only instinctual factors are in part determined by heredity, but also the apparatus of the ego underlying the functions just mentioned. We speak of the primary autonomous functions of the ego. It is true that analysis is, due to its method, directly dealing with environmental factors and with reactions to them, but this has never implied a denial on principle, of heredity. It is in this sense that we speak of a drive constitution, and today also of constitutional elements in the ego, and of the role of maturational factors in the typical sequence of developmental phases.

To those noninstinctual functions that we attribute to the ego belongs also what one can call the centralized functional control which integrates the different parts of personality with each other and with outer reality. This function (synthetic function or organizing function) is in a way similar to what, since Cannon, we call homeostasis, and may represent one level of it.

The ego is, then, a substructure of personality and is defined by its functions. The instinctual aspect of personality is today conceptualized as the id. Through the development of the ego it becomes possible that the pleasure principle, dominant with the instinctual drives, can be modified to that consideration of reality, in thinking and action, that makes adaptation possible and is termed, as I said before, the reality principle. Through recent work, the relation between adaptation to outer reality and the state of integration of inner reality has become more accessible. This development in psychoanalytic theory has thus led to an improved understanding of man's relations to his environment, and to the most significant part of it, his fellowmen—which is, however, not to say that the socio-cultural aspects of mental functions and development had been overlooked in earlier analysis. Psychoanalysis, in contradistinction to some other schools of psychology, has never considered "innerpsychic" processes only, but also, and not only accidentally, includes the consideration of the individual's interactions with the environment. At any rate, the study of object relations in human development has more recently become one of the most fruitful centers of analytic interest ("new environmentalism," Kris, 25). Ego psychology represents a more balanced consideration of the biological and the social and cultural aspects of human behavior. We may say that in analysis cultural phenomena are often studied in their biological context and significance and biological phenomena in relation to the socio-cultural environment (Hartmann, 19). But this aspect will be discussed more fully later.

Some of the functions of the ego have, in the course of development, to be wrested from the influence of the drives. Gradually, they then reach, through a change of function, a certain degree of independence from instinctual origins and of resistance against reinvolvement with the drives (secondary autonomy—see Hartmann, 15, 17). A similar concept, though less specific in relation to psychoanalytic propositions, has been introduced by G.

Allport (2). This relative independence of the ego is also energically conceptualized, with respect to the sources of energy at the disposal of ego functions. The necessity to distinguish function from genesis more clearly is one of the main implications of the structural viewpoint.

The third unit of functions, considered a substructure of personality, is called the superego. To it we attribute the functions of self-criticism, conscience and the formation of ideals. The acceptance of moral standards is considered a natural step in ontogenesis. Moral conflict, and the guilt feelings that are an expression of it, are, from the time when the superego has been instituted, one fundamental aspect of human behavior. The superego has a biological root in the comparatively long dependency and helplessness of the child of the human species, which also means increased importance of the parents for its development. The superego develops out of identification with them, to which, in subsequent layers of development, identifications with others are added. Also obvious in its genesis is a socio-cultural factor, which accounts for an important segment of tradition formation. The acceptance of certain moral demands, the rejection of others, the degree of severity of the superego and its capacity to enforce its demands can very frequently be traced in clinical investigation.

Structural hypotheses are in many ways more comprehensive, but also, if I may say so, more elegant than earlier formulations of partly the same problems. They have also a considerable value in clinical thinking, because they are particularly fit to account for what has remained dominant in clinical work, that is, the various forms of typical conflict situations. Actually, the demarcation lines of those units of functions, or systems, or substructures of personality are so drawn that they correspond to the main conflicts of man, which we now describe as conflicts between ego and id, superego and ego, and ego and reality. It was in this respect that Freud found the older topographical model, the layer model (conscious - preconscious - unconscious), disappointing, though in other respects it still retains a certain degree of significance. Defenses as well as drives can be unconscious; thus differences between conscious and unconscious processes cannot be used to account for these conflicts.

I thought it advisable to begin by giving a picture of certain fundamentals of psychoanalytic theory, and of the degree of its comprehensiveness, by indicating at least some of its dimensions, and also the relations between different parts of these theories. Its comprehensiveness means also its actual or potential importance in many neighboring fields. My survey shows also at least some of the points at which questions can be raised from the viewpoint of a philosophy of science. There would have been an alternative to the way of presentation I chose. I could have shown how, in the analysis of a symptom or a dream, our observations lead to anticipations, and how the various levels of our conceptual tools are brought to bear on them; also, how in this process theoretical thinking is constantly brought back to the observables. But this alternative would inevitably demand the introduction of a great number of variables and a discussion of the analytic method and the analytic situation much broader than I am able to give here. Of course, a sector of psychoanalytic propositions can be tested outside analysis, and some have been tested in this way; but it is still true that it is, in the field of analysis, extremely difficult to assay the suitability of the hypotheses for the purposes for which they have been primarily devised without the use, in the analytic situation, of the analytic method.

Generally, Freud's views on introspection have not always been clearly appreciated. They are, though, evident already in the kind of psychoanalytic thinking that is comparatively close to observational data, as in Freud's ideas on the psychopathology of everyday life. In a slip of the tongue, for instance, when, in place of a word we consciously intended to use, another one, not consciously intended, appears, we use the behavioral aspect in evaluating the psychological situation—we use it, that is, in taking the word actually spoken as an indication of an unconscious motivation that takes precedence over the conscious one.

The data gathered in the psychoanalytic situation with the help of the psychoanalytic method are primarily behavioral data; and the aim is clearly the exploration of human behavior. The data are mostly the patient's verbal behavior, but include other kinds of action. They include his silences, his postures (F. Deutsch,7), and his movements in general, more specifically his expressive movements. While analysis aims at an explanation of human behavior, those data, however, are interpreted in analysis in terms of mental processes, of motivation, of "meaning"; there is, then, a clear-cut difference between this approach and the one usually called "behavioristic," and this difference is even more marked if we consider the beginnings of behaviorism, rather than its more recent formulations.

As to the data, it is hard to give, outside the analytic process itself, an impression of the wealth of observational data collected in even one single "case." One frequently refers to the comparatively small number of cases studied in analysis and tends to forget the very great number of actual observations on which we base, in every individual case, the interpretations of an aspect of a person's character, symptoms and so on.*

By keeping certain variables in the analytic situation, if not constant, as close to constancy as the situation allows, it becomes easier to evaluate the significance of other variables that enter the picture. The best-studied example of this is what is called the "passivity" of the analyst, in contradistinction to the considerably more pronounced activity of the psychotherapist. This is not to claim that psychoanalysis is an experimental discipline. However, there are situations where it comes close to it. At any rate, there is sufficient evidence for the statement that our observations in the psychoanalytic situation, set in the context of psychoanalytic experience and hypotheses, make predictions possible —predictions of various degrees of precision or reliability, but as a rule superior to any others that have been attempted in the psychology of personality. Due to the emphasis on the genetic viewpoint, many predictions are what has been called "predictions of the past," (Hartmann, Kris, 20) that is, reconstructions of the past which can often be confirmed in astonishing detail (Bonaparte, 6). One obvious limitation of our predictive potential is, of course, the great number of factors determining, according

to psychoanalytic theory, every single element of behavior—what Freud has termed "overdetermination." Still, our technique is constantly directed by tentative predictions of the patient's reaction. Also, studies in developmental psychology by means of direct child observation, such as have been conducted by E. Kris and other psychoanalysts (M. Kris, 26), are guided by the formulation of expectations and their checking in individual cases. Here I just want to point to one way in which psychoanalytic hypotheses can be used vis-à-vis individual cases and how they may be confirmed in clinical experience. I may mention here that problems of validation of psychoanalytic hypotheses ought not to be equated, as has too often been done, with the problem of therapeutic success.

A further difficulty results from the fact that psychoanalytic theory has also to deal with the relation between observer and observed in the analytic situation. There are personality layers, if you will excuse this term, that in the average case the observed cannot reach without the help of the observer and his method of observation. But the insight of the observer ought not to be confused with the insight of the observed. Some of these problems belong in a theory of psychoanalytic technique. But there is also the problem of the "personal equation" (Hartmann, 18; Kris, 25). The field of observation includes not only the patient, but also the observer who interacts with the former ("participant observation"). The interaction of analyst and analysand are accounted for in the theories of transference and countertransference. As to the potential handicaps of observations traceable to the mental processes of the observer, they are subject to the constant scrutiny of the analyst. Some such handicaps of psychological observation can certainly be eliminated by the personal analysis of the observer, and this is one of the reasons that a didactic analysis is an essential element in the training of our students of analysis. Thus, what I want to say here is not that in the psychology of personality objectivity is impossible. It is rather that psychoanalysis has discovered potential sources of error and found a way to combat them.

Another aspect of the clinical origins of psychoanalytic theory is the fact that more was found, in the beginning, about

---

*Thus every single clinical "case" represents, for research, hundreds of data of observed regularities, and in hundreds of respects.

pathological than about normal behavior. The etiology of neurosis was studied before the etiology of health, though psychoanalysis has, on principle, always aimed at a comprehensive general psychology. Also, as I mentioned, more became known, in the first attempts to deal with the field, about the instinctual drives, especially about sexuality and its development, than about the forces opposing the drives in the typical ego-id conflicts. This, however, has changed in the last two or three decades, and analysis thus has today come closer to what it always was intended to be, though not every aspect and not every implication of its very comprehensive conceptual frame has so far been actually developed.

In clinical work, one is used to being guided by signs and symptoms in forming an opinion on the presence or absence of a pathological process. But the question of the significance and the use of signs for purposes of explanation is, of course, logically of much wider relevance. Different meanings can be attributed to the terms sign, signal, expressive sign, symbol, and so on, and these differences are important also in psychoanalysis. However, I don't propose to deal with this problem here. Suffice it to say that a considerable part of psychoanalytic work can be described as the use of signs—a series of associations, a dream, an affect vis-à-vis the analyst—as indications of mental processes. In this sense one speaks of the psychoanalytic method as a method of interpretation (Hartmann, 14; Bernfeld, 4; Loewenstein, 28). This has both a cognitive and a therapeutic aspect. They partly coincide, that is, in so far as a therapeutic agent of foremost significance in analysis is making the patient aware of, and capable of integrating, previously unconscious and, through defense, splitoff processes. Some of those signs, for example, some of the symbols we find in dreams, have a rather ubiquitous meaning, while the interpretation of others requires a closer scrutiny of the individual under observation. At any rate, there are many situations in which the relation between a sign and what it signifies becomes easily recognizable, for instance in the associations immediately following the observation of some detail of behavior. In others, various levels of theory have to be introduced to explain the connection. Such sign systems are used today not only in the psychoanalytic situation, but also in the study by analysts, by means of direct observation, of child development. Many childhood situations of incisive significance for the formation of the adult personality have a low probability of direct manifestation. One tries to learn about the sign function of data of child behavior for a recognition of the central, and often unconscious, development that we know from the psychoanalytic interview (Hartmann, 18). At this point it is possible, or even likely, that a misunderstanding may occur of what I have said about a low probability of manifestation outside analysis of certain processes investigated in analysis. I want, then, to add explicitly that this was not meant to be a general statement. Many phenomena first studied in the analytic situation could later be studied also in the direct observation of psychotics, in so-called applied psychoanalysis, or in the direct observation of children. What I want to emphasize in this context is that the comparative study of reconstructive data and data of direct observation of children leads, on the one hand, to the confirmation of analytical propositions; on the other hand it leads to the formulation of more specific hypotheses.

The essential importance of constructs for the coherence of the psychoanalytic system (or whatever we choose to call it) can be gathered already from the brief outline I have given in the first part of this discussion. Theories, or hypotheses of a different order, connect them with observational data. That these constructs, which are introduced because of their explanatory value, cannot be directly defined in terms of observational data, but that inferences from the constructs can be tested by observation, has long been known in psychoanalysis (Hartmann, 14). Still, some of these constructs seem particularly suspect to many critics of analysis. An occasional lack of caution in the formulation of its propositions, or Freud's liking for occasional striking metaphors, has led to the accusation against analysis of an anthropomorphization of its concepts. But in all those cases a more careful formulation can be substituted which will dispel this impression.

There is, then, the question whether and in what sense such constructs are considered "real"; and, more specifically, the question has often been asked whether and in what sense Freud considered constructs like libido, the "system unconscious," and the substructures of personality in the sense of structural psychology, as real. He said that the basic concepts of science form rather the roof than the foundation of science and ought to be changed when they no longer seem able to account for experience; also that they have the character of conventions. But he certainly thought that what he meant to cover by these basic concepts had effects which could be observed. He was in no danger of confusing concepts with realities; he was a "realist" in a different sense. He does not seem to have thought that "real" means just "the simplest theoretical presentation of our experiences," but rather that those basic concepts pointed to something real in the ordinary sense of the word.

As to the genetic propositions of analysis, the direct observation of children has not only become a rich source of information, but also given us the possibility to make our hypotheses more specific and to check their validity. A great number of Freud's hypotheses on childhood could be confirmed by direct observation of children. But to validate more completely our genetic propositions, "systematic observations of life histories from birth on" are necessary. "If the longitudinal observation in our own civilization were to be systematized and the study of life histories were to be combined with that of the crucial situations in Freud's sense, many hunches might be formulated as propositions, and others might be discarded" (Hartmann and Kris, 20).

The literature on experimental research, both in animals and in man, devised for the purpose of testing propositions derived from psychoanalysis has become very extensive. It has been repeatedly reviewed (Sears, 31; Kris, 24; Benjamin, 3; Frenkel-Brunswik, 10; and others), and I do not think I should go into it in any detail here. The following remarks are, then, random remarks and do not attempt to be in any way systematic. The classical animal experiments of Hunt, Levy, Miller, Masserman are probably known to many of you. Many of the animal experiments were conducted with considerable insight and great skill. Where the experimental set-up is adequate, the frequency of

"confirmation" is impressive. Or, as Hilgard (22) states, "It has been possible to parallel many psychoanalytic phenomena in the laboratory. When this is done, the correspondence between predictions according to psychoanalytic theory and what is found is on the whole very satisfactory."

References

1. Adrian, E. D., "The Mental and the Physical Origins of Behavior," *International Journal of Psychoanalysis*, XXVII, 1946.
2. Allport, G., *Personality*. New York: Henry Holt, 1937.
3. Benjamin, J., "Methodological Considerations in the Validation and Elaboration of Psychoanalytical Personality Theory." *American Journal of Orthopsychiatry, 20,* 1950.
4. Bernfeld, S., "Der Begriff der Deutung in der Psychoanalyse," *Zeitschrift für Angewandte Psychologie*, XLII, 1932.
5. ————, "Freud's Earliest Theories and the School of Helmholtz," *Psychoanalytic Quarterly*, XIII, 1944.
6. Bonaparte, M., "Notes on the Analytical Discovery of a Primal Scene," *Psychoanalytic Study of the Child*, I, 1945.
7. Deutsch, F., "Analytic Posturology." *Psychoanalytic Quarterly*, XXI, 1952.
8. Dollard, J. and Miller, N. E., *Personality and Psychotherapy*. New York: McGraw-Hill, 1950.
9. Ellis, A., *An Introduction to the Principles of Scientific Psychoanalysis*, Genetic Psychology Monograph, *41,* 1950.
10. Frenkel-Brunswik, E., *Psychoanalysis and the Unity of Science*, Proceedings of the American Academy of Arts and Sciences, *80,* 1954.
11. Freud, A., "The Contributions of Psychoanalysis to Genetic Psychology," *American Journal of Orthopsychiatry*, XXI, 1951.
12. Freud, S., *The Claim of Psychoanalysis to Scientific Interest*. London: Hogarth Press, Standard Edition, Vol. XIII.
13. ————, *Psycho-Analysis*. London: Hogarth Press, Standard Edition, Vol. XVIII.
14. Hartmann, H., *Die Grundlagen der Psychoanalyse*. Leipzig, 1927.
15. ————, "Ichpsychologie und Anpassungsproblem," *Internationale Zeitschrift für Psychoanalyse*, XXIV, 1939. Partly translated in: D. Rapaport, *Organization and Pathology of Thought*. New York: Columbia University Press, 1951.
16. ————, "Comments on the Psychoanalytic Theory of Instinctual Drives," *Psychoanalytic Quarterly*, XVII, 1948.
17. ————, "Comments on the Psychoanalytic Theory of the Ego," *Psychoanalytic Study of the Child*, V. 1950.
18. ————, "Psychoanalysis and Developmental Psychology." *Psychoanalytic Study of the Child*, V, 1950.
19. ————, "The Development of the Ego Con-

cept in Freud's Work," *International Journal of Psychoanalysis,* XXXVII, 1956.

20. —————— and Kris, E., "The Genetic Approach in Psychoanalysis," *Psychoanalytic Study of the Child,* I, 1945.

21. ——————, Kris, E. and Loewenstein, R., "Comments on the Formation of Psychic Structure," *Psychoanalytic Study of the Child,* II, 1946.

22. Hilgard, E., "Experimental Approaches to Psychoanalysis," in: *Psychoanalysis as Science,* ed. E. Pumpian-Mindlin. Stanford University Press, 1952.

23. Klein, G., "Cognizant Style and Motivation," in: *Assessment of Human Motives,* ed. G. Lindzey. New York: Rinehart, 1958.

24. Kris, E., "The Nature of Psychoanalytic Propositions and their Validation," in: *Freedom and Experience,* ed. S. Hook and M. R. Konvitz, Cornell University Press, 1947.

25. ——————, "Notes on the Development and on some Current Problems of Psychoanalytic Child Psychology," *Psychoanalytic Study of the Child,* V, 1950.

26. Kris, M., "The Use of Prediction in a Longitudinal Study," *Psychoanalytic Study of the Child,* XII, 1957.

27. Kubie, L., "Problems and Techniques of Psychoanalytic Validation and Progress," in: *Psychoanalysis as Science,* ed. E. Pumpian-Mindlin. Stanford University Press, 1952.

28. Loewenstein, R., "Some Thoughts on Interpretation in the Theory and Practice of Psychoanalysis," *Psychoanalytic Study of the Child,* XII, 1957.

29. Mises, R. v., *Kleines Lehrbuch des Positivismus.* The Hague, 1939.

30. Rapaport, D., "The Structure of Psychoanalytic Theory (A Systematizing Attempt)," in: *Psychology: A Study of a Science,* ed. S. Koch. New York: McGraw-Hill, 1958, Vol. III.

31. Sears, R., "Survey of Objectives Studies of Psychoanalytic Concepts," Social Sciences Research Council *Bulletin,* 1943, 51.

32. Wisdom, J., *Philosophy and Psycho-Analysis.* New York: Philosophical Library, 1953.

ETIOLOGY AND DEVELOPMENT

The key to the development of pathological behavior, according to the intrapsychic theorist, can be found in faulty experiences in early life. Each child is born with a variety of drives or instincts which require nourishment and stimulation. Deprivation or conflicts associated with these needs result in feelings of anxiety and insecurity. In an effort to handle these feelings, the child adopts a variety of defensive maneuvers which ultimately lead to maladaptive behavior.

Carl Jung, an early disciple of Freud who broke from the main stream of psychoanalysis, retained Freud's focus on the role of unconscious processes. He posited the existence of a collective unconscious to represent a hypothetical pattern of inborn dispositions bequeathed by the ancestral past of mankind. Failure to find adequate expression for these dispositions was viewed by Jung to be the crux of psychopathology. In the paper presented here, Jung discusses in detail the pros and cons for a psychological interpretation of schizophrenia. His article can be viewed as a companion piece to the paper presented earlier by Eugen Bleuler. It represents, in part, a rebuttal to Bleuler's conviction that the basic etiology of schizophrenia is organic.

Erik Erikson, one of the major contemporary figures in "ego psychology," has formulated a model for ego development which parallels Freud's conception of the stages of psychosexual development. In the selection reprinted here, he outlines, with a clarity rare among intrapsychic writers, the major phases of early interpersonal experience. Disruptions in the sequence of this developmental pattern often lead to pathological development, according to Erikson.

13. On the Psychogenesis of Schizophrenia

CARL G. JUNG

It is just twenty years ago that I read a paper on the "Problem of Psychogenesis in Mental Disease" before this Society. William McDougall, whose recent death we all deplore, was in the chair. What I then said about psychogenesis could be safely repeated to-day, for it has left no visible traces, or other noticeable consequences, either in text-books or in clinics. Although I hate to repeat myself, it is almost impossible to say something wholly new and different about a subject which has not changed its face in the many years that have gone by. My experience, however, has increased and some of my views have matured, but I could not say that my standpoint has had to undergo any radical change. I am therefore in the somewhat uncomfortable situation of one who, on the one hand, believes that he

From *J. of Mental Science 85:* 993–1011, 1939, by permission of the Royal Medico-Psychological Association.

has a well-founded conviction, but, on the other hand, is afraid to indulge in the habit of repeating old stories. Although psychogenesis has been discussed long ago, it is still a modern, even an ultra-modern, problem.

There is little doubt nowadays about the psychogenesis of hysteria and other neuroses, although thirty years ago some brain enthusiasts still cherished vague suspicions that at bottom "there was something organically wrong even with neuroses." But the *consensus doctorum* in their vast majority has admitted the psychical causation of hysteria and similar neuroses. Concerning mental diseases, however, and especially concerning schizophrenia, they agreed unanimously upon an essentially organic aetiology, although for a long time specific destruction of the brain-matter could not be proved. Even in our days the question of how far schizophrenia itself can destroy brain-cells is not satisfactorily answered; much less the more specific question of how far primary organic disintegrations account for the symptomatology of schizophrenia. I quite agree with Bleuler that the great majority of symptoms are of a secondary nature and are chiefly due to psychical causes. For the primary symptoms, however, Bleuler assumes the existence of an organic cause. As the *primary symptom* he points to a peculiar disturbance of the association process which is difficult to describe. According to his description it is a matter of a sort of disintegration, inasmuch as the associations seem to be peculiarly mutilated and disjointed. He refuses to adopt Wernicke's concept of *sejunctio* on account of its anatomical implications. He prefers to term it "schizophrenia", obviously understanding by this concept a more *functional* disturbance. Such disturbances, or at least very similar ones, can be observed in delirious conditions of various kinds. Bleuler himself points out the remarkable likeness between schizophrenic associations and the association phenomena in dreams and half-waking conditions. From his description it becomes sufficiently clear, that the primary symptom coincides with the condition which Pierre Janet has formulated as *abaissement du niveau mental*. It is due to a peculiar *faiblesse de la volonté*. If we are permitted to call the main guiding and controlling force of

our mental life *will-power*, then one can agree that Janet's concept of the *abaissement* explains a psychical condition in which a train of thought is not carried through to its logical end, or where it is interrupted by strange contents insufficiently inhibited. Though Bleuler does not refer to Janet, I hold that Janet's notion of the *abaissement* aptly formulates Bleuler's views on the primary symptoms.

It is true, however, that Janet uses his hypothesis chiefly in order to explain the symptomatology of hysteria and other neuroses, which are indubitably psychogenic and different from schizophrenia. Yet there are certain noteworthy analogies between the neurotic and the schizophrenic mental condition. If you study the association tests of neurotics, for instance, you find that the normal associations are disturbed by the spontaneous interference of complex contents typical of an *abaissement*. The dissociation can even go so far as the creation of one, or of several, secondary personalities with an apparently complete segregation of consciousness. But the fundamental difference from schizophrenia consists in the maintenance of the potential unity of the personality. Despite the fact that consciousness can be split up into several personal consciousnesses, the unity of all the dissociated fragments is not only visible to the professional eye, but it can also be re-established by means of hypnosis. This is not the case with schizophrenia. The general picture of an association test of a schizophrenic may be very similar to the test of a neurotic, but a close exploration reveals the fact that in a schizophrenic patient the connection between the ego and certain complexes is more or less completely lost. The split is not relative, it is rather absolute. A hysterical patient might suffer from a sort of persecution mania very similar to a real paranoia, but the difference is that in the case of hysteria one can bring the delusion back under the control of consciousness, whereas it is impossible to do this in paranoia. A neurosis, it is true, is characterized by a relative autonomy of its complexes, but in schizophrenia the complexes have become disjointed and autonomous fragments, which either do not reintegrate to the psychical totality, or, in the case of a remission, are unexpectedly joined together, as if nothing had happened before.

The dissociation in schizophrenia is not only far more serious, but very often it is also irreversible. The dissociation is no longer *liquid and changeable,* as it is in a neurosis, but is more like a mirror broken up into splinters. The unity of personality which lends a humanly understandable character to its own secondary personalities in a case of hysteria is definitely severed into fragments. In a hysterical multiple personality there is an almost smooth, even a tactful, co-operation between the different persons, who neatly keep their role and, if possible, do not bother each other. One feels the presence of an invisible *spiritus rector,* or a central manager, who arranges the stage for the different figures in an almost rational way, often in the form of a more or less sentimental drama. Each figure has a suggestive name and an admissible character, and they are just as nicely hysterical and as sentimentally biased as the patient's consciousness.

The picture of a personality dissociation in schizophrenia is quite a different matter. The split-off figures assume banal, grotesque or highly exaggerated names and characters and are often objectionable in many ways. They do not, moreover, co-operate with the patient's consciousness. They are not tactful and they have no respect for sentimental values. On the contrary, they break in and make a disturbance at any time, they torture the ego in a hundred ways; all and sundry are objectionable and shocking either in their noisy and impertinent behaviour, or in their grotesque cruelty and obscenity. There is an apparent chaos of inconsistent visions, voices and characters of an overwhelmingly strange and incomprehensible nature. If there is a drama at all, it is certainly far beyond the patient's understanding. In most cases it transcends even the physician's mind, so much so that he is inclined to suspect anybody's mental sanity who sees anything more than mere madness in the ravings of a lunatic.

The autonomous figures have liberated themselves from the control of the ego so thoroughly that their original participation in the patient's mental make-up has vanished beyond recognition. The *abaissement* has reached a degree unheard of in the sphere of neuroses. A hysterical dissociation is bridged-over by a unity of the personality which still functions, whereas in schizophrenia the very foundations of the personality are injured. The *abaissement* causes:

1. A loss of whole regions of normally controlled contents.
2. It thus produces split-off fragments of the personality.
3. It hinders the normal train of thought from being consistently carried through and completed.
4. It decreases the responsibility and the adequate reaction of the ego.
5. It causes incomplete realizations and thus produces insufficient and inadequate emotional reactions.
6. It lowers the threshold of consciousness and thus allows normally inhibited contents of the unconscious mind to enter consciousness in the form of autonomous intrusions.

We meet all these effects of the *abaissement* in neuroses as well as in schizophrenia. But in neuroses the unity of personality is at least potentially preserved, whereas in schizophrenia it is more or less damaged. On account of this fundamental injury the cleavage between dissociated psychical elements amounts to a real destruction of their former connections.

Psychogenesis of schizophrenia, therefore, in the first place means the question: Can the primary symptom, viz. the extreme *abaissement* be considered as an effect of psychological conflicts and other disorders of an emotional nature or not? I do not think that it is necessary to discuss at length the question of whether *secondary symptoms,* as Bleuler describes them, owe their existence and their specific form to psychological determination or not. Bleuler himself is fully convinced that they derive their form and contents, i.e. their individual phenomenology, entirely from emotional complexes. I agree with Bleuler, whose experience of the psychogenesis of secondary symptoms coincides with my own, for we were collaborating in the years which preceded his famous book on dementia praecox. As a matter of fact I began as early as 1903 to analyse cases of schizophrenia for theoretical purposes. There can, indeed, be no doubt about the psychological determination of secondary symptoms. Their structure and derivation is in no way different from those of neurotic symptoms, with, of course, the significant exception that they exhibit all the characteristics of mental contents no longer subordinated to the supreme control of a complete personality. There is, as a matter of fact, hardly one secondary symptom which does not show signs of the typical *abaissement* in some ways. This character, however, does not depend upon psychogenesis, but it derives entirely from the primary symptom. Psychological causes, in other words, produce secondary symptoms exclusively on the basis of the primary condition.

In dealing with the question of psychogenesis in schizophrenia we can dismiss the secondary symptoms altogether. There is only one problem, viz., the psychogenesis of the primary condition, i. e., the extreme *abaissement,* which is, from the psychological point of view, the root of the schizophrenic disorder. We ask therefore: Is there any reason to believe that such an *abaissement* can be due to causes which are strictly psychological? An *abaissement* can be produced—as we well know—by many causes: by fatigue, normal sleep, intoxication, fever, anaemia, intense affects, shocks, organic diseases of the central nervous system, induction through mob psychology or primitive mentality or religious and political fanaticism, etc. It can also be due to constitutional and hereditary factors.

The general and more frequent form of *abaissement* does not touch the unity of the personality, at least not seriously. Thus all dissociations and other psychical phenomena derived from this general form of *abaissement* carry the seal of the integral personality.

Neuroses are specific consequences of an *abaissement;* as a rule they derive from a habitual or chronic form of it. Where they appear to be the effect of an acute form, a more or less latent psychological disposition always existed previous to the *abaissement,* so that the latter does not mean more than a conditional cause.

Now there is no doubt that an *abaissement* which leads to a neurosis is produced either by exclusively psychological factors or by those in conjunction with other, perhaps more physical, conditions. Any *abaissement,* particularly one that leads to a neurosis, means in itself that there is a weakening of the supreme control. A neurosis is a relative dissociation, a conflict between the ego and a resistant force based upon unconscious contents. Those contents are relatively severed from the connection with the psychical totality. They form parts, and the loss of them means a depotentiation of the conscious personality. The intense conflict on the other side, however, expresses an equally acute desire to re-establish the severed connection. There is no cooperation, but there is at least a violent conflict, which functions instead of a positive connection. Every neurotic fights for the maintenance and supremacy of his ego-consciousness and for the subjugation of the resistant unconscious forces. But a patient who allows himself to be swayed by the intrusions of strange contents from the unconscious, a case that does not fight, that even identifies with the morbid elements, immediately exposes himself to the suspicion of schizophrenia. His *abaissement* has reached the fatal extreme degree, where the ego loses all power of resistance against the inimical onslaught of an apparently more powerful unconscious.

Neurosis lies this side of the critical point, schizophrenia is beyond it. We do not doubt that psychological motives can bring about an *abaissement* which eventually results in a neurosis. A neurosis approaches the danger line, yet it somehow manages to remain on the hither side. If it should transgress the lines it would cease to be a neurosis. Yet are we quite certain that neurosis never steps beyond the danger line? You know that there are such cases, neuroses to all appearances for many years, and then it suddenly happens that the patient steps beyond the line and clearly transforms himself into a real psychotic.

Now, what do we say in such a case? We say that it has always been a psychosis, a "latent" one, or one concealed or camouflaged by an apparent neurosis. But what has really happened? For many years the patient fought for the maintenance of his ego, for the supremacy of his control and for the unity of his personality. But at last he gave out—he succumbed to the invader, whom he could suppress no longer. He is not merely overcome by a violent emotion, he is really drowned in a flood of insurmountably strong forces and thought forms, which are far beyond any ordinary emotion, no matter how violent. These unconscious forces and contents existed long ago and he had wrestled with them successfully for years. As a matter of fact such strange contents are not confined to the patient alone, they exist in other peoples' unconscious just as well, who, however, are fortunate enough to be profoundly ignorant of them. These forces did not originate in our patient out of the nowhere. They are most emphatically not the result of poisoned brain-cells, but are normal constituents of our unconscious minds. They appeared in numberless dreams, in the same or a similar form, at a time of life when seemingly nothing was wrong. And they appear even in the dreams of normal people, who never get anywhere near to a psychosis. But if such a normal individual should suddenly undergo a dangerous *abaissement,* his dreams would instantly seize upon him and make him think, feel and act exactly like a lunatic. And he would be one, like the man in one of Andreyev's stories, who thought he could safely bark at the moon, because he knew that he was perfectly normal. But when he barked he lost consciousness of the little difference between normal and crazy, and thus the other side overwhelmed him and he became mad.

What happened to our case was an attack of weakness—in reality it is often just a sudden panic—it made him hopeless or desperate, and then all the suppressed material welled up and drowned him.

In my experience of almost forty years I have seen quite a number of cases who developed either a psychotic interval or a lasting psychosis out of a neurotic condition. Let us assume for the time being that they really suffered from a *latent psychosis* concealed in the cloak of a neurosis. What, then, is a latent psychosis exactly? It is obviously nothing but the possibility that an individual may become mentally deranged at some period of his life. The existence of strange unconscious material proves nothing of all. You find the same with neurotics, modern artists and poets, and also with fairly normal people, who have submitted to a careful investigation of their dreams. Moreover, you find most suggestive parallels in the mythology and symbolism of all races and times. The possibility of a future psychosis has nothing to do with the peculiar contents of the unconscious

mind. But it has everything to do with the question of whether the individual can stand a certain panic, or the chronic strain of a psyche at war with itself. Very often it is merely the question of a little bit too much, i. e. of the drop that falls into a vessel already full, or of the spark that incidentally lands upon a heap of gunpowder.

Under the effect of an extreme *abaissement* the psychical totality falls asunder and splits up into complexes, and the ego-complex ceases to play the important role among these. It is just one among several or many complexes which are equally important, or perhaps even more important, than the ego is. All these complexes assume a certain personal character, although they remain fragments. It is understandable that people get panicky or that they eventually become demoralized under a chronic strain or that they despair of their hopes and expectations. It is also comprehensible when their willpower weakens and their self-control becomes slack and begins to lose its grip upon circumstances, moods and thoughts. It is quite consistent with such a state of mind when some particularly unruly parts of the patient's psyche assume a certain amount of autonomy.

Thus far schizophrenia does not behave in any way differently from a merely psychological disorder. We should search in vain for anything characteristic of our ailment in this part of the symptomatology. The real trouble begins with the disintegration of the personality and the divestment of the ego-complex from its habitual supremacy. As I have already pointed out, not even multiple personality, or certain religious or "mystical" phenomena, can be compared to what happens in schizophrenia. The primary symptom seems to have no analogy with any kind of functional disturbance. It is just as if the very basis of the psyche were giving way, as if an explosion or an earthquake were tearing asunder the structure of a normally built house. I use this allegory on purpose, because it is suggested through the symptomatology of the initial stages. Sollier has given us a vivid description of these *"troubles cénesthésiques,"* which are compared to explosions, pistol-shots and other violent noises in the head. Their projected appearance are earthquakes, cosmic catastrophes, such as the fall of the stars, the splitting of the sun, the falling asunder of the moon, the transformation of people into corpses, the freezing of the universe, and so on.

I have just said that the primary symptom appears to have no analogy with any kind of functional disturbance, yet I have omitted to mention the phenomena of the *dream*. Dreams can produce similar pictures of great catastrophes. They can show all stages of personal disintegration, so it is no exaggeration when we say that the dreamer is normally insane, or that insanity is a dream which has replaced normal consciousness. To say that insanity is a dream which has become real is no metaphor. The phenomenology of the dream and of schizophrenia is almost identical, with certain difference of course; for the one state occurs normally under the condition of sleep, while the other upsets the waking or conscious state. Sleep is also an *abaissement du niveau mental* which leads into a more or less complete oblivion of the ego. The psychical mechanism, therefore, which is destined to bring about the normal extinction and disintegration on consciousness, is a normal function which almost obeys our will. It seems as if this function were set in motion in order to bring about that sleep-like condition in which consciousness becomes reduced to the level of dreams, or where dreams are intensified to a degree paramount to that of consciousness.

Yet even if we knew that the primary symptom is produced by the aid of an always present normal function, we should still have to explain why a pathological condition ensues instead of the normal effect, viz. sleep. It must, however, be emphasized that it is precisely not sleep which is produced, but something which disturbs sleep, namely, the dream. Dreams are due to an incomplete extinction of consciousness, or to a somewhat excited state of the unconscious which interferes with sleep. Sleep is bad if too many remnants of consciousness go stirring; or if there are unconscious contents with too much energic charge, for they then rise above the threshold and create a relatively conscious state. Thus it is better to explain many dreams from the remnants of conscious impressions, while others derive directly from unconscious sources which have never existed in consciousness. The former dreams have a personal character and agree with the rules of a personalistic psychology; the latter have a collective character, inasmuch as they exhibit a peculiarly mythological, legendary or generally archaic imagery. One must turn to historical or primitive symbology in order to explain such dreams.

Both types of dream mirror themselves in the symptomatology of schizophrenia. There is a mixture of personal and collective material just as there is in dreams. But in contradistinction to normal dreams the collective material seems to prevail. This is particularly obvious in the so-called "dream states" or delirious intervals, and in paranoid conditions. It seems also to prevail in katatonic phases, in so far as we can succeed in getting a certain insight into the inner experiences of such patients. Whenever collective material prevails under normal conditions it is matter of important dreams. Primitives call them "big dreams" and consider them of tribal importance. You find the same in the Greek and Roman civilizations, where such dreams were reported to the Areopagos or to the Senate. One meets these dreams frequently in the decisive moments or periods of life: in childhood from the 3rd to the 6th year, at the time of puberty, from 14 to 16, of maturity from 20 to 25, in the middle of life from 35 to 40, and before death. They occur also when it is a matter of particularly important psychological situations. It seems that such dreams come chiefly at the moments or periods where antique or primitive mentality deemed it necessary to celebrate certain religious or magic rites, in order to produce favourable issues, or to propitiate the gods for the same end.

We may safely assume that important personal matters and worries. account sufficiently for personal dreams. We are not so sure of our ground, however, when we come to collective dreams with their often weird and archaic imagery, which it is impossible to trace back to personal sources. Yet historical symbology yields the most surprising and most enlightening parallels, without which we could never follow up the often remarkable meaning of such dreams.

This fact lets one feel how inadequate the psychological training of the alienist is. It is, of course, impossible to appreciate the importance of comparative psychology for the theory of delusions without a detailed knowledge of historical and ethnical symbology. No sooner did we begin with the qualitative analysis of schizophrenic conditions at the Psychiatric Clinic in Zürich than we realized the need of such additional information. We naturally started with an entirely personalistic medical psychology, mainly as presented by Freud. But we soon came up against the fact that, in its basic structure, the human psyche is as little personalistic as the body. It is rather an inherited and universal affair. The logic of our mind, the *"raison du coeur,"* the emotions, the instincts, the basic images and forms of imagination, have in a way more resemblance to Kant's table of *a priori* categories or to Plato's *eida*, than to the scurrilities, circumstantialities, whims and tricks of our personal mind. It is especially schizophrenia that yields an immense harvest of collective symbology, neuroses yield far less, for, with a few exceptions, they show a predominantly personal psychology. The fact that schizophrenia upsets the foundations accounts for the abundance of collective symbolism, because it is the latter material that constitutes the basic structure of personality.

From this point of view we might conclude that the schizophrenic state of mind, in so far as it yields archaic material, has all the characteristics of a "big dream"—in other words, that it is an important event, exhibiting the same "numinous" quality which primitive civilizations attribute to the corresponding magic ritual. As a matter of fact, the insane person has always enjoyed the prerogative of being the one possessed by spirits or haunted by a demon, which is, by the way, a correct rendering of his psychical condition, for he is invaded by autonomous figures and thought-forms. The primitive evaluation of insanity, moreover, points out a certain characteristic which we should not overlook: it ascribes personality, initiative and wilful intention to the unconscious—again a true interpretation of the obvious facts. From the primitive standpoint it is perfectly clear that the unconscious, out of its own volition, has taken possession of the ego. According to this view the ego is not primarily enfeebled, on the contrary, it is the unconscious that is strengthened through the presence of a demon. The primitive theory, therefore, does not seek the reason for insanity in a primary weakness of consciousness, but rather in an inordinate strength of the unconscious.

I must admit it is exceedingly difficult to decide the intricate question of whether it is a matter of primary weakness and a corresponding dissociability of consciousness or of a primary strength of the unconscious. The latter possibility cannot easily be dismissed, since it is not unthinkable that the abundant archaic material might be the expression of a still existing infantile, as well as primitive, mentality. It might be a question of *atavism*. I seriously consider the possibility of a so-called *"developpement arrêté,"* where a more than normal amount of primitive psychology remains intact and does not become adapted to modern conditions. It is natural that under such conditions a considerable part of the psyche should not catch up with the normal progress of consciousness. In the course of years the distance between the unconscious and the conscious mind increases and produces a latent conflict at first. But when a particular effort at adaptation is needed, and when consciousness should draw upon its unconscious instinctive resources, the conflict becomes manifest; and the hitherto latent primitive mind suddenly bursts forth with contents that are too incomprehensible and too strange for assimilation to be possible. As a matter of fact, such a moment marks the beginning of the psychosis in a great number of cases.

But one should not disregard the fact that many patients seem to be quite capable of producing a modern and sufficiently developed consciousness, sometimes of a particularly concentrated, rational and obstinate kind. However one must add quickly that such a consciousness shows early signs of a self-defensive nature. This is a symptom of weakness, not of strength.

It may be that a normal consciousness is confronted with an unusually strong unconscious; it may also be that the consciousness is just weak and therefore unable to succeed in keeping back the inflow of unconscious material. Practically I must allow for the existence of two groups of schizophrenia: the one with a weak consciousness and the other with a strong unconscious. We have here a certain analogy with neuroses, where we also find plenty of cases with a markedly weak consciousness and little willpower, and other patients, who enjoy a remarkable energy, but who are confronted with an almost overwhelmingly strong unconscious determination. This is particularly the case where creative (artistic or otherwise) impulses are coupled with unconscious incompatibilities.

If we return now to our original question, viz. the psychogenesis of schizophrenia, we reach the conclusion that the problem itself is rather complicated. At all events we ought to make it clear, that the term "psychogenesis" consists of two different things: (1) It means an exclusive psychological origin. (2) It means a number of psychological and psychical conditions. We have dealt with the second point, but we have not yet touched upon the first. This point envisages psychogenesis from the standpoint of the *causa efficiens*. The question is: Is the sole and absolute reason for a schizophrenia a psychological one or not?

In the whole field of medicine such a question is, as you know, more than awkward. Only in a very few cases can it be answered positively. The usual aetiology consists of a competition of various conditions. It has been urged, therefore, that the word causality or cause should be struck off the medical vocabulary and replaced by the term "conditionalism." I am absolutely in favour of such a measure, since it is well-nigh impossible to prove, even approximately, that schizophrenia is an organic disease to begin with. It is equally impossible to make an exclusively psychological origin evident. We may have strong suspicions as to the organic aspect of the primary symptom, but we cannot omit the well-established fact that there are many cases which developed out of an emotional shock, a disappointment, a difficult situation, a reverse of fortune, etc., and also that many relapses as well as improvements are due to psychological conditions. What shall we say about a case like this: A young student experiences a great disappointment in a love affair. He has a katatonic attack, from which he recovers after months. He then finishes his studies and becomes a successful academical man. After a number of years he returns to Zürich, where he had experienced his love affair. Instantly he is seized by a new and very similar attack.

He says that he believes he saw the girl somewhere. He recovers and avoids Zürich for several years. Then he returns and in a few days he is back in the clinic with a katatonic attack, again because he is under the impression that he has seen the girl, who by that time is married and has children.

My teacher, Eugen Bleuler, used to say that a psychological cause can only release the symptoms of the disease, but not the disease itself. This statement may be profound or the reverse. At all events it shows the alienist's perplexity. One could say, for instance, that our patient returned to Zürich when he felt the disease coming on, and one thinks that one has said something clever. He denies it—naturally, you will say. But it is a fact that this man is still deeply in love with his girl. He never went near another woman and his thoughts kept on returning to Zürich. What could be more natural than that once in a while he should give way to his unconquered longing to see the streets, the houses, the walks again, where he had met her, insanity or not? We do not know, moreover, what ecstasies and adventures he experienced during insanity and what unknown expectation tempted him to seek the experience once more. I once treated a schizophrenic girl who told me that she hated me because I had made it impossible for her to return into her beautiful psychosis. . . .

I admit that I cannot imagine, how "merely" psychical events can cause an *abaissement* which destroys the unity of personality, only too often beyond repair. But I know from long experience not only that the overwhelming majority of symptoms are due to psychological determination, but also that the beginning of an unlimited number of cases is influenced by, or at least coupled with, psychical facts which one would not hesitate to declare as causal in a case of neurosis. Statistics in this respect prove nothing to me, for I know that even in a neurotic case one runs the risk of only discovering the true anamnesis after months of careful analysis. Psychiatric anamnesis often suffers from a lack of psychological knowledge which is sometimes appalling. I do not say that physicians in general should have a knowledge of psychology, but if the alienist aims at psychotherapy at all he certainly ought to have a proper psychological education. What we call "medical psychology" is unfortunately a very one-sided affair. It may give you some knowledge of every-day complexes, but it knows far too little beyond the medical department. Psychology does not consist of medical rules of thumb, it has far more to do with the history of civilisation, of philosophy, or religion and quite particularly with primitive mentality. The pathological mind is a vast, almost un-explored, area and little has been done in this field, whereas the biology, anatomy and physiology of schizophrenia have had all the attention they want. And with all this work, what exact knowledge have we about heredity or the nature of the primary symptom? I should say: Let us discuss the question of psychogenesis once more when the psychical side of schizophrenia has had a fair deal.

14. Growth and Crises

ERIK H. ERIKSON

BASIC TRUST VERSUS BASIC MISTRUST

For the first component of a healthy personality I nominate a sense of *basic trust,* which I think is an attitude toward oneself and the world derived from the experiences of the first year of life. By "trust" I mean what is commonly implied in reasonable trustfulness as far as others are concerned and a simple sense of trustworthiness as far as oneself is concerned. When I say "basic," I mean that neither this component nor any of those that follow are, either in childhood or in adulthood, especially conscious. In fact, all of these criteria, when developed in childhood and when integrated in adulthood, blend into the total personality. Their crises in childhood, however, and their impairment in adulthood are clearly circumscribed.

In describing this growth and its crises as a development of a series of alternative basic attitudes, we take recourse to the term *"a sense of."* Like a "sense of health" or a "sense of not being well," such "senses" pervade surface and depth, consciousness and the unconscious. They are ways of conscious *experience,* accessible to introspection (where it develops); ways of *behaving,* observable by others; and unconscious *inner states* determinable by test and analysis. It is important to keep these three dimensions in mind, as we proceed.

In *adults* the impairment of basic trust is expressed in a *basic mistrust.* It characterizes individuals who withdraw into themselves in particular ways when at odds with themselves and with others. These ways, which often are not obvious, are more strikingly represented by individuals who regress into psychotic states in which they sometimes close up, refusing food and comfort and becoming oblivious to companionship. In so far as we hope to assist them with psychotherapy, we must try to reach them again in specific ways in order to convince them that they can trust the world and that they can trust themselves (Fromm-Reichmann, 1950).

It is from the knowledge of such radical regressions and of the deepest and most infantile layers in our not-so-sick patients that we have learned to regard basic trust as the cornerstone of a healthy personality. Let us see what justifies our placing the crisis and the ascendancy of this component at the beginning of life.

As the newborn infant is separated from his symbiosis with the mother's body, his inborn and more or less coordinated ability to take in by mouth meets the mother's more or less coordinated ability and intention to feed him and to welcome him. At this point he lives through, and loves with, his mouth; and the mother lives through, and loves with, her breasts.

For the mother this is a late and com-

From *Psychological Issues,* edited by G. S. Klein, pages 54–94, International Universities Press, 1959, by permission of the publisher. The original version of this paper appeared in *Symposium on the Healthy Personality,* Supplement II; Problems of Infancy and Childhood, Transactions of Fourth Conference, March, 1950, M. J. E. Senn, ed., New York: Josiah Macy, Jr. Foundation.

plicated accomplishment, highly dependent on her development as a woman; on her unconscious attitude toward the child; on the way she has lived through pregnancy and delivery; on her and her community's attitude toward the act of nursing—and on the response of the newborn. To him the mouth is the focus of a general first approach to life—the *incorporative* approach. In psychoanalysis this stage is usually referred to as the "oral" stage. Yet it is clear that, in addition to the overwhelming need for food, a baby is, or soon becomes receptive in many other respects. As he is willing and able to suck on appropriate objects and to swallow whatever appropriate fluids they emit, he is soon also willing and able to "take in" with his eyes whatever enters his visual field. His tactual senses, too, seem to "take in" what feels good. In this sense, then, one could speak of an *"incorporative stage,"* one in which he is, relatively speaking, receptive to what he is being offered. Yet many babies are sensitive and vulnerable, too. In order to ensure that their first experience in this world may not only keep them alive but also help them to coordinate their sensitive breathing and their metabolic and circulatory rhythms, we must see to it that we deliver to their senses stimuli as well as food in the proper intensity and at the right time; otherwise their willingness to accept may change abruptly into diffuse defense—or into lethargy.

Now, while it is quite clear what *must* happen to keep a baby alive (the minimum supply necessary) and what *must not* happen, lest he be physically damaged or chronically upset (the maximum early frustration tolerable), there is a certain leeway in regard to what *may* happen; and different cultures make extensive use of their prerogatives to decide what they consider workable and insist upon calling necessary. Some people think that a baby, lest he scratch his own eyes out, must necessarily be swaddled completely for the better part of the day and throughout the greater part of the first year; also, that he should be rocked or fed whenever he whimpers. Others think that he should feel the freedom of his kicking limbs as early as possible, but also that he, as a matter of course, be forced to cry "please" for his meals until he literally gets blue in the face. All of this (more or less consciously) seems related to the culture's general aim

and system. I have known some old American Indians who bitterly decried the way in which we often let our small babies cry because we believe that "it will make their lungs strong." No wonder (these Indians said) that the white man, after such an initial reception, seems to be in a hurry to get to the "next world." But the same Indians spoke proudly of the way their infants (breast fed into the second year) became blue in the face with fury when thumped on the head for "biting" the mother's nipples; here the Indians, in turn, believed that "it's going to make good hunters of them."

There is some intrinsic wisdom, some unconscious planning and much superstition in the seemingly arbitrary varieties of child training: what is "good for the child," what *may* happen to him, depends on what he is supposed to become and where.

At any rate, it is already in his earliest encounters that the human infant meets up with the basic modalities of his culture. The simplest and the earliest modality is *"to get,"* not in the sense of *"go and get"* but in that of receiving and accepting what is given; and this sounds easier than it is. For the groping and unstable newborn's organism learns this modality only as he learns to regulate his readiness to get with the methods of a mother who, in turn, will permit him to coordinate his means of getting as she develops and coordinates her means of giving. The mutuality of relaxation thus developed is of prime importance for the first experience of friendly otherness: from psychoanalysis one receives the impression that in thus *getting what is given,* and in learning to *get somebody to do* for him what he wishes to have done, the baby also develops the necessary groundwork to *get to be* the giver, to "identify" with her.

Where this *mutual regulation* fails, the situation falls apart into a variety of attempts to control by duress rather than by reciprocity. The baby will try to get by random activity what he cannot get by central suction; he will activate himself into exhaustion or he will find his thumb and damn the world. The mother's reaction may be to try to control matters by nervously changing hours, formulas, and procedures. One cannot be sure what this does to a baby; but it certainly is our clinical impression that in some sensitive individuals (or in individuals whose early frustration was never compensated for) such a situation can be a model for a radical disturbance in their relationship to the "world," to "people," and especially to loved or otherwise significant people.

There are ways of maintaining reciprocity by giving to the baby what he can get through other forms of feeding and by making up for what is missed orally through the satiation of other than oral receptors: his pleasure in being held, warmed, smiled at, talked to, rocked, and so forth. Besides such *"horizontal"* compensation (compensation during the same stage of development) there are many *"longitudinal"* compensations in life: compensations emerging from later stages of the life cycle.[1]

During the "second oral" stage the ability and the pleasure in a more active and more directed incorporative approach ripen. The teeth develop and with them the pleasure in biting *on* hard things, in biting *through* things, and in biting *off* things. This *active-incorporative* mode characterizes a variety of other activities (as did the first incorporative mode). The eyes, first part of a passive system of accepting impressions as they come along, have now learned to focus, to isolate, to "grasp" objects from the vaguer background and to follow them. The organs of hearing similarly have learned to discern significant sounds, to localize them, and to guide an appropriate change in position (lifting and turning the head, lifting and turning the upper body). The arms have learned to reach out determinedly and the hands to grasp firmly. We are more interested here in the over-all *configuration and final integration* of developing approaches to the world than in the *first appearance of specific abilities* which are

so well described in the child-development literature.[2]

With all of this a number of interpersonal patterns are established which center in the social modality of *taking* and *holding on to* things—things which are more or less freely offered and given, and things which have more or less a tendency to slip away. As the baby learns to change positions, to roll over, and very gradually to establish himself on the throne of his sedentary kingdom, he must perfect the mechanisms of grasping and appropriating, holding and chewing all that is within his reach.

The *crisis* of the oral stage (during the second part of the first year) is difficult to assess and more difficult to verify. It seems to consist of the coincidence in time of three developments: (1) a physiological one: the general tension associated with a more violent drive to incorporate, appropriate, and observe more actively (a tension to which is added the discomfort of "teething" and other changes in the oral machinery); (2) a psychological one: the infant's increasing awareness of himself as a distinct person; and (3) an environmental one: the mother's apparent turning away from the baby toward pursuits which she had given up during late pregnancy and postnatal care. These pursuits include her full return to conjugal intimacy and may soon lead to a new pregnancy.

Where breast feeding lasts into the biting stage (and, generally speaking, this has been the rule) it is now necessary to learn how to continue sucking without biting, so that the mother may not withdraw the nipple in pain or anger. Our clinical work indicates that this point in the individual's early history provides him with some sense of basic loss, leaving the general impression that once upon a time one's unity with a material matrix was destroyed. Weaning, therefore, should not mean sudden loss of the breast and loss of the mother's reassuring presence too, unless, of course, other women can be depended upon to sound

---

[1] My participation in the longitudinal research of the Institute of Child Welfare at the University of California (see Macfarlane, 1938; Erikson, 1951b) has taught me the greatest respect for the resiliency and resourcefulness of individual children who, with the support of an expanding economy and of a generous social group, learned to compensate for grievous early misfortunes of a kind which in our clinical histories would suffice to explain malfunctioning rather convincingly. The study gave me an opportunity to chart a decade of the life histories of about fifty (healthy) children, and to remain somewhat informed about the further fortunes of some of them. However, only the development of the identity concept . . . has helped me to approach an understanding of the mechanisms involved. I hope to publish my impressions.

---

[2] The reader trained in child development may want to pay special attention to the fact that one can think of a stage as the time when a capacity *first appears* (or appears in testable form) or as that period when it is so well *established* and integrated (has become an available apparatus for the ego, as we would say) that the next step in development can safely be initiated.

and feel much like the mother. A drastic loss of accustomed mother love without proper substitution at this time can lead (under otherwise aggravating conditions) to acute infantile depression (Spitz, 1945) or to a mild but chronic state of mourning which may give a depressive undertone to the whole remainder of life. But even under more favorable circumstances, this stage seems to introduce into the psychic life a sense of division and a dim but universal nostalgia for a lost paradise.

It is against the combination of these impressions of having been deprived, of having been divided, and of having been abandoned, all of which leave a residue of basic mistrust, that basic trust must be established and maintained.[3]

What we here call "trust" coincides with what Therese Benedek has called "confidence." If I prefer the word "trust," it is because there is more naiveté and more mutuality in it: an infant can be said to be trusting, but it would be assuming too much to say that he "has confidence." The general state of trust, furthermore, implies not only that one has learned to rely on the sameness and continuity of the outer providers but also that one may trust oneself and the capacity of one's own organs to cope with urges; that one is able to consider oneself trustworthy enough so that the providers will not need to be on guard or to leave.

In the psychiatric literature we find frequent references to an "oral character," which is a characterological deviation based on the unsolved conflicts of this stage. Wherever oral pessimism becomes dominant and exclusive, infantile fears, such as that of "being left empty," or simply of "being left," and also of being "starved of stimulation," can be discerned in the depressive forms of "being empty" and of "being no good." Such fears, in turn, can give orality that particular avaricious quality which in psychoanalysis is called "oral sadism," that is, a cruel need to get and to take in ways harmful to others. But there is an optimistic oral character, too, one which has learned to make giving and receiving the most important thing in life; and there is "orality" as a normal substratum in all individuals, a lasting residuum of this first period of dependency on powerful providers. It normally expresses itself in our dependencies and nostalgias, and in our all too hopeful and all too hopeless states. The integration of the oral stage with all the following ones results, in adulthood, in a combination of faith and realism.

The pathology and irrationality of oral trends depend entirely on the degree to which they are integrated with the rest of the personality and the degree to which they fit into the general cultural pattern and use approved interpersonal techniques for their expression.

Here, as elsewhere, we must therefore consider as a topic for discussion the expression of *infantile urges* in *cultural patterns* which one may (or may not) consider a pathological deviation in the total economic or moral system of a culture or a nation. One could speak, for example, of the invigorating belief in "chance," that traditional prerogative of American trust in one's own resourcefulness and in Fate's store of good intentions. This belief, at times, can be seen to degenerate—in large-scale gambling, or in "taking chances" in the form of an arbitrary and often suicidal provocation of Fate, or in the insistence that one has not only the right to an equal chance but also the privilege of being preferred over all other investors in the same general enterprise. In a similar way all the pleasant reassurances which can be derived (especially in good company) from old and new

---

[3]One of the chief misuses of the schema presented here is the connotation that the sense of trust (and all the other *positive* senses to be postulated) is an *achievement,* secured once and for all at a given stage. In fact, some writers are so intent on making an *achievement scale* out of these stages that they blithely omit all the *negative* senses (basic mistrust, etc.) which are and remain the dynamic counterpart of the positive senses throughout life. (See, for example, the "maturation chart" distributed at the National Congress of Parents and Teachers in Omaha, Nebraska [1958], which omits any reference to crises, and otherwise 'adapts" the stages presented here.)

What the child acquires at a given stage is a certain *ratio* between the positive and the negative which, if the balance is toward the positive, will help him to meet later crises with a better chance for unimpaired total development. The idea that at any stage a *goodness* is achieved which is impervious to new conflicts within and changes without is a projection on child development of that success ideology which so dangerously pervades our private and public daydreams and can make us inept in the face of a heightened struggle for a meaningful existence in our time.

Only in the light of man's inner division and social antagonism is a belief in his essential resourcefulness and creativity justifiable and productive.

taste sensations, from inhaling and im-
bibing, from munching and swallowing
and digesting, can turn into mass
addictions neither expressive of, nor conducive to, the kind of basic trust which
we have in mind.

Here we are obviously touching on
phenomena the analysis of which would
call for a comprehensive approach both to
personality and to culture. This would be
true also for an epidemiological approach
to the problem of the more or less malignant elaboration of the oral character in
"schizoid" characters and the mental diseases seemingly expressive of an underlying weakness in oral reassurance and
basic trust. A related problem is the belief
(reflected in much of contemporary ob-
stetric and pediatric concern with the
methods of child care) that the establishment of a basic sense of trust in earliest
childhood makes adult individuals less dependent on mild or malignant forms of addiction, on self-delusion, and on avaricious appropriation. Of this, little is
known; and the question remains whether
healthy orality makes for a healthy culture
or a healthy culture makes for healthy
orality—or both.

At any rate, the psychiatrists,
obstetricians, pediatricians, and anthropologists, to whom I feel closest, today would agree that the *firm establishment of enduring patterns for the balance
of basic trust over basic mistrust* is the
first task of the budding personality and
therefore first of all a task for maternal
care. But it must be said that the *amount
of trust* derived from earliest infantile experience does not seem to depend on
absolute *quantities of food or dem-
onstrations of love* but rather on the
quality of the maternal relationship.
Mothers create a sense of trust in their
children by that kind of administration
which in its quality combines sensitive
care of the baby's individual needs and a
firm sense of personal trustworthiness
within the trusted framework of their community's life style. (This forms the basis
in the child for a sense of identity which
will later combine a sense of being "all
right," of being oneself, and of becoming
what other people trust one will become.)
Parents must not only have certain ways
of guiding by prohibition and permission;
they must also be able to represent to the
child a deep, an almost somatic conviction
that there is a meaning to what they are

doing. In this sense a traditional system
of child care can be said to be a factor
making for trust, even where certain items
of that tradition, taken singly, may seem
irrational or unnecessarily cruel. Here
much depends on whether such items are
inflicted on the child by the parent in the
firm traditional belief that this is the only
way to do things or whether the parent
misuses his administration of the baby and
the child in order to work off anger, alleviate fear, or win an argument, with the
child or with somebody else (mother-
in-law, doctor, or priest).

In times of change—and what other
times are there, in our memory?—one
generation differs so much from another
that items of tradition often become disturbances. Conflicts between mother's
ways and one's own self-made ways,
conflicts between the expert's advice and
mother's ways, and conflicts between the
expert's authority and one's own self-
willed ways may disturb a mother's
trust in herself. Furthermore, all the
mass transformations in American life
(immigration, migration, and Americanization; industrialization, urbanization,
mechanization, and others) are apt to
disturb young mothers in those tasks
which are so simple yet so far-reaching.
No wonder, then, that the first section
of the first chapter of Benjamin Spock's
(1945) book is entitled "Trust Yourself." But while it is true that the expert obstetrician and pediatrician can do
much to replace the binding power of
tradition by giving reassurance and
guidance, he does not have the time to
become the father-confessor for all the
doubts and fears, angers and arguments
which can fill the minds of lonely young
parents. Maybe a book like Spock's needs
to be read in study groups where the true
psychological spirit of the town meeting
can be created; that is, where matters are
considered to be agreed upon not because
somebody said so, but because the free
airing of opinions and emotions, of prejudices and of errors has led to a general
area of relative consent and of tolerant
good will.

This chapter has become unduly long.
In regard to the matters discussed here
it is too bad that one must begin with the
beginning. We know so little of the beginning, of the deeper strata of the human
mind. But since we have already embarked on general observations, a word

must be said about one cultural and traditional institution which is deeply related to the matter of trust, namely, religion.

It is not the psychologist's job to decide whether religion should or should not be confessed and practiced in particular words and rituals. Rather the psychological observer must ask whether or not in any area under observation religion and tradition are living psychological forces creating the kind of faith and conviction which permeates a parent's personality and thus reinforces the child's basic trust in the world's trustworthiness. The psychopathologist cannot avoid observing that there are millions of people who cannot really afford to be without religion, and whose pride in not having it is that much whistling in the dark. On the other hand, there are millions who seem to derive faith from other than religious dogmas, that is, from fellowship, productive work, social action, scientific pursuit, and artistic creation. And again, there are millions who profess faith, yet in practice mistrust both life and man. With all of these in mind, it seems worth while to speculate on the fact that religion through the centuries has served to restore a sense of trust at regular intervals in the form of faith while giving tangible form to a sense of evil which it promises to ban. All religions have in common the periodical childlike surrender to a Provider or providers who dispense earthly fortune as well as spiritual health; the demonstration of one's smallness and dependence through the medium of reduced posture and humble gesture; the admission in prayer and song of misdeeds, of misthoughts, and of evil intentions; the admission of inner division and the consequent appeal for inner unification by divine guidance; the need for clearer self-delineation and self-restriction; and finally, the insight that individual trust must become a common faith, individual mistrust a commonly formulated evil, while the individual's need for restoration must become part of the ritual practice of many, and must become a sign of trustworthiness in the community.

Whosoever says he has religion must derive a faith from it which is transmitted to infants in the form of basic trust; whosoever claims that he does not need religion must derive such basic faith from elsewhere.

AUTONOMY VERSUS SHAME AND DOUBT

A survey of some of the items discussed in Spock's book under the headings "The One-Year-Old" and "Managing Young Children" will enable those of us who, at this time, do not have such inquisitive creatures in our homes to remember our skirmishes, our victories, and our defeats:

> Feeling his oats.
> The passion to explore.
> He gets more dependent and more independent at the same time.
> Arranging the house for a wandering baby.
> Avoiding accidents.
> Now's the time to put poisons out of reach.
> How do you make him leave certain things alone?
> Dropping and throwing things.
> Children learn to control their own aggressive feelings.
> Biting humans.
> Keeping bedtime happy.
> The small child who won't stay in bed at night.

My selection is intended to convey the inventory and range of problems described though I cannot review here either the doctor's excellent advice or his good balance in depicting the remarkable ease and matter-of-factness with which the nursery may be governed at this as at any other stage. Nevertheless, there is an indication of the sinister forces which are leashed and unleashed, especially in the guerilla warfare of unequal wills; for the child is often unequal to his own violent drives, and parent and child unequal to each other.

The over-all significance of this stage lies in the maturation of the muscle system, the consequent ability (and doubly felt inability) to coordinate a number of highly conflicting action patterns such as "holding on" and "letting go," and the enormous value with which the still highly dependent child begins to endow his autonomous will.

Psychoanalysis has enriched our vocabulary with the word "anality" to designate the particular pleasurableness and willfulness which often attach to the eliminative organs at this stage. The whole procedure of evacuating the bowels and the bladder as completely as possible is, of course, enhanced from the beginning by a premium of "feeling good" which says in effect, "well done." This premium, at the beginning of life, must make up for quite frequent discomfort and tension suffered as the bowels learn to do their daily work. Two developments gradually give these anal experiences the necessary volume: the arrival of better formed stool and the general coordination of the muscle system which permits the development of voluntary release, of dropping and throwing away. This new dimension of approach to things, however, is not restricted to the sphincters. A general ability, indeed, a violent need, develops to drop and to throw away and to alternate withholding and expelling at will.

As far as anality proper is concerned, at this point everything depends on whether the cultural environment wants to make something of it. There are cultures where the parents ignore anal behavior and leave it to older children to lead the toddler out to the bushes so that his compliance in this matter may coincide with his wish to imitate the bigger ones. Our Western civilization, and especially certain classes within it, have chosen to take the matter more seriously. It is here that the machine age has added the ideal of a mechanically trained, faultlessly functioning, and always clean, punctual, and deodorized body. In addition it has been more or less consciously assumed that early and rigorous training is absolutely necessary for the kind of personality which will function efficiently in a mechanized world which says "time is money" and which calls for orderliness, punctuality, and thrift. Indications are that in this, we have gone too far; that we have assumed that a child is an animal which must be broken or a machine which must be set and tuned—while, in fact, human virtues can grow only by steps. At any rate our clinical work suggests that the neurotics of our time include the "over-compulsive" type, who is stingy, retentive, and meticulous in matters of affection, time, and money, as well as in matters concerning his bowels. Also, bowel and bladder training has become the most obviously disturbing item of child training in wide circles of our society.

What, then, makes the anal problem potentially important and difficult?

The anal zone lends itself more than any other to the expression of stubborn insistence on conflicting impulses because, for one thing, it is the model zone for two contradictory modes which must become alternating; namely, *retention* and *elimination*. Furthermore, the sphincters are only part of the muscle system with its general ambiguity of rigidity and relaxation, of flexion and extension. This whole stage, then, becomes a battle for *autonomy*. For as he gets ready to stand on his feet more firmly, the infant delineates his world as "I" and "you," "me" and "mine." Every mother knows how astonishingly pliable a child may be at this stage, if and when he has made the decision that he *wants* to do what he is supposed to do. It is impossible, however, to find a reliable formula for making him want to do just that. Every mother knows how lovingly a child at this stage will snuggle and how ruthlessly he will suddenly try to push the adult away. At the same time the child is apt both to hoard things and to discard them, to cling to possessions and to throw them out of the windows of houses and vehicles. All of these seemingly contradictory tendencies, then, we include under the formula of the retentive-eliminative modes.

The matter of mutual regulation between adult and child now faces its severest test. If outer control by too rigid or too early training insists on robbing the child of his attempt *gradually* to control his bowels and other functions willingly and by his free choice, he will again be faced with a double rebellion and a double defeat. Powerless in his own body (sometimes afraid of his bowels) and powerless outside, he will again be forced to seek satisfaction and control either by regression or by fake progression. In other words, he will return to an earlier, oral control, that is, by sucking his thumb and becoming whiny and demanding; or he will become hostile and willful, often using his feces (and, later, dirty words) as ammunition; or he will pretend an autonomy and an ability to do without anybody to lean on which he has by no means really gained.

This stage, therefore, becomes decisive for the ratio between love and hate, for that between cooperation and willfulness, and for that between the freedom of self-expression and its suppression. From a sense of *self-control without loss of self-esteem* comes a lasting sense of autonomy and pride; from a sense of muscular and anal impotence, of loss of self-control, and of parental overcontrol comes a lasting sense of doubt and shame.

To develop autonomy, a firmly developed and a convincingly continued stage of early trust is necessary. The infant must come to feel that basic faith in himself and in the world (which is the lasting treasure saved from the conflicts of the oral stage) will not be jeopardized by this sudden violent wish to have a choice, to appropriate demandingly, and to eliminate stubbornly. *Firmness* must protect him against the potential anarchy of his as yet untrained sense of discrimination, his inability to hold on and to let go with circumspection. Yet his environment must back him up in his wish to "stand on his own feet" lest he be overcome by that sense of having exposed himself prematurely and foolishly which we call shame, or that secondary mistrust, that "doubletake," which we call doubt.

Shame is an infantile emotion insufficiently studied. Shame supposes that one is completely exposed and conscious of being looked at—in a word, self-conscious. One is visible and not ready to be visible; that is why we dream of shame as a situation in which we are stared at in a condition of incomplete dress, in night attire, "with one's pants down." Shame is early expressed in an impulse to bury one's face, or to sink, right then and there, into the ground. This potentiality is abundantly utilized in the educational method of "shaming" used so exclusively by some primitive peoples, where it supplants the often more destructive sense of guilt to be discussed later. The destructiveness of shaming is balanced in some civilizations by devices for *"saving face."* Shaming exploits an increasing sense of being small, which paradoxically develops as the child stands up and as his awareness permits him to note the relative measures of size and power.

Too much shaming does not result in a sense of propriety but in a secret determination to try to get away with things when unseen, if, indeed, it does not result in deliberate *shamelessness.* There is an impressive American ballad in which a murderer to be hanged on the gallows before the eyes of the community, instead of feeling appropriately afraid or ashamed, begins to berate the onlookers, ending every salvo of defiance with the words, "God damn your eyes." Many a small child, when shamed beyond endurance, may be in a mood (although not in possession of either the courage or the words) to express defiance in similar terms. What I mean by this sinister reference is that there is a limit to a child's and an adult's individual endurance in the face of demands which force him to consider himself, his body, his needs, and his wishes as evil and dirty, and to believe in the infallibility of those who pass such judgment. Occasionally he may be apt to turn things around, to become secretly oblivious to the opinion of others, and to consider as evil only the fact that they exist: his chance will come when they are gone, or when he can leave them.

Many a defiant child, many a young criminal, is of such makeup, and deserves at least an investigation into the conditions which caused him to become that way.

To repeat: muscular maturation sets the stage for experimentation with two simultaneous sets of social modalities —*holding on* and *letting go.* As is the case with all of these modalities, their basic conflicts can lead in the end either to hostile or to benign expectations and attitudes. Thus, "to hold" can become a destructive and cruel retaining or restraining, and it can become a pattern of care: "to have and to hold." To "let go," too, can turn into an inimical letting loose of destructive forces, or it can become a relaxed "to let pass" and "to let be." Culturally speaking, these modalities are neither good nor bad; their value depends on whether their hostile implications are turned against enemy or fellow man—or against the self.

The last-named danger is the one best known to psychiatry. Denied the gradual and well-guided experience of the autonomy of free choice, or weakened by an initial loss of trust, the sensitive child may turn against himself all his urge to discriminate and to manipulate. He will *overmanipulate himself,* he will develop a *precocious conscience.* Instead of taking possession of things in order to test them by repetitive play, he will become obssessed by his own repetitiveness; he will want to have everything "just so," and only in a given sequence and tempo. By such infantile obsessiveness, by dawdling, for example, or by becoming a stickler for certain rituals, the child then learns to gain power over his parents and nurses in areas where he could not find large scale mutual regulation with them. Such hollow victory, then, is the infantile model for a compulsion neurosis. As for the consequences of this for adult character, they can be observed in the classical compulsive character which we have mentioned. We must add to this the character dominated by the wish to "get away with" things—yet unable to get away even with the wish. For while he learns evasion from others, his precocious conscience does not let him really get away with anything, and he goes through life habitually ashamed, apologetic, and afraid to be seen; or else, in a manner which we call "overcompensatory," he evinces a defiant kind of autonomy. Real inner autonomy, however, is not carried on the sleeve.

But it is time to return from these considerations of the abnormal to a study of the headings which transmit the practical and benevolent advice of the children's doctor. They all add up to this: be firm and tolerant with the child at this stage, and he will be firm and tolerant with himself. He will feel pride in being an autonomous person; he will grant autonomy to others; and now and again he will even let himself get away with something.

Why, then, if we know how, do we not tell parents in detail what to do to develop this intrinsic, this genuine autonomy? The answer is: because when it comes to human values, nobody knows how to fabricate or manage the fabrication of the genuine article. My own field, psychoanalysis, having studied particularly the excessive increase of guilt feelings beyond any normal rhyme or reason, and the consequent excessive estrangement of the child from his own body, attempted at least to formulate what should *not* be done to children. These formulations, however, often aroused superstitious inhibitions in those who were inclined to make anxious rules out of vague warnings. Actually, we are learning only gradually

what exactly *not* to do with *what kind* of children at *what age*.

People all over the world seem convinced that to make the right (meaning *their*) kind of human being, one must consistently introduce the senses of shame, doubt, guilt and fear into a child's life. Only the patterns vary. Some cultures begin to restrict early in life, some late, some abruptly, others more gradually. Until enough comparative observations are available, we are apt to add further superstitions, merely because of our wish to *avoid* certain pathological conditions, without even knowing definitely all the factors which are responsible for these conditions. So we say: Don't wean too early; don't train too early. But what is too early and what is too late seem to depend not only on the pathologies we wish to avoid but also on the values we wish to create, or, to put it more honestly, on the values we wish to live by. For no matter what we do in detail, the child will feel primarily what we live by, what makes us loving, cooperative, and firm beings, and what makes us hateful, anxious, and divided in ourselves.

There are of course a few matters of necessary avoidance which become clear from our basic epigenetic point of view. It will be remembered that every new development carries with it its own specific vulnerability. For example, at around eight months the child seems to be somehow more aware, as it were, of his *separateness;* this prepares him for the impending sense of autonomy. At the same time he becomes more cognizant of his mother's features and presence and of the strangeness of others. Sudden or prolonged separation from his mother at that time apparently can cause a sensitive child to experience an aggravation of the experience of division and abandonment, arousing violent anxiety and withdrawal. Again, in the first quarter of the second year, if everything has gone well, the infant just begins to become aware of the autonomy discussed in this chapter. The introduction of bowel training at this time may cause him to resist with all his strength and determination, because he seems to feel that his budding will is being "broken." To avoid this feeling is certainly more important than to insist on his being trained just then because there is a time for the stubborn ascendancy of autonomy and there is a time for the partial sacrifice of secure autonomy, but obviously the time for a meaningful sacrifice is *after* one has acquired and reinforced a core of autonomy and has also acquired more insight.

The more exact localization in time of the most critical growth periods of the personality is becoming established only now. Often, the unavoidable cause of trouble is not one event but the coincidence in time of a number of changes which upset the child's orientation. He may have been involved in a special growth period when the family moved to a new place. Perhaps he was forced to conceive of his first words all over again when the grandmother who had taught him these words suddenly died. A trip on the part of the mother may have exhausted her because she happened to be pregnant at the time, and thus unable, on returning, to make proper amends. Given the right spirit toward life and its vicissitudes, a parent can usually handle such matters, if necessary with the help of the pediatrician or guidance expert. The expert's job, however, should be (to quote Frank Fremont-Smith) *"to set the frame of reference within which choice is permissible and desirable."* For in the last analysis (as comparative studies in child training have convinced many of us) the kind and degree of a sense of autonomy which parents are able to grant their small children depends on the dignity and the sense of personal independence which they derive from their own lives. Again, just as the sense of trust is a reflection of the parent's sturdy and realistic faith, so is the sense of autonomy a reflection of the parents' dignity as individuals.

As was the case with "oral" personality, the compulsive personality (often referred to as "anal" in the psychiatric literature) has its normal aspects and its abnormal exaggerations. If well integrated with other compensatory traits, some compulsiveness is useful in the administration of matters in which order, punctuality, and cleanliness are essential. The question is always whether we remain the masters of the rules by which we want to make things more manageable (not more complicated) or whether the rules master the ruler. But it often happens, in the individual as well as in group life, that the letter of the rules kills the spirit which created them.

We have related basic trust to the institution of religion. The basic need of the individual for a delineation of his *autonomy* in the adult order of things seems, in turn, to be taken care of by the *principle of "law and order,"* which in daily life as well as in the high courts of law apportions to each his privileges and his limitations, his obligations and his rights. The sense of autonomy which arises, or should arise, in the second stage of childhood, is fostered by a handling of the small individual which expresses a sense of rightful dignity and lawful independence on the part of the parents and which gives him the confident expectation that the kind of autonomy fostered in childhood will not be frustrated later. This, in turn, necessitates a relationship of parent to parent, of parent to employer, and of parent to government which reaffirms the parent's essential dignity within the hierarchy of social positions. It is important to dwell on this point because much of the shame and doubt, much of the indignity and uncertainty which is aroused in children is a consequence of the parents' frustrations in marriage, in work, and in citizenship. Thus, the sense of autonomy in the child (a sense richly fostered in American childhood in general) must be backed up by the preservation in economic and political life of a high sense of autonomy and of self-reliance.

Social organization assigns with the power of government certain privileges of leadership and certain obligations of conduct; while it imposes on the ruled certain obligations of compliance and certain privileges of remaining autonomous and self-determining. Where this whole matter becomes blurred, however, the matter of individual autonomy becomes an issue of mental health, as well as one of economic reorientation. Where large numbers of people have been prepared in childhood to expect from life a high degree of personal autonomy, pride, and opportunity, and then in later life find themselves ruled by superhuman organizations and machinery too intricate to understand, the result may be deep chronic disappointment not conducive to healthy personalities willing to grant each other a measure of autonomy. All great nations (and all the small ones) are increasingly challenged by the complication and mechanization of modern life, and are being enveloped in the problems of the organization of larger units, larger spheres, and larger interdependencies which by necessity redefine the role of the individual. It is important for the spirit of this country, as it is for that of the world, that an increased consciousness of equality and individuality may grow out of the necessity for divided function within the increasing complexity of organization; for otherwise a number of fears are aroused which find expression in anxiety on a large scale, often individually slight and hardly conscious, but nevertheless strangely upsetting to people who seemingly, on the surface, have what they want or what they seem to have a right to expect. Besides irrational fears of losing one's autonomy—"don't fence me in"—there are fears of being sabotaged in one's free will by inner enemies; of being restricted and constricted in one's autonomous initiative; and, paradoxically enough, at the same time of not being completely controlled enough, of not being told what to do. While many such fears are, of course, based on the realistic appraisal of dangers inherent in complex social organizations and in the struggle for power, safety, and security, they seem to contribute to psychoneurotic and psychosomatic disturbances on the one hand, and, on the other, to the easy acceptance of slogans which seem to promise alleviation of conditions by excessive and irrational conformity.

INITIATIVE VERSUS GUILT

Having found a firm solution of his problem of autonomy, the child of four and five is faced with the next step—and with the next crisis. Being firmly convinced that he *is* a person, the child must now find out *what kind* of a person he is going to be. And here he hitches his wagon to nothing less than a star: he wants to be like his parents, who to him appear very powerful and very beautiful, although quite unreasonably dangerous. He "identifies with them," he plays with the idea of how it would be to be them. Three strong developments help at this stage, yet also serve to bring the child closer to his crisis: (1) he learns to *move around* more freely and more violently and therefore establishes a wider and, so it seems to him, an unlimited radius of goals; (2) his sense of *language* becomes perfected to the point where he understands and can ask about many things just enough to misunderstand them thoroughly; and (3) both language and locomotion permit him to expand his *imagination* over so many things that he cannot avoid frightening himself with what he himself has dreamed and thought up. Nevertheless, out of all this he must emerge with a sense of *unbroken initiative* as a basis for a high and yet realistic sense of ambition and independence.

One may ask here—one may, indeed—what are the criteria for such an unbroken sense of initiative? The criteria for all the senses discussed here are the same: a crisis, beset with fears, or at least a general anxiousness or tension, seems to be resolved, in that the child suddenly seems to "grow together" both psychologically and physically. He seems to be "more himself," more loving and relaxed and brighter in his judgment (such as it is at this stage). Most of all, he seems to be, as it were, self-activated; he is in the free possession of a certain surplus of energy which permits him to forget failures quickly and to approach what seems desirable (even if it also seems dangerous) with undiminished and better aimed effort. In this way the child and his parents face the next crisis much better prepared.

We are now approaching the end of the third year, when walking is getting to be a thing of ease, or vigor. The books tell us that a child "can walk" much before this; but from the point of view of personality development he cannot really walk as long as he is only able to accomplish the feat more or less well, with more or fewer props, for short spans of time. He has made walking and running an item in his sphere of mastery when gravity is felt to be *within*, when he can forget that he is doing the walking and instead can find out what he can do *with it.* Only then do his legs become an unconscious part of him instead of being an external and still unreliable ambulatory appendix. Only then will he find out with advantage what he now *may* do, along with what he *can* do.

To look back: the first way-station was prone relaxation. The trust based on the experience that the basic mechanisms of breathing, digesting, sleeping, and so forth have a consistent and familiar relation to the foods and comforts offered gives zest to the developing ability to raise oneself to a sitting and then to a standing position. The second way-station (accomplished only securely but, as it were, untiringly, a feat which permits the muscle system gradually to be used for finer discrimination and for more autonomous ways of selecting and discarding, of piling things up—and of throwing them away with a bang.

The third way-station finds the child able to move independently and vigorously. He is ready to visualize himself as being as big as the perambulating grown-ups. He begins to make comparisons and is apt to develop untiring curiousity about differences in sizes in general, and sexual differences in particular. He tries to comprehend possible future roles, or at any rate to understand what roles are worth imitating. More immediately, he can now associate with those of his own age. Under the guidance of older children or special women guardians, he gradually enters into the infantile politics of nursery school, street corner, and barnyard. His learning now is eminently intrusive and vigorous: it leads away from his own limitations and into future possibilities.

The *intrusive mode,* dominating much of the behavior of this stage, characterizes a variety of configurationally "similar" activities and fantasies. These include the intrusion into other bodies by physical attack; the intrusion into other people's ears and minds by aggressive talking; the intrusion into space by vigorous locomotion; the intrusion into the unknown by consuming curiosity.

This is also the stage of infantile sexual curiosity, genital excitability, and occasional preoccupation and over-concern with sexual matters. This "genitality" is, of course, rudimentary, a mere promise of things to come; often it is not particularly noticeable as such. If not specifically provoked into precocious manifestation by especially strict and pointed prohibitions ("if you touch it, the doctor will cut it off") or special customs (such as sex play in groups), it is apt to lead to no more than a series of fascinating experiences which soon become frightening and pointless enough to be repressed. This leads to the ascendancy of that human specialty which Freud called the

"latency" period, that is, the long delay separating infantile sexuality (which in animals is followed by maturity) and physical sexual maturation.

The sexual orientation of the boy is focused on the phallus and its sensations, purposes, and meanings. While erections undoubtedly occur earlier (either reflexively or in response to things and people who make the child feel intensively), a focused interest may now develop in the genitalia of both sexes, as well as an urge to perform playful sex acts, or at least acts of sexual investigation. The increased locomotor mastery and the pride in being big now and *almost* as good as father and mother receives its severest setback in the clear fact that in the genital sphere one is vastly inferior; furthermore, it receives an additional setback in the fact that not even in the distant future is one ever going to be father in sexual relationship to mother, or mother in sexual relationship to father. The very deep emotional consequences of this insight and the magic fears associated with it make up what Freud has called the oedipus complex.

Psychoanalysis verifies the simple conclusion that boys attach their first genital affection to the maternal adults who have otherwise given comfort to their bodies and that they develop their first sexual rivalry against the persons who are the sexual owners of those maternal persons. The little girl, in turn, becomes attached to her father and other important men and jealous of her mother, a development which may cause her much anxiety, for it seems to block her retreat to that self-same mother, while it makes the mother's disapproval ever so much more magically dangerous because unconsciously "deserved."

Girls often have a difficult time at this stage, because they observe sooner or later that, although their locomotor, mental, and social intrusiveness is increased equally with, and is as adequate as, that of the boys, thus permitting them to become perfect tomboys, they lack one item: the penis; and with it, important prerogatives in some cultures and classes. While the boy has this visible, erectable, and comprehensible organ to which he can attach dreams of adult bigness, the girl's clitoris only poorly sustains dreams of sexual equality. She does not even have breasts as analogously tangible tokens of her future, her maternal drives are relegated to play fantasy or baby tending. On the other hand, where mothers dominate households, the boy, in turn, can develop a sense of inadequacy because he learns at this stage that while a boy can do well in play and work, he will never boss the house, the mother, and the older sisters. His mother and sisters, in fact, might get even with him for vast doubts in themselves by making him feel that a boy (with his snails and puppy-dog tails) is really an inferior if not a repulsive creature. Both the girl and the boy are now extraordinarily appreciative of any convincing promise of the fact that someday they will be as good as father or mother—perhaps better; and they are grateful for sexual enlightenment, a little at a time, and patiently repeated at intervals. Where the necessities of economic life and the simplicity of its social plan make the male and female roles and their specific powers and rewards comprehensible, the early misgivings about sexual differences are, of course, more easily integrated in the culture's design for the differentiation of sexual roles.

This stage adds to the inventory of basic social modalities in both sexes that of "making" in the older and today slangier sense of "being on the make." There is no simpler, stronger word to match the social modalities previously enumerated. The word suggests enjoyment of competition, insistence on goal, pleasure of conquest. In the boy the emphasis remains on "making" by head-on attack; in the girl it may change to "making" by making herself attractive and endearing. The child thus develops the prerequisites for *masculine* and *feminine initiative,* that is, for the selection of social goals and perseverance in approaching them. Thus the stage is all set for entrance into life, except that life must first be school life. The child here must repress or forget many of his fondest hopes and most energetic wishes, while his exuberant imagination is tamed and he learns the necessary self-restraint and the necessary interest in impersonal things —even the three R's. This often demands a change of personality that is sometimes too drastic for the good of the child. This change is not only a result of education but also of an inner reorientation, and it is based on a biological fact

(the delay of sexual maturation) and a psychological one (the repression of childhood wishes). For those sinister oedipal wishes (so simply and so trustingly expressed in the boy's assurance that he will marry mother and make her proud of him and in the girl's that she will marry father and take much better care of him), in consequence of vastly increased imagination and, as it were, the intoxication of increased locomotor powers, seem to lead to secret fantasies of terrifying proportions. The consequence is a deep sense of *guilt*—a strange sense, for it forever seems to imply that the individual has committed crimes and deeds which, after all, were not only not committed but also would have been biologically quite impossible.

While the struggle for autonomy at its worst concentrated on keeping rivals out, and was therefore more an expression of *jealous rage* most often directed against encroachments by *younger* siblings, initiative brings with it *anticipatory rivalry* with those who were there first and who may therefore occupy with their superior equipment the field toward which one's initiative is directed. Jealousy and rivalry, those often embittered and yet essentially futile attempts at demarcating a sphere of unquestioned privilege, now come to a climax in a final contest for a favored position with one of the parents; the inevitable and necessary failure leads to guilt and anxiety. The child indulges in fantasies of being a giant and a tiger, but in his dreams he runs in terror for dear life. This, then, is the stage of fear for life and limb, including the fear of losing (or on the part of the girl the conviction that she may have lost) the male genital as punishment for the fantasies attached to infantile genital excitement.

All of this may seem strange to readers who have only seen the sunnier side of childhood and have not recognized the potential powerhouse of destructive drives which can be aroused and temporarily buried at this stage, only to contribute later to the inner arsenal of a destructiveness so ready to be used when opportunity provokes it. By using the words "potential," "provoke" and "opportunity," I mean to emphasize that there is little in these inner developments which cannot be harnessed to constructive and peaceful initiative if only we learn to understand the conflicts and anxieties of childhood and the importance of child-hood for mankind. But if we should choose to overlook or belittle the phenomena of childhood, or to regard them as "cute" (even as the individual forgets the best and the worst dreams of his childhood), we shall forever overlook one of the eternal sources of human anxiety and strife.

It is at this stage of initiative that the great governor of initiative, namely, *conscience,* becomes firmly established. Only as a dependent does man develop conscience, that dependence on himself which makes him, in turn, dependable; and only when thoroughly dependable with regard to a number of fundamental values can he become independent and teach and develop tradition.

The child now feels not only ashamed when found out but also afraid of being found out. He now hears, as it were, God's voice without seeing God. Moreover, he begins automatically to feel guilty even for mere thoughts and for deeds which nobody has watched. This is the cornerstone of morality in the individual sense. But from the point of view of mental health, we must point out that if this great achievement is overburdened by all too eager adults, it can be bad for the spirit and for morality itself. For the conscience of the child *can* be primitive, cruel, and uncompromising, as may be observed in instances where children learn to constrict themselves to the point of over-all inhibition; where they develop an obedience more literal than the one the parent wishes to exact; or where they develop deep regressions and lasting resentments because the parents themselves do not seem to live up to the new conscience which they have fostered in the child. One of the deepest conflicts in life is the hate for a parent who served as the model and the executor of the conscience but who (in some form) was found trying to "get away with" the very transgressions which the child can no longer tolerate in himself. These transgressions often are the natural outcome of the existing inequality between parent and child. Often, however, they represent a thoughtless exploitation of such inequality; with the result that the child comes to feel that the whole matter is not one of universal goodness but of arbitrary power. The suspiciousness and evasiveness which is thus mixed in with the all-

or-nothing quality of the superego, that organ of tradition, makes moralistic man a great potential danger to himself and to his fellow men. It is as if morality, to him, became synonymous with vindictiveness and with the suppression of others.

It is necessary to point to the source of such moralism (not to be mistaken for morality) in the child of this age because infantile moralism is a stage to be lived through and worked through. The consequences of the guilt aroused at this stage (guilt expressed in a deep-seated conviction that the child as such, or drive as such, is essentially bad) often do not show until much later, when conflicts over initiative may find expression in a self-restriction which keeps an individual from living up to his inner capacities or to the powers of his imagination and feeling (if not in relative sexual impotence or frigidity). All of this, of course, may in turn be "overcompensated" in a great show of tireless initiative, in a quality of "go-at-itiveness" at all cost. Many adults feel that their worth as people consists entirely in *what they are doing,* or rather in *what they are going to do next,* and not in what they are, as individuals. The strain consequently developed in their bodies, which are always "on the go," with the engine racing, even at moments of rest, is a powerful contribution to the much-discussed psychosomatic diseases of our time.

Pathology, however, is only the sign that valuable human resources are being neglected, that they have been neglected first of all in childhood. The problem is again one of mutual regulation. Where the child, now so ready to overrestrict himself, can gradually develop a sense of responsibility, where he can gain some simple feeling for the institutions, functions, and roles which will permit him to anticipate his responsible participation as an adult, he will soon find pleasurable accomplishment in wielding miniature tools and weapons, in manipulating meaningful toys, and in taking care of himself—and of younger children.

For such is the wisdom of the ground plan that at no time is the individual more ready to learn quickly and avidly, to become big in the sense of sharing obligation, discipline, and performance rather than power, in the sense of *making things, instead of "making" people,* than during this period of his development. He is also eager and able to *make things together,* to combine with other children for the purpose of constructing and planning, instead of trying to boss and coerce them; and he is able and willing to profit fully by the association with teachers and ideal prototypes.

Parents often do not realize why some children suddenly seem to think less of them and seem to attach themselves to teachers, to the parents of other children, or to people representing occupations which the child can grasp: firemen and policemen, gardeners and plumbers. The point is that children do not wish to be reminded of the principal inequality with the parent of the same sex. They remain identified with this same parent; but for the present they look for opportunities where superficial identification seems to promise a field of initiative without too much conflict or guilt.

Often, however (and this seems more typical of the American home than of any other in the world), the child can be guided by the parent himself into a second, a more realistic identification based on the spirit of equality experienced in doing things together. In connection with comprehensible technical tasks, a companionship may develop between father and son, an experience of essential *equality in worth,* in spite of the *inequality in time schedules*. Such companionship is a lasting treasure not only for parent and child but for mankind, which so sorely needs an alleviation of all those hidden hatreds which stem from the exploitation of weakness because of mere size or schedule.

Only a combination of early prevention and alleviation of hatred and guilt in the growing being, and the consequent handling of hatred in the free collaboration of people who feel *equal in worth although different in kind or function or age,* permits a peaceful cultivation of initiative, a truly free sense of enterprise. And the word "enterprise" was deliberately chosen. For a comparative view of child training suggests that it is the prevalent economic ideal, or some of its modifications, which is transmitted to the child at the time when, in identification with his parent, he applies the dreams of early childhood to the as yet dim goals of an active adult life.

INDUSTRY VERSUS INFERIORITY

One might say that personality at the first stage crystallizes around the conviction "I am what I am given," and that of the second, "I am what I will." The third can be characterized by "I am what I can imagine I will be." We must now approach the fourth: "I am what I learn." The child now wants to be shown how to get busy with something and how to be busy with others.

This trend, too, starts much earlier, especially in some children. They want to watch how things are done and to try doing them. If they are lucky they live near barnyards or on streets around busy people and around many other children of all ages, so that they can watch and try, observe and participate as their capacities and their initiative grow in tentative spurts. But now it is time to *go to school*. In all cultures, at this stage, children receive some systematic instruction, although it is by no means always in the kind of school which literate people must organize around teachers who have learned how to teach literacy. In preliterate people much is learned from adults who become teachers by acclamation rather than by appointment; and very much is learned from older children. What is learned in more primitive surroundings is related to the basic skills of *technology* which are developed as the child gets ready to handle the utensils, the tools, and the weapons used by the big people: he enters the technology of his tribe very gradually but also very directly. More literate people, with more specialized careers, must prepare the child by teaching him things which first of all make him literate. He is then given the widest possible basic education for the greatest number of possible careers. The greater the specialization, the more indistinct the goal of initiative becomes; and the more complicated the social reality, the vaguer the father's and mother's role in it. Between childhood and adulthood, then, our children go to school; and school seems to be a world all by itself, with its own goals and limitations, its achievements and disappointments.

Grammar-school education has swung back and forth between the extreme of making early school life an extension of grim adulthood by emphasizing self-restraint and a strict sense of duty in doing what one is *told* to do, and the other extreme of making it an extension of the natural tendency in childhood to find out by playing, to learn what one must do by doing steps which one *likes* to do. Both methods work for some children at times but not for all children at all times. The first trend, if carried to the extreme, exploits a tendency on the part of the preschool and grammar-school child to become entirely dependent on prescribed duties. He thus learns much that is absolutely necessary and he develops an unshakable sense of duty; but he may never unlearn again an unnecessary and costly self-restraint with which he may later make his own life and other people's lives miserable, and in fact spoil his own children's natural desire to learn and to work. The second trend, when carried to an extreme, leads not only to the well-known popular objection that children do not learn anything any more but also to such feelings in children as are expressed in the by now famous remark of a metropolitan child who apprehensively asked one morning: "Teacher, *must* we do today what we *want* to do?" Nothing could better express the fact that children at this age *do* like to be mildly but firmly coerced into the adventure of finding out that one can learn to accomplish things which one would never have thought of by oneself, things which owe their attractiveness to the very fact that they are *not* the product of play and fantasy but the product of reality, practicality, and logic; things which thus provide a token sense of participation in the real world of adults. In discussions of this kind it is common to say that one must steer a middle course between play and work, between childhood and adulthood, between old-fashioned and progressive education. It is always easy (and it seems entirely satisfactory to one's critics) to say that one plans to steer a middle course, but in practice it often leads to a course charted by avoidances rather than by zestful goals. Instead of pursuing, then, a course which merely avoids the extremes of easy play or hard work, it may be worth while to consider what play is and what work is, and then learn to dose and alternate each in such a way that *play is play and work is work*. Let us review briefly what play may mean at various stages of childhood and adulthood.

The adult plays for purposes of recreation. He steps out of his reality into imaginary realities for which he has made up arbitrary but nonetheless binding rules. But an adult rarely gets away with being a playboy. Only he who works shall play —if, indeed, he can relax his competitiveness.

The playing child, then, poses a problem: whoever does not work shall not play. Therefore, to be tolerant of the child's play the adult must invent theories which show either that childhood play is really the child's work or that it does not count. The most popular theory, and the easiest on the observer, is that the child is nobody yet and that the nonsense of his play reflects it. According to Spencer, play uses up surplus energy in the young of a number of mammalians who do not need to feed or protect themselves because their parents do it for them. Others say that play is either preparation for the future or a method of working off past emotion, a means of finding imaginary relief for past frustrations.

It is true that the content of individual play often proves to be the infantile way of thinking over difficult experiences and of *restoring a sense of mastery,* comparable to the way in which we repeat, in ruminations and in endless talk, in daydreams and in dreams during sleep, experiences that have been too much for us. This is the rationale for play observation, play diagnosis, and play therapy. In watching a child play, the trained observer can get an impression of what it is the child is "thinking over," and what faulty logic, what emotional dead end he may be caught in. As a diagnostic tool such observation has become indispensable.

The small world of manageable toys is a harbor which the child establishes, returning to it when he needs to overhaul his ego. But the thing-world has its own laws: it may resist rearrangement or it may simply break to pieces; it may prove to belong to somebody else and be subject to confiscation by superiors. Thus, play may seduce the child into an unguarded expression of dangerous themes and attitudes which arouse anxiety and lead to sudden *disruption of play*. This is the counterpart, in waking life, of the anxiety dream; it can keep children from trying to play just as the fear of night terror can keep them from going to sleep. If thus frightened or disappointed, the child may regress into daydreaming, thumb sucking, masturbating. On the other hand, if the first use of the thing-world is successful and guided properly, the *pleasure of mastering toy things* becomes associated with the *mastery of the conflicts* which were projected on them and with the *prestige* gained through such mastery.

Finally, at nursery-school age playfulness reaches into the world *shared with others*. At first these others are treated as things; they are inspected, run into, or forced to "be horsie." Learning is necessary in order to discover what potential play content can be admitted only to fantasy or only to play by and with oneself; what content can be successfully represented only in the world of toys and small things; and what content can be shared with others and even forced upon them.

What is infantile play, then? We saw that it is not the equivalent of adult play, that it is not recreation. The playing adult steps sideward into another, an artificial reality; the playing child advances forward to new stages of *real mastery*. This new mastery is not restricted to the technical mastery of toys and *things;* it also includes an infantile way of mastering *experience* by meditating, experimenting, planning, and sharing.

While all children at times need to be left alone in solitary play (or later in the company of books and radio, motion pictures and video, all of which, like the fairy tales of old, at least *sometimes* seem to convey what fits the needs of the infantile mind), and while all children need their hours and days of make-believe in games, they all, sooner or later, become dissatisfied and disgruntled without a sense of being useful, without a sense of being able to make things and make them well and even perfectly: this is what I call the *sense of industry*. Without this, the best entertained child soon acts exploited. It is as if he knows and his society knows that now that he is psychologically already a rudimentary parent, he must begin to be somewhat of a worker and potential provider before becoming a biological parent. With the oncoming latency period, then, the normally advanced child forgets, or rather "sublimates" (that is, applies to more useful pursuits and approved goals) the necessity of "making" people by direct attack or the desire to become father or mother in a hurry: he now learns to win recognition by *producing things*. He develops industry, that is, he adjusts himself to the inorganic laws of the tool world. He can become an eager and absorbed unit of a productive situation. To bring a productive situation to completion is an aim which gradually supersedes the whims and wishes of his idiosyncratic drives and personal disappointments. As he once untiringly strove to walk well, and to throw things away well, he now wants to make things well. He develops the pleasure of *work completion* by steady attention and persevering diligence.

The danger at this stage is the development of a sense of *inadequacy and inferiority*. This may be caused by an insufficient solution of the preceding conflict: he may still want his mummy more than knowledge; he may still rather be the baby at home than the big child in school; he still compares himself with his father, and the comparison arouses a sense of guilt as well as a sense of anatomical inferiority. Family life (small family) may not have prepared him for school life, or school life may fail to sustain the promises of earlier stages in that nothing that he has learned to do well already seems to count one bit with the teacher. And then, again, he may be potentially able to excel in ways which are dormant and which, if not evoked now, may develop late or never.

Good teachers, healthy teachers, relaxed teachers, teachers who feel trusted and respected by the community, understand all this and can guide it. They know how to alternate play and work, games and study. They know how to recognize special efforts, how to encourage special gifts. They also know how to give a child time, and how to handle those children to whom school, for a while, is not important and rather a matter to endure than to enjoy; or the child to whom, for a while, other children are much more important than the teacher.

Good parents, healthy parents, relaxed parents feel a need to make their children trust their teachers, and therefore to have teachers who can be trusted. It is not my job here to discuss teacher selection, teacher training, and the status and payment of teachers in their communities—all of which is of direct importance for the development and the maintenance in children of a *sense of industry* and of a positive identification with those who *know* things and know how to *do* things. Again and again I have observed in the lives of especially gifted and inspired people that one teacher, somewhere, was able to kindle the flame of hidden talent.

The fact that the majority of teachers in the elementary school are women must be considered here in passing, because it often leads to a conflict with the "ordinary" boy's masculine identification, as if knowledge were feminine, action masculine. Both boys and girls are apt to agree with Bernard Shaw's statement that those who can, do, while those who cannot, teach. The selection and training of teachers, then, is vital for the avoidance of the dangers which can befall the individual at this stage. There is, first, the above-mentioned sense of inferiority, the feeling that one will never be any good—a problem which calls for the type of teacher who knows how to emphasize what a child *can* do, and who knows a psychiatric problem when she sees one. Second, there is the danger of the child's identifying too strenuously with a too virtuous teacher or becoming the teacher's pet. What we shall presently refer to as his sense of identity can remain prematurely fixed on being nothing but a good little worker or a good little helper, which may not be all he *could* be. Third, there is the danger (probably the most common one) that throughout the long years of going to school he will never acquire the enjoyment of work and the pride of doing at least one kind of thing well. This is particularly of concern in relation to that part of the nation who do not complete what schooling is at their disposal. It is always easy to say that they are born that way; that there must be less educated people as background for the superior ones; that the market needs and even fosters such people for its many simple and unskilled tasks. But from the point of the healthy personality (which, as we proceed, must now include the aspect of playing a constructive role in a healthy society), we must consider those who have had just enough schooling to appreciate what more fortunate people are learning to do but who, for one reason or another, have lacked inner or outer support of their stick-to-itiveness.

It will have been noted that, regarding the period of a developing sense of industry, I have referred to *outer* hindrances but not to any crisis (except a deferred inferiority crisis) coming from the inventory of basic human drives. This stage differs from the others in that it does not consist of a swing from a violent inner upheaval to a new mastery. The reason why Freud called it the latency stage is that violent drives are normally dormant at that time. But it is only a lull before the storm of puberty.

On the other hand, this is socially a most decisive stage: since industry involves doing things beside and with others, a first sense of *division of labor* and of *equality of opportunity* develops at this time. When a child begins to feel that it is the color of his skin, the background of his parents, or the cost of his clothes rather than his wish and his will to learn which will decide his social worth, lasting harm may ensue for the *sense of identity,* to which we must now turn.

IDENTITY VERSUS IDENTITY DIFFUSION

With the establishment of a good relationship to the world of skills and to those who teach and share the new skills, childhood proper comes to an end. Youth begins. But in puberty and adolescence all sameness and continuities relied on earlier are questioned again because of a rapidity of body growth which equals that of early childhood and because of the entirely new addition of physical genital maturity. The growing and developing young people, faced with this physiological revolution within them, are now primarily concerned with attempts at consolidating their social roles. They are sometimes morbidly, often curiously, preoccupied with what they appear to be in the eyes of others as compared with what they feel they are and with the question of how to connect the earlier cultivated roles and skills with the ideal prototypes of the day. In their search for a new sense of continuity and sameness, some adolescents have to refight many of the crises of earlier years, and they are never ready to install lasting idols and ideals as guardians of a final identity.

The integration now taking place in the form of the ego identity is more than the sum of the childhood identifications. It is the inner capital accrued from all those experiences of each successive stage, when successful identification led to a successful alignment of the individual's *basic drives* with his *endowment* and his *opportunities*. In psychoanalysis we ascribe such successful alignments to "ego synthesis"; I have tried to demonstrate that the ego values accrued in childhood culminate in what I have called a *sense of ego identity*. The sense of ego identity, then, is the accrued confidence that one's ability to maintain inner sameness and continuity (one's ego in the psychological sense) is matched by the sameness and continuity of one's meaning for others. Thus, self-esteem, confirmed at the end of each major crisis, grows to be a conviction that one is learning effective steps toward a tangible future, that one is developing a defined personality within a social reality which one understands. The growing child must, at every step, derive a vitalizing sense of reality from the awareness that his individual way of mastering experience is a successful variant of the way other people around him master experience and recognize such mastery.

In this, children cannot be fooled by empty praise and condescending encouragement. They may have to accept artificial bolstering of their self-esteem in lieu of something better, but what I call their accruing ego identity gains real strength only from wholehearted and consistent recognition of real accomplishment, that is, achievement that has meaning in their culture. On the other hand, should a child feel that the environment tries to deprive him too radically of all the forms of expression which permit him to develop and to integrate the next step in his ego identity, he will resist with the astonsihing strength encountered in animals who are suddenly forced to defend their lives. Indeed, in the social jungle of human existence, there is no feeling of being alive without a sense of ego identity. To understand this would be to understand the trouble of adolescents better, especially the trouble of all those who cannot just be "nice" boys and girls, but are desperately seeking for a satisfactory sense of belonging, be it in cliques and gangs here in our country or in inspiring mass movements in others.

Ego identity, then, develops out of a gradual integration of all identifications, but here, if anywhere, the whole has a different quality than the sum of its parts.

Under favorable circumstances children have the nucleus of a separate identity in early life; often they must defend it against any pressure which would make them over-identify with one of their parents. This is difficult to learn from patients, because the neurotic ego has, by definition, fallen prey to overidentification and to faulty identifications with disturbed parents, a circumstance which isolated the small individual both from his budding identity and from his milieu. But we can study it profitably in the children of minority-group Americans who, having successfully graduated from a marked and well-guided stage of autonomy, enter the most decisive stage of American childhood: that of initiative and industry.

Minority groups of a lesser degree of Americanization (Negroes, Indians, Mexicans, and certain European groups) often are privileged in the enjoyment of a more sensual early childhood. Their crises come when their parents and teachers, losing trust in themselves and using sudden correctives in order to approach the vague but pervasive Anglo-Saxon ideal, create violent discontinuities; or where, indeed, the children themselves learn to disavow their sensual and over-protective mothers as temptations and a hindrance to the formation of a more American personality.

On the whole, it can be said that American schools successfully meet the challenge of training children of play-school age and of the elementary grades in a spirit of self-reliance and enterprise. Children of these ages seem remarkably free of prejudice and apprehension preoccupied as they still are with growing and learning and with the new pleasures of association outside their families. This, to forestall the sense of individual inferiority, must lead to a hope for "industrial association," for equality with all those who apply themselves wholeheartedly to the same skills and adventures in learning. Many individual successes, on the other hand, only expose the now overly encouraged children of mixed backgrounds and somewhat deviant endowments to the shock of American adolescence: the standardization of individuality and the intolerance of "differences."

The emerging ego identity, then, bridges the early childhood stages, when the body and the parent images were given their specific meanings, and the later stages, when a variety of social roles becomes available and increasingly coercive. A lasting ego identity cannot begin to exist without the trust of the first oral stage; it cannot be completed without a promise of fulfillment which from the dominant image of adulthood reaches down into the baby's beginnings and which creates at every step an accruing sense of ego strength.

The danger of this stage is *identity diffusion;* as Biff puts it in Arthur Miller's *Death of a Salesman,* "I just can't take hold, Mom, I can't take hold of some kind of a life." Where such a dilemma is based on a strong previous doubt of one's ethnic and sexual identity, delinquent and outright psychotic incidents are not uncommon. Youth after youth, bewildered by some assumed role, a role forced on him by the inexorable standardization of American adolescence, runs away in one form or another; leaving schools and jobs, staying out all night, or withdrawing into bizarre and inaccessible moods. Once "delinquent," his greatest need and often his only salvation, is the refusal on the part of older friends, advisers, and judiciary personnel to type him further by pat diagnoses and social judgments which ignore the special dynamic conditions of adolescence. For if diagnosed and treated correctly, seemingly psychotic and criminal incidents do not in adolescence have the same fatal significance which they have at other ages. Yet many a youth, finding that the authorities expect him to be "a bum" or "a queer," or "off the beam," perversely obliges by becoming just that.

In general it is primarily the inability to settle on an occupational identity which disturbs young people. To keep themselves together they temporarily overidentify, to the point of apparent complete loss of identity, with the heroes of cliques and crowds. On the other hand, they become remarkably clannish, intolerant, and cruel in their exclusion of others who are "different," in skin color or cultural background, in tastes and gifts, and often in entirely petty aspects of dress and gesture arbitrarily selected as *the* signs of an in-grouper or out-grouper. It is important to understand (which does not mean condone or participate in) such intolerance as the necessary *defense against a sense of identity diffusion,* which is unavoidable at a time of life when the body changes its proportions radically, when genital maturity floods body and imagination with all manners of drives, when intimacy with the other sex approaches and is, on occasion, forced on the youngster, and when life lies before one with a variety of conflicting possibilities and choices. Adolescents help one another temporarily through such discomfort by forming cliques and by stereotyping themselves, their ideals, and their enemies.

It is important to understand this because it makes clear the appeal which simple and cruel totalitarian doctrines have on the minds of the youth of such countries and classes as have lost or are losing their group identities (feudal, agrarian, national, and so forth) in these times of worldwide industrialization, emancipation, and wider intercommunication. The dynamic quality of the tempestuous adolescences lived through in patriarchal and agrarian countries (countries which face the most radical changes in political structure and in economy) explains the fact that their young people find convincing and satisfactory identities in the simple totalitarian doctrines of race, class, or nation. Even though we may be forced to win wars against their leaders, we still are faced with the job of winning the peace with these grim youths by convincingly demonstrating to them (by living it) a democratic identity which can be strong and yet tolerant, judicious and still determined.

But it is increasingly important to understand this also in order to treat the intolerances of our adolescents at home with understanding and guidance rather than with verbal stereotypes or prohibitions. It is difficult to be tolerant if deep down you are not quite sure that you are a man (or a woman), that you will ever grow together again and be attractive, that you will be able to master your drives, that you really know who you are,[4] that you know what you want to be, that you know what you look like to others, and that you will know how to make the right decisions without, once for all, committing yourself to the wrong friend, sexual partner, leader, or career.

---

[4]On the wall of a cowboys' bar in the wide-open West hangs a saying: "I ain't what I ought to be, I ain't what I'm going to be, but I ain't what I was."

Democracy in a country like America poses special problems in that it insists on *self-made identities* ready to grasp many chances and ready to adjust to changing necessities of booms and busts, of peace and war, of migration and determined sedentary life. Our democracy, furthermore, must present the adolescent with ideals which can be shared by youths of many backgrounds and which emphasize autonomy in the form of independence and initiative in the form of enterprise. These promises, in turn, are not easy to fulfill in increasingly complex and centralized systems of economic and political organization, systems which, if geared to war, must automatically neglect the "self-made" identities of millions of individuals and put them where they are most needed. This is hard on many young Americans because their whole upbringing, and therefore the development of a healthy personality, depends on a certain degree of *choice,* a certain hope for an individual *chance,* and a certain conviction in freedom of *self-determination.*

We are speaking here not only of high privileges and lofty ideas but also of psychological necessities. Psychologically speaking, a gradually accruing ego identity is the only safeguard against the *anarchy of drives* as well as the *autocracy of conscience,* that is, the cruel overconscientiousness which is the inner residue in the adult of his past inequality in regard to his parent. Any loss of a sense of identity exposes the individual to his own childhood conflicts—as could be observed, for example, in the neuroses of World War II among men and women who could not stand the general dislocation of their careers or a variety of other special pressures of war. Our adversaries, it seems, understand this. Their psychological warfare consists in the determined continuation of general conditions which permit them to indoctrinate mankind within their orbit with the simple and yet for them undoubtedly effective identities of class warfare and nationalism, while they know that the psychology, as well as the economy, of free enterprise and of self-determination is stretched to the breaking point under the conditions of long-drawn-out cold and lukewarm war. It is clear, therefore, that we must bend every effort to present our young men and women with the tangible and trustworthy promise of opportunities for a rededication to the life for which the country's history, as well as their own childhood, has prepared them. Among the tasks of national defense, this one must not be forgotten.

I have referred to the relationship of the problem of trust to matters of adult faith; to that of the problem of autonomy to matters of adult independence in work and citizenship. I have pointed to the connection between a sense of initiative and the kind of enterprise sanctioned in the economic system, and between the sense of industry and a culture's technology. In searching for the social values which guide identity, one confronts the problem of aristocracy, in its widest possible sense which connotes the conviction that the best people rule and that that rule develops the best in people. In order not to become cynically or apathetically lost, young people in search of an identity must somewhere be able to convince themselves that those who succeed thereby shoulder the obligation of being the best, that is, of personifying the nation's ideals. In this country, as in any other, we have those successful types who become the cynical representatives of the "inside track," the "bosses" of impersonal machinery. In a culture once pervaded with the value of the self-made man, a special danger ensues from the idea of a synthetic personality: as if you are what you can appear to be, or as if you are what you can buy. This can be counteracted only by a system of education that transmits values and goals which determinedly aspire beyond mere "functioning" and "making the grade."

PATHOLOGICAL PATTERNS

Intrapsychic theorists recognize that pathological behavior represents, in large measure, an adaptive strategy developed by patients in response to feelings of anxiety and threat. The bizarre and maladaptive behavior they display is not viewed as functionless or random, but as an intricate, albeit self-defeating, maneuver to relieve oneself of anguish, humiliation, and insecurity. In childhood, a youngster will cope with anxiety by a variety of spontaneous strategies; he may be submissive, hostile, ambitious, avoidant, exploitive, or independent, shifting from one to the other at different times. Eventually, a dominant pattern of adaptive behavior emerges. The excerpts from the works of Karen Horney and Erich Fromm, two of the better known neo-Freudians, illustrate the typical characteristics of several of these ingrained adaptive personality patterns.

15. Culture and Neurosis

KAREN HORNEY

In the psychoanalytic concept of neuroses a shift of emphasis has taken place: whereas originally interest was focussed on the dramatic symptomatic picture, it is now being realized more and more that the real source of these psychic disorders lies in character disturbances, that the symptoms are a manifest result of conflicting character traits, and that without uncovering and straightening out the neurotic character structure we cannot cure a neurosis. When analyzing these character traits, in a great many cases one is struck by the observation that, in marked contrast to the divergency of the symptomatic pictures, character difficulties invariably center around the same basic conflicts.

These similarities in the content of conflicts present a problem. They suggest, to minds open to the importance of cultural implications, the question of whether and to what extent neuroses are moulded by cultural processes in essentially the same way as "normal" character forma-

tion is determined by these influences; and, if so, how far such a concept would necessitate certain modifications in Freud's views of the relation between culture and neurosis.

In the following remarks I shall try to outline roughly some characteristics typically recurring in all our neuroses. The limitations of time will allow us to present neither data—good case histories—nor method, but only results. I shall try to select from the extremely complex and diversified observational material the essential points.

There is another difficulty in the presentation. I wish to show how these neurotic persons are trapped in a vicious circle. Unable to present in detail the factors leading up to the vicious circle, I must start rather arbitrarily with one of the outstanding features, although this in itself is already a complex product of several interrelated, developed mental factors. I start, therefore, with the problem of competition.

The problem of competition, or rivalry, appears to be a never-failing center of neurotic conflicts. How to deal

From *Amer. Sociol. Review 1*:221–230, 1936, by permission of the American Sociological Association.

with competition presents a problem for everyone in our culture; for the neurotic, however, it assumes dimensions which generally surpass actual vicissitudes. It does so in three respects:

(1) There is a constant measuring-up with others, even in situations which do not call for it. While striving to surpass others is essential for all competitive situations, the neurotic measures up even with persons who are in no way potential competitors and have no goal in common with him. The question as to who is the more intelligent, more attractive, more popular, is indiscriminately applied towards everyone.

(2) The content of neurotic ambitions is not only to accomplish something worth while, or to be successful, but to be absolutely best of all. These ambitions, however, exist in fantasy mainly—fantasies which may or may not be conscious. The degree of awareness differs widely in different persons. The ambitions may appear in occasional flashes of fantasy only. There is never a clear realization of the powerful dramatic roles these ambitions play in the neurotic's life, or of the great part they have in accounting for his behavior and mental reactions. The challenge of these ambitions is not met by adequate efforts which might lead to realization of the aims. They are in queer contrast to existing inhibitions towards work, towards assuming leadership, towards all means which would effectually secure success. There are many ways in which these fantastic ambitions influence the emotional lives of the persons concerned: by hypersensitivity to criticism, by depressions or inhibitions following failures, etc. These failures need not necessarily be real. Everything which falls short of the realization of the grandiose ambitions is felt as failure. The success of another person is felt as one's own failure.

This competitive attitude not only exists in reference to the external world, but is also internalized, and appears as a constant measuring-up to an ego-ideal. The fantastic ambitions appear on this score as excessive and rigid demands towards the self, and failure in living up to these demands produces depressions and irritations similar to those produced in competition with others.

(3) The third characteristic is the amount of hostility involved in neurotic ambition. While intense competition implicitly contains elements of hostility —the defeat of a competitor meaning victory for oneself—the reactions of neurotic persons are determined by an insatiable and irrational expectation that no one in the universe other than themselves should be intelligent, influential, attractive, or popular. They become infuriated, or feel their own endeavors condemned to futility, if someone else writes a good play or a scientific paper or plays a prominent role in society. If this attitude is strongly accentuated, one may observe in the analytical situation, for example, that these patients regard any progress made as a victory on the part of the analyst, completely disregarding the fact that progress is of vital concern to their own interests. In such situations they will disparage the analyst, betraying, by the intense hostility displayed, that they feel endangered in a position of paramount importance to themselves. They are as a rule completely unaware of the existence and intensity of this "no one but me" attitude, but one may safely assume and eventually always uncover this attitude from reactions observable in the analytical situation, as indicated above.

This attitude easily leads to a fear of retaliation. It results in a fear of success and also in a fear of failure: "If I want to crush everyone who is successful, then I will automatically assume identical reactions in others, so that the way to success implies exposing me to the hostility of others. Furthermore: if I make any move towards this goal and fail, then I shall be crushed." Success thus becomes a peril and any possible failure becomes a danger which must at all costs be avoided. From the point of view of all these dangers it appears much safer to stay in the corner, be modest and inconspicuous. In other and more positive terms, this fear leads to a definite recoiling from any aim which implies competition. This safety device is assured by a constant, accurately working process of automatic self-checking.

This self-checking process results in inhibitions, particularly inhibitions towards work, but also towards all steps necessary to the pursuit of one's aims, such as seizing opportunities, or revealing to others that one has certain goals or capacities. This eventually results in an incapacity to stand up for one's own wishes. The peculiar nature of these inhibitions is best demonstrated by the fact that these persons may be quite capable of fighting for the needs of others or for an impersonal cause. They will, for instance, act like this:

When playing an instrument with a poor partner, they will instinctively play worse than he, although otherwise they may be very competent. When discussing a subject with someone less intelligent than themselves, they will compulsively descend below his level. They will prefer to be in the rank and file, not to be identified with the superiors, not even to get an increase in salary, rationalizing this attitude in some way. Even their dreams will be dictated by this need for reassurance. Instead of utilizing the liberty of a dream to imagine themselves in glorious situations, they will actually see themselves, in their dreams, in humble or even humiliating situations.

This self-checking process does not restrict itself to activities in the pursuit of some aim, but going beyond that, tends to undermine the self-confidence, which is a prerequisite for any accomplishment, by means of self-belittling. The function of self-belittling in this context is to eliminate oneself from any competition. In most cases these persons are not aware of actually disparaging themselves, but are aware of the results only as they feel themselves inferior to others and take for granted their own inadequacy.

The presence of these feelings of inferiority is one of the most common psychic disorders of our time and culture. Let me say a few more words about them. The genesis of inferiority feelings is not always in neurotic competition. They present complex phenomena and may be determined by various conditions. But that they do result from, and stand in the service of, a recoiling from competition, is a basic and ever-present implication. They result from a recoiling inasmuch as they are the expression of a discrepancy between high-pitched ideals and real accomplishment. The fact, however, that these painful feelings at the same time fulfill the important function of making secure the recoiling attitude itself, becomes evident through the vigor with which this position is defended when attacked. Not only will no evidence of competence or attractiveness ever convince these persons, but they may actually become scared or angered by any attempt to convince them of their positive qualities.

The surface pictures resulting from this situation may be widely divergent. Some persons appear thoroughly convinced of their unique importance and may be anxious to demonstrate their superiority on every occasion, but betray their insecurity in an excessive sensitivity to every criticism, to every dissenting opinion, or every lack of responsive admiration. Others are just as thoroughly convinced of their incompetence or unworthiness, or of being unwanted or unappreciated; yet they betray their actually great demands in that they react with open or concealed hostility to every frustration of their unacknowledged demands. Still others will waver constantly in their self-estimation between feeling themselves all-important and feeling, for instance, honestly amazed that anyone pays any attention to them.

If you have followed me thus far, I can now proceed to outline the particular vicious circle in which these persons are moving. It is important here, as in every complex neurotic picture, to recognize the vicious circle, because, if we overlook it and simplify the complexity of the processes going on by assuming a simple cause-effect relation, we either fail to get an understanding of the emotions involved, or attribute an undue importance to some one cause. As an example of this error, I might mention regarding a highly emotion-charged rivalry attitude as derived directly from rivalry with the father. Roughly, the vicious circle looks like this:

The failures, in conjunction with a feeling of weakness and defeat, lead to a feeling of envy towards all persons who are more successful, or merely more secure or better contented with life. This envy may be manifest or it may be repressed under the pressure of the same anxiety which led to a repression of, and a recoiling from, rivalry. It may be entirely wiped out of consciousness and represented by the substitution of a blind admiration; it may be kept from awareness by a disparaging attitude towards the person concerned. Its effect, however, is apparent in the incapacity to grant to others what one has been forced to deny oneself. At any rate, no matter to what degree the envy is repressed or expressed, it implies an increase in the existing hostility against people and consequently an increase in the anxiety, which now takes the particular form of an irrational fear of the envy of others.

The irrational nature of this fear is shown in two ways: (1) it exists regardless of the presence or absence of envy in the given situation; and (2) its intensity is out of proportion to the dangers menacing from the side of the envious competitors. This irrational side of the fear of envy always remains unconscious, at least in nonpsychotic persons, therefore it is never corrected by a reality-testing process, and is all the more effective in the direction of reinforcing the existing tendencies to recoil.

Consequently the feeling of own insignificance grows, the hostility against people grows, and the anxiety grows. We thus return to the beginning, because now the fantasies come up, with about this content: "I wish I were more powerful, more attractive, more intelligent than all the others, then I should be safe, and besides, I could defeat them and step on them." Thus we see an ever-increasing deviation of the ambitions towards the stringent, fantastic, and hostile.

This pyramiding process may come to a standstill under various conditions, usually at an inordinate expense in loss of expansiveness and vitality. There is often some sort of resignation as to personal ambitions, in turn permitting the diminution of anxieties as to competition, with the inferiority feelings and inhibitions continuing.

It is now time, however, to make a reservation. It is in no way self-evident that ambition of the "no-one-but-me" type must necessarily evoke anxieties. There are persons quite capable of brushing aside or crushing everyone in the way of their ruthless pursuit of personal power. The question then is: Under what special condition is anxiety invoked in neurotically competitive people?

The answer is that they at the same time want to be loved. While most persons who pursue an asocial ambition in life care little for the affection or the opinion of others, the neurotics, although possessed by the same kind of competitiveness, simultaneously have a boundless craving for affection and appreciation. Therefore, as soon as they make any move towards self-assertion, competition, or success, they begin to dread losing the affection of others, and must automatically check their aggressive impulses. This conflict between ambition and affection is one of the gravest and most typical dilemmas of the neurotics of our time.

Why are those two incompatible strivings so frequently present in the same individual? They are related to each other in more than one way. The briefest formulation of this relationship would perhaps be that they both grow out of the same sources, namely, anxieties, and they both serve as a means of reassurance against the anxieties. Power and affection may both be safeguards. They generate each other, check each other, and reinforce each other. These interrelations can be observed most accurately within the analytic situation, but sometimes are obvious from only a casual knowledge of the life history.

In the life history may be found, for instance, an atmosphere in childhood lacking in warmth and reliability, but rife with frightening elements—battles between the parents, injustice, cruelty, oversolicitousness—generation of an increased need for affection—disappointments—development of an outspoken competitiveness—inhibition—attempts to get affection on the basis of weakness, helplessness, or suffering. We sometimes hear that a youngster has suddenly turned to ambition after an acute disappointment in his need for affection, and then given up the ambition on falling in love.

Particularly when the expansive and aggressive desires have been severely curbed in early life by a forbidding atmosphere, the excessive need for reassuring affection will play a major role. As a guiding principle for behavior this implies a yielding to the wishes or opinions of others rather than asserting one's own wishes or opinions; an overvaluation of the significance for one's own life of expressions of fondness from others, and a dependence on such expressions. And similarly, it implies an overvaluation of signs of rejection and a reacting to such signs with apprehension and defensive hostility. Here again a vicious circle begins easily and reinforces the single elements: In diagram it looks somewhat like this:

Anxiety plus repressed hostility
Need for reassuring affection
Anticipation of, sensitivity to, rejection
Hostile reactions to feeling rejected

These reactions explain why emotional contact with others that is attained on the basis of anxiety can be at best only a very shaky and easily shattered bridge between individuals, and why it always fails to bring them out of their emotional isolation. It may, however, serve to cope with anxieties and even get one through life rather smoothly, but only at the expense of growth and personality development, and only if circumstances are quite favorable.

Let us ask now, which special features in our culture may be responsible for the frequent occurrence of the neurotic structures just described?

We live in a competitive, individualistic culture. Whether the enormous economic and technical achievements of our culture were and are possible only on the basis of the competitive principle is a question for the economist or sociologist to decide. The psychologist, however, can evaluate the personal price we have paid for it.

It must be kept in mind that competition not only is a driving force in economics activities, but that it also pervades our personal life in every respect. The character of all our human relationships is moulded by a more or less outspoken competition. It is effective in the family between siblings, at school, in social relations (keeping up with the Joneses), and in love life.

In love, it may show itself in two ways: the genuine erotic wish is often overshadowed or replaced by the merely competitive goal of being the most popular, having the most dates, love letters, lovers, being seen with the most desirable man or woman. Again, it may pervade the love relationship itself. Marriage partners, for example, may be living in an endless struggle for supremacy, with or without being aware of the nature or even of the existence of this combat.

The influence on human relations of this competitiveness lies in the fact that it creates easily aroused envy towards the stronger ones, contempt for the weaker, distrust towards everyone. In consequence of all these potentially hostile tensions, the satisfaction and reassurance which one can get out of human relations are limited and the individual becomes more or less emotionally isolated. It seems that here, too, mutually reinforcing interactions take place, so far as insecurity and dissatisfaction in human relations in turn compel people to seek gratification and security in ambitious strivings, and vice versa.

Another cultural factor relevant to the structure of our neurosis lies in our attitude towards failure and success. We are inclined to attribute success to good personal qualities and capacities, such as competence, courage, enterprise. In religious terms this attitude was expressed by saying that success was due to God's grace. While these qualities may be effective—and in certain periods, such as the pioneer days, may have represented the only conditions necessary—this ideology omits two essential facts: (1) that the possibility for success is strictly limited; even external conditions and personal qualities being equal, only a comparative few can possibly attain success; and (2) that other factors than those mentioned may play the decisive role, such as, for example, unscrupulousness or fortuitous circumstances. Inasmuch as these factors are overlooked in the general evaluation of success, failures, besides putting the persons concerned in a factually disadvantageous position, are bound to reflect on his self-esteem.

The confusion involved in this situation is enhanced by a sort of double moral. Although, in fact, success meets with adoration almost without regard to the means employed in securing it, we are at the same time taught to regard modesty and an undemanding, unselfish attitude as social or religious virtues, and are rewarded for them by praise and affection. The particular difficulties which confront the individual in our culture may be summarized as follows: for the competitive struggle he needs a certain amount of available aggressiveness; at the same time, he is required to be modest, unselfish, even self-sacrificing. While the competitive life situation with the hostile tensions involved in it creates an enhanced need of security, the chances of attaining a feeling of safety in human relations—love, friendship, social contacts—are at the same time diminished. The estimation of one's personal value is all too dependent on the degree of success attained, while at the same time the possibilities for success are limited and the success itself is dependent, to a great extent, on fortuitous circumstances or on personal qualities of an asocial character.

Perhaps these sketchy comments have suggested to you the direction in which to explore the actual relationship of our culture to our personality and its neurotic deviations. Let us now consider the relation of this conception to the views of Freud on culture and neurosis.

The essence of Freud's views on this subject can be summarized, briefly, as follows: Culture is the result of a sublimation of biologically given sexual and aggressive drives—"sexual" in the extended connotation Freud has given the term. Sublimation presupposes unwitting suppression of these instinctual drives. The more complete the suppression of these drives, the higher the cultural development. As the capacity for sublimating is limited, and as the intensive suppression of primitive drives without sublimation may lead to neurosis, the growth of civilization must inevitably imply a growth of neurosis. Neuroses are the price humanity has to pay for cultural development.

The implicit theoretical presupposition underlying this train of thought is the belief in the existence of biologically determined human nature, or, more precisely, the belief that oral, anal, genital, and aggressive drives exist in all

human beings in approximately equal quantities.[1] Variations in character formation from individual to individual, as from culture, are due, then, to the varying intensity of the suppression required, with the addition that this suppression can affect the different kinds of drives in varying degrees.

This viewpoint of Freud's seems actually to encounter difficulties with two groups of data. (1) Historical and anthropological findings[2] do not support the assumption that the growth of civilization is in a direct ratio to the growth of instinct suppression. (2) Clinical experience of the kind indicated in this paper suggests that neurosis is due not simply to the quantity of suppression of one or the other instinctual drives, but rather to difficulties caused by the conflicting character of the demands which a culture imposes on its individuals. The differences in neuroses typical of different cultures may be understood to be conditioned by the amount and quality of conflicting demands within the particular culture.

In a given culture, those persons are likely to become neurotic who have met these culturally determined difficulties in accentuated form, mostly through the medium of childhood experiences; and who have not been able to solve their difficulties, or have solved them only at great expense to personality.

---

[1] I pass over Freud's recognition of individual constitutional difference.

[2] Ruth Benedict, *Patterns of Culture;* Margaret Mead, *Sex and Temperament in Three Savage Societies.*

16.   Non-Productive Character Orientations

ERICH FROMM

Freud tried to account for this dynamic nature of character traits by combining his characterology with his libido theory. In accordance with the type of

materialistic thinking prevalent in the natural sciences of the late nineteenth century, which assumed the energy in natural and psychical phenomena to be a substantial not a relational entity, Freud believed that the sexual drive was the source of energy of the character. By a number of complicated and brilliant assumptions he explained different char-

---

acter traits as "sublimations" of, or "reaction formations" against, the various forms of the sexual drive. He interpreted the *dynamic nature* of character traits as an expression of their *libidinous source*.

The progress of psychoanalytic theory led, in line with the progress of the natural and social sciences, to a new concept which was based, not on the idea of a primarily isolated individual, but on the *relationship* of man to others, to nature, and to himself. It was assumed that this very relationship governs and regulates the energy manifest in the passionate strivings of man. H. S. Sullivan, one of the pioneers of this new view, has accordingly defined psychoanalysis as a "study of interpersonal relations."

The theory presented in the following pages follows Freud's characterology in essential points: in the assumption that character traits underlie behavior and must be inferred from it; that they constitute forces which, though powerful, the person may be entirely unconscious of. It follows Freud also in the assumption that the fundamental entity in character is not the single character trait but the total character organization from which a number of single character traits follow. These character traits are to be understood as a syndrome which results from a particular organization or, as I shall call it, orientation of character. I shall deal only with a very limited number of character traits which follow immediately from the underlying orientation. A number of other character traits could be dealt with similarly, and it could be shown that they are also direct outcomes of basic orientations or mixtures of such primary traits of character with those of temperament. However, a great number of others conventionally listed as character traits would be found to be not character traits in our sense but pure temperament or mere behavior traits.

The main difference in the theory of character proposed here from that of Freud is that the fundamental basis of character is not seen in various types of libido organization but in specific kinds of a person's relatedness to the world. In the process of living, man relates himself to the world (1) by acquiring and assimilating things, and (2) by relating himself to people (and himself). The former I shall call the process of assimilation; the latter, that of socialization. Both forms of relatedness are "open" and not, as with the animal, instinctively determined. Man can acquire things by receiving or taking them from an outside source or by producing them through his own effort. But he must acquire and assimilate them in some fashion in order to satisfy his needs. Also, man cannot live alone and unrelated to others. He has to associate with others for defense, for work, for sexual satisfaction, for play, for the upbringing of the young, for the transmission of knowledge and material possessions. But beyond that, it is necessary for him to be related to others, one with them, part of a group. Complete isolation is unbearable and incompatible with sanity. Again man can relate himself to others in various ways: he can love or hate, he can compete or cooperate; he can build a social system based on equality or authority, liberty or oppression; but he must be related in some fashion and the particular form of relatedness is expressive of his character.

These orientations, by which the individual relates himself to the world, constitute the core of his character; character can be defined as the *(relatively permanent) form in which human energy is canalized in the process of assimilation and socialization*. This canalization of psychic energy has a very significant biological function. Since man's actions are not determined by innate instinctual patterns, life would be precarious, indeed, if he had to make a deliberate decision each time he acted, each time he took a step. On the contrary, many actions must be performed far more quickly than conscious deliberation allows. Furthermore, if all behavior followed from deliberate decision, many more inconsistencies in action would occur than are compatible with proper functioning. According to behavioristic thinking, man learns to react in a semiautomatic fashion by developing habits of action and thought which can be understood in terms of conditioned reflexes. While this view is correct to a certain extent, it ignores the fact that the most deeply rooted habits and opinions which are characteristic of a person and resistant to change grow from his character structure: they are expressive of the particular form in which energy has been canalized in the character structure. The character system can be considered the human substitute for the instinctive apparatus of the animal. Once energy is canalized in a certain way, action takes place "true to character." A particular character may be undesirable ethically, but at least it permits a person to act fairly consistently and to be relieved of the burden of having to make a new and deliberate decision every time. He can arrange his life in a way which is geared to his character and thus create a certain degree of compatibility between the inner and the outer situation. Moreover, character has also a selective function with regard to a person's ideas and values. Since to most people ideas seem to be independent of their emotions and wishes and the result of logical deduction, they feel that their attitude toward the world is confirmed by their ideas and judgments when actually these are as much a result of their character as their actions are. This confirmation in turn tends to stabilize their character structure since it makes the latter appear right and sensible.

Not only has character the function of permitting the individual to act consistently and "reasonably"; it is also the basis for his adjustment to society. The character of the child is molded by the character of its parents in response to whom it develops. The parents and their methods of child training in turn are determined by the social structure of their culture. The average family is the "psychic agency" of society, and by adjusting himself to his family the child acquires the character which later makes him adjusted to the tasks he has to perform in social life. He acquires that character which makes him want to do what he has to do and the core of which he shares with most members of the same social class or culture. The fact that most members of a social class or culture share significant elements of character and that one can speak of a "social character" representing the core of a character structure common to most people of a given culture shows the degree to which character is formed by social and cultural patterns. But from the social character we must differentiate the individual character in which one person differs from another within the same culture. These differences are partly due to the differences of the personalities of the parents and to the differences, psychic and material, of the specific social environment in which the child grows up. But they are also due to the constitutional differences of each individual, particularly those of temperament. Genetically, the formation of individual character is determined by the impact of its life experiences, the individual ones and those which follow from the culture, on temperament and physical constitution. Environment is never the same for two people, for the difference in constitution makes them experience the same environment in a more or less different way. Mere habits of action and thought which develop as the result of an individual's conforming with the cultural pattern and which are not rooted in the character of a person are easily changed under the influence of new social patterns. If, on the other hand, a person's behavior is rooted in his character, it is charged with energy and changeable only if a fundamental change in a person's character takes place.

In the following analysis *nonproductive orientations* are differentiated from the *productive orientation*. It must be noted that these concepts are "ideal-types," not descriptions of the character of a given individual. Furthermore, while, for didactic purposes, they are treated here separately, the character of any given person is usually a blend of all or some of these orientations in which one, however, is dominant. Finally, I want to state here that in the description of the nonproductive orientations only their negative aspects are presented.

THE RECEPTIVE ORIENTATION

In the receptive orientation a person feels "the source of all good" to be outside, and he believes that the only way to get what he wants—be it something material, be it affection, love, knowledge, pleasure—is to receive it from that outside source. In this orientation the problem of love is almost exclusively that of "being loved" and not that of loving. Such people tend to be indiscriminate in the choice of their love objects, because being loved by anybody is such an overwhelming experience for them that they "fall for" anybody who gives them love or what looks like love. They are exceedingly sensitive to any withdrawal or rebuff they experience on the part of the loved person. Their orientation is the same in the sphere of thinking: if intelligent, they make the best listeners, since their orientation is one of receiving, not of producing, ideas; left to themselves, they feel paralyzed. It is characteristic of these people that their first thought is to find somebody else to give them needed information rather than to make even the smallest effort of their own. If religious, these persons have a concept of God in which they expect everything from God and nothing from their own activity. If not religious, their relationship to persons or institutions is very much the same; they are always in search of a "magic helper." They show a particular kind of loyalty, at the bottom of which is the gratitude for the hand that feeds them and the fear of ever losing it. Since they need many hands to feel secure, they have to be loyal to numerous people. It is difficult for them to say "no," and they are easily caught between conflicting loyalties and promises. Since they cannot say "no," they love to say "yes" to everything and everybody, and the resulting paralysis of their critical abilities makes them increasingly dependent on others.

They are dependent not only on authorities for knowledge and help but on people in general for any kind of support. They feel lost when alone because they feel that they cannot do anything without help. This helplessness is especially important with regard to those acts which by their very nature can only be done alone—making decisions and taking responsibility. In personal relationships, for instance, they ask advice from the very person with regard to whom they have to make a decision.

This receptive type has great fondness for food and drink. These persons tend to overcome anxiety and depression by eating or drinking. The mouth is an especially prominent feature, often the most expressive one; the lips tend to be open, as if in a state of continuous expectation of being fed. In their dreams, being fed is a frequent symbol of being loved; being starved, an expression of frustration or disappointment.

By and large, the outlook of people of this receptive orientation is optimistic and friendly; they have a certain confidence in life and its gifts, but they become anxious and distraught when their "source of supply" is threatened. They often have a genuine warmth and a wish to help others, but doing things for others also assumes the function of securing their favor.

THE EXPLOITATIVE ORIENTATION

The exploitative orientation, like the receptive, has as its basic premise the feeling that the source of all good is outside, that whatever one wants to get must be sought there, and that one cannot produce anything oneself. The difference between the two, however, is that the exploitative type does not expect to receive things from others as gifts, but to take them away from others by force or cunning. This orientation extends to all spheres of activity.

In the realm of love and affection these people tend to grab and steal. They feel attracted only to people whom they can take away from somebody else. Attractiveness to them is conditioned by a person's attachment to somebody else; they tend not to fall in love with an unattached person.

We find the same attitude with regard to thinking and intellectual pursuits. Such people will tend not to produce ideas but to steal them. This may be done directly in the form of plagiarism or more subtly by repeating in different phraseology the ideas voiced by others and insisting they are new and their own. It is a striking fact that frequently people with great intelligence proceed in this way, although if they relied on their own gifts they might well be able to have ideas of their own. The lack of original ideas or independent production in otherwise gifted people often has its explanation in this character orientation, rather than in any innate lack of originality. The same statement holds true with regard to their orientation to material things. Things which they can take away from others always seem better to them than anything they can produce themselves. They use and exploit anybody and anything from whom or from which they can squeeze something. Their motto is: "Stolen fruits are sweetest." Because they want to use and exploit people, they "love" those who, explicitly or implicitly, are promising objects of exploitation, and get "fed up" with persons whom they have squeezed out. An extreme example is the kleptomaniac who enjoys things only if he can steal them, although he has the money to buy them.

This orientation seems to be symbolized by the biting mouth which is often a prominent feature in such people. It is not a play upon words to point out that they often make "biting" remarks about others. Their attitude is colored by a mixture of hostility and manipulation. Everyone is an object of exploitation and is judged according to his usefulness. Instead of the confidence and optimism which characterizes the receptive type, one finds here suspicion and cynicism, envy and jealousy. Since they are satisfied only with things they can take away from others, they tend to overrate what others have and underrate what is theirs.

THE HOARDING ORIENTATION

While the receptive and exploitative types are similar inasmuch as both expect to get things from the outside world, the hoarding orientation is essentially different. This orientation makes people have little faith in anything new they might get from the outside world; their security is based upon hoarding and saving, while spending is felt to be a threat. They have surrounded themselves, as it were, by a protective wall, and their main aim is to bring as much as possible into this fortified position and to let as little as possible out of it. Their miserliness refers to money and material things as well as to feelings and thoughts. Love is essentially a possession; they do not give love but try to get it by possessing the "beloved." The hoarding person often shows a particular kind of faithfulness toward people and even toward memories. Their sentimentality makes the past appear as golden; they hold on to it and indulge in the memories of bygone feelings and experiences. They know everything but are sterile and incapable of productive thinking.

One can recognize these people too by facial expressions and gestures. Theirs is the tight-lipped mouth; their gestures are characteristic of their withdrawn attitude. While those of the receptive type are inviting and round, as it were, and the gestures of the exploitative type are aggressive and pointed, those of the hoarding type are angular, as if they wanted to emphasize the frontiers between themselves and the outside world. Another characteristic element in this attitude is pedantic orderliness. The hoarder will be orderly with things, thoughts, or feelings, but again, as with memory, his orderliness is sterile and rigid. He cannot endure things out of place and will automatically rearrange them. To him the outside world threatens to break into his fortified position; orderliness signifies mastering the world outside by putting it, and keeping it, in its proper place in order to avoid the danger intrusion. His compulsive cleanliness is another expression of his need to undo contact with the outside world. Things beyond his own frontiers are felt to be dangerous and "unclean"; he annuls the menacing contact by compulsive washing, similar to a religious washing ritual prescribed after contact with unclean things or people. Things have to be put not only in their proper place but also into their proper time; obsessive punctuality is characteristic of the hoarding type; it is another form of mastering the outside world. If the outside world is experienced as a threat to one's fortified position, obstinacy is a logical reaction. A constant "no" is the almost automatic defense against intrusion; sitting tight, the answer to the danger of being pushed. These people tend to feel that they possess only a fixed quantity of strength, energy, or mental capacity, and that this stock is diminished or exhausted by use and can never be replenished. They cannot understand the self-replenishing function of all living substance and that activity and the use of one's powers increase strength while stagnation paralyzes; to them, death and destruction have more reality than life and growth. The act of creation is a miracle of which they hear but in which they do not believe. Their highest values are order and security; their motto: "There is nothing new under the sun." In their relationship to others intimacy is a threat; either remoteness or possession of a person means security. The hoarder tends to be suspicious and to have a particular sense of justice which in effect says: "Mine is mine and yours is yours."

THE MARKETING ORIENTATION

The marketing orientation developed as a dominant one only in the modern era. In order to understand its nature one must consider the economic function of the market in modern society as being not only analogous to this character orientation but as the basis and the main condition for its development in modern man.

Barter is one of the oldest economic mechanisms. The traditional local market, however, is essentially different from the market as it has developed in modern capitalism. Bartering on a local market offered an opportunity to meet for the purpose of exchanging commodities. Producers and customers became acquainted; they were relatively small groups; the demand was more or less known, so that the producer could produce for this specific demand.

The modern market is no longer a meeting place but a mechanism characterized by abstract and impersonal demand. One produces for this market, not for a known circle of customers; its verdict is based on laws of supply and demand; and it determines whether the commodity can be sold and at what price. No matter what the *use value* of a pair of shoes may be, for instance, if the supply is greater than the demand, some shoes will be sentenced to economic death; they might as well not have been produced at all. The market day is the "day of judgment" as far as the exchange *value* of commodities is concerned.

The reader may object that this description of the market is oversimplified. The producer does try to judge the demand in advance, and under monopoly conditions even obtains a certain degree of control over it. Nevertheless, the regulatory function of the market has been, and still is, predominant enough to have a profound influence on the character formation of the urban middle class and, through the latter's social and cultural influence, on the whole population. The market concept of value, the emphasis on exchange value rather than on use value, has led to a similar concept of value with regard to people and particularly to oneself. The character orientation which is rooted in the experience of oneself as a commodity and of one's value as exchange value I call the marketing orientation.

In our time the marketing orientation has been growing rapidly, together with the development of a new market that is a phenomenon of the last decades—the "personality market." Clerks and salesmen, business executives and doc-

tors, lawyers and artists all appear on this market. It is true that their legal status and economic positions are different: some are independent, charging for their services; others are employed, receiving salaries. But all are dependent for their material success on a personal acceptance by those who need their services or who employ them.

The principle of evaluation is the same on both the personality and the commodity market: on the one, personalities are offered for sale; on the other, commodities. Value in both cases is their exchange value, for which use value is a necessary but not a sufficient condition. It is true, our economic system could not function if people were not skilled in the particular work they have to perform and were gifted only with a pleasant personality. Even the best bedside manner and the most beautifully equipped office on Park Avenue would not make a New York doctor successful if he did not have a minimum of medical knowledge and skill. Even the most winning personality would not prevent a secretary from losing her job unless she could type reasonably fast. However, if we ask what the respective weight of skill and personality as a condition for success is, we find that only in exceptional cases is success predominantly the result of skill and of certain other human qualities like honesty, decency, and integrity. Although the proportion between skill and human qualities on the one hand and "personality" on the other hand as prerequisites for success varies, the "personality factor" always plays a decisive role. Success depends largely on how well a person sells himself on the market, how well he gets his personality across, how nice a "package" he is; whether he is "cheerful," "sound," "aggressive," "reliable," "ambitious"; furthermore what his family background is, what clubs he belongs to, and whether he knows the right people. The type of personality required depends to some degree on the special field in which a person works. A stockbroker, a salesman, a secretary, a railroad executive, a college professor, or a hotel manager must each offer different kinds of personality that, regardless of their differences, must fulfill one condition: to be in demand.

The fact that in order to have success it is not sufficient to have the skill and equipment for performing a given task but that one must be able to "put across" one's personality in competition with many others shapes the attitude toward oneself. If it were enough for the purpose of making a living to rely on what one knows and what one can do, one's self-esteem would be in proportion to one's capacities, that is, to one's use value; but since success depends largely on how one sells one's personality, one experiences oneself as a commodity or rather simultaneously as the seller *and* the commodity to be sold. A person is not concerned with his life and happiness, but with becoming salable. This feeling might be compared to that of a commodity, of handbags on a counter, for instance, could they feel and think. Each handbag would try to make itself as "attractive" as possible in order to attract customers and to look as expensive as possible in order to obtain a higher price than its rivals. The handbag sold for the highest price would feel elated, since that would mean it was the most "valuable" one; the one which was not sold would feel sad and convinced of its own worthlessness. This fate might befall a bag which, though excellent in appearance and usefulness, had the bad luck to be out of date because of a change in fashion.

Like the handbag, one has to be in fashion on the personality market, and in order to be in fashion one has to know what kind of personality is most in demand. This knowledge is transmitted in a general way throughout the whole process of education, from kindergarten to college, and implemented by the family. The knowledge acquired at this early stage is not sufficient, however; it emphasizes only certain general qualities like adaptability, ambition, and sensitivity to the changing expectations of other people. The more specific picture of the models for success one gets elsewhere. The pictorial magazines, newspapers, and newsreels show the pictures and life stories of the successful in many variations. Pictorial advertising has a similar function. The successful executive who is pictured in a tailor's advertisement is the image of how one should look and be, if one is to draw down the "big money" on the contemporary personality market.

The most important means of transmitting the desired personality pattern to the average man is the motion picture. The young girl tries to emulate the facial expression, coiffure, gestures of a high-priced star as the most promising way to success. The young man tries to look and be like the model he sees on the screen. While the average citizen has little contact with the life of the most successful people, his relationship with the motion-picture stars is different. It is true that he has no real contact with them either, but he can see them on the screen again and again, can write them and receive their autographed pictures. In contrast to the time when the actor was socially despised but was nevertheless the transmitter of the works of great poets to his audience, our motion-picture stars have no great works or ideas to transmit, but their function is to serve as the link an average person has with the world of the "great." Even if he can not hope to become as successful as they are, he can try to emulate them; they are his saints and because of their success they embody the norms for living.

Since modern man experiences himself both as the seller and as the commodity to be sold on the market, his self-esteem depends on conditions beyond his control. If he is "successful," he is valuable; if he is not, he is worthless. The degree of insecurity which results from this orientation can hardly be overestimated. If one feels that one's own value is not constituted primarily by the human qualities one possesses, but by one's success on a competitive market with ever-changing conditions, one's self-esteem is bound to be shaky and in constant need of confirmation by others. Hence one is driven to strive relentlessly for success, and any setback is a severe threat to one's self-esteem; helplessness, insecurity, and inferiority feelings are the result. If the vicissitudes of the market are the judges of one's value, the sense of dignity and pride is destroyed.

But the problem is not only that of self-evaluation and self-esteem but of one's experience of oneself as an independent entity, of one's *identity with oneself*. The mature and productive individual derives his feeling of identity from the experience of himself as the agent who is one with his powers; this feeling of self can be briefly expressed as meaning *"I am what I do."* In the marketing orientation man encounters his own powers as commodities alienated from him. He is not one with them but they are masked from him because what matters is not his self-realization in the process of using them but his success in the process of selling them. Both his powers and what they create become estranged, something different from himself, something for others to judge and to use; thus his feeling of identity becomes as shaky as his self-esteem; it is constituted by the sum total of roles one can play: *"I am as you desire me."*

Intrapsychic Theories

THERAPY

Pathological behavior, according to the intrapsychic theorists, reflects the operation of unconscious anxieties and defensive maneuvers which have persisted from early childhood. The task of therapy, then, is to bring these residues of the past into consciousness where they can be reevaluated and reworked in a constructive fashion. The excerpt chosen from Lewis Wolberg's excellent book, The Technique of Psychotherapy, summarizes the logic and the technical procedures utilized to accomplish this goal. Harry Stack Sullivan, one of the outstanding theorists of the intrapsychic persuasion, presents in the excerpt reproduced here a detailed statement of the roles and activities assumed by patient and therapist in the treatment of schizophrenia. This paper is especially important in light of the fact that many critics suggest that the psychoanalytic approach is of little value in the therapy of psychotic patients.

17.   Technique of Reconstructive Therapy

LEWIS R. WOLBERG

Freud contended that the essence of a neurosis was a repression of infantile fears and experiences which continually forced the individual to act in the present as if he were living in the past. The neurotic seemed to be dominated by past anxieties that, split off, operated autonomously and served no further function in reality.

Internal dangers were constantly threatened by the efforts of the id to discharge accumulated tension. Such discharge was opposed by the mental force of the super-ego in the form of repression to prevent the release of tension. Repression was a dynamic force which attempted to seal off internal dangers. However, the maintenance of repression required an enormous expenditure of energy. The ego derived this energy from the id in a subversive manner. Thus, an idea or tendency invested with libido (cathexis) would be stripped of libido and this energy used to oppose the idea or tendency (anti-cathexis).

Subtle mechanisms such as symbolization, condensation, distortion and displacement were employed to evade repressive forces and to provide a substitutive discharge of repressed energy, and a consequent relief of tension. Fantasies, dreams and symptoms were expressions of such mechanisms. Where the substitutive expression was in harmony with social values and super-ego ideals, it provided a suitable means of relief (sublimation). Where it was not in harmony, conflict resulted and repressive mechanisms were again invoked. If repression proved ineffective in mediating tension, a regression to earlier modes of adaptation was possible. This happened particularly where the individual was confronted by experiences similar to, or representative of, those which initiated anxiety in childhood. The ego reacted automatically to these experiences, as if the reality conditionings of later years had had no corrective effect on the original danger situation. It responded with essentially the

From Lewis R. Wolberg *Technique of Psychotherapy,* pages 58–63, Grune & Stratton, Inc., 1954, by permission of the publisher and author.

170

same defenses of childhood, even though these were now inappropriate.

A retention of a relationship to reality at the expense of an intrapsychic balance produced a psychoneurotic disturbance. The existing conflict here was between the ego and the id. If an intrapsychic balance developed at the expense of reality relationships, the consequence was psychosis. The latter resulted when the ego was overwhelmed by id forces, the conflict being between the ego and the environment.

In addition to the libido theory described above, Freud elaborated the theory of the death instinct to account for phenomena not explicable in terms of libido. He postulated that an instinct existed in the id which prompted aggressive and destructive drives. This instinct manifested itself in a "repetition compulsion" to undo the forward evolutionary development of the organism, and to its primordial inorganic state. The death instinct, though sometimes libidinized (sadism) was totally different from the sexual instinct.

Freudian psychoanalytic therapy is based on the libido theory described above. It rests on the hypothesis that neurotic illness is nurtured by the repression of vital aspects of the self and its experiences; particularly oral, anal and sexual (including Oedipal) experiences in relation to important parental agencies. This repression is sponsored by fear of the loss of love or of punishment from the parents, which has been internalized in the super-ego. Repressed feelings, attitudes and fears, and the early experiences associated with them, continue to strive for conscious recognition, but are kept from awareness by dread of repetition of parental loss of love or punishment now invested in the super-ego. The removal from the mainstream of consciousness makes it impossible for the individual to come to grips with basic conflicts. These remain in their pristine state, uncorrected by reality and by later experiences. The energy required to maintain repression, as well as to sustain other defenses against anxiety, robs the individual of energy that could be utilized to nurture psychosexual development.

Therapy, of necessity, consists of restoring to consciousness that which was removed by repression, and which has been draining off energies needed to foster personality growth. In therapy, the relationship with the therapist helps strengthen the ego to a point where it can eventually cope with anxiety, mobilized by the return of the repressed to awareness. It is essential that the patient recognize the derivatives of the repressed, since these represent in an attenuated form, the warded-off material. To minimize the distortion of these derivatives, the obtrusion of current situations and other reality influences must be kept at a minimum. This is fostered by certain technical procedures, such as "free association," the assumption of the couch position, passivity of the therapist, encouragement of transference, the use of dreams, and the focusing of the interview away from reality considerations.

The basis of Freudian psychoanalysis lies in what is perhaps Freud's most vital discovery, that of transference. As has previously been indicated, Freud found that the patient, if not interfered with, inevitably projected into the therapeutic situation, feelings and attitudes that were parcels of his past. Sometimes transference manifestations became so intense that the patient actually reproduced and reenacted with the therapist important conflictual situations and traumatic experiences (transference neurosis) which had been subject to infantile amnesia. By recovering and recognizing these repressed experiences and conflictual situations that had never been resolved, and by living them through with a new, less neurotic and nonpunitive parental agency, the super-ego was believed to undergo modification. The individual became tolerant of his id, and more capable of altering ego defenses that had crippled his adaptation. There occurred, finally, a mastery of his early conflicts and a liberation of fixated libido which could then enter into the development of a mature personality.

Since the Oedipus complex is considered by Freud to be the nucleus of every neurosis, its analysis and resolution in transference constitutes a primary focus. Where the Oedipus complex is not revealed, where its pathologic manifestations are not thoroughly analyzed and worked through, and where forgotten memories of early childhood experiences are not restored, treatment is considered incomplete.

Because Freudian psychoanalysis *is* transference analysis, all means of facilitating transference are employed. These include the assumption by the therapist of an extremely passive role, the verbalization by the patient of a special kind of communication—"free association"—the analysis of dream material, the maintenance of an intense contact with the patient on the basis of no less than five visits weekly, and the employment of the recumbent couch position.

Passivity on the part of the therapist is judiciously maintained even through long periods of silence. The therapist also refrains from reacting emotionally, or responding positively or negatively to any verbalized or non-verbalized attitude or feeling expressed by the patient. Strict anonymity is observed, no personal information being supplied to the patient irrespective of how importunate he may become. A non-judgmental, non-punitive, non-condoning attitude by the therapist is adhered to, dogmatic utterances of any kind being forbidden.

The only "rule" the patient is asked to obey is the "basic rule" or "fundamental rule" of verbalizing whatever comes to his mind, however fleeting, repulsive or seemingly inconsequential it may seem (free association). This undirected kind of thinking is a most important means of tapping the unconscious, and of reviving unconscious conflicts and the memories that are related to their origin. Most importantly, free association, like passivity, enhances the evolution of transference. So long as the patient continues to associate freely, the therapist keeps silent, even though entire sessions may pass without a comment. The therapist fights off all temptations toward "small talk" or impulses to expound on theory. Only when resistances to free association develop, does he interfere, and only until the patient proceeds with his verbalizations.

Dream analysis is utilized constantly as another means of penetrating the unconscious. By activating repressed material and working on defenses as they are revealed in dream structure, the therapist aids the development of transference.

The frequency of visits in Freudian psychoanalysis is important. To encourage transference, no fewer than five visits weekly are required. In some cases four visits may suffice. Fewer visits than this encourage "acting-out" and other resistances to transference.

The use of the recumbent couch position enables the patient to concentrate on the task of free association with as few encumbrances of reality as possible. It helps the therapist, also, to focus on the unconscious content underlying the patient's verbalizations without having to adjust himself to the demands such as would exist in a face-to-face position. Concentrating on his inner life rather than on external reality, helps to bring on the phenomenon of transference.

During the early stages of analysis, the main task is to observe—from his free associations and dreams—unconscious conflicts, and the types of defenses employed by the patient, which form a kind of blueprint of the unconscious problems of the patient. This blueprint is utilized later at the stage of transference. Since repression is threatened by the operation of exploring the unconscious, anxiety is apt to appear, stimulating defensive mechanisms. These function as resistances to productivity, and even to verbalization. Free association may consequently cease, and the patient may exhibit other manifestations that oppose cooperation with the treatment endeavor. Such resistances are dealt with by interpretation. Through interpretation the patient is brought to an awareness of how and why he is resisting, and the conflicts that make resistance necessary.

Sooner or later the patient will "transfer" past attitudes and feelings into the present relationship with the analyst. Observance of the "basic rule," the attack on his resistances through interpretation, and the consideration of unconscious material in dreams and free associations, remove habitual protective devices and facades that permit the patient to maintain a conventional relationship. Toward the therapist he is most apt to express strivings rooted in past experiences, perhaps even reproducing his past in the present. Thus, a revival of pathogenic past conflicts develops. Unlike supportive and reeducative therapy, in which transference may be utilized as a therapeutic vehicle, the transference is interpreted to the patient in order to expose its nature. This is the chief means of resolving resistance, of bringing the individual to an awareness of the warded off content, and of realizing the historical origin of his conflicts.

The development of transference may occur insidiously and manifest itself indirectly, or it may suddenly break out in stark form. It often shows itself in changes in the content of free associations, from inner feelings and past relationships with parents, to more innocuous topics, like current events and situations. This shift is evidence of resistance to deeper material activated by the erupting transference feelings. Sometimes free association may cease entirely, with long stubborn silences prevailing which are engendered by an inability to talk about feelings in relation to the therapist. The purpose of superficial talk or silence is to keep from awareness repressed emotions and forgotten memories associated with early childhood, particularly the Oedipus complex. Until these can be brought out into the open, the emotions relating to them discharged, and the associated memories revived, the conflictual base of neurosis will remain. The transference neurosis offers an opportunity for this revival, since, in the relationship with the therapist, the patient will "act-out" his loves, fears and hates, which were characteristic of his own experiences during the Oedipal period.

Transference, however, acts as a source of powerful resistances that impede therapeutic progress. Once the patient is in the grip of such resistances, he is usually determined to cling to them at the expense of any other motivation, including that of getting well. On the positive side, transference is important diagnostically, since it reveals a most accurate picture of the patient's inner conflicts. Additionally, it induces a coming to grips with and a working-through in a much more favorable setting of those unresolved conflicts that have blocked maturation. The resolution of transference is felt by Freudian psychoanalysts to be the most powerful vehicle known today for producing structural alterations in the personality.

Active interpretations of the transference are essential to its resolution. These include the interpretation of its manifestations, its origin, and its original and present purposes. The working-through of transference is accompanied by a recollection of forgotten infantile and childhood experiences—a recounting of distortions in relationships with parents or parental surrogates. Interpretations will usually be denied at first as part of the resistance manifestation. Acknowledgment of the unreal nature of transference is usually opposed by the patient, because this either constitutes too great a threat for him, or because he does not want to relinquish transference gratifications which are deemed essential to life itself. So long as he continues to accept transference as factual, the analysis will remain interminable, unless forcefully terminated by either participant. With persistence on the part of the therapist, interpretations usually take hold, and the patient is rewarded with greater insight, an increased sense of mastery, liberation from neurotic symptoms, and a genuine growth in maturity.

The therapist must also constantly guard against manifestations of counter-transference, which may be both disguised and varied, and which are mobilized by unresolved problems and pressing needs within the therapist himself. Common forms of counter-transference are subtle sadistic attacks on the patient, impulses to be pompous and omnipotent, or desires to reject the patient or to detach oneself from the relationship. Because of counter-transference, a personal analysis is considered essential for the analyst in order that he can deal with his own unconscious tendencies and resistances precipitated by his contact with his patients.

As the ego of the patient is strengthened by an alliance with the therapist, it becomes more and more capable of tolerating less and less distorted derivatives of unconscious conflict. The continued interpretation by the therapist of the patient's unconscious feelings and attitudes, as well as the defensive devices that he employs against them, enables the patient to work-through his problems by seeing how they condition every aspect of his life. In the medium of the therapeutic relationship, the individual is helped to come to grips with early fears and misconceptions, resolving these by living them through in the transference. The patient is finally able to resolve libidinal fixations, and to liberate energy that should originally have gone into the formation of a mature sexual organization.

Disagreement with certain psychoanalytic concepts is legion. Even those analysts who consider themselves to be "orthodox" Freudians are not in complete accord with Freud in theory and method. For instance, there are many analysts who challenge the death instinct hypothesis. Insofar as technique is concerned, practically every analyst implements psychoanalytic methods in his own specific way. An extensive questionnaire distributed by Glover to a representative group of practicing psychoanalysts demonstrated that deviations from orthodox techniques were extensive. There were differences in the form, timing, amount and depth of interpretation. The degree of adherence to free association varied, as did the assumption of passivity and anonymity, the use of reassurance, and the management of transference. Variation in methods of doing psychoanalysis was indicated by the fact that out of eighty-two questions, there was general agreement on only six, and even here there was not complete conformity.

Criticism of Freudian psychoanalysis is voiced both by those who have had no intimate contact with the psychoanalytic technique, as well as by well-trained psychoanalysts who have been thoroughly schooled in Freudian principles. Lines of disagreement will be discussed in the next section on non-Freudian psychoanalysis. One commonly voiced criticism of the Freudian method is that some analysts insist upon wedging their patients into a preconceived theoretic structure. When the patient does not produce appropriate material that substantiates accepted notions of dynamics, or when he refuses to accept interpretations, he is credited as being in an obstinate state of resistance. Another criticism expressed by non-Freudians is that, in their eagerness to smuggle "deep" insights into patients, certain "orthodox" analysts make dogmatic interpretations which the patient feels obliged to accept. These may mobilize intense anxiety, which disorganizes patients with weak ego structures. A third criticism is that many Freudian analysts are intolerant toward those who practice any therapies other than Freudian psychoanalysis, considering these to be superficial and of little real value. Accordingly, they are inclined to depreciate the results of treatment by non-analysts, as well as by analysts of non-Freudian orientation.

Freudian psychoanalysis is taught extensively in this country, being sponsored by the American Psychoanalytic Association and by most of the current schools of psychoanalytic training.

18.   The Modified Psychoanalytic Treatment of Schizophrenia

HARRY STACK SULLIVAN

In this presentation, an attempt will be made to contribute some factual material bearing on the nature of the schizophrenic mental disorders, and on their treatment by a procedure rather intimately related to the psychoanalytic method of Sigmund Freud. No argument will be offered as to the propriety of the use of "psychoanalytic" in referring to a definite variation from Dr. Freud's

From *Amer. J. Psychiat.* 88:519–540, 1931–1932, by permission of the American Psychiatric Association.

technique, nor will a review of the orthodox Freudian contributions to the schizophrenia problem be undertaken. The former cannot but remain a matter of personal opinion. For the latter we may await a presently forthcoming study by Dr. William V. Silverberg. Since a session of our current meeting has been devoted to the subject of schizophrenia, and since some of the views expressed therein are doubtless not consonant with those of the present writer, some attention must also be devoted to the meaning of schizophrenia as hereinafter used. No importance is attached, however, to the magnificent expression of my personal prejudices in these matters.[1]

Firstly, it is held that if there is any difference between the "schizoid" and the "schizophrenic" mental disturbances, the difference is wholly one of degree, and not one of kind. The writer is no more entertained by "thobbing" about an essential organic disorder in schizophrenia, than is he by tedious speculation as to the relations of organic anomaly or defect to particular psychoses with mental deficiency. In contradistinction, for example, to Schilder's contribution at the earlier session,* this paper is intended to deal with consensually valid information about actual patients and actual procedures of therapy, rather than with ingenuity of thinking about hypotheses concerning possibilities of an unknown order of probability. It must follow the tedious scientific rather than the spectacular philosophic road, and its verbiage must be so carefully organized and so adequately elucidated as to provide the psychiatric reader with a formulation useful to himself and his patients. It does not set up any new frame of reference by use of which one can achieve a high percentage of "hits" at the game of prognostic prophecy: to the writer, the future of any particular person is a highly contingent matter, unless the subject-person be psychobiologically an adult—and in the latter case, unless also he be approaching the *senium,* the degree of contingency of his future is *distinct* if not still *high.* Had we persisted for many generations in an agrarian culture, and had this, improbably, been accompanied by extensive, well-integrated psychobiological research, so that we came to know a great deal about the living of our people, then, perchance, we would have come to a fair acquaintance with the actualities of *human probability.* Translated, however, in a few generations from such a culture to the unprecedented industrial situation, we are now in a state of almost complete ignorance of these facts of living, and

therefore without any basis for prophecy as to the outcome of this or that poorly envisaged complex of more or less important but partly unrecognized factors. The future of each physico-chemical organism may subsist in some reality underlying our hypothetical time-dimension, but the future of each *person* must be recognized as a function of the eternally changing configuration of the cultural-social present. Conceivably, the identical germ plasm evolving in monozygotic twins may be representative in the present of a path in the future such that the twins shall arrive synchronously at a physico-chemical fiasco in the shape of appendicial inflammation. Conceivably, it was in some ultimately comprehensible fashion ordained at the moment of the writer's conception that he shall cease to live owing to rupture of the middle meningeal artery at the age of 57 years, three months and five days, plus or minus less than 100 hours. But that the present fact of his condemning what Dr. Gregory Stragnell has so aptly dubbed the scholasticism of certain psychoanalytically inclined psychiatrists—in this particular case Paul Schilder about real and pseudoschizophrenia —that this activity was determined more remotely than the occasion of the last meeting of the Association for Research in Nervous and Mental Diseases, is not true.[2]

---

[1]The reader is respectfully referred to the perhaps redundant but no less relevant "Thobbing" of Henshaw Ward (New York: Bobbs-Merrill, 1926). To *thob* is to *th*ink out something, which *o*pinion is glorified as an extravasation of one's personality, and most vigorously *b*elieved and "defended," thereafter.

[*Paul Schilder, "Scope of Psychotherapy in Schizophrenia," *Amer. J. Psychiatry* (1931–32) *88*:1181–1187.]

---

[2]The most signicant determining factors in this particular situation, *so far as the writer is chiefly concerned,* may be "dated" as follows: March 12, 1931, psychiatric meeting at which the protagonist "presented" a case illustrating the alleged relations of the organic and the functional; March 18, 1931, dinner discussion; April 10, 1931, psychiatric meeting, as previous; April 24, 1931, psychiatric meeting, as previous; April 28, 1931, protagonist's discussion of "The Pathogenesis of Schizophrenia" by Dr. Gregory Zilboorg, New York Psychoanalytic Society; May 13, 1931, reading of summary of protagonist's paper in the program of the current meeting; May 17, 1931, realization that someone must be made a "goat" for illustrating pseudopsychiatric contributions; May 21, 1931, conclusion that the ends justified the risk of this sort of illustration before so kindly and democratic an audience as the present one.

The *situation* under discussion is *interpersonal;* involving, as major nexus, (a) the writer variously expanded, (b) his "impersonal" hearers and readers, (c) the person, Paul Schilder as protagonist, auditor, reader, and reactor, and secondarily those who "side" with him in the alleged "controversy" which many conceive all psychiatric criticism to be, (d) the body of valid and other information that is the psychiatry of schizophrenia; and so forth.

No one could conceivably demonstrate any preordination of the effect on the protagonist's future of this situation, prior to the date first named. That which at least two people cannot demonstrate cannot be utilized in scientific procedure. It seems therefore fairly proven that the effects of the current interpersonal situation on the future of Dr. Paul Schilder, arise *de novo* from the configuration of the present; this in turn, in so far as it is focused in the writer, arising from configurations *actually existing* at particular moments on certain dates in the recent past; these, in further turn, arising from streams of events so complex in themselves, and so complex in their interrelations, that any prophecy of the current situation, on a date more distant than six months ago, would have been fantastic in the extreme.[3]

To return now to the crux of this point: *either no one* of the acutely schizophrenic young men received by the research service of the Sheppard and Enoch Pratt Hospital in the past two years was in fact schizophrenic but instead all were "schizoid"—in which case we might perhaps assume that schizophrenia *the* disease is not shown by native-born males before the age of 25—*or* there is no great importance to be attached to the organic substratum of personality in young

acute schizophrenics, but rather great stress to be laid on the socio-psychiatric treatment to which they are exposed, in our studying of the factors relevant to outcome. It is my opinion that a consensus of qualified observers can be secured in support of the latter conclusion. The question of an "organic disorder" is therefore irrelevant to this consideration of schizophrenia.[4]

Secondly, in further delimitation of the term, schizophrenia, it is held that these disorders have not been defined psychoanalytically. It is necessary, before adumbrating the original communication herein attempted, to discountenance any conclusion that the writer's study of schizophrenia has "proven" or "disproven" psychoanalytic theory, or any part or parcel thereof, other than the doctrine of narcissistic neurosis. The psychoanalytic terms hereinafter utilized are terms as to the meaning of which, in the writer's opinion, a consensus of competent observers could be obtained. That these consensually defined meanings would be identical with or quite different from the most orthodox Freudian definitions, is unknown. Psychoanalytic formulations are extremely individualistic, in the sense that they are largely Prof. Freud's opinions about his experience with his patients, in the formation of which opinions—as in the great part of all psychiatric opinions—the social and cultural aspects of the thinker's opinion-formation have mostly been ignored. There could not be a meaningful use of the term schizophrenia in regard of a man who had grown from birth into adolescence in utter detachment from any person or personally organized culture. Again, it is possible so to organize a society that the living of its persons, normal to each other, would be regarded as schizophrenic by psychiatrists who

---

[3]The best that could have been ventured is something as follows: The present writer, being deeply interested in schizophrenia, and having amassed consensually valid information which he interprets as evidence convincing to any intelligent observer to the effect that *no such illness of acute onset is apt to manifest a dependable sign of bad outcome regardless of treatment,* being moreover activated by a drive to insure the active attention of all concerned to the importance of early care in determining the outcome of schizophrenic disorders, being also interested in the growth of psychiatric knowledge and its refinement from fantasy, *will to a considerable probability,* sooner or later, subject the views of the protagonist to more or less effective criticism. If suitable occasion arise, this will doubtless occur in the course of a psychiatric meeting. Since the writer will be activated to reach the largest audience, it will probably occur at a meeting of The American Psychiatric Association. After reading the program of the current meeting—a prophecy the more probable in that it is but a few weeks "ahead of" the events—an astute prognostician might have said, "It is *quite probable* that this situation will arise on June 3 or 5, 1931." Even if, on May 27, he had read this paper, he would have had clearly in mind the fact that the occurrence of the present situation *continued to be contingent* on many actually unpredictable factors.

[4]The acuteness or insidiousness of *onset of the observed psychosis,* however, may finally give the question of underlying organic state new relevance. It is quite *possible,* in the writer's opinion, that an ultimately measurable something of great prognostic signicance may be found to underlie these insidious disintegrations of personality attended by more or less of schizophrenic phenomena, that are now lumped with disorders of acute *observed onset.* Statistics of the Sheppard expreience indicate so great a difference in course of the two groups, that one cannot but wish that effort might be directed to the comparative study of individuals of acute *versus* insidious observed onset.

studied any one of its members in sufficiently alien surroundings. In brief, schizophrenia is meaningful only in an *interpersonal context;* its characteristics can only be established by a study of the interrelation of the schizophrenic with schizophrenic, less schizophrenic, and nonschizophrenic others. A "socially recovered" schizophrenic is often still psychotic, but is certainly *less* schizophrenic than is a patient requiring active institutional supervision. To isolate the *non*schizophrenic individual, however, is no small problem. It implies criteria of presence or absence of these processes, of which criteria there seems to be a marked dearth. One might use the following as a fundamental basis for classification: the nonschizophrenic individual, in his interaction with other persons, behaves and thinks in complete consonance with their mutual cultural make-up. Then, to the extent that one's behavior and thought in dealing with another diverges from the mutual culture—traditions, conventions, fashions—to that extent he would be schizophrenic. This seems to be a good working hypothesis, but it has not yet ensued in much consensually valid information. There is, as yet, no measuring of mutual culture; we know that being exposed to culture does not necessarily imply its incorporation in a personality; we know that there are certain personality differentials that greatly affect the incorporation of cultural entities; but we have not paid much attention to evolving techniques for distinguishing the cultural aspects of individual personalities.[5]

There is, however, an indirect approach to this problem—one, moreover, that has seemed to be of practical application. We know that the dream-life of the individual is to a very great degree, purely personal. This consideration applies to a lesser extent to the waking fantasy-life. While there is probably very little indeed of the waking fantasy that is uninfluenced by environing persons or personal entities not wholly of the self, we can assume that certain "primitive" dreams are almost entirely without ex-

ternal reference. We therefore conclude that the more like the dream of deep sleep a given content is, the more purely of the self it is. We can then surmise that a rough approximation to our basis for division into the schizophrenic and the non-schizophrenic can be hypothecated on the consideration of the more purely personal *versus* the consensually valid apperception of a given interpersonal situation. If the "contact" with external reality is wholly unintelligible *per se* to the presumably fairly sane observer, then the subject-individual manifests a content indistinguishable from a dream, and is either in a state of serious disorder of the integrating systems, or is schizophrenic. An individual manifesting behavior when not fully awake would thus be clearly schizophrenic. An individual suffering the disorder of interest manifested in severe fatigue would likewise come under this rubric.

A psychiatrist's initial reaction to this formulation can scarcely be one of instant acceptance. He knows of people who "awaken" in nightmares and have trouble in throwing off the content of the dream. He knows that most of these folk are comparatively normal, in their daily life. He is not ready to identify their transitory disturbance of consciousness on occasional nights with the mental disorder shown 18 hours or so per day, day in and day out by the "dementia praecox" patients in the wards of the mental hospital. It is the writer's opinion that neither phenomenologically nor dynamically can distinction be shown between the two situations. Schizophrenics, in the first hours or days of the frank illness, show just as abrupt transitions among distinguishable states as does our troubled dreamer. The dream-state in their case tends to become habitual, or at least frequently recurrent, and whenever this occurs, the individual is definitely schizophrenic.[6]

The questions that would seem to require answers before acceptance of this formulation of schizophrenia are somewhat as follows: How does it happen that most of us are able to sort out our dreams

---

[5]The development of this topic—*viz.,* the cultural entities built into and going to make up the individual personality—is to be found in the writer's forthcoming text, "The Sickness of The Modern Mind: The Psychopathology of Interpersonal Relations" [probably Personal Psychopathology].

[6]That this conception of schizophrenia is broad enough to include the clinical entity, *hysteria,* has not escaped the writer. This is not the occasion on which to develop the implications of a classification of levels of consciousness, nor of the dynamics underlying major and minor dissociations.

and our waking experience with a very high degree of success, while the schizophrenic fails in this? Why do only some of those who have night-terror or nightmares progress into chronic schizophrenic states? And, from the organicist, why, if this definition is approximately correct, should not a treatment by alternation of rest and the use of a powerful cerebral stimulant like caffeine bring about at least a suspension of the schizophrenic state? As to the first of these questions, the actual sorting out of *some little* of our dream-life from waking experience is a difficult or impossible task. The little that is "hard to locate" as to whether dream or "reality" is often quite transparently related to important but none too well recognized tendency systems within the personality concerned. We come thus to the answer of questions one and two: To the extent that important tendency systems of the personality *have* to discharge themselves in sleep, to that extent the dream-processes tend to exaggerate personal importance, and to augmented "reality value." That which permits tendency systems no direct manifestation except during sleep and other states of altered consciousness is their condition of *dissociation* by other tendency systems of the personality—systems apparently invariably represented in the self. At this point, a digression must be made anent a fairly popular psychoanalytic "thob" about the "strength" *versus* "weakness" of the ego. We learn that the superego is "weak" in the schizophrenic; also, that it is "strong" in the schizophrenic; that the ego and the ideal of ego are weak or strong; that the feeble ego is ground between the powerful id of instinctual cravings and the superego; and so forth. Leaving aside the fact that there is plenty of clinical material to be observed by anyone seriously interested in *finding out* what this is all about—there being at least 250,000 patients diagnosed as schizophrenic in the hospitals of the United States—the writer would point out that no night-terror, nightmare, or schizophrenic disorder *can occur* unless there is a waking dissociation of some one powerful tendency system by another powerful tendency system. And, by direct implication of the formula, a continued dream-state, schizophrenia, cannot occur unless there is continued an approximation to a dynamic balance between the

tendency system manifesting in the conscious self and the one dissociated from such manifestation.[7] As to the chemotherapeutic employment of agents to provide rest alternating with cerebral stimulants of the caffeine group, it may be noted that this very program, applied during the first hours of schizophrenic collapse, does delay the disaster. The cerebrum and the other areas responding to caffeine stimulation, however, are not solely the province of the conscious self, and the raised threshold of function is not solely at the service of the *dissociating* system. This topic, together with that of delirifacient drugs and of ethyl alcohol, has been discussed by the writer, elsewhere.

It appears, then, that no well-integrated personality—in whom there is no dissociation of an important tendency system—can show schizophrenic processes of more than momentary duration; and that any personality in whom there is a chronic dissociation of a powerful tendency system may show persisting schizophrenia after any event that destroys the balance by strengthening the dissociated tendency system, or by enfeebling the dissociating system. Physiological maturation and toxic-exhaustive states are frequent factors in this connection.

The partition of time to the schizophrenic processes—whether they occupy but moments during the time ordinarily devoted to sleep, or instead persist days on end in active psychosis—is determined by the balance between the dissociated and the dissociating systems. The "healing" process that ordinarily occurs in night-terror and nightmare is the source of an important insight into this matter. One "recovers" from the failing dissociation manifesting more or less lucidly in the nightmare, by reintegrating one's consciousness of circumambient reality, including one's "place," status, etc. If the pressure of the dissociated system is great, one "knows better" than to return to sleep until one has strengthened the dissociating system by a readjustment of interest and attention to one's waking world. In night-terror, the healing process

---

[7]Since it is not the present purpose to discuss the strength or weakness of the ego and so forth, no comment will be made on, for example, the highly relevant data provided by psychopathic personalities.

is less conscious, but usually more directly *interpersonal*. In any case, in the writer's opinion, the restoration of balance in favor of the dissociating system is achieved by some *adjustment of interpersonal relations*. On the other hand, a persisting dream-state represents a failure of interpersonal adjustment, such that the tendency system previously dissociated is now as powerful in integrating interpersonal situations as is the previously successful dissociating system. The augmentation of the one may alternate somewhat with that of the other; the *degree* of consciousness may vary, but conflict and a consciously perceived threat of eruption of the dissociated system is sustained. It is evident that these dynamics may lead to the phenomena delineated in the paper of Dr. Mary O'Malley earlier in the program. It is equally clear that the "retreat" from the personal realities of others, the "seclusiveness" and the inaccessibility to easy personal contacts that are so classically schizophrenic are but the avoidance of accentuated conflict between the tendency systems, which integrate or "strive" to integrate the sufferer into mutually incongruous interpersonal relations, with the appearance of most distressing interests and attention.

We proceed from this theoretic formulation of the facts of schizophrenia to consideration of the treatment of these disorders. It is to be noted that the basic formula of all psychotherapy is that of interpersonal relations, and their effects on the further growth of tendency systems within the patient-personality. Observation of the processes shown in improvements and aggravations of personality disorder is clearly in line with this formulation. One sees that there is no *essential* difference between psychotherapeutic achievement and achievements in other forms of education. There is, in each, an alteration in the cultural-social part of the affected personality, to a state of better adaptation to the physico-chemical, social, and cultural environment. No essential difference exists between the better integration of a personality to be achieved by way of psychoanalytic personality study, and the better integration to be achieved by an enlightened teacher of physics in demonstrating to his student the properties of matter. There are several differences in the technique re-

quired, but these are superficial rather than fundamental, and are to be regarded as determined by actual early training of the patient, in the end reducible to the common denominator of *experience incorporated into the self*. The principal factors responsible for the apparent gap between the ordinary good educative techniques and the orthodox psychoanalytic procedures are to be found in the peculiar characteristics of very early experience—*viz.,* that of the first 18 to 30 months of extrauterine life.[8] Since the characteristics of this material are discussed in various psychoanalytic contributions—including that of Dr. Gregory Zilboorg in this session—and since the purpose of this paper is to present the necessary steps preliminary to dealing with the infantile and early childhood experience, we shall proceed immediately to a consideration of the *interpersonal requirements* for the successful therapy of the schizophrenic.

Psychotherapy, like all experience, functions by promoting personality growth, *with or without* improvement of personality integration. Pure suggestion therapy, if such there be, merely adds experience to one or more of the important tendency systems of the personality, thereby perhaps altering the dynamic summation manifested in behavior and thought. Even such a therapy could perhaps be useful in preschizophrenic personalities and, conceivably, even in acute psychosis. A purely rational therapy would be directed to the better integration of the personality systems, as well as to the provision of additional experience. Since it could apply only at the level of verbal communication, it should scarcely be expected to produce great affect in the field of extra-conscious processes. Hortatory therapy would generally be directed to the augmentation of the superego aspects of personality. This includes persuasion and the all too prevalent "bucking up" treatment. None of these procedures is in line with the information which we have secured as to the growth and function of personality.

Treatment in states of reduced consciousness, notably under hypnosis, could

---

[8]Consideration of these factors is not directly relevant to the contribution herein attempted, and has been outlined elsewhere [*Personal Psychopathology*].

be more nearly adjusted to the total personality. Unfortunately, however, the integration of the treatment situation implied by the occurrence of the hypnotic or even the hypnoid states imposes a great responsibility on the physician. Unless he is expert indeed in dealing with the earlier experience incorporated in each personality, the net result of the treatment is sadly disappointing. Either there is little more achieved than could have been secured by a fairly rational exhortation, or there is disturbance of the superego functions and an increased severity of conflict. The integration of the hypnosis situation in the incipient or acute schizophrenic is difficult in extreme. This manipulation of the personality is therefore for us chiefly of theoretic importance. The attempt at hypnotizing distressed preschizophrenics should perhaps be emphatically discouraged, as the mandatory—even if self-determined—submission to the other personality is almost certain to cause a severe emotional upheaval, with the hypnotist thereafter in an unenviable role as chief personification of the goal of the dissociated system.

The only tools that have shown results that justify any enthusiasm in regard of the treatment of schizophrenia are the *psychoanalytic* procedures and the *sociopsychiatric* program which the writer has evolved from them. Before taking up these procedures, however, it may be well to note that the process of benefit by psychoanalysis seems none too clearly envisaged by many of its practitioners. One might be led to assume from the literature that a "cure" is achieved by a releasing of the libido from its "point of the fixation" existing somewhere in the past of the individual. A steadily increasing complexity of the map of possible fixation points is leading some of the outstanding thinkers in this field to doubt the importance of the doctrine of fixation. The writer has long since indicated his inability to discover anything corresponding to a point of fixation in schizophrenia, and has come to believe that "releasing the libido from its fixations" is but a figure of speech for something that occurs in recovery under analysis. Observation shows that psychoanalytic therapy consists of two major processes, the combination of which leads to growth and improved integration of personality. These are, firstly, a retrospective survey of the experiential

basis of tendencies that conflict with the simple adaptation of the person to others with resulting growth to a more adult character; and secondly, the provision of experience that facilitates the reorganization of the undeveloped or warped tendencies such that adaptation becomes more successful. The achievement of this double process requires the establishment between the physician and patient of the situation called by Freud the "transference."

There has been a good deal written about "transference," and many peculiarities of technique have been originated with view to its cultivation and management. There seems to the writer to be nothing other than *the purpose* of the interpersonal situation which distinguishes the psychoanalytic transference relation from other situations of interpersonal intimacy. In other words, it seems to be a special case of interpersonal adaptation, distinguished chiefly by the role of subordination to an enlightened physician skilled in penetrating the self-deceptions to which man is uniquely susceptible, with a mutually accepted purpose of securing the patient an increased skill in living. Like almost all other situations tending towards intimacy the early stages of the psychoanalytic situation include a great body of fantasy processes that are not directly helpful to the achievement of the goal of the physician. Like all other interpersonal relations, this one includes a good deal of intercommunication by channels other than that of spoken propositions. As it is ordinarily applied, the psychoanalytic situation involves a patient the organization of whose self is not satisfactory, and whose self-regard is inadequate. This is very much the case in preschizophrenic and incipiently and acutely (catatonic) schizophrenic patients. By reason of the extreme distress caused by any threatened (or fantasied) reduction of the already distressingly small self-regard of these patients, and also by reason of specific painful experience with all previously significant persons, these patients are extremely uneasy about any situation in which the favorable cooperation of another is required for its resolution. The appearance of strong positive tendency towards the physician is thus attended by an extraordinary augmentation of attention for unfavorable signs, and very slight provocation may lead to a reversal of the tendency—from positive to negative, love to hate.

Before proceeding to develop the implications of these facts for the actual management of these patients, reemphasis must be made of the writer's distinction of schizophrenia from hebephrenic deterioration and from paranoid maladjustments. In brief, the patients to whom therapy may be applied with high probability of success are, firstly, patients in whom there has been a rather rapid change from a state of partial adjustment, to one of apparent psychosis, a matter of weeks, not months or years—this transition being the incipient schizophrenic state; secondly, patients who have not progressed into that regression of interests to early childhood or late infancy levels, to which we refer as the hebephrenic; and thirdly, patients who have not made a partial recovery by massive projection and transfer of blame, the "paranoid schizophrenic," or paranoid state with more or less of residual schizophrenic phenomena. The case of the chronic catatonic state is of potentially good outcome, this seeming to be but a chronic continuation of the purely schizophrenic state, but the actual duration in illness is a factor that is not to be ignored.

The procedure of treatment begins with removing the patient from the situation in which he is developing difficulty, to a situation in which he is encouraged to renew efforts at adjustment with others. This might well be elsewhere than to an institution dealing with a cross-section of the psychotic population; certainly, it should not be to a large ward of mental patients of all sorts and ages. The subprofessional personnel with whom the patient is in contact must be aware of the principal difficulty—*viz.*, the extreme sensitivity underlying whatever camouflage the patient may use. They must be activated by a well-integrated purpose of helping in the redevelopment or development *de novo* of self-esteem as an individual *attractive* to others. They must possess sufficient insight into their own personality organization to be able to avoid masked or unconscious sadism, jealousies, and morbid expectations of results. They must be free from the more commonplace ethical delusions and superstitions. Admittedly, this is no small order, and the creation of this

sort of situation is scarcely to be expected either from chance or from the efforts of a commonplace administrative agent.

Given the therapeutic environment, the first stage of therapy by the physician takes the form of providing an orienting experience. After the initial, fairly searching, interview, the patient is introduced to the new situation in a matter-of-fact fashion, with emphasis on the personal elements. In other words, he is made to feel that he is now one of a group, composed partly of sick persons—the other patients—and partly of well folk—the physician and all the others concerned. Emphasis is laid on the fact that something is the matter with the patient, and—once this is at least clearly understood to be the physician's view—that regardless of the patient's occasional or habitual surmise to the contrary, everyone who is well enough to be a help will from thenceforth be occupied in giving him a chance to get well. From the start, he is treated as a *person among persons*.

There is never to be either an acceptance of his disordered thought and behavior as *outré* or "crazy," or a "never-mind" technique that ignores the obvious. Everyone is to regard the outpouring of thought or the doing of acts as at least *valid* for the patient, and to be considered seriously as something that at least he should understand. The individualism of the patient's performances is neither to be discouraged nor encouraged, but instead, when they seem clearly morbid, to be noted and perhaps questioned. The questioning must not arise from ethical grounds, nor from considerations of mere convenience, but from a desire to center the patient's attention on the discovery of the factors concerned. If there is violence, it is to be discouraged, *unemotionally,* and in the clearly expressed interest of the general or special good. If, as is often the case, violence arises from panic, the situation must be dealt with by the physician. If, however, the patient seems obviously to increase in comfort without professional attention after the introduction to care, the physician can profitably await developments. A considerable proportion of these patients proceed in this really human environment to the degree of social recovery that permits analysis, without much contact with the supervising physician. Moreover, in the process, they become aware of their need for insight into their previous difficulties, and somewhat cognizant of the nature of the procedures to be used to that end. They become not only ready but prepared for treatment.

If the patient does not respond in so gratifying a fashion to the special environment, the physician must discover the difficulty. In some cases, the previously dissociated tendency system is integrating personal situations that precipitate panic or panicky states. This requires reassurance by a technique of realistic acceptance of the underlying tendencies, a bringing out into the open of the cause for the fear experienced by the self, with the resulting beneficent effects of a new feeling of group solidarity in that the harsh appraisal of the tendency incorporated in the patient's personality is temporarily suspended or enfeebled, by acquaintance with people to whom the situation is a commonplace of life. In all too many cases, the ideal-organization is such that the appearance of this solidarity-reaction is judged by the self to be ominous, and the attempt to diminish the violence of reaction to the previously dissociated tendency system fails. It is necessary, however, that the conflict be abated, otherwise the development of interpersonal security that is absolutely necessary for a social recovery cannot be achieved. In such cases, recourse is had to chemotherapeutic agencies, notably ethyl alcohol, which impair the highly discriminative action of the more lately acquired tendency systems, and permit the at least rudimentary functioning of the more primitive, without much stress. After from three to ten days of continuous mild intoxication, almost all such patients, in the writer's experience, have effected a considerable readjustment. The *modus operandi* may be indicated roughly by remarking that these patients discover by actual experience that the personal environment is not noxious, and, having discovered this, have great difficulty in subsequently elaborating convictions of menace, plots, fell purposes, etc. It is the rule to have several interviews with the patient during the period of intoxication, and in them to carry out the reassuring technique above indicated.

Occasionally, an acute schizophrenic, showing a marked tendency to paranoid maladjustment, proceeds all the more rapidly in this direction under the type of care thus far outlined. Several devices have been used in combating the process, but the results are not yet satisfactory. It has become clear that this eventuality requires an extraordinary intervention, if the patient is to be saved; and some pioneering work has been done in this connection. The principle involved, however, is one sufficiently startling to justify hesitancy in reporting but two patients. For the present, it must suffice that patients who show progressively deepening paranoid developments or those who are received in florid paranoid states should not remain with the group under active treatment.

As the patient improves, and as his acceptance of the need for help grows, the efforts of the physician become more direct in their application. Energy is expended chiefly in *reconstructing the actual chronology of the psychosis.* All tendencies to "smooth over" the events are discouraged, and free-associational technique is introduced at intervals to fill in "failures of memory." The role of significant persons and their doings is emphasized, the patient being constantly under the influence of the formulation above set forth—*viz.,* that however mysteriously the phenomena originated, everything that has befallen him is related to his actual living among a relatively small number of significant people, in a relatively simple course of events. Psychotic phenomena recalled from the more disturbed periods are subjected to study as to their relation to these people. Dreams are studied under this guide. During this phase of the work, the patient may or may not grasp the dynamics of his difficulty as they become apparent to the physician. Interpretations are never to be forced on him, and preferably none are offered excepting as statistical findings. In other words, if the patient's actual insight seems to be progressing at a considerable pace, it can *occasionally* be offered that thus-and-so has, in some patients, been found to be the result of this-and-that, with a request for his associations to this comment.

One of perhaps three situations now develops. Firstly, if the patient is doing very well, the family insist on taking him home, and generally ignore advice as to further treatment. Secondly, the chronology of the course of recent events running into the psychosis is rather well recovered, and the patient is found to have great difficulty in coming to insight. He is then discharged into regular treatment at the hands of a suitable psychoanalyst, experienced in the psychiatry of schizophrenia—and not too rigid in devotion to technique. Thirdly, the stage of chronology-perfecting is accompanied by so much growth of insight that it is shifted gradually to a close approximation to regular analytic sessions that follow a liberal variant of the orthodox technique.

In the writer's experience, covering some 11 years, there have been regrettable events to be charged off to precipitate and to rigid techniques of psychotherapy. From these mistakes and from the singular opportunities provided by patients themselves, the sociopsychiatric technique above indicated has finally evolved. When physical facilities were made available, it was tried out rather thoroughly. The condition of no patient was aggravated by its use, and the social and real recovery rates obtained were extremely gratifying. It would seem that, for the group as defined above, schizophrenia is an illness of excellent prognosis. The treatment required, however, is obviously far from widely available, and the schizophrenia problem therefore continues to be very urgently one of prevention.

Certain considerations bearing on the professional personnel for working with schizophrenics may not be amiss. In the first place, it seems quite clearly demonstrated in the Sheppard experience that the therapeutic situations must be integrated between individuals of the same sex. Two male patients treated by woman physicians did remarkably badly, while "cooperating" much better than the average. A number of women, treated by the writer, also "cooperated" nicely, as they progressed into deterioration or paranoid maladjustments. Male patients treated by the writer are not as comfortable in the treatment situation as were these women. But they are correspondingly more successful in achieving actual rather than fantastic results.

In the second place, the unanalyzed psychiatrist and the psychiatrist filled with the holy light of his recent analysis are in general not to be considered for this work. The former have generally a rigid system of taboos and compromises which are rather obvious to the schizophrenic intuition, so that the patient comes early to be treating the physician, and to be fearing him. The analytic zealot knows so many things that are not so that the patient never makes a beginning.

Thirdly, the philosophical type of person is a poor candidate for success as a therapist of schizophrenics; they too love philosophizing—it is so much safer to "think" than to go through the mill of observation and understanding. Also, most of these people get systematized so early that they are blind to experience less than a personal psychosis.

Fourthly, those elsewhere identified as the "resistant homosexual types" are poor material for schizophrenia therapists; they are too busy finding "homosexual components" in everyone to note the facts flowing past them.

Fifthly, the reformer element, who "know" how life should be lived, and what is good and bad, if they must do psychiatric work, should keep far from the schizophrenic. Perhaps the manic-depressive psychosis is their ideal field.

Sixthly, perhaps of all the people least fitted for this work are those that are psychiatrists because it gives them powers and principalities over their fellows; to them should go the obsessional neurotics.

Lastly, sadly enough, those to whom life has brought but a pleasant flood of trifling problems without any spectacular disturbances, who have grown up in quiet backwashes far from the industrial revolution, within the tinted half-lights of the passing times—these are afield in undertaking the schizophrenia problem. It is one up to the last minute in its ramifications, and can but bring them a useless gloom and pessimism about youth and the times. There are some ecclesiasts who find joy in tinkering with the mild mental disorders, in Church Healing Missions and the like. These folk might learn much from, for example, the Rev. Anton Boisen, Chaplain of the Worcester State Hospital, who has come by the tedious and often deeply disturbing road of observation and experimentation to a sane grasp of the relations of religious thoughts and techniques to the schizophrenia problem.

In conclusion, it may be restated that, at least in the case of the male, fairly young schizophrenic patients whose divorcement from fairly conventional behavior and thought has been rather abrupt, when received under care before they have progressed either into hebephrenic dilapidation or durable paranoid maladjustments, are to be regarded as of good outlook for recovery and improvement of personality, if they can be treated firstly to the end of socialization, and thereafter by more fundamental reorganization of personality.

Intrapsychic Theories

CRITICAL EVALUATION

Intrapsychic theorists have created a highly complicated superstructure of concepts and propositions to amplify their notions. Although the intricacies of man's behavior are infinite, intrapsychic theorists appear to incorporate an excessive number of principles and terms to account for them. Critics are especially prone to note the rather shoddy empirical foundation upon which these concepts are based. They contend that the line of reasoning connecting dubious clinical observations to the theory progresses through a series of highly tenuous and obscure steps. In short, not only is the source of intrapsychic data suspect, but the sequence of reasoning which ties it to the conceptual system seems excessively involved and imprecise. The papers by B. F. Skinner, the well-known behaviorist, and N. S. Lehrman, a practicing therapist, articulate these points persuasively.

19. Critique of Psychoanalytic Concepts and Theories

B. F. SKINNER

Freud's great contribution to Western thought has been described as the application of the principle of cause and effect to human behavior. Freud demonstrated that many features of behavior hitherto unexplained—and often dismissed as hopelessly complex or obscure—could be shown to be the product of circumstances in the history of the individual. Many of the causal relationships he so convincingly demonstrated had been wholly unsuspected—unsuspected, in particular, by the very individuals whose behavior they controlled. Freud greatly reduced the sphere of accident and caprice in our considerations of human conduct. His achievement in this respect appears all the more impressive when we recall that he was never able to appeal to the quantitative proofs characteristic of other sciences. He carried the day with sheer persuasion—with the massing of instances and the delineation of surprising parallels and analogies among seemingly diverse materials.

This was not, however, Freud's own view of the matter. At the age of seventy he summed up his achievement in this way: "My life has been aimed at one goal only: to infer or guess how the mental apparatus is constructed and what forces interplay and counteract in it." (2) It is difficult to describe the mental apparatus he refers to in noncontroversial terms, partly because Freud's conception changed from time to time and partly because its very nature encouraged misinterpretation and misunderstanding. But it is perhaps not too wide of the mark to indicate its principal features as follows: Freud conceived of some realm of the mind, not necessarily having physical extent, but nevertheless capable of topographic description and of subdivision into regions of the conscious, co-conscious, and unconscious. Within this space, various mental events—ideas, wishes, memories, emotions, instinctive tendencies, and so on—interacted and combined in many complex ways. Systems of these mental events came to be conceived of almost as subsidiary personalities and were given proper names: the id, the ego, and the superego. These systems divided among themselves

From the *Scientific Monthly* 79:300–305, November, 1954, by permission of the American Association for the Advancement of Science and the author.

185

a limited store of psychic energy. There were, of course, many other details.

No matter what logicians may eventually make of this mental apparatus, there is little doubt that Freud accepted it as real rather than as a scientific construct or theory. One does not at the age of seventy define the goal of one's life as the exploration of an explanatory fiction. Freud did not use his "mental apparatus" as a postulate system from which he deduced theorems to be submitted to empirical check. If there was any interaction between the mental apparatus and empirical observations, such interaction took the form of modifying the apparatus to account for newly discovered facts. To many followers of Freud the mental apparatus appears to be equally as real as the newly discovered facts, and the exploration of such an apparatus is similarly accepted as the goal of a science of behavior. There is an alternative view, however, which holds that Freud did not discover the mental apparatus but rather invented it, borrowing part of its structure from a traditional philosophy of human conduct but adding many novel features of his own devising.

There are those who will concede that Freud's mental apparatus was a scientific construct rather than an observable empirical system but who, nevertheless, attempt to justify it in the light of scientific method. One may take the line that metaphorical devices are inevitable in the early stages of any science and that although we may look with amusement today upon the "essences," "forces," "phlogistons," and "ethers," of the science of yesterday, these nevertheless were essential to the historical process. It would be difficult to prove or disprove this. However, if we have learned anything about the nature of scientific thinking, if mathematical and logical researches have improved our capacity to represent and analyze empirical data, it is possible that we can avoid some of the mistakes of adolescence. Whether Freud could have done so is past demonstrating, but whether we need similar constructs in the future prosecution of a science of behavior is a question worth considering.

Constructs are convenient and perhaps even necessary in dealing with certain complicated subject matters. As Frenkel-Brunswik shows (1), Freud was aware of the problems of scientific

methodology and even of the metaphorical nature of some of his own constructs. When this was the case, he justified the constructs as necessary or at least highly convenient. But awareness of the nature of the metaphor is no defense of it, and if modern science is still occasionally metaphorical, we must remember that, theorywise, it is also still in trouble. The point is not that metaphor or construct is objectionable but that particular metaphors and constructs have caused trouble and are continuing to do so. Freud recognized the damage worked by his own metaphorical thinking, but he felt that it could not be avoided and that the damage must be put up with. There is reason to disagree with him on this point.

Freud's explanatory scheme followed a traditional pattern of looking for a cause of human behavior inside the organism. His medical training supplied him with powerful supporting analogies. The parallel between the excision of a tumor, for example, and the release of a repressed wish from the unconscious is quite compelling and must have affected Freud's thinking. Now, the pattern of an inner explanation of behavior is best exemplified by doctrines of animism, which are primarily concerned with explaining the spontaneity and evident capriciousness of behavior. The living organism is an extremely complicated system behaving in an extremely complicated way. Much of its behavior appears at first blush to be absolutely unpredictable. The traditional procedure has been to invent an inner determiner, a "demon," "spirit," "homunculus," or "personality" capable of spontaneous change of course or of origination of action. Such an inner determiner offers only a momentary explanation of the behavior of the outer organism, because it must, of course, be accounted for also, but it is commonly used to put the matter beyond further inquiry and to bring the study of a causal series of events to a dead end.

Freud, himself, however, did not appeal to the inner apparatus to account for spontaneity or caprice because he was a thoroughgoing determinist. He accepted the responsibility of explaining, in turn, the behavior of the inner determiner. He did this by pointing to hitherto unnoticed external causes in the environmental and genetic history of the individual. He did not, therefore, need the traditional explanatory system for traditional purposes; but he was unable to eliminate the pattern from his thinking. It led him to represent each of the causal relationships he had discovered as a series of three events. Some environmental condition, very often in the early life of the individual, leaves an effect upon the inner mental apparatus, and this in turn produces the behavioral manifestation or symptom. Environmental event, mental state or process, behavioral symptom—these are the three links in Freud's causal chain. He made no appeal to the middle link to explain spontaneity or caprice. Instead he used it to bridge the gap in space and time between the events he had proved to be causally related.

A possible alternative, which would have had no quarrel with established science, would have been to argue that the environmental variables leave *physiological* effects that may be inferred from the behavior of the individual, perhaps at a much later date. In one sense, too little is known at the moment of these physiological processes to make them useful in a legitimate way for this purpose. On the other hand, too much is known of them, at least in a negative way. Enough is known of the nervous system to place certain dimensional limits upon speculation and to clip the wings of explanatory fiction. Freud accepted, therefore, the traditional fiction of a mental life, avoiding an out-and-out dualism by arguing that eventually physiological counterparts would be discovered. Quite apart from the question of the existence of mental events, let us observe the damage that resulted from this maneuver.

We may touch only briefly upon two classical problems that arise once the conception of a mental life has been adopted. The first of these is to explain how such a life is to be observed. The introspective psychologists had already tried to solve this problem by arguing that introspection is only a special case of the observation upon which all science rests and that man's experience necessarily stands between him and the physical world with which science purports to deal. But it was Freud himself who pointed out that not all of one's mental life was accessible to direct observation—that many events in the mental apparatus were necessarily inferred. Great as this discovery was, it would have been still greater if Freud had

taken the next step, advocated a little later by the American movement called Behaviorism, and insisted that conscious, as well as unconscious, events were inferences from the facts. By arguing that the individual organism simply reacts to its environment, rather than to some inner experience of that environment, the bifurcation of nature into physical and psychic can be avoided.*

A second classical problem is how the mental life can be manipulated. In the process of therapy, the analyst necessarily acts upon the patient only through physical means. He manipulates variables occupying a position in the first link of Freud's causal chain. Nevertheless, it is commonly assumed that the mental apparatus is being directly manipulated. Sometimes it is argued that processes are initiated within the individual himself, such as those of free association and transference, and that these in turn act directly upon the mental apparatus. But how are these mental processes initiated by physical means? The clarification of such a causal connection places a heavy and often unwelcome burden of proof upon the shoulders of the dualist.

The important disadvantages of Freud's conception of mental life can be described somewhat more specifically. The first of these concerns the environmental variables to which Freud so convincingly pointed. The cogency of these variables was frequently missed because the variables were transformed and obscured in the course of being represented in mental life. The physical world of the organism was converted into conscious and unconscious experience, and these experiences were further transmuted as they combined and changed in mental processes. For example, early punishment of sexual behavior is an observable fact that undoubtedly leaves behind a changed organism. But when this change is represented as a state of conscious or unconscious anxiety or guilt, specific details of the punishment are lost.

---

*Although it was Freud himself who taught us to doubt the face of introspection, he appears to have been responsible for the view that another sort of direct experience is required if certain activities in the mental apparatus are to be comprehended. Such a requirement is implied in the modern assertion that only those who have been psychoanalyzed can fully understand the meaning of transference or the release of a repressed fear.

When, in turn, some unusual characteristic of the sexual behavior of the adult individual is related to the supposed guilt, many specific features of the relationship may be missed that would have been obvious if the same features of behavior had been related to the punishing episode. Insofar as the mental life of the individual is used as Freud used it to represent and to carry an environmental history, it is inadequate and misleading.

Freud's theory of the mental apparatus had an equally damaging effect upon his study of behavior as a dependent variable. Inevitably, it stole the show. Little attention was left to behavior per se. Behavior was relegated to the position of a mere mode of expression of the activities of the mental apparatus or the symptoms of an underlying disturbance. Among the problems not specifically treated in the manner that was their due, we may note five.

1. The nature of the act as a unit of behavior was never clarified. The simple *occurrence* of behavior was never well represented. "Thoughts" could "occur" to an individual; he could "have" ideas according to the traditional model; but he could "have" behavior only in giving expression to these inner events. We are much more likely to say that "the thought occurred to me to ask him his name" than that "the act of asking him his name occurred to me." It is in the nature of thoughts and ideas that they occur to people, but we have never come to be at home in describing the emission of behavior in a comparable way. This is especially true of verbal behavior. In spite of Freud's valuable analysis of verbal slips and of the techniques of wit and verbal art, he rejected the possibility of an analysis of verbal behavior in its own right rather than as the expression of ideas, feelings, or other inner events, and therefore missed the importance of this field for the analysis of units of behavior and the conditions of their occurrence.

The behavioral nature of perception was also slighted. To see an object as an object is not mere passing sensing; it is an act, and something very much like it occurs when we see an object although no object is present. Fantasy and dreams were for Freud not the perceptual *behavior* of the individual but pictures painted by an inner artist in some atelier of the mind which the individual then con-templated and perhaps then reported. This division of labor is not essential when the behavioral component of the act of seeing is emphasized.

2. The dimensions of behavior, particularly its dynamic properties, were never adequately represented. We are all familiar with the fact that some of our acts are more likely to occur upon a given occasion than others. But this likelihood is hard to represent and harder to evaluate. The dynamic changes in behavior that are the first concern of the psychoanalyst are primarily changes in probability of action. But Freud chose to deal with this aspect of behavior in other terms—as a question of "libido," "cathexis," "volume of excitation," "instinctive or emotional tendencies," "available quantities of psychic energy," and so on. The delicate question of how probability of action is to be quantified was never answered, because these constructs suggested dimensions to which the quantitative practices of science in general could not be applied.

3. In his emphasis upon the genesis of behavior, Freud made extensive use of processes of learning. These were never treated operationally in terms of changes in behavior but rather as the acquisition of ideas, feelings, and emotions later to be expressed by, or manifested in, behavior. Consider, for example, Freud's own suggestion that sibling rivalry in his own early history played an important part in his theoretical considerations as well as in his personal relationships as an adult.

An infant brother died when Freud himself was only one and a half years old, and as a young child Freud played with a boy somewhat older than himself and presumably more powerful, yet who was, strangely enough, in the nominally subordinate position of being his nephew. To classify such a set of circumstances as sibling rivalry obscures, as we have seen, the many specific properties of the circumstances themselves regarded as independent variables in a science of behavior. To argue that *what was learned* was the effect of these circumstances upon unconscious or conscious aggressive tendencies or feelings of guilt works a similar misrepresentation of the dependent variable. An emphasis upon behavior would lead us to inquire into the specific acts plausibly assumed to be engendered by these childhood episodes. In very specific terms, how was the behavior of the young Freud *shaped* by the special reinforcing contingencies arising from the presence of a younger child in the family, by the death of that child, and by later association with an older playmate who nevertheless occupied a subordinate family position? What did the young Freud *learn to do* to achieve parental attention under these difficult circumstances? How did he avoid aversive consequences? Did he exaggerate any illness? Did he feign illness? Did he make a conspicuous display of behavior that brought commendation? Was such behavior to be found in the field of physical prowess or intellectual endeavor? Did he learn to engage in behavior that would in turn increase the repertoires available to him to achieve commendation? Did he strike or otherwise injure young children? Did he learn to injure them verbally by teasing? Was he punished for this, and if so, did he discover other forms of behavior that had the same damaging effect but were immune to punishment?

We cannot, of course, adequately answer questions of this sort at so late a date, but they suggest the kind of inquiry that would be prompted by a concern for the *explicit shaping of behavioral repertoires* under childhood circumstances. What has survived through the years is not aggression and guilt, later to be manifested in behavior, but rather patterns of behavior themselves. It is not enough to say that this is "all that is meant" by sibling rivalry or by its effects upon the mental apparatus. Such an expression obscures, rather than illuminates, the nature of the behavioral changes taking place in the childhood learning process. A similar analysis could be made of processes in the fields of motivation and emotion.

4. An explicit treatment of behavior as a datum, of probability of response as the principal quantifiable property of behavior, and of learning and other processes in terms of changes of probability is usually enough to avoid another pitfall into which Freud, in common with his contemporaries, fell. There are many words in the layman's vocabulary that suggest the activity of an organism yet are not descriptive of behavior in the narrower sense. Freud used many of these freely; for example, the individual is said to discriminate, remember, infer, repress,

decide, and so on. Such terms do not refer to specific acts. We say that a man discriminates between two objects when he behaves differently with respect to them; but discriminating is not itself behavior. We say that he represses behavior which has been punished when he engages in other behavior *just because* it displaces the punished behavior; but repressing is not action. We say that he decides upon a course of conduct either when he enters upon one course to the exclusion of another, or when he alters some of the variables affecting his own behavior in order to bring this about; but there is no other "act of deciding." The difficulty is that when one uses terms which suggest an activity, one feels it necessary to invent an actor, and the subordinate personalities in the Freudian mental apparatus do, indeed, participate in just these activities rather than in the more specific behavior of the observable organism.

Among these activities are conspicuous instances involving the process of self-control—the so-called "Freudian mechanisms." These need not be regarded as activities of the individual or any subdivision thereof—they are not, for example, what happens when a skillful wish evades a censor—but simply as ways of representing relationships among responses and controlling variables. I have elsewhere tried to demonstrate this by restating the Freudian mechanisms without reference to Freudian theory (3).

5. Since Freud never developed a clear conception of the behavior of the organism and never approached many of the scientific problems peculiar to that subject matter, it is not surprising that he misinterpreted the nature of the observation of one's own behavior. This is admittedly a delicate subject, which presents problems that no one, perhaps, has adequately solved. But the act of self-observation can be represented within the framework of physical science. This involves questioning the reality of sensations, ideas, feelings, and other states of consciousness which many people regard as among the most immediate experiences of their life. Freud himself prepared us for this change. There is, perhaps, no experience more powerful than that which the mystic reports of his awareness of the presence of God. The psychoanalyst explains this in other ways. He himself, however, may insist upon the reality of

certain experiences that others wish to question. There are other ways of describing what is actually seen or felt under such circumstances.

Each of us is in particularly close contact with a small part of the universe enclosed within his own skin. Under certain limited circumstances, we may come to react to that part of the universe in unusual ways. But it does not follow that that particular part has any special physical or nonphysical properties or that our observations of it differ in any fundamental respect from our observations of the rest of the world. I have tried to show elsewhere (3) how self-knowledge of this sort arises and why it is likely to be subject to limitations that are troublesome from the point of view of physical science. Freud's representation of these events was a particular personal contribution influenced by his own cultural history. It is possible that science can now move on to a different description of them. If it is impossible to be wholly nonmetaphorical, at least we may improve upon our metaphors.

The crucial issue here is the Freudian distinction between the conscious and unconscious mind. Freud's contribution has been widely misunderstood. The important point was not that the individual was often unable to describe important aspects of his own behavior or identify important causal relationships, but that his ability to describe them was irrelevant to the occurrence of the behavior or to the effectiveness of the causes. We begin by attributing the behavior of the individual to events in his genetic and environmental history. We then note that because of certain cultural practices, the individual may come to describe some of that behavior and some of those causal relationships. We may say that he is conscious of the parts he can describe and unconscious of the rest. But the act of self-description, as of self-observation, plays no part in the determination of action. It is superimposed upon behavior. Freud's argument that we need not be aware of important causes of conduct leads naturally to the broader conclusion that awareness of cause has nothing to do with causal effectiveness.

In addition to these specific consequences of Freud's mental apparatus in obscuring important details among the variables of which human behavior is a function and in leading to the neglect of important problems in the analysis of behavior as a primary datum, we have to note the most unfortunate effect of all. Freud's methodological strategy has prevented the incorporation of psychoanalysis into the body of science proper. It was inherent in the nature of such an explanatory system that its key entities would be unquantifiable in the sense in which entities in science are generally quantifiable, but the spatial and temporal dimensions of these entities have caused other kinds of trouble.

One can sense a certain embarrassment among psychoanalytic writers with respect to the primary entities of the mental apparatus. There is a predilection for terms that avoid the embarrassing question of the spatial dimensions, physical or otherwise, of terms at the primary level. Although it is occasionally necessary to refer to mental events and their qualities and to states of consciousness, the analyst usually moves on in some haste to less committal terms such as *forces, processes, organizations, tensions, systems,* and *mechanisms.* But all these imply terms at a lower level. The notion of a conscious or unconscious "force" may be a useful metaphor, but if this is analogous to force in physics, what is the analogous mass that is analogously accelerated? Human behavior is in a state of flux and undergoing changes that we call "processes," but what is changing in what direction when we speak of, for example, an affective process? Psychological "organization," "mental systems," "motivational interaction"—these all imply arrangements or relationships among *things,* but what are the things so related or arranged? Until this question has been answered the problem of the dimensions of the mental apparatus can scarcely be approached. It is not likely that the problem can be solved by working out independent units appropriate to the mental apparatus, although it has been proposed that such a step be undertaken in an attempt to place psychoanalysis on a scientific footing.

Before one attempts to work out units of transference, or scales of anxiety, or systems of mensuration appropriate to the regions of consciousness, it is worth asking whether there is not an alternative program for a *rapprochement* with physical science that would make such a task unnecessary. Freud could hope for an eventual union with physics or physiology only through the discovery of neurological mechanisms that would be the analogues of, or possibly only other aspects of, the features of his mental apparatus. Since this depended upon the prosecution of a science of neurology far beyond its current state of knowledge, it was not an attractive future. Freud appears never to have considered the possibility of bringing the concepts and theories of a psychological science into contact with the rest of physical and biological science by the simple expedient of an operational definition of terms. This would have placed the men-

tal apparatus in jeopardy as a life goal, but it would have brought him back to the observable, manipulable, and pre-eminently physical variables with which, in the last analysis, he was dealing.

References

1. Frenkel-Brunswik, Else. "Meaning of Psycho-analytic Concepts and Confirmation of Psychoanalytic Theories," *Scientific Monthly*, 79:293–300 (1954).
2. Jones, E. *Life and Work of Sigmund Freud*, Vol. 1. New York: Basic Bks., 1953.
3. Skinner, B. F. *Science and Human Behavior*. New York: Macmillan, 1953.

20. Precision in Psychoanalysis

N. S. LEHRMAN

The purpose of this paper is: (a) to show that precise definition of terms is necessary if psychoanalysis is to become more scientific and useful, and (b) to demonstrate two contrascientific trends within classical psychoanalysis resulting from its lack of precision: a refusal to face facts, and a tendency to retreat to a therapeutically-nihilistic "elite" status (1). These retreating trends tend to evoke hopeless abandonment of the interpersonal search for the cause and cure of mental illness, thereby leaving the field to chemists, geneticists and physiologists whose tools, though refined, appear unsuited for the analysis of human feelings and mental illness.

We shall first attempt to define the word "scientific," and to indicate the role of precision in scientific work. Second, we shall examine a recent classical psychoanalytic conceptualization to demonstrate its lack of precision and its unverifiability. Third, we shall try to show that a scientific reformulation of this conceptualization may make experimental and clinical verification possible. Fourth, we shall examine Freud's metaphorical

method to show that it lacked precision and frequently confused reiterated hypotheses for proved facts. Finally, we shall examine Freud's unscientific justification of his opposition to precise definitions, and shall seek the consequences in American classical psychoanalysis today.

WHAT DOES "SCIENTIFIC" MEAN?

The Merriam-Webster Unabridged Dictionary defines "scientific" as "conducted . . . strictly according to the principles and practice . . . of exact science, especially as designed to establish incontestably sound conclusions and generalizations by absolute accuracy of investigation."

The phrase "incontestably sound" includes the basic concept of verifiability. Descartes' scientific concept of how the brain worked, as the neurophysiologist H. S. Magoun notes (2), "was so clearly put as to possess the danger of permitting easy determination of its truth."

If "scientific" means "conducted according to the principles and practice . . . of exact science," we can examine the practice and principles of an exact science

From *Amer. J. Psychiat.* 116:1097–1103, 1960, by permission of the American Psychiatric Association and the author.

for guidance. Nobel Laureate Robert A. Millikan (3), writes:

The first principle of the physicist, when he uncovers a new phenomenon, is to determine *what* he is to measure; the next is to devise *means* to measure it(3a) . . . All scientific investigations which have led to real progress have begun . . . by the treatment of simple and specific problems with quantitative exactness, not by making deductions from general philosophical schemes or *a priori* principles(3b).

One of the cardinal principles of scientific work, therefore, is precision, both in definitions and in measurements.

A RECENT VAGUE PSYCHOANALYTIC CONCEPTUALIZATION

Percival Bailey's recent Academic Lecture (4) criticizing classical psychoanalysis drew an almost definitive reply from Ostow (1), one of the ablest of the classical psychoanalysts. Let us apply the principles of scientific methodology which Millikan has just described to one of Ostow's key statements.

As a hypothesis, Ostow offers the psychoanalytic proposition that *"every man has a tendency to enjoy a physical, sexual relationship with his mother."* Verification of this statement requires, as Millikan indicates, determining *what* is to be measured, and then determining *how* it is to be measured.

As is unfortunately so frequent in psychoanalytic statements, many words in Ostow's hypothesis have rather vague meanings. His use of the word "every" would mean the proposition disproved if one man on earth lacked this tendency. Does the word "man" mean an adult male, or does it mean *all* human males, or does it mean all young human males, *i.e.,* boys? I believe Ostow is really referring to boys rather than to men.

But the key word in Ostow's hypothesis is "tendency"; what does it mean? The total proposition cannot be scientifically examined until we know *what* this "tendency" is which we are measuring and against what yardstick.

The word "tendency" itself is an example of the fuzziness of definition so frequently seen in psychoanalytic writings. A "tendency" has a self-initiated efferent quality quite similar to that present in the psychoanalytic concepts of wishes, drives, impulses and instincts. But all these efferent concepts have two separate aspects: that which is either innately or experientially responsive to stimuli, and that which is mystically self-propelled, as were Freud's life and death instincts. Failure to distinguish between the responsive and self-initiated aspects makes Ostow's meaning rather unclear.

For the sake of discussion, let us assume we know what Ostow's "tendency" means. How do we verify its existence?

We are usually told that the hypothesis is validly confirmed by patients' productions in psychoanalytic treatment. But Grinker (5) denies that such confirmation is valid. He says:

Using the tools of psychoanalysis, (psychoanalysts) find what they search for and little else. . . . The patient is the psychoanalyst's biased collaborator. Each interpretation may be a hypothesis . . . but there are no alternatives and little possibility that the patient-collaborator will refute it, although theoretically much is made of the patient's behavior as an index of correctness or refutation of interpretations. We have demonstrated in our experiments . . . (that) the patient-subject interprets almost everything that the psychiatrist states as having therapeutic meaning. The patient is not an unbiased scientific colleague.

Verification of a psychoanalyst's hypothesis by his patients' responses is, therefore, not a scientifically valid, independent confirmation of the hypothesis, particularly when the analyst determines whether the student-patient progresses in his course of psychoanalytic training. Instead, it may well be part of a closed philosophical system.

What other means are there of direct verification of hypotheses such as Ostow's? Is selecting (4a) "from a mass of data of observation those items which support (one's) thesis" worth while? Such a selection is valid in the formulation of hypotheses, but not valid in proving them.

Isaac Newton (6) pointed to the lack of validity of "proofs" arrived at by such selection of data. He wrote:

The best and safest method of philosophizing certainly seems to be, first, to inquire diligently into the properties of things, and to establish these properties by experiments.

Psychoanalysis has had relatively few such experiments. Newton continues:

Then, [one should] proceed more slowly to hypotheses for the explanation of them. For *hypotheses* ought to be used only in explaining the properties of things, and ought not to be assumed for determining them, *except where they are able to furnish experiments.* For if from the possibility of *hypotheses* alone, anyone makes a conjecture concerning the true nature of things, I do not see by what means it is possible to determine certainty in any science, since it is always possible to devise any number of hypotheses, which will seem to overcome new difficulties.

Hence, selection of data to fit a hypothesis by no means proves it; confirming a hypothesis is more important than, and should precede, elaborations upon it.

Is the "general opinion" of the correctness of psychoanalytic concepts proof of its validity? If this were so, the earth suddenly became spheroidal in 1492, after having previously been flat, and no one needed psychoanalytic aid before Freud appeared. "General opinion" therefore lacks validity as scientific proof. Consequently we must conclude that there are no direct proofs for the validity of Ostow's imprecisely formulated psychoanalytic hypothesis.

The only indirect proof for the classical psychoanalytic hypotheses lies in the value of the procedure in helping patients. Yet Teuber (7), discussing the Cambridge-Somerville experiment, points out that "the burden of proof is on anyone who claims specific results for a given form of therapy." But when the American Psychoanalytic Association examined its members' treatment results, it could not prove the value of the classical psychoanalytic treatment. Weinstock, chairman of the survey committee, stated (8), "It is not that the figures can be used to prove analytic therapy effective or ineffective." Hence indirect therapeutic proof of the classical psychoanalytic hypotheses is also lacking.

Consequently, there is no proof, direct or indirect, for Ostow's imprecisely formulated psychoanalytic Oedipal hypothesis.

A VERIFIABLE REFORMULATION OF THE OEDIPAL HYPOTHESIS

Is there sexual attraction (a more precise formulation than "a tendency to enjoy a sexual relationship") between a boy and his mother? I believe there is, because there are apparently inborn sexual responses in all of us to members of the opposite sex which may well be mediated outside of conscious awareness, and at least partly through the sense of smell (9). Since the mother is the female with whom the boy has most contact, his inborn sexual responses will probably be directed mostly toward her, but there may well be a corresponding unconscious sexual response on her part toward him as well. These concepts, unlike classical formulations such as Ostow's, can perhaps be experimentally tested and quantitatively measured. But until such testing confirms them, they must be regarded as hypotheses only, no matter how many times our patients may confirm them, unless, perhaps, it can be clearly shown that using them is statistically helpful in accomplishing cure.

AN EXAMPLE OF FREUD'S METAPHORICAL VAGUENESS

Let us now examine an example of Freud's metaphorical method, to see the lack of precision characterizing much of his work. That this led to later mysticism, with life and death instincts in eternal unverifiable conflict, is well known. We shall, however, take an example from the more scientific early part of his career.

In his "Interpretation of Dreams," he discusses the behavior of a hungry infant, and states (10), "nothing prevents us from assuming that there was a primitive state of the psychical apparatus . . . in which wishing ended in hallucinating." In this connection, let us recall Newton's statement (6) that "it is always possible to devise any number of hypotheses which will *seem* to overcome new difficulties."

Freud maintains, essentially, that since the baby has been fed before, when he is again hungry, the memory image of the previous feeding might be experienced as a hallucination. But there is quantitatively a far cry between the memory trace of a previous feeding in a two-day-old baby, and the relatively adult quality of a hallucination. An hallucination of milk involves the anticipatory differentiation of milk from non-milk, something utterly beyond the capacity of a two-day-old infant. Moreover, while perhaps (10) "nothing prevents us from assuming" this hallucination, scientific method demands, as Newton (6) points out, that such hypotheses "ought *not* to be assumed for determining (the properties of things), *except where they are able to furnish experiments.''* In the 59 years since Freud's assumption of infantile hallucinations, what experiments have been made to prove or disprove them? Yet this and many other unprovable assumptions continue to be accepted in psychoanalytic thinking because one great man postulated them.

But here, and elsewhere as well, Freud's lack of precision led him down an unverifiable and therefore unscientific path. Was this imprecision accidental? Perhaps it was at first, but it was later explicitly justified.

We have seen how Millikan insisted that hypotheses cannot be verified until *after* they have been rigorously defined, and that hypotheses cannot themselves be defined until their fundamental terms and basic concepts have previously been rigorously defined. But psychoanalysis consciously and explicitly declines to define its terms rigorously; it is as if Freud's statements are, *ipso facto,* sometimes exempted from the scientific requirement for objective verification. In reality, however, it is a long way from "nothing prevents us from assuming" to proven fact.

FREUD'S JUSTIFICATION FOR "ELASTIC" DEFINITIONS

The question of "clear and sharply defined basal concepts" is discussed in Freud's 1915 paper, "Instincts and Their Vicissitudes" (11). His concept of scientific method differs quite sharply from that of the exact scientists already quoted. It also differs sharply from Osler (12), who wrote that "the leaven of science gives to men habits of mental accuracy . . . which enlarge the mental vision."

In his 1915 paper, Freud correctly points out that concepts are changed as a science progresses. Continued investigation reveals conceptual imperfections, and the concepts and definitions are therefore changed accordingly. Because, at the beginning of a scientific investigation, we do not know its final concepts with *absolute* accuracy, Freud incorrectly denied the necessity of precise definition of the *relatively* accurate conceptual tools with which the investigation begins.

When we deal with precisely defined concepts such as Newton's or Descartes', we can fairly easily determine the accuracies and inaccuracies within them. Such determinations result in more precise formulations, which are then subjected to the same evaluative process, leading to still greater precision.

When, however, we have no firm definitions with which to work, we find ourselves without a valid starting point. We are consequently attempting to dissect warm air with empty hands. The fact that concepts and definitions become altered as the result of investigation is very different from the idea that *working* definitions, like scissors, should be elastic.

Hence Freud's statement (11) that "the progress of science demands a certain elasticity even in . . . definitions" is unscientific. Working definitions are points of reference, but not rubber bands; they can be and are changed, but they are not elastic. They become *different* definitions after their alteration, rather than merely being somewhat stretched. A sexually altered dog is sexually quite different from what it used to be; there is no question of elasticity whatsoever. Just as an oak is quite different from the acorn from which it has grown, so is an hallucination quite different from an infantile memory trace.

But, it might be said, psychoanalysis differs from physics and mathematics inasmuch as it deals with the unconscious, with feelings and with instincts. Ernst Mach (13) categorically rejected abdication of scientific method to the "instinctive." He wrote:

Instinctive knowledge is very frequently the starting-point of investigations. . . . This by no means compels us, however, to create a new mysticism out of the instinctive in science and to regard this factor as infallible. That it is not infallible, we very easily discover. . . . The instinctive is just as fallible as the distinctly conscious.

Freud failed to separate meticulously the mystical, self-initiatory aspects in his concept of instinct from its scientific responsive aspects. This failure, continued by some of his followers, has helped lead to the pessimistic religious trend which has pervaded much of classical psychoanalysis for so long. Indeed, the psychologist Joseph Lyons (14) recently noted that

If there is one all-pervading faith that binds twentieth century western man, it may be found in his uncritical acceptance of the value of psychotherapy. If there is a universal answer offered in these times for the anxiety that is supposed to be the mark of the age, it lies in the role of the patient in psychotherapy. It is our new religion, arising out of and efficiently tailored to the moral crisis of the day.

THE RESULTS OF IMPRECISION IN CLASSICAL PSYCHOANALYSIS TODAY

Freud's refusal, continued by his followers, to define terms meticulously has led, in part, to the rather poor estimation other scientists hold of psychoanalysis. James R. Newman (15), author of *The World of Mathematics,* recently reviewed a new psychological and psychoanalytic dictionary. Referring to these fields, he wrote:

A discipline cannot live without words, but words can corrupt and destroy it. This explains the importance of good science dictionaries, which are as much works of criticism as they are guides to usage. No subjects are in greater need for such services than psychology and psychoanalysis. The vocabularies of both these wildly flourishing branches of study are plagued by amateurishness, pretentiousness and a general professional weakness for fancy terms. As Goethe wrote in Faust, "When ideas fail, words come in very handy."

This is one example of an exact scientist's view of psychoanalysis today.

Percival Bailey (4a), the distinguished neurosurgeon happily turned psychiatrist, wrote:

I know that there are attempts to prove that psychoanalysis is a science. They do not convince me and have convinced very few objective observers(4b). Even Freud(4c) admitted that it is only a sort of post-dictive science, lacking in power of synthesis and prediction. Science cannot be built on the insights of visionaries or on the mutual titillation of interdisciplinary minds at Palo Alto, or elsewhere. Science can be built only by the cautious, laborious verification, step by step, of one's hypotheses, establishing each one solidly before passing on to the next. As Jones says(4d), Freud had no patience with such a method.

There is another example of an exact scientist's view of psychoanalysis today.

TWO UNFORTUNATE PSYCHOANALYTIC RESPONSES

Two important contra-scientific trends can be seen within classical psychoanalysis in response to its general scientific vagueness and to its specific failure to prove its therapeutic effectiveness. The first trend declines to reveal the data about its lack of therapeutic effectiveness, and seeks to rationalize away this anti-scientific suppression of data. The second trend maintains that only a psychoanalytic "elite" are capable of meaningfully evaluating both themselves and their results.

The first trend is exemplified in Weinstock's explanation of the American Psychoanalytic's decision not to publish its survey results. "The material on which either opinion is based (whether or not psychoanalysis is therapeutically effective) is inadequately established, and controversial publicity on such material cannot be of benefit in any way." This fear of "controversial publicity" includes refusal to allow investigators who are not members of the American Psychoanalytic even to see the report unless they pledge in advance to keep the material "confidential." This is material which has already been circularized to the membership of the American Psychoanalytic, and which has already been described in detail in the *New York Herald Tribune.*

How scientific is this point of view?

Avoidance of "controversy" (*i.e.,* disagreement) and suppression of data because they might support the "wrong" side still occur in politics, but have not been in style in astronomy, for example, for about 350 years. At that time, Tycho Brahe spent 25 years making astronomical observations to destroy the Copernican heliocentric theory. His observations were, however, available to Kepler, who used them to prove the Copernican doctrine, and to place it on a firm foundation.

It would appear to me that the general public and the healing professions in particular would greatly benefit from the publication of the results of treatment at the hands of members of the American Psychoanalytic Association. The Bible says, "The truth shall make you free." It seems to me that the only people to whom "publicity on such material cannot be of benefit in any way" (8) would be individuals who, for some reason, may be afraid of what the truth will show. But science itself is more important than the reputation of any individual scientific worker, or of any particular group of workers.

The second unfortunate trend in classical psychoanalysis maintains that only the psychoanalytic "elite" (1) are capable of meaningfully evaluating both themselves and their results.

The analyzed are an elite . . . in the sense that they have had certain filters removed from their visual apparatus so that they can now see clearly what they previously could not see at all, or could see only with serious distortion(1).

While training analyses are often helpful, ascription of such crystal-clear thinking only to the products of "authentic" psychoanalysis (which Ostow contrasts with the "shoddy perversions and dilutions that usurp its name"), suggests a defensive device more than a statement of scientific fact.

For Ostow's statement to be completely accurate and for all the filters to be removed, a perfect training analyst would be required. But no human being is perfect.

Indeed, there are data suggesting that the training analysis may even *add* visual filters not previously present. Edward Glover, as "authentic" an analyst as there is, writes (16),

Training analysts' methods of analyzing candidates are influenced by their own character formations and peculiarities, and by the training they (themselves) have undergone. These peculiarities they, in their turn, are quite likely to transvey to their pupils.

I have known several analysts both before their training analyses began and since they have finished them. It seems to me, as an observant friend, that most of them are stiffer, less courageous and less human after their supposedly successful analyses than they were before. Some are members of the "authentic" American Psychoanalytic, and some are not. From my own small sample (hardly enough for a hypothesis, and certainly not for an assertion), those who have been "authentically" analyzed by training analysts of the "approved" New York institutes seem, in general, to be less warm, less spontaneous, less human and far more arrogant than those friends whose analyses were conducted under the aegis of one or another of "the shoddy perversions and dilutions that usurp the name" of psychoanalysis.

If classical psychoanalysts wish to make a secular religious cult of themselves, nobody can stop them, even if the consequences affect our entire society. It is also their privilege disdainfully to flee the epidemic of mental illness which Dr. Gunnar Gundersen, President of the American Medical Association, describes as sweeping our country.

But, as "authentic" Allen Wheelis writes (17), "Knowledgeable moderns put their backs to the couch, and in so doing may fail occasionally to put their shoulders to the wheel." Might not those who "authentically" worship Freud's great courage be more useful if they emulated it as well?

The more widespread the classical psychoanalytic retreat from American psychiatric realities, the more the classical analysts leave the field of investigation of mental illness to chemists, geneticists and physiologists, whose tools are not designed for the best available understanding of human feelings. There is some danger that this classical psychoanalysts' retreat from reality will tend toward the abandonment of perhaps the greatest contribution by Freud to psychiatry: his recognition that mental illness arises from distorted interpersonal relationships, beginning with the family of origin.

This retreat of some classical psychoanalysts also abandons the most potent tool there is in the field, a tool scientifically defined by Freud's genius, and used, although in part incorrectly, by him and his followers: the emotional interaction between patient and doctor. This retreat also abandons one of the most effective curative techniques yet devised in psychiatry: free association into the past to discover the "reminiscences" still plaguing patients.

All of these potent contributions to human welfare would be jettisoned should all of classical psychoanalysis withdraw to sulk in elite secrecy. It could then perhaps join other self-proclaimed aristocracies, such as Virginia Woolf's "aristocracy of sensibility." But is not retreat into such "elitism" an abdication of the physician's responsibility to the patients needing his aid?

I believe the science of interpersonal relationships which Freud founded can, when properly modified, lay open the causes and nature of functional mental illness. I believe that only psychoanalysis has forged the scientific tools able to overcome the effects of man's inhumanity to man, perhaps the prime cause of human fear and mental illness.

Fortunately, despite the negative trends mentioned above, psychoanalysis is far from dead. The incisive work of Ackerman (18) and others on intra-family interactions, the distinguished studies which Spitz (19) has made on insufficiently fondled children, Ferenczi's (20) demonstration that the analyst's warmth is a necessary condition for cure, and Fromm-Reichmann's (21) brilliant sensitivity with schizophrenics all encourage the hope that precise knowledge of the effects of interpersonal warmth at the breast, in the home and role-appropriate warmth in the office can help us fulfill our task of preventing and curing mental illness. But for us to do so, we must also return to scientific precision, even in the presence of human warmth.

SUMMARY

Scientific precision has far too often been consciously excluded from classical psychoanalysis, because Freud rejected it. In consequence, classical psychoanalysis has assumed many of the trappings of a religion, and lost many of the essential characteristics of a science. Two anti-scientific trends in the field, defensive secrecy and arrogant "elitism," seem to have occurred in part as a result of perpetuation of this lack of precision.

References

1. Ostow, M.: Am. J. Psychiat., *113*: 844, 1957.
2. Margoun, H. W.: The Waking Brain. Springfield, Ill.: C. C Thomas, 1958, p. 11.
3. Millikan, R. A., Roller, W., and Watson, E. C.: Mechanics, Molecular Physics, Heat and Sound: Boston: Ginn and Co., 1937. a. p. 3. b. plate 4, following p. 35.
4. Bailey, P.: Am. J. Psychiat., *113*: 387, 1956. a. p. 394. b. Sears, R. R.: Survey of Objective Studies of Psychoanalytic Concepts. New York: Social Science Research Council, 1943 (Bailey reference #146). c. Freud, S.: The Psychogenesis of a Case of Homosexuality in a Woman. Collected Papers, II. London, 1933 (Bailey reference #56). d. Jones, E.: The Life and Work of Sigmund Freud. New York: Basic Books, 1945-46. Vol. I, pp. 34, 40 (Bailey reference #100).
5. Grinker, R. R.: A Philosophical Appraisal of Psychoanalysis. *In* Masserman, J. H.: Science and Psychoanalysis. New York: Grune and Stratton, 1958, p. 137.
6. Newton, Isaac: Philosophical Transactions, *7*: 5014, 1672. Quoted in Millikan *et al.* (3), p. 52.
7. Teuber, H. L., and Powers, E.: Res. Publ. Assoc. Nerv. Ment. Dis., *31*: 138, 1953.
8. Ubell, Earl: Psychiatric Treatment Results Are Measured. New York Herald Tribune, July 7, 1958, p. 1.
9. Bieber, Irving: Olfaction in Sexual Development and Sexual Organization. Papers read before Academy of Psychoanalysis, New York, December 7, 1958. To be published.
10. Freud, S.: The Interpretation of Dreams. Translated by James Strachey. N.Y.: Basic Books, 1955, p. 566.
11. Freud, S.: Instincts and Their Vicissitudes. *In* Collected Papers of Sigmund Freud. London: Hogarth Press, 1949. Vol. 4, p. 61.
12. Osler, W.: Aequanimitas. Philadelphia: Blakiston, 1932, p. 93.
13. Mach, E.: The Science of Mechanics. The Open Court Publishing Co., 1893, pp. 26-27. Quoted in Millikan *et al.* (3), p. 64.
14. Lyons, Joseph: Midstream, *5*: 46, Spring 1959.
15. Newman, J. R.: Unsigned Book Review of "A Comprehensive Dictionary of Psychological and Psychoanalytic Terms," by H. B. and A. C. English. Scient. Am., *199*: 146, Oct. 1958.
16. Glover, E.: Technique of Psychoanalysis. New York: International Universities Press, 1955, p. 6.
17. Wheelis, Allen: J. Am. Psychoanal. Assn., *4*: 289, 1956.
18. Ackerman, N. W.: Psychodynamics of Family Life. New York: Basic Books, 1958.
19. Spitz, R.: Child Development, *20*: 146, Sept. 1949.
20. Ferenczi, S.: Further Contributions to the Theory and Technique of Psychoanalysis. London: Hogarth Press, 1926.
21. Fromm-Reichmann, F.: Principles of Intensive Psychotherapy. Chicago: University of Chicago Press, 1950.

Part III

Phenomeno-logical Theories

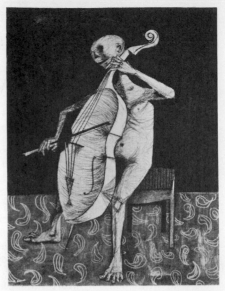

Marco Prassinos — *Cellist*. (The Museum of Modern Art, Gift of Victor S. Risenfeld.)

INTRODUCTION

Phenomenologists stress that the individual reacts to the world only in terms of his unique perception of it. No matter how transformed or unconsciously distorted this perception may be, it is the person's way of perceiving events which determines his behavior. Concepts and propositions must be formulated, therefore, not in terms of objective realities or unconscious processes, but in accordance with how events actually are consciously perceived by the individual; concepts must not disassemble these experiences into depersonalized or abstract categories.

The phenomenon of consciousness is one of the most controversial topics in both psychological and philosophical literature. No one doubts that self-awareness exists, but how can phenomenological reality as experienced by another person be categorized, measured, or even sensed? At best, observers must adopt an emphatic attitude, a sensing in one's self of what another may be experiencing. But this method is justly suspect, fraught with the distortions and insensitivities of the observer. To obviate this difficulty, phenomenologists assume that the verbal statements of the individual accurately reflect his phenomenal reality. Any datum which represents the individual's portrayal of his experience is grist, therefore, for the phenomenologist's mill. They contend that an individual's verbal reports reveal the most important influences upon his behavior. Is it not simple efficiency to ask a person directly what is disturbing him and how this disturbance came to pass? Is his report more prone to error than an observer's speculations gathered from the odds and ends of a case history study? Is it less reliable than deductions which are drawn from dreams and free-associations? The fact that some verbal recollections and feelings are misleading is not reason to dismiss them as useless; they summarize events in terms closest to the individual's experience of them and often embody knowledge that is not otherwise available.

Phenomenological Theories

ORIENTATION

Phenomenologists believe that the distinctive characteristics of each individual's conscious experience should be the primary focus of clinical science. The selection by Rollo May, the primary exponent of the "existential" school in America, represents a direct and convincing application of phenomenological philosophy to the study of mental disorders. In it, he draws upon his own experiences to illustrate the central phenomenological concepts of anxiety and self. George Kelly, originator of the "personal construct" theory, provides a detailed exposition of the essential themes of his position. In the paper published here, he argues clearly for the view that psychological science can best develop from a framework of systematic phenomenological principles and hypotheses.

21. Existential Psychology

ROLLO MAY

Existentialism means centering upon the *existing* person; it is the emphasis on the human being as he is *emerging, becoming*. The word "existence" comes from the root *ex-sistere,* meaning literally "to stand out, emerge." Traditionally in Western culture, *existence* has been set over against *essence,* the latter being the emphasis upon immutable principles, truth, logical laws, etc. that are supposed to stand above any given existence. In endeavoring to separate reality into its discrete parts and to formulate abstract laws for these parts, Western science has by and large been *essentialist* in character; mathematics is the ultimate, pure form of this essentialist approach. In psychology, the endeavors to see human beings in terms of forces, drives, conditioned reflexes, and so on, illustrate the approach via essences.

The emphasis on essences was dominant in Western thought and science— with such notable exceptions, to name only a few, as Socrates, Augustine, and Pas-

cal—until roughly a hundred years ago. The "peak" was reached, the most systematic and comprehensive expression of "essentialism," in Hegel's panrationalism, an endeavor to encompass all reality in a system of concepts that identified reality with abstract thought. It was against Hegel that Kierkegaard, and later Nietzsche, revolted so strenuously.

But in the decades since World War I, the existential approach has emerged from the status of stepchild of Western culture to a dominant position in the center of Western art, literature, theology, and philosophy. It has gone hand in hand with the new developments in science, particularly the physics of Bohr and Heisenberg.

The extreme of the existentialist position is found in Jean Paul Sartre's statement that "existence precedes essence," the assertion that only as we affirm our existence do we have any essence at all. This is a consistent part of Sartre's great emphasis on decision: "We *are* our choices."

My own position, and that of most psychologists who appreciate the great value of this existential revolution, is not so extreme as Sartre's. "Essences" must not be ruled out—they are presupposed in logic, mathematical forms, and other aspects of truth which are not dependent upon any individual's decision or whim. But that is not to say that you can adequately describe or understand a living human being, or any living organism, on an "essentialist" basis. *There is no such thing as truth or reality for a living human being except as he participates in it, is conscious of it, has some relationship to it.* We can demonstrate at every moment of the day in our psychotherapeutic work that only the truth that comes alive, becomes more than an abstract idea, and is "felt on the pulse," only the truth that is genuinely experienced on all levels of being, including what is called subconscious and unconscious and never excluding the element of conscious decision and responsibility—only this truth has the power to change a human being.

The existentialist emphasis in psychology does not, therefore, deny the validity of the approaches based on conditioning, the formulation of drives, the study of discrete mechanisms, and so on. It only holds that you can never explain or understand any *living* human being on that basis. And the harm arises when the image of man, the presuppositions about man himself are exclusively based on such methods. There seems to be the following "law" at work: the more accurately and comprehensively you can describe a given mechanism, the more you lose the existing person. *The more absolutely and completely you formulate the forces or drives, the more you are talking about abstractions and not the existing, living human being.* For the living person (who is not hypnotized or drugged or in some other way placed in an artificial position, such as in a laboratory, in which his element of decision and his responsibility for his own existence are temporarily suspended for the purposes of the experiment) always transcends the given mechanism and always experiences the "drive" or "force" in his unique way. The distinction is whether the "person has meaning in terms of the mechanism" or the "mechanism has meaning in terms of the person." The existential emphasis is firmly on the latter. And it holds that the former can be integrated within the latter.

True, the term "existentialist" is dubious and confused these days, associated as it is with the beatnik movement at one extreme and with esoteric, untranslatable, Germanic, philosophical concepts at the other. True also, the movement collects the "lunatic fringe" groups—to which existential psychology and psychiatry are by no means immune. I often ask myself whether in some quarters the term has become so dubious as to be no longer useful. But "existence" does have the important historical meanings outlined above and probably, therefore, can and ought to be saved from its deteriorated forms.

In psychology and psychiatry, the term demarcates an *attitude,* an approach to human beings, rather than a special school or group. It is doubtful whether it makes sense to speak of "*an* existential psychologist or psychotherapist" in contradistinction to other schools; it is not a system of therapy but an attitude toward therapy, not a set of new techniques but a concern with the understanding of the structure of the human being and his experience that must underlie all techniques. This is why it makes sense, if I may say so without being misunderstood, to say that every psychotherapist is existential to the extent that he is a good therapist, i.e., that he is able to grasp the patient in his reality and is characterized by the kinds of understanding and presence that will be discussed below.

I wish, after these sallies at definition, to *be* existentialist in this essay and to speak directly from my own experience as a person and as a practicing psychoanalytic psychotherapist. Some fifteen years ago, when I was working on my book, *The Meaning of Anxiety*, I spent a year and a half in bed in a tuberculosis sanatorium. I had a great deal of time to ponder the meaning of anxiety—and plenty of first hand data in myself and my fellow patients. In the course of this time, I studied the only two books written on anxiety till our day, *The Problem of Anxiety* by Freud and *The Concept of Dread* by Kierkegaard. I valued Freud's formulations: namely, his first theory, that anxiety is the re-emergence of repressed libido, and his second, that anxiety is the ego's reaction to the threat of the loss of the loved object. Kierkegaard, on the other hand, described anxiety as the struggle of the living being against non-being—which I could immediately experience there in my struggle with death or the prospect of being a life-long invalid.

He went on to point out that the real terror in anxiety is not this death as such, but the fact that each of us within himself is on both sides of the fight, that "anxiety is a desire for what one dreads," as he put it; thus, like an "alien power it lays hold of an individual, and yet one cannot tear one's self away."

What struck me powerfully then, was that Kierkegaard was writing about *exactly what my fellow patients and I were going through*. Freud was not; he was writing on a different level, giving formulations of the psychic mechanisms by which anxiety comes about. Kierkegaard was portraying what is immediately experienced by human beings in crisis. It was, specifically, the crisis of life against death, which was completely real to us patients, but he was writing about a crisis that I believe is not in its essential form different from the various crises of people who come for therapy, or the crises that all of us experience in much more minute form a dozen times a day, even though we push the ultimate prospect of death far from our minds. Freud was writing on the technical level, where his genius was supreme; perhaps more than any man up to his time, he *knew about anxiety*. Kierkegaard, a genius of a different order, was writing on the existential, ontological level; he *knew anxiety*.

This is not a value dichotomy; obviously both are necessary. Our real problem, rather, is given us by our cultural-historical situation. We in the Western world are the heirs of four centuries of technical achievement in power over nature and now over ourselves; this is our greatness and, at the same time it is also our greatest peril. We are not in danger of repressing the technical emphasis (of which Freud's tremendous popularity in this country is proof if any were necessary). But rather we repress the opposite. If I may use terms which I shall be discussing and defining more fully later, we repress the *sense of being*, the *ontological sense*. One consequence of this repression of the sense of being is that modern man's image of himself, his experience and concept of himself as a responsible individual have likewise disintegrated.

I make no apologies in admitting that I take very seriously, as will have been evident already, the dehumanizing dangers in our tendency in modern science to make man over into the image of the machine, into the image of the techniques by which we study him. This tendency is not the fault of any "dangerous" men or "vicious" schools; it is rather a crisis brought upon us by our particular historical predicament. Karl Jaspers, both psychiatrist and existentialist philosopher, holds that we are actually in process of losing self-consciousness and that we may well be in the last age of historical man. William Whyte, in his *Organization Man*, cautions that modern man's enemies may turn out to be a "mild-looking group of therapists, who . . . would be doing what they did to help you." He refers here to the tendency to use the social sciences in support of the social ethic of our historical period; and thus the process of helping people may actually make them conform and tend toward the destruction of individuality. We cannot brush aside the cautions of such men as unintelligent or antiscientific; to try to do so would make *us* the obscurantists. There is a real possibility that we may be helping the individual adjust and be happy at the price of loss of his being.

One may agree with my sentiments here but hold that the existentialist approach, with these terms "being" and "non-being," may not be of much help. Some readers will already have concluded that their suspicion was only too right, that this so-called existential approach to psychology is hopelessly vague and horribly muddled. Carl Rogers remarks in a later chapter that many American psychologists must find these terms abhorrent because they sound so general, so philosophical, so untestable. Rogers goes on to point out, however, that he had no difficulty in putting the existential principles in therapy into empirically testable hypotheses.

But I would go further and hold that *without* some concepts of "being" and "non-being" we cannot even understand our most commonly used psychological mechanisms. Take for example, *repression, resistance,* and *transference*. The usual discussions of these terms hang in midair, it seems to me, unconvincing and psychologically unreal, precisely because we have lacked an underlying structure on which to base them. The term "repression," for example, obviously refers to a phenomenon we observe all the time, a dynamism which Freud clearly, and in many forms, described. The mechanism is generally explained by saying that the child represses into unconsciousness certain impulses, such as sex and hostility, because the culture, in the form of parental figures, disapproves, and the child must protect his own security with those figures. But this culture which assumedly disapproves is made up of the very same people who do the repressing. Is it not an illusion, therefore, and much too simple to speak of the culture over against the individual in such fashion and to make it our whipping boy? Furthermore, where did we get the idea that children or adults are so concerned with security and libidinal satisfactions? Are these not carryovers from our work with the *neurotic, anxious* child and the *neurotic* adult?

Certainly the neurotic, anxious child *is* compulsively concerned with security, for example; and certainly the neurotic adult, and we who study him, read our later formulations back into the unsuspecting mind of the child. But is not the normal child just as truly interested in moving out into the world, exploring, following his curiosity and sense of adventure—going out "to learn to shivver and to shake," as the nursery rhyme puts it? And if you block these needs of the child, do you not get a traumatic reaction from him just as you do when you take away his security? I, for one, believe we vastly overemphasize the human being's concern with security and survival satisfactions because they so neatly fit our cause-and-effect way of thinking. I believe Nietzsche and Kierkegaard were more accurate when they described man as *the organism who makes certain values—prestige, power, tenderness, love— more important than pleasure and even more important than survival itself.*†

---

†This is the point Binswanger is making in the case of *Ellen West,* translated in the volume *Existence.* By means of the discussion of the psychological illness and suicide of Ellen West, he asks whether there are times when an existence, in order to fulfill itself, must destroy its existence. In this case, Binswanger, like so many of his European psychiatric and psychological colleagues, discusses a case for the purpose of delving into the understanding of some problem about human beings rather than for the purpose of illustrating how the case should or should not be managed therapeutically. In presenting the case, we assumed, as editors of *Existence,* that it, like the other cases,

The implication of our argument here is that we can understand such a mechanism as repression, for example, only on the deeper level of the meaning of the human beings' potentialities. In this respect, "being" is to be defined as the *individual's unique pattern of potentialities*. These potentialities will be partly shared with other individuals but will in every case form a unique pattern for this particular person.

We must ask these questions, therefore, if we are to understand repression in a given person: What is this person's relation to his own potentialities? What goes on that he chooses, or is forced to choose, to block off from his awareness something that he knows, and on another level *knows that he knows?* In my own work in psychotherapy, there appears more and more evidence that anxiety in our day arises not so much out of fear of lack of libidinal satisfactions or security, but rather out of the patient's fear of his own powers and the conflicts that arise from that fear. This may well be the particular "neurotic personality of our time"—the neurotic pattern of contemporary "outer-directed," organizational man.

The "unconscious," then, is not to be thought of as a reservoir of impulses, thoughts, and wishes that are culturally unacceptable. I define it rather as *those potentialities for knowing and experiencing that the individual cannot or will not actualize*. On this level, we shall find that the simple mechanism of repression, which we blithely started with, is infinitely less simple than it looks; that it involves a complex struggle of the individual's *being* against the possibility of

would be understood on the basis of the purposes and assumptions of its authors in writing it; this was an unrealistic assumption. The case is almost universally discussed—and from that point of view justly criticized—in this country from the point of view of what therapy should have been given Ellen West. If it had been Binswanger's purpose to discuss techniques of therapy, he would not have taken a case from the archives of four and a half decades ago in his sanatorium. He seeks, rather, to ask this most profound of all questions: Does the human being have needs and values that transcend its own survival, and are there not situations when the existence, in order to fulfill itself, needs to destroy itself? The implication of this question is in the most radical way to question simple adaptation, length of life, and survival as ultimate goals. It is similar to Nietzsche's point referred to above, and also similar to Maslow's emphasis when he brings out that the "self-actualizing personalities" that he studied resist acculturation.

non-being; that it cannot be adequately comprehended in "ego" and "not-ego" terms, or even "self" and "not-self"; and that it inescapably raises the question of the human being's freedom with respect to his own potentialities. This margin of freedom must be assumed if one is to deal with an existing person. In this margin resides the individual's responsibility for himself, which even the therapist cannot take away.

Thus, every mechanism or dynamism, every force or drive, presupposes an underlying structure that is infinitely greater than the mechanism, drive, or force itself. And note that I do not say it is the "sum total" of the mechanisms, et cetera. It is not the "sum total," though it includes all the mechanisms, drives, or forces: it is the underlying structure from which they derive their meaning. This structure is, to use one definition proposed above, the *pattern of potentiality* of the living individual man *of whom* the mechanism is one expression; the given mechanism is one of a multitude of ways in which he actualizes his potentiality. Surely, you can abstract a given mechanism like "repression" or "regression" for study and arrive at formulations of forces and drives which seem to be operative; but your study will have meaning only if you say at every point, "I am abstracting such and such a form of behavior," and if you also make clear at every point *what* you are abstracting *from,* namely the living man who *has* these experiences, the man *to whom* these things happen.

In a similar vein, I have, for a number of years, been struck, as a practicing therapist and teacher of therapists, by how often our concern with trying to understand the patient in terms of the mechanisms by which his behavior takes place blocks our understanding of what he really is experiencing. Here is a patient, Mrs. Hutchens, who comes into my office for the first time, a suburban woman in her middle thirties, who tries to keep her expression poised and sophisticated. But no one could fail to see in her eyes something of the terror of a frightened animal or a lost child. I know, from what her neurological specialists have already told me, that her presenting problem is hysterical tenseness of the larynx, as a result of which she can talk only with a perpetual hoarseness. I have been given the

hypothesis from her Rorschach that she has felt all her life, "If I say what I really feel, I'll be rejected; under these conditions it is better not to talk at all." During this first hour with her, I also get some hints of the genetic *why* of her problem as she tells me of her authoritarian relation with her mother and grandmother and of *how* she learned to guard firmly against telling any secrets at all.

But if, as I sit here, I am chiefly thinking of these *whys* and *hows* of the way the problem came about, I will have grasped everything *except the most important thing of all, the existing person.* Indeed, I will have grasped everything except the only real source of data I have, namely, this experiencing human being, this person now emerging, becoming, "building world," as the existential psychologists put it, immediately in this room with me.

This is where *phenomenology,* the first stage in the existential psychotherapeutic movement, has been a helpful breakthrough for many of us. Phenomenology is the endeavor to take the phenomena as given. It is the disciplined effort to clear one's mind of the presuppositions that so often cause us to see in the patient only our own theories or the dogmas of our own systems, the effort to experience instead the phenomena in their full reality as they present themselves. It is the attitude of openness and readiness to hear—aspects of the art of listening in psychotherapy that are generally taken for granted and sound so easy but are exceedingly difficult.

Note that we say *experience* the phenomena and not *observe;* for we need to be able, as far as possible, to catch what the patient is communicating on many different levels; these include not only the words he utters but his facial expressions, his gestures, the distance from us at which he sits, various feelings which he will have and communicate subtly to the therapist and will serve as messages even though he cannot verbalize them directly, ad infinitum. And there is always a great deal of subliminal communication on levels below what either the patient or therapist may be conscious of at the moment. This points toward a controversial area in therapy which is most difficult in the training and practice of therapists, but which is unavoidable because it is so important, namely, subliminal, empathetic "telepathic" communication. We shall not go into it here; I wish only to say this experiencing of the communications of the patient on many different levels at once is one aspect of what the existential psychiatrists like Binswanger call *presence*.

Phenomenology requires an "attitude of disciplined naïveté," in Robert Mac-Leod's phrase. And commenting on this phrase, Albert Wellek adds his own, "an ability to *experience critically*." It is not possible, in my judgment, to listen to any words or even to give one's attention to anything without some assumed concepts, some constructs in one's own mind by which he hears, by which he orients himself in his world at that moment. But the important terms "disciplined" in Mac-Leod's phrase and "critically" in Wellek's refer, I take it, to the difficult attainment of objectivity—that while one must have constructs as he listens, one's aim in therapy is to make one's own constructs sufficiently flexible so that he can listen in terms of the patient's constructs and hear in the patient's language.

Phenomenology has many complex ramifications, particularly as developed by Edmund Husserl, who decisively influenced not only the philosophers Heidegger and Sartre but also the psychiatrists Minkowski, Straus, and Binswanger, the psychologists Buytendijk, Merleau-Ponty, and many others. We shall not go into these ramifications here.

Sometimes the phenomenological emphasis in psychotherapy is used as a disparagement of the learning of technique or as a reason for not studying the problems of diagnosis and clinical dynamics. I think this is an error. What is important, rather, is to apprehend the fact that the technical and diagnostic concerns are on a different level from the understanding that takes place in the immediate encounter in therapy. The mistake is in confusing them or letting one absorb the other. The student and practicing psychologist must steer his course between the Scylla of letting knowledge of techniques be a substitute for direct understanding and communication with the patient and the Charybdis of assuming that he acts in a rarified atmosphere of clinical purity without any constructs at all.

Certainly it is true that students learn-

ing therapy often become preoccupied with techniques; this is the strongest anxiety-allaying mechanism available to them in the turmoil-fraught encounters in psychotherapy. Indeed, one of the strongest motivations for dogmatism and rigid formulations among psychotherapeutic and analytic schools of all sorts lies right here—the technical dogma protects the psychologist and psychiatrist from their own anxiety. But to that extent, the techniques also protect the psychologist or psychiatrist from understanding the patient; they block him off from the full presence in the encounter which is essential to understanding what is going on. One student in a case seminar on existential psychotherapy put it succinctly when he remarked that the chief thing he had learned was that "understanding does not follow knowledge of dynamics."

There is, however, a danger of "wild eclecticism" in these phenomenological and existential approaches to therapy when they are used without the rigorous clinical study and thought which precedes any expertness. Knowledge of techniques and the rigorous study of dynamics in the training of the psychotherapist should be presupposed. Our situation is analogous to the artist: long and expert training is necessary, but if, at the moment of painting, the artist is preoccupied with technique or technical questions—a preoccupation every artist knows arises exactly at those points at which some anxiety overtakes him—he can be sure nothing creative will go on. Diagnosis is a legitimate and necessary function, particularly at the beginning of therapy; but it is a function different from the therapy itself and requires a different attitude and orientation to the patient. There is something to be said for the attitude that once one gets into therapy with a patient and has decided on the general direction, one forgets for the time being the diagnostic question. By the same token, questions of technique will arise in the therapist's mind from time to time as the therapy proceeds, and one of the characteristics of existential psychotherapy is that the technique changes. These changes will not be hit and miss, however, but will depend on the needs of the patient at given times.

If this discussion sounds unconcluded and gives the appearance of straddling the issue of "technique" on one side and "understanding" on the other, the appearance is indeed correct. The whole topic of the "technical-objective" versus the "understanding-subjective" attitude has been on a false dichotomized basis in our psychological and psychiatric discussions. It needs to be restated on the basis of the concept of the existence of the patient as *being-in-the-world,* and the therapist as existing in and participating in this world. I shall not essay such a restatement here, but I wish only to state my conviction that such a reformulation is possible and gives promise of taking us out of our present dichotomy on this topic. And in the meantime, I wish as a practical expedient to take my stand against the nascent antirational tendencies in the existential approach. Though I believe that therapists are born and not made, it inheres in one's integrity to be cognizant of the fact that there also is a great deal we can learn!

Another question that has perennially perplexed many of us in psychology has already been implied above, and we now turn to it explicitly. What are the presuppositions which underlie our science and our practice? I do not say "scientific method" here; already a good deal of attention has been paid, and rightly, to the problem of methodology. But every method is based on certain presuppositions—assumptions about the nature of man, the nature of his experience, and so forth. These presuppositions are partially conditioned by our culture and by the particular point in history at which we stand. As far as I can see, this crucial area is almost always covered over in psychology: we tend to assume uncritically and implicitly that our particular method is true for all time. The statement that science has built-in self-corrective measures—which is partially true—cannot be taken as a reason for overlooking the fact that our particular science is culturally and historically conditioned and is thereby limited even in its self-corrective measures.

At this point, the existential insistence is that, because every psychology, every way of understanding man, is based upon certain presuppositions, the psychologist must continually analyze and clarify his own presuppositions. One's presuppositions always limit and constrict what one sees in a problem, experiment, or therapeutic situation; from this aspect of our human "finiteness" there is no escape. The

naturalist perceives in man what fits his naturalistic spectacles; the positivist sees the aspects of experience that fit the logical forms of his propositions; and it is well known that different therapists of different schools will see in the same dream of a single patient the dynamics that fit the theory of their particular school. The old parable of the blind men and the elephant is writ large on the activities of men in the enlightened twentieth century as well as those of earlier, more "benighted" ages. Bertrand Russell puts the problem well with respect to physical science: "Physics is mathematical not because we know so much about the physical world but because we know so little; it is only its mathematical properties that we can discover."

No one, physicist, psychologist, or anyone else, can leap out of his historically conditioned skin. But the one way we can keep the presuppositions underlying our particular method from undue biasing effect is to know consciously what they are and so not to absolutize or dogmatize them. Thus we have at least a chance of refraining from forcing our subjects or patients upon our "procrustean couches" and lopping off, or refusing to see, what does not fit.

In Ludwig Binswanger's little book relating his conversations and correspondence with Freud, *Sigmund Freud: Reminiscences of a Friendship,* there are some interesting interchanges illustrating this point. The friendship between Freud, the psychoanalyst, and Binswanger, a leading existential psychiatrist of Switzerland, was lifelong and tender, and it marks the only instance of Freud's continuing friendship with someone who differed radically with him.

Shortly before Freud's eightieth birthday, Binswanger wrote an essay describing how Freud's theory had radically deepened clinical psychiatry, but he added that Freud's own existence as a person pointed beyond the deterministic presuppositions of his theory. "Now [with Freud's psychoanalytic contribution] man is no longer merely an animated organism but a 'living being' who has origins in the finite life process of this earth, and who dies its life and lives its death; illness is no longer an externally or internally caused disturbance of the 'normal' course of a life on the way to its death." But Binswanger went on to point out that as a result of his interest in existential analysis, he believed that in Freud's theory man is not yet man in the full sense of the word:

. . . for to be a man does not mean merely to be a creature begotten by living-dying life, cast into it and beaten about, and put in high spirits or low spirits by it; it means to be a being that looks its own and mankind's fate in the face, a being that is "steadfast," i.e., one taking its own stance, or one standing on its own feet. . . . The fact that our lives are determined by the forces of life, is only one side of the truth; the other is that we determine these forces as our fate. Only the two sides together can take in the full problem of sanity and insanity. Those who, like Freud, have forged their fates with the hammer—the work of art he has created in the medium of language is sufficient evidence of this—can dispute this fact least of all.

Then, on the occasion of Freud's eightieth birthday, the Viennese Medical Society invited Binswanger, along with Thomas Mann, to deliver papers at the anniversary celebration. Freud himself did not attend, not being in good health and also, as he wrote Binswanger, not being fond of anniversary celebrations. ("They seem to be on the American model.") Binswanger spent two days with Freud in Vienna at the time of this birthday and remarked that in these conversations he was again impressed by how far Freud's own largeness and depth of humanity as a man surpassed his scientific theories.

In his paper at the celebration, Binswanger gave credit to Freud for having enlarged and deepened our insight into human nature more, perhaps, than anyone since Aristotle. But he went on to point out that these insights wore "a theoretic-scientific garb that as a whole appeared to me too 'one-sided' and narrow." He held that Freud's great contribution was in the area of *homo natura,* man in relation to nature (*Umwelt*)—drives, instincts, and similar aspects of experience. And as a consequence, Binswanger believed that in Freud's theory there was only a shadowy, epiphenomenal understanding of man in relation to his fellowmen (*Mitwelt*) and that the area of man in relation to himself (*Eigenwelt*) was omitted entirely.

Binswanger sent a copy of the paper to Freud and a week later received a letter from him containing the following sentences:

As I read it I was delighted with your beautiful language, your erudition, the vastness of your horizon, your tactfulness in contradicting me. As is well known, one can put up with vast quantities of praise. . . . *Naturally, for all that you have failed to convince me.** I have always confined myself to the ground floor and basement of the edifice. You maintain that by changing one's point of view, one can also see the upper story, in which dwell such distinguished guests as religion, art, etc. . . . I have already found a place for religion, but putting it under the category of "the neurosis of mankind." But probably we are speaking at cross purposes, and our differences will be ironed out only after centuries. In cordial friendship, and with greetings to your charming wife, your Freud.

Binswanger then adds in his book —and this is the central reason we quote the interchange—"As can be seen from the last sentence, Freud looked upon our differences as something to be surrounded by empirical investigation, not as something bearing upon the transcendental** conceptions that underly all empirical research."

In my judgment, Binswanger's point is irrefutable. One can gather empirical data, let us say on religion and art, from now till doomsday, and one will never get any closer to understanding these activities if, to start with, his presuppositions shut out what the religious person is dedicated to and what the artist is trying to do. Deterministic presuppositions make it possible to understand everything about art except the creative act and the art itself; mechanistic naturalistic presuppositions may undercover many facts about religion, but, as in Freud's terms, religion will always turn out to be more or less a neurosis, and what the genuinely religious person is concerned with will never get into the picture at all.

The point we wish to make in this discussion is the necessity of analyzing the presuppositions one assumes and of making allowance for the sectors of reality—which may be large indeed—that one's particular approach necessarily leaves out. In my judgment, we in

---

*Binswanger's italics.

**By "transcendental," Binswanger of course does not refer to anything ethereal or magical: he means the underlying presuppositions which "point beyond" the given fact, the presuppositions which determine the goals of one's activity.

psychology have often truncated our understanding and distorted our perception by failure consciously to clarify these presuppositions.

I vividly recall how, back in my graduate days in psychology some twenty years ago, Freud's theories tended to be dismissed as "unscientific" because they did not fit the methods then in vogue in graduate schools of psychology. I maintained at the time that this missed the point: Freud had uncovered realms of human experience of tremendous importance, and if they did not fit our methods, so much the worse for our methods; the problem was to devise new ones. In actual fact, the methods did catch up—perhaps, one should add, with a vengeance, until, as Rogers has stated, Freudianism is now the dogma of American clinical psychology. Remembering my own graduate-school days, I am therefore inclined to smile when someone says that the concepts of existential psychology are "unscientific" because they do not fit the particular methods *now* in vogue.

It is certainly clear that the Freudian mechanisms invite the separation into discrete cause-and-effect formulations which fit the deterministic methodology dominant in American psychology. But what also needs to be seen is that this making of Freudianism into the dogma of psychology has been accomplished at the price of omitting essential and vitally important aspects of Freud's thought. There is at present a three-cornered liaison, in tendency and to some extent in actuality, between Freudianism, behaviorism in psychology, and positivism in philosophy. An example of the first side of the liaison is the great similarity between Hull's drive-reduction theory of learning and Freud's concept of pleasure, the goal of behavior, as consisting of the reduction of stimuli. An example of the second is the statement of the philosopher Herman Feigl in his address at a recent annual convention of the American Psychological Association, that Freud's specific mechanisms could be formulated and used scientifically, but such concepts as the "death instinct" could not be.

But the trouble there is that such concepts as the "death instinct" in Freud were precisely what saved him from the full mechanistic implications of his system; these concepts always point beyond the deterministic limitations of his theory. They are, in the best sense of the word, a mythology. Freud was never content to let go of this mythological dimension to his thinking despite his great effort at the same time to formulate psychology in terms of his nineteenth-century biological presuppositions. In my judgment, his mythology is fundamental to the greatness of his contribution and essential to his central discoveries, such as "the unconscious." It was likewise essential to his radical contribution to the new image of man, namely, man as pushed by demonic, tragic, and destructive forces. I have tried elsewhere to show that Freud's tragic concept of the Oedipus is much closer to the truth than our tendency to interpret the Oedipus complex in terms of discrete sexual and hostile relationships in the family. The formulation of the "death instinct" as a biological instinct makes no sense, of course, and in this sense is rightly rejected by American behaviorism and positivism. But as a psychological and spiritual statement of the tragic nature of man, the idea has very great importance indeed and transcends any purely biological or mechanistic interpretation.

Methodology always suffers from a cultural lag. Our problem is to open our vision to more of human experience, to develop and free our methods so that they will as far as possible do justice to the richness and breadth of man's experience.

22. Personal Construct Theory

GEORGE A. KELLY

Who can say what nature is? Is it what now exists about us, including all the tiny hidden things that wait so patiently to be discovered? Or is it the vista of all that is destined to occur, whether tomorrow or in some distant eon of time? Or is nature, infinitely more varied than this, the myriad trains of events that might ensue if we were to be so bold, ingenious, and irreverent as to take a hand in its management?

Personal construct theory neither offers nor demands a firm answer to any of these questions, and in this respect it is unique. Rather than depending upon bedrock assumptions about the inherent nature of the universe, or upon fragments of truth believed to have been accumulated, it is a notion about how man may launch out from a position of admitted ignorance, and how he may aspire from one day to the next to transcend his own dogmatisms. It is, then, a theory of man's personal inquiry—a psychology of the human quest. It does not say what has or will be found, but proposes rather how we might go about looking for it.

PHILOSOPHICAL POSITION

Like other theories, the psychology of personal constructs is the implementation of a philosophical assumption. In this case the assumption is that whatever nature may be, or howsoever the quest for truth will turn out in the end, the events we face today are subject to as great a variety of constructions as our wits will enable us to contrive. This is not to say that one construction is as good as any other, nor is it to deny that at some infinite point in time human vision will behold reality out to the utmost reaches of existence. But it does remind us that all our present perceptions are open to question and reconsideration, and it does broadly suggest that even the most obvious occurrences of everyday life might appear utterly transformed if we were inventive enough to construe them differently.

This philosophical position we have called *constructive alternativism,* and its implications keep cropping up in the psychology of personal constructs. It can be constrasted with the prevalent epistemological assumption of *accumulative fragmentalism,* which is that truth is collected piece by piece. While constructive alternativism does not argue against the collection of information, neither does it measure truth by the size of the collection. Indeed it leads one to regard a large accumulation of facts as an open invitation to some far-reaching reconstruction which will reduce them to a mass of trivialities.

A person who spends a great deal of his time hoarding facts is not likely to be happy at the prospect of seeing them converted into rubbish. He is more likely to want them bound and preserved, a memorial to his personal achievement. A scientist, for example, who thinks this way, and especially a psychologist who does so, depends upon his facts to furnish the ultimate proof of his propositions. With these shining nuggets of truth in his grasp it seems unnecessary for him to take responsibility for the conclusions he claims they thrust upon him. To suggest to him at this point that further human reconstruction can completely alter the appearance of the precious fragments he has accumulated, as well as the direction of their arguments, is to threaten his scientific conclusions, his philosophical position, and even his moral security. No wonder, then, that in the eyes of such a conservatively minded person, our assumption that all facts are subject—are wholly subject—to alternative constructions looms up as culpably subjective and dangerously subversive to the scientific establishment.

THE MEANING OF EVENTS

Constructive alternativism stresses the importance of events. But it looks to man to propose what the character of their import shall be. The meaning of an event

Excerpted from J. Mancuso, *Readings for a Cognitive Theory of Personality,* New York: Holt, Rinehart and Winston, 1970, pp. 27–47. Reprinted by permission of Mrs. Gladys T. Kelly; copyright, Gladys T. Kelly.

—that is to say, the meaning we ascribe to it—is anchored in its antecedents and its consequents. Thus meaning displays itself to us mainly in the dimension of time. This is much more than saying that meanings are rehearsals of outcomes, a proposition implicit in behavioristic theory, or that the ends justify the means—the ethical statement of the same proposition.

Besides including anticipated outcomes, meaning includes also the means by which events are anticipated. This is to suggest that different meanings are involved when identical events are correctly anticipated by different sets of inferences. It suggests also the implication of quite different meanings when the basic assumptions are different, even when the chains of inference are otherwise more or less similar.

In all of this we look to events to confirm our predictions and to encourage our venturesome constructions. Yet the same events may confirm different constructions, and different, or even incompatible, events may appear to validate the same construction. So, for each of us, meaning assumes the shape of the arguments which lead him to his predictions, and the only outside check on his personal constructions are the events which confirm or disconfirm his expectations. This is a long way from saying that meaning is revealed by what happens, or that meaning is something to be discovered in the natural course of events, or that events shape men and ideas. Thus in constructive alternativism events are crucial, but only man can devise a meaning for them to challenge.

When we place a construction of our own upon a situation, and then pursue its implications to the point of expecting something to happen, we issue a little invitation to nature to intervene in our personal experience. If what we expect does happen, or appears to happen, our expectation is confirmed and we are likely to think that we must have had a pretty good slant on the trend of affairs, else we would have lost our bet. But if we think the matter over carefully we may begin to have doubts. Perhaps a totally different interpretation would have led to an equally successful prediction; and it may, besides, have been more straightforward, or more consistent with our conscience. Or perhaps our vivid expectations overlaid our perception of what actually happened.

So, on second thought, even when events are reconciled with a construction, we cannot be sure that they have proved it true. There are always other constructions, and there is the lurking likelihood that some of them will turn out to be better. The best we can ever do is project our anticipations with frank uncertainty and observe the outcomes in terms in which we have a bit more confidence. But neither anticipation nor outcome is ever a matter of absolute certainty from the dark in which we mortals crouch. And, hence, even the most valuable construction we have yet contrived—even our particular notion of God Himself—is one for which we shall have to continue to take personal responsibility—at least until someone turns up with a better one. And I suspect he will! This is what we mean by *constructive alternativism*. Our view might even be called a philosophical position of *epistemological responsibility*.

BASIC POSTULATE

A person's processes are psychologically channelized by the ways in which he anticipates events. This is what we have proposed as a fundamental postulate for the psychology of personal constructs. The assumptions of constructive alternativism are embedded in this statement, although it may not be apparent until later in our exposition of the theme just how it is that they are.

We start with a *person*. Organisms, lower animals, and societies can wait. We are talking about someone we know, or would like to know—such as you, or myself. More particularly, we are talking about that person as an event—the processes that express his personality. And, since we enter the system we are about to elaborate at the point of a process—or life—rather than at the point of a body or a material substance, we should not have to invoke any special notions, such as dynamics, drives, motivation, or force to explain why our object does not remain inert. As far as the theory is concerned, it never was inert. As we pursue the theoretical line emerging from this postulate I think it becomes clear also why we do not need such notions to account for the direction of movement—any more than we need them to explain the movement itself.

This is to be a psychological theory. Mostly this is a way of announcing in the basic postulate that we make no commitment to the terms of other disciplines, such as physiology or chemistry. Our philosophical position permits us to see those other disciplines as based on manmade constructions, rather than as disclosures of raw realities, and hence there is no need for the psychologist to accept them as final, or to limit his proposals to statements consistent with them. In addition, I think the theory sounds more or less like the other theories that are known as psychological. This gives me an inclusive, as well as an exclusive reason for calling it a psychological theory, although this is more or less a matter of taste rather than of definition. Certainly I have no intention of trying to define psychology; there are just too many things called psychological that I do not care to take responsibility for.

Some have suggested that personal construct theory not be called a psychological theory at all, but a metatheory. That is all right with me. It suggests that it is a theory about theories, and that is pretty much what I have in mind. But I hope that it is clear that it is not limited to being a metatheory of formal theories, or even of articulate ones.

There is also the question of whether or not it is a cognitive theory. Some have said that it was; other have classed it as existential. Quite an accomplishment; not many theories have been accused of being both cognitive and existential! But this, too, is all right with me. As a matter of fact, I am delighted. There are categorical systems in which I think the greater amount of ambiguity I stir up, the better. Cognition, for example, strikes me as a particularly misleading category, and, since it is one designed to distinguish itself from affect and conation, those terms, too, might well be discarded as inappropriately restrictive.

Personal construct theory has also been categorized by responsible scholars as an emotional theory, a learning theory, a psychoanalytic theory (Freudian, Adlerian, and Jungian—all three), a typically American theory, a Marxist theory, a humanistic theory, a logical positivistic theory, a Zen Buddhistic theory, a Thomistic theory, a behavioristic theory, an Apollonian theory, a pragmatistic theory, a reflexive theory, and no theory at all. It has also been classified as nonsense, which indeed, by its own admission, it will likely some day turn out to be. In each case there were some convincing arguments offered for the categorization, but I have forgotten what most of them were. I fear that no one of these categorizations will be of much help to the reader in understanding personal construct theory, but perhaps having a whole lap full of them all at once will suggest what might be done with them.

The fourth term in the postulate —channelized—was chosen as one less likely than others to imply dynamics. This is because there is no wish to suggest that we are dealing with anything not already in motion. What is to be explained is the direction of the processes, not the transformation of states into processes. We see states only as an *ad interim* device to get time to stand still long enough for us to see what is going on. In other words, we have assumed that a process can be profitably regarded as more basic than an inert substance. We have had to do this notwithstanding the commitments of the centuries to quite another kind of language system. There are some disadvantages that come with this notion of what is basic, but we are willing to accept them for the time being in order to explore the heraclitean implications more fully than psychologists have ever done before.

In specifying *ways of anticipating events* as the directive referent for human processes we cut ourselves free of the stimulus-response version of nineteenth century scientific determinism. I am aware that this is a drastic step indeed, and I suspect that others who claim to have taken similar steps have not always seriously taken stock of the difficulties to be encountered. For one thing the very syntax of the language we must employ to voice our protest is built on a world view that regards objects as agents and outcomes as the products of those agents.

In our present undertaking the psychological initiative always remains a property of the person—never the property of anything else. What is more, neither past nor future events are themselves ever regarded as basic determinants of the course of human action—not even the events of childhood.

But one's way of anticipating them, whether in the short range or in the long view—this is the basic theme in the human process of living. Moreover, it is that events are anticipated, not merely that man gravitates toward more and more comfortable organic states. Confirmation and disconfirmation of one's predictions are accorded greater psychological significance than rewards, punishments, or the drive reduction that reinforcements produce.

There are, of course, some predictions we would like to see disconfirmed, as well as some we hope will indeed materialize. We should not make the mistake of translating personal construct theory back into stimulus-response theory and saying to ourselves that confirmation is the same as a positive reinforcement, and that disconfirmation nullifies the meaning of an experience. Disconfirmation, even in those cases where it is disconcerting, provides grounds for reconstruction—or of repentance, in the proper sense of that term —and it may be used to improve the accuracy and significance of further anticipations. Thus we envision the nature of life in its outreach for the future, and not in its perpetuation of its prior conditions or in its incessant reverberation of past events.

Personal construct theory is elaborated by a string of eleven corollaries which may be loosely inferred from its basic postulate. Beyond these are certain notions of more limited applicability which fall in line with personal construct thinking—notions about such matters as anxiety, guilt, hostility, decision making, creativity, the strategy of psychological research, and other typical concerns of professional psychologists. These latter notions need not be considered part of the formal structure of the theory, although our theoretical efforts may not come to life in the mind of the reader until he has seen their applicability to the daily problems he faces.

CONSTRUCTION COROLLARY

A person anticipates events by construing their replications. Since events never repeat themselves, else they would lose their identity, one can look forward to them only by devising some construction which permits him to perceive two of them in a similar manner. His construction must also permit him to be selective about which two are to be perceived similarly. Thus the same construction that serves to infer their similarity must serve also to differentiate them from others. Under a system that provides only for the identification of similarities the world dissolves into homogeneity; under one that provides only for differentiation it is shattered into hopelessly unrelated fragments.

Perhaps it is true that events, as most of us would like to believe, really do repeat aspects of previous occurrences. But unless one thinks he is precocious enough to have hit upon what those aspects will ultimately turn out to be, or holy enough to have had them revealed to him, he must modestly concede that the appearance of replication is a reflection of his own fallible construction of what is going on. Thus the recurrent themes that make life seem so full of meaning are the original symphonic compositions of a man bent on finding the present in his past, and the future in his present.

INDIVIDUALITY COROLLARY

Persons differ from each other in their constructions of events. Having assumed that construction is a personal affair, it seems unlikely that any two persons would ever happen to concoct identical systems. I would go further now than when I originally proposed this corollary and suggest that even particular constructions are never identical events. And I would extend it the other way too, and say that I doubt that two persons ever put their construction systems together in terms of the same logical relationships. For myself, I find this a most encouraging line of speculation, for it seems to open the door to more advanced systems of thinking and inference yet to be devised by man. Certainly it suggests that scientific research can rely more heavily on individual imagination than it usually dares.

ORGANIZATION COROLLARY

Each person characteristically evolves, for his convenience in anticipat-

ing events, a construction system embracing ordinal relationships between constructs. If a person is to live actively within his construction system it must provide him with some clear avenues of inference and movement. There must be ways for him to resolve the more crucial contradictions and conflicts that inevitably arise. This is not to say that all inconsistencies must be resolved at once. Some private paradoxes can be allowed to stand indefinitely, and, in the face of them, one can remain indecisive or can vacillate between alternative expectations of what the future holds in store for him.

So it seems that each person arranges his constructions so that he can move from one to another in some orderly fashion, either by assigning priorities to those which are to take precedence when doubts or contradictions arise, or by arranging implicative relationships, as in boolean algebra, so that he may infer that one construction follows from another. Thus one's commitments may take priority over his opportunities, his political affiliations may turn him from compassion to power, and his moral imperatives may render him insensitive to the brute that tugs at his sleeve. These are the typical prices men pay to escape inner chaos.

DICHOTOMY COROLLARY

A person's construction system is composed of a finite number of dichotomous constructs. Experience has shown me that this is the point where many of my readers first encounter difficulty in agreeing with me. What I am saying is that a construct is a "black and white" affair, never a matter of shadings, or of "grays." On the face of it, this sounds bad, for it seems to imply categorical or absolutistic thinking rather than any acceptance of relativism or conditionalism. Yet I would insist that there is nothing categorical about a construct.

When we look closely the initial point of difficulty in following personal construct theory usually turns out to lie in certain unrecognized assumptions made earlier while reading the exposition, or even carried over from previous habits of thought. Let us see if we can get the matter straightened out before any irreparable damage is done.

Neither our constructs nor our construing systems come to use from nature, except, of course, from our own nature. It must be noted that this philosophical position of constructive alternativism has much more powerful epistemological implications than one might at first suppose. We cannot say that constructs are essences distilled by the mind out of available reality. They are imposed *upon* events, not abstracted *from* them. There is only one place they come from; that is from the person who is to use them. He devises them. Moreover, they do not stand for anything or represent anything, as a symbol, for example, is supposed to do.

So what are they? They are reference axes, upon which one may project events in an effort to make some sense out of what is going on. In this sense they are like cartesian coordinates, the x, y and z axes of analytic geometry. Events correspond to the point plotted within cartesian space. We can locate the points and express relations between points by specifying x, y and z distances. The cartesian axes *do not represent* the points projected upon them, but serve as guidelines for locating those points. That, also, is what constructs do for events, including ones that have not yet occurred. They help us locate them, understand them, and anticipate them.

But we must not take the cartesian analogy too literally. Des Cartes' axes were lines or scales, each containing in order an infinite number of imaginary points. Certainly his x- or y-axis embodied well enough the notion of shadings or a succession of grays. Yet a construct is not quite such an axis.

A construct is the basic contrast between two groups. When it is imposed it serves both to distinguish between its elements and to group them. Thus constructs refer to the nature of the distinction one attempts to make between events, not to the array in which his events appear to stand when he gets through applying the distinction between each of them and all the others.

Suppose one is dealing with the construct of good versus bad. Such a construct is not a representation of all things that are good, and an implicit exclusion of all that are bad. Nor is it a representation of all that are bad. It is not even a representation of all things that can be called either good or bad. The construct, of itself, is the kind of contrast one perceives and not in any way a representation of objects. As far as the construct is concerned there is no good-better-best scale, or any bad-worse-worst array.

But, while constructs do not represent or symbolize events, they do enable us to cope with events, which is a statement of quite a different order. They also enable us to put events into arrays or scales, if we wish. Suppose, for example, we apply our construct to elements, say persons, or to their acts. Consider three persons. One may make a good-bad distinction between them which will say that two of them are good in relation to the third, and the third is bad in relation to the two good ones. Then he may, in turn, apply his construct between the two good ones and say one of them is good with respect to the other formerly "good" one and the one already labeled "bad."

This, of course, makes one of the persons, or acts, good in terms of one cleavage that has been made and bad in relation to the other. But this relativism applies only to the objects; the construct of good versus bad is itself absolute. It may not be accurate, and it may not be stable from time to time, but, as a construct, it has to be absolute. Still, by its successive application to events one may create a scale with a great number of points differentiated along its length. Now a person who likes grays can have them—as many as he likes.

But let us make no mistake: A scale, in comparison to a construct, is a pretty concrete affair. Yet one can scarcely have himself a scale unless he has a construct working for him. Only if he has some basis for discrimination and association can he get on with the job of marking off a scale.

Now note something else. We have really had to fall back on our philosophical position of constructive alternativism in order to come up with this kind of an abstraction. If we had not first disabused ourselves of the idea that events are the source of our construct, we would have had a hard time coming around to the point where we could envision the underlying basis of discrimination and association we call the construct.

CHOICE COROLLARY

A person chooses for himself that alternative in a dichotomized construct through which he anticipates the greater possibility for the elaboration of his system. It seems to me to follow that if a person makes so much use of his constructs, and is so dependent upon them, he will make choices which promise to develop their usefulness. Developing the usefulness of a construction system involves, as far as I can see, two things: defining it and extending it. One defines his system, by extension at least, by making it clear how its construct components are applied to objects or are linked with each other. He amplifies his system by using it to reach our for new fields of application. In the one case he consolidates his position and in the other he extends it.

Note that the choice is between alternatives expressed in the construct, not, as one might expect, between objects divided by means of the construct. There is a subtle point here. Personal construct theory is a psychological theory and therefore has to do with the behavior of man, not with the intrinsic nature of objects. A construct governs what the man does, not what the object does. In a strict sense, therefore, man makes decisions which initially affect himself, and which affect other objects only subsequently—and then only if he manages to take some effective action. Making a choice, then, has to do with involving oneself, and cannot be defined in terms of the external object chosen. Besides, one does not always get the object he chooses to gain. But his anticipation does have to do with his own processes, as I tried to say in formulating the basic postulate.

So when a man makes a choice what he does is align himself in terms of his constructs. He does not necessarily succeed, poor fellow, in doing anything to the objects he seeks to approach or avoid. Trying to define human behavior in terms of the externalities sought or affected, rather than the seeking process, gets the psychologist pretty far off the track. It makes more of a physicist of him than a psychologist, and a rather poor one, at that. So what we must say is that a person, in deciding whether to believe or do something, uses his construct system to proportion his field, and then moves himself strategically and tactically within its presumed domain.

Men change things by changing themselves first, and they accomplish their objectives, if at all, only by paying the price of altering themselves—as some have found to their sorrow and others to their salvation. The choices that men make are choices of their own acts, and the alternatives are distinguished by their own constructs. The results of the choices, however, may range all the way from nothing to catastrophe, on the one hand, or to consummation, on the other.

EXPERIENCE COROLLARY

A person's construction system varies as he successively construes the replications of events. The tendency is for personal constructs to shift when events are projected upon them. The distinctions they implement are likely to be altered in three ways: (1) The construct may be applied at a different point in the galaxy, (2) it may become a somewhat different kind of distinction, and (3) its relations to other constructs may be altered.

In the first of these shifts it is a matter of a change in the location of the construct's application, and hence not exactly an intrinsic change in the construct itself. In the second case, however, it is the abstraction itself which is altered, although the change may not be radical enough for the psychologist to say a new construct has been substituted. Finally, in the third case, the angular relations with other constructs are necessarily affected by the transition, unless, by some chance, the construct system were rotated as a whole. But that is not a very likely contingency.

The first kind of shift might be observed when a person moves to an urban community. Some of the actions he once regarded as aloof and unneighborly he may come to accept as relatively friendly in the new social context. But he may also rotate the axis of his construct as he gains familiarity with city life, and, as a result, come to see "aloofness" as a neighborly respect for his privacy, something he had never had very clearly in mind before. This would be an example of the second kind of shift. The third kind of shift comes when he alters his notion of respect as a result of the experience, perhaps coming to sense it not so much a matter of subservience or adulation but more a matter of empathy and consideration. As a matter of fact, we might regard the whole transition as leading him in the direction of greater maturity.

Keeping in mind that events do not actually repeat themselves and that the replication we talk about is a replication of ascribed aspects only, it begins to be clear that the succession we call experience is based on the constructions we place on what goes on. If those constructions are never altered, all that happens during a man's years is a sequence of parallel events having no psychological impact on his life. But if he invests himself—the most intimate event of all —in the enterprise, the outcome, to the extent that it differs from his expectation or enlarges upon it, dislodges the man's construction of himself. In recognizing the inconsistency between his anticipation and the outcome, he concedes a discrepancy between what he was and what he is. A succession of such investments and dislodgements constitutes the human experience.

A subtle point comes to light at this juncture. Confirmation may lead to reconstruing quite as much as disconfirmation—perhaps even more. A confirmation gives one an anchorage in some area of his life, leaving him free to set afoot adventuresome explorations nearby, as, for example, in the case of a child whose security at home emboldens him to be the first to explore what lies in the neighbor's yard.

The unit of experience is, therefore, a cycle embracing five phases: anticipation, investment, encounter, confirmation or disconfirmation, and constructive revision. This is followed, of course, by new anticipations, as the first phase of a subsequent experiential cycle gets underway. Certainly in personal construct theory's line of reasoning experience is not composed of encounters alone.

Stated simply, the amount of a man's experience is not measured by the number of events with which he collides, but by the investments he has made in his anticipations and the revisions of his constructions that have followed upon his facing up to consequences. A man whose only wager in life is upon reaching heaven by immunizing himself against the miseries of his neighbors, or upon following a bloody party-line straight to utopia, is prepared to gain little experience until he arrives—either there, or somewhere else clearly recognized as not the place he was looking for. Then, if he is not too distracted by finding that his architectural specifications have been blatantly disregarded, or that the wrong kind of people have started moving in, I suppose he may begin to think of some other investments he might better have been making in the meantime. Of course, a little hell along the way, if taken more to heart than most heaven-bound people seem to take it, may have given him a better idea of what to expect, before it was too late to get a bit of worthwhile experience and make something out of himself.

ETIOLOGY AND DEVELOPMENT

Phenomenologists stress that every individual is the center of his changing world of experiences; experiences must be viewed, therefore, only in terms of their relevance to the individual. As the individual matures, a portion of his experience becomes differentiated into a conscious perception of the self-as-object. Once this self-concept is established, it influences the perceptions, memories, and thoughts of the individual. If experiences are inconsistent with the self-image, they are ignored or disowned.

Carl Rogers, the major American exponent of "self theory," details this process of growth and indicates the points at which "breakdown and disorder" arise. Rogers contends that psychopathology occurs when the individual abandons his inherent potentials and feelings and adopts values that are imposed upon him by others. Abraham Maslow's paper argues strongly for the healthy potential that exists within each individual, believing that if the child is encouraged to "actualize" his inherent potentials, he will develop into a mature and well-integrated adult.

23. A Theory of Personality

CARL R. ROGERS

In endeavoring to order our perceptions of the individual as he appears in therapy, a theory of the development of personality, and of the dynamics of behavior, has been constructed. It may be well to repeat the warning previously given, and to note that the initial propositions of this theory are those which are furthest from the matrix of our experience and hence are most suspect. As one reads on, the propositions become steadily closer to the experience of therapy. As before, the defined terms and constructs are italicized, and are to be understood as previously defined.

From "A Theory of Therapy, Personality, and Interpersonal Relationships, as Developed in the Client-centered Framework," pages 221–231. In *Psychology: A Study of a Science* edited by S. Koch, Vol. 3, copyright 1959, used by permission of McGraw-Hill Book Company.

A. POSTULATED CHARACTERISTICS OF THE HUMAN INFANT

It is postulated that the individual, during the period of infancy, has at least these attributes.

1. He perceives his *experience* as reality. His *experience* is his reality.
    a. As a consequence he has greater potential *awareness* of what reality is for him than does anyone else, since no one else can completely assume his *internal frame of reference*.
2. He has an inherent tendency toward *actualizing* his organism.
3. He interacts with his reality in terms of his basic *actualizing* tendency. Thus his behavior is the goal-directed attempt of the organism to satisfy the experienced needs for *actualization* in the reality as *perceived*.

4. In this interaction he behaves as an organized whole, as a gestalt.

5. He engages in an *organismic valuing process,* valuing *experience* with reference to the *actualizing tendency* as a criterion. *Experiences* which are *perceived* as maintaining or enhancing the organism are valued positively. Those which are *perceived* as negating such maintenance or enhancement are valued negatively.

6. He behaves with adience toward positively valued *experiences* and with avoidance toward those negatively valued.

Comment. In this view as formally stated, the human infant is seen as having an inherent motivational system (which he shares in common with all living things) and a regulatory system (the valuing process) which by its "feedback" keeps the organism "on the beam" of satisfying his motivational needs. He lives in an environment which for theoretical purposes may be said to exist only in him, or to be of his own creation.

This last point seems difficult for some people to comprehend. It is the perception of the environment which constitutes the environment, regardless as to how this relates to some "real" reality which we may philosophically postulate. The infant may be picked up by a friendly, affectionate person. If his perception of the situation is that this is a strange and frightening experience, it is this perception, not the "reality" or the "stimulus" which will regulate his behavior. To be sure, the relationship with the environment is a transactional one, and if his continuing experience contradicts his initial perception, then in time his perception will change. But the effective reality which influences behavior is at all times the perceived reality. We can operate theoretically from this base without having to resolve the difficult question of what "really" constitutes reality.

Another comment which may be in order is that no attempt has been made to supply a complete catalogue of the equipment with which the infant faces the world. Whether he possesses instincts, or an innate sucking reflex, or an innate need for affection, are interesting questions to pursue, but the answers seem peripheral rather than essential to a theory of personality.

B. THE DEVELOPMENT OF THE SELF

1. In line with the tendency toward differentiation which is a part of the *actualizing tendency,* a portion of the individual's *experience* becomes differentiated and *symbolized* in an *awareness* of being, *awareness* of functioning. Such awareness may be described as *self-experience.*

2. This representation in *awareness* of being and functioning, becomes elaborated, through interaction with the environment, particularly the environment composed of significant others, into a *concept of self,* a perceptual object in his *experiential field.*

Comment. These are the logical first steps in the development of the self. It is by no means the way the construct developed in our own thinking, as has been indicated in the section of definitions.

C. THE NEED FOR POSITIVE REGARD

1. As the awareness of self emerges, the individual develops a *need for positive regard.* This need is universal in human beings, and in the individual, is pervasive and persistent. Whether it is an inherent or learned need is irrelevant to the theory. Standal, who formulated the concept, regards it as the latter.

   a. The satisfaction of this need is necessarily based upon inferences regarding the experiential field of another.

     (1) Consequently it is often ambiguous.

   b. It is associated with a very wide range of the individual's *experiences.*

   c. It is reciprocal, in that when an individual discriminates himself as satisfying another's need for *positive regard,* he necessarily experiences satisfaction of his own need for *positive regard.*

     (1) Hence it is rewarding both to satisfy this need in another, and to experience the satisfaction of one's own need by another.

d. It is potent, in that the *positive regard* of any social other is communicated to the total *regard complex* which the individual associates with that social other.

(1) Consequently the expression of positive regard by a significant social other can become more compelling than the *organismic valuing process,* and the individual becomes more adient to the *positive regard* of such others than toward *experiences* which are of positive value in *actualizing* the organism.

D. THE DEVELOPMENT OF THE NEED FOR SELF-REGARD

1. The positive regard satisfactions or frustrations associated with any particular *self-experience* or group of *self-experiences* come to be *experienced* by the individual independently of *positive regard* transactions with social others. *Positive regard experienced* in this fashion is termed *self-regard.*

2. A *need for self-regard* develops as a learned need developing out of the association of *self-experiences* with the satisfaction or frustration of the *need for positive regard.*

3. The individual thus comes to *experience positive regard* or loss of *positive regard* independently of transactions with any social other. He becomes in a sense his own significant social other.

4. Like *positive regard, self-regard* which is *experienced* in relation to any particular *self-experience* or group of *self-experiences,* is communicated to the total *self-regard complex.*

E. THE DEVELOPMENT OF CONDITIONS OF WORTH

1. When *self-experiences* of the individual are discriminated by significant others as being more or less worthy of *positive regard,* then *self-regard* becomes similarly selective.

2. When a *self-experience* is avoided (or sought) solely because it is less (or

more) worthy o dividual is said to h *dition of worth.*

3. If an individual sh only *unconditional positive* no *conditions of worth* woul *self-regard* would be uncondition needs for *positive regard* and *self-re* would never be at variance with *orga mic evaluation,* and the individual woul continue to be *psychologically adjusted,* and would be fully functioning. This chain of events is hypothetically possible, and hence important theoretically, though it does not appear to occur in actuality.

Comment. This is an important sequence in personality development, stated more fully by Standal. It may help to restate the sequence in informal, illustrative, and much less exact terms.

The infant learns to need love. Love is very satisfying, but to know whether he is receiving it or not he must observe his mother's face, gestures, and other ambiguous signs. He develops a total gestalt as to the way he is regarded by his mother and each new experience of love or rejection tends to alter the whole gestalt. Consequently each behavior on his mother's part such as a specific disapproval of a specific behavior tends to be experienced as disapproval in general. So important is this to the infant that he comes to be guided in his behavior not by the degree to which an experience maintains or enhances the organism, but by the likelihood of receiving maternal love.

Soon he learns to view himself in much the same way, liking or disliking himself as a total configuration. He tends, quite independently of his mother or others, to view himself and his behavior in the same way they have. This means that some behaviors are regarded positively which are not actually experienced organismically as satisfying. Other behaviors are regarded negatively which are not actually experienced as unsatisfying. It is when he behaves in accordance with these introjected values that he may be said to have acquired conditions of worth. He cannot regard himself positively, as having worth, unless he lives in terms of these conditions. He now reacts with adience or avoidance toward certain behaviors solely because of these introjected conditions of self-regard, quite

*f self-regard, the in-
ve acquired a con-
uld experience
regard, then
l develop,
nal, the
gard
is-*

on-
hat
cted
con-

that
ifant
were
ome
con-
This
ed if
f this
ng it
r (or

to defecate when and where you please,
or to destroy things) and I love you and
am quite willing for you to have those feelings. But I am quite willing for me to have
my feelings, too, and I feel very distressed
when your brother is hurt, (or annoyed or
sad at other behaviors) and so I do not
let you hit him. Both your feelings and my
feelings are important, and each of us can
freely have his own.'' If the child were
thus able to retain his own organismic
evaluation of each experience, then his life
would become a balancing of these
satisfactions. Schematically he might feel,
''I enjoy hitting baby brother. It feels
good. I do not enjoy mother's distress.
That feels dissatisfying to me. I enjoy
pleasing her.'' Thus his behavior would
sometimes involve the satisfaction of hitting his brother, sometimes the satisfaction of pleasing mother. But he would
never have to disown the feelings of satisfaction or dissatisfaction which he experienced in this differential way.

F. THE DEVELOPMENT OF INCONGRUENCE BETWEEN SELF AND EXPERIENCE

1. Because of the need for *self-*
regard, the individual *perceives* his *experience* selectively, in terms of the *conditions of worth* which have come to exist
in him.

   a. Experiences which are in accord with his *conditions of
   worth* are *perceived* and *symbolized* accurately in *awareness.*

   b. Experiences which run contrary to the *conditions of
   worth* are *perceived* selective-

ly and distortedly as if in accord with the *conditions of
worth,* or are in part or whole,
denied to awareness.

2. Consequently some experiences
now occur in the organism which are not
recognized as *self-experiences,* are not
accurately *symbolized,* and are not
organized into the *self-structure* in
accurately symbolized form.

3. Thus from the time of the first
selective *perception* in terms of *conditions
of worth,* the states of *incongruence between self and experience,* of *psychological maladjustment* and of *vulnerability,*
exist to some degree.

Comment. It is thus because of the
distorted perceptions arising from the conditions of worth that the individual departs
from the integration which characterizes
his infant state. From this point on his
concept of self includes distorted
perceptions which do not accurately represent his experience, and his experience
includes elements which are not included
in the picture he has of himself. Thus he
can no longer live as a unified whole person, but various part functions now
become characteristic. Certain experiences tend to threaten the self. To
maintain the self-structure defensive
reactions are necessary. Behavior is reg-
ulated at times by the self and at times
by those aspects of the organisms's experience which are not included in the
self. The personality is henceforth divided, with the tensions and inadequate
functioning which accompany such lack of
unity.

This, as we see it, is the basic
estrangement in man. He has not been
true to himself, to his own natural organismic valuing of experience, but for the
sake of preserving the positive regard of
others has now come to falsify some of
the values he experiences and to perceive
them only in terms based upon their value
to others. Yet this has not been a conscious choice, but a natural—and tragic
—development in infancy. The path of
development toward psychological maturity, the path of therapy, is the undoing of this estrangement in man's functioning, the dissolving of conditions of
worth, the achievement of a self which is
congruent with experience, and the restoration of a unified organismic valuing
process as the regulator of behavior.

G. THE DEVELOPMENT OF DISCREPANCIES IN BEHAVIOR

1. As a consequence of the incongruence between self and experience described in *F,* a similar incongruence arises in the behavior of the individual.

 a. Some behaviors are consistent with the *self-concept* and maintain and actualize and enhance it.

   (1) Such behaviors are *accurately symbolized* in *awareness.*

 b. Some behaviors maintain, enhance, and actualize those aspects of the experience of the organism which are not assimilated into the *self-structure.*

   (1) These behaviors are either unrecognized as *self-experiences* or *perceived* in distorted or selective fashion in such a way as to be *congruent* with the *self.*

H. THE EXPERIENCE OF THREAT AND THE PROCESS OF DEFENSE

1. As the organism continues to *experience,* an *experience* which is incongruent with the self-structure (and its incorporated *conditions of worth,* is *subceived* as *threatening*).

2. The essential nature of the *threat* is that if the *experience* were *accurately symbolized* in *awareness,* the *self-concept* would no longer be a consistent gestalt, the *conditions of worth* would be violated, and the *need for self-regard* would be frustrated. A state of *anxiety* would exist.

3. The process of *defense* is the reaction which prevents these events from occurring.

 a. This process consists of the selective *perception* or *distortion* of the *experience* and/or the *denial to awareness* of the *experience* or some portion thereof, thus keeping the total *perception* of the *experience* consistent with the individual's *self-structure,* and consistent with his *conditions of worth.*

4. The general consequences of the process of *defense,* aside from its pres-

ervation of the above consistencies, are a rigidity of *perception,* due to the necessity of distorting *perceptions,* an inaccurate *perception* of reality, due to distortion and omission of data, and *intensionality.*

Comment. Section G describes the psychological basis for what are usually thought of as neurotic behaviors, and Section *H* describes the mechanisms of these behaviors. From our point of view it appears more fundamental to think of defensive behaviors (described in these two sections) and disorganized behaviors (described below). Thus the defensive behaviors include not only the behaviors customarily regarded as neurotic—rationalization, fantasy, projection, compulsions, phobias, and the like—but also some of the behaviors customarily regarded as psychotic, notably paranoid behaviors and perhaps catatonic states. The disorganized category includes many of the "irrational" and "acute" psychotic behaviors, as will be explained below. This seems to be a more fundamental classification than those usually employed, and perhaps more fruitful in considering treatment. It also avoids any concept of neurosis and psychosis as entities in themselves, which we believe has been an unfortunate and misleading conception.

Let us consider for a moment the general range of the defensive behaviors from the simplest variety, common to all of us, to the more extreme and crippling varieties. Take first of all, rationalization. ("I didn't really make that mistake. It was this way. . . .") Such excuses involve a perception of behavior distorted in such a way as to make it congruent with our concept of self (as a person who doesn't make mistakes). Fantasy is another example. ("I am a beautiful princess, and all the men adore me.") Because the actual experience is threatening to the concept of self (as an adequate person, in this example), this experience is denied, and a new symbolic world is created which enhances the self, but completely avoids any recognition of the actual experience. Where the incongruent experience is a strong need, the organism actualizes itself by finding a way of expressing this need, but it is perceived in a way which is consistent with the self. Thus an individual whose self-concept involves no "bad" sexual thoughts may feel or express the thought "I am pure, but you are trying to make me think filthy thoughts." This would be thought of as projection or as a paranoid idea. It involves the expression of the organism's need for sexual satisfactions, but it is expressed in such a fashion that this need may be denied to awareness and the behavior perceived as consistent with the self. Such examples could be continued, but perhaps the point is clear that the incongruence between self and experience is handled by the distorted perception of experience or behavior, or by the denial of experience in awareness (behavior is rarely denied, though this is possible), or by some combination of distortion and denial.

I. THE PROCESS OF BREAKDOWN AND DISORGANIZATION

Up to this point the theory of personality which has been formulated applies to every individual in a lesser or greater degree. In this and the following section certain processes are described which occur only when certain specified conditions are present.

1. If the individual has a large or significant degree of *incongruence between self and experience* and if a significant experience demonstrating this *incongruence* occurs suddenly, or with a high degree of obviousness, then the organism's process of *defense* is unable to operate successfully.

2. As a result *anxiety* is *experienced* as the *incongruence* is subceived. The degree of *anxiety* is dependent upon the extent of the *self-structure* which is *threatened*.

3. The process of *defense* being unsuccessful, the *experience* is *accurately symbolized* in *awareness,* and the gestalt of the *self-structure* is broken by this *experience* of the *incongruence* in *awareness.* A state of disorganization results.

4. In such a state of disorganization the organism behaves at times in ways which are openly consistent with experiences which have hitherto been distorted or denied to awareness. At other times the self may temporarily regain regnancy, and the organism may behave in ways consistent with it. Thus in such a

state of disorganization, the tension between the concept of self (with its included distorted perceptions) and the experiences which are not accurately symbolized or included in the concept of self, is expressed in a confused regnancy, first one and then the other supplying the "feedback" by which the organism regulates behavior.

Comment. This section, as will be evident from its less exact formulation, is new, tentative, and needs much more consideration. Its meaning can be illuminated by various examples.

Statements 1 and 2 above may be illustrated by anxiety-producing experiences in therapy, or by acute psychotic breakdowns. In the freedom of therapy, as the individual expresses more and more of himself, he finds himself on the verge of voicing a feeling which is obviously and undeniably true, but which is flatly contradictory to the conception of himself which he has held. Anxiety results, and if the situation is appropriate (as described under *J*) this anxiety is moderate, and the result is constructive. But if, through overzealous and effective interpretation by the therapist, or through some other means, the individual is brought face to face with more of his denied experiences than he can handle, disorganization ensues and a psychotic break occurs, as described in statement 3. We have known this to happen when an individual has sought "therapy" from several different sources simultaneously. It has also been illustrated by some of the early experience with sodium pentathol therapy. Under the drug the individual revealed many of the experiences which hitherto he had denied to himself, and which accounted for the incomprehensible elements in his behavior. Unwisely faced with the material in his normal state he could not deny its authenticity, his defensive processes could not deny or distort the experience, and hence the self-structure was broken, and a psychotic break occurred.

Acute psychotic behaviors appear often to be describable as behaviors which are consistent with the denied aspects of experience rather than consistent with the self. Thus the person who has kept sexual impulses rigidly under control, denying them as an aspect of self, may now make open sexual overtures to those with whom he is in contact. Many of the so-called irrational behaviors of psychosis are of this order.

Once the acute psychotic behaviors have been exhibited, a process of defense again sets in to protect the organism against the exceedingly painful awareness of incongruence. Here I would voice my opinion very tentatively as to this process of defense. In some instances perhaps the denied experiences are now regnant, and the organism defends itself against the awareness of the self. In other instances the self is again regnant, and behavior is consistent with it, but the self has been greatly altered. It is now a self concept which includes the important theme, "I am a crazy, inadequate, unreliable person who contains impulses and forces beyond my control." Thus it is a self in which little or no confidence is felt.

It is hoped that this portion of the theory may be further elaborated and refined and made more testable in the future.

J. THE PROCESS OF REINTEGRATION

In the situations described under sections *G* and *H*, (and probably in situations of breakdown as described under *I*, though there is less evidence on this) a process of reintegration is possible, a process which moves in the direction of increasing the *congruence* between *self* and *experience*. This may be described as follows:

1. In order for the process of *defense* to be reversed—for a customarily *threatening experience* to be *accurately symbolized* in *awareness* and assimilated into the *self-structure*, certain conditions must exist.

    a. There must be a decrease in the *conditions of worth.*

    b. There must be an increase in *unconditional self-regard.*

2. The communicated *unconditional positive regard* of a significant other is one way of achieving these conditions.

    a. In order for the *unconditional positive regard* to be communicated, it must exist in a context of *empathic* understanding.

    b. When the individual *perceives* such *unconditional positive regard*, existing *conditions of worth* are weakened or dissolved.

    c. Another consequence is the increase in his own *unconditional positive self-regard.*

    d. Conditions *2a* and *2b* above thus being met, *threat* is reduced, the process of *defense is reversed,* and *experiences* customarily *threatening* are *accurately symbolized* and integrated into the *self concept.*

3. The consequences of 1 and 2 above are that the individual is less likely to encounter *threatening experiences;* the process of *defense* is less frequent and its consequences reduced; *self* and *experience* are more *congruent; self-regard* is increased; *positive regard* for others is increased; *psychological adjustment* is increased; the *organismic valuing process* becomes increasingly the basis of regulating behavior; the individual becomes nearly fully functioning.

Comment. This section is simply the theory of therapy which we presented earlier, now stated in a slightly more general form. It is intended to emphasize the fact that the reintegration or restoration of personality occurs always and only (at least so we are hypothesizing) in the presence of certain definable conditions. These are essentially the same whether we are speaking of formal psychotherapy continued over a considerable period, in which rather drastic personality changes may occur or whether we are speaking of the minor constructive changes which may be brought about by contact with an understanding friend or family member.

One other brief comment may be made about item *2a,* above. Empathic understanding is always necessary if unconditional positive regard is to be fully communicated. If I know little or nothing of you, and experience an unconditional positive regard for you, this means little because further knowledge of you may reveal aspects which I cannot so regard. But if I know you thoroughly, knowing and empathically understanding a wide variety of your feelings and behaviors, and still experience an unconditional positive regard, this is very meaningful. It comes close to being fully known and fully accepted.

24. Defense and Growth

ABRAHAM H. MASLOW

This chapter is an effort to be a little more systematic in the area of growth theory. For once we accept the notation of growth, many questions of detail arise. Just how does growth take place? Why do children grow or not grow? How do they know in which direction to grow? How do they get off in the direction of pathology?

After all, the concepts of self-actualization, growth and self are all high-level abstractions. We need to get closer to actual processes, to raw data, to concrete, living happenings.

These are far goals. Healthily growing infants and children don't live for the sake of far goals or for the distant future; they are too busy enjoying themselves and spontaneously living for the moment. They are *living,* not *preparing* to live. How can they manage, just being, spontaneously, not *trying* to grow, seeking only to enjoy the present activity, nevertheless to move forward step by step? i.e., to grow in a healthy way? to discover their real selves? How can we reconcile the facts of Being with the facts of Becoming? Growth is not in the pure case a goal out ahead, nor is self-actualization, nor is the discovery of Self. In the child, it is not specifically purposed; rather it just happens. He doesn't so much search as find. The laws of deficiency-motivation and of purposeful coping do not hold for growth, for spontaneity, for creativeness.

The danger with a pure Being-psychology is that it may tend to be static, not accounting for the facts of movement, direction and growth. We tend to describe states of Being, of self-actualization as if they were Nirvana states of perfection. Once you're there, you're there, and it seems as if all you could do is to rest content in perfection.

The answer I find satisfactory is a simple one, namely, that growth takes place when the next step forward is subjectively more delightful, more joyous, more intrinsically satisfying than the last; that the only way we can ever know what is right for us is that it feels better subjectively than any alternative. The new

experience validates *itself* rather than by an outside criterion. It is self-justifying, self-validating.

We don't do it because it is good for us, or because psychologists approve, or because somebody told us to, or because it will make us live longer, or because it is good for the species, or because it will bring external rewards, or because it is logical. We do it for the same reason that we choose one dessert over another. I have already described this as a basic mechanism for falling in love, or for choosing a friend, i.e., kissing one person gives more delight than kissing the other, being friends with *a* is more satisfying subjectively than being friends with *b.*

In this way, we learn what we are good at, what we really like or dislike, what our tastes and judgments and capacities are. In a word, this is the way in which we discover the Self and answer the ultimate questions Who am I? What am I?

The steps and the choices are taken out of pure spontaneity, from within outward. The healthy infant or child, just Being, as *part* of his Being, is randomly, and spontaneously curious, exploratory, wondering, interested. Even when he is non-purposeful, non-coping, expressive, spontaneous, not motivated by any deficiency of the ordinary sort, he tends to try out his powers, to reach out, to be absorbed, fascinated, interested, to play, to wonder, to manipulate the world. *Exploring, manipulating, experiencing,* being interested, choosing, delighting, *enjoying* can all be seen as attributes of pure Being, and yet lead to Becoming, though in a serendipitous way, fortuitously, unplanned, unanticipated. Spontaneous, creative experience can and does happen without expectations, plans, foresight, purpose, or goal.[1] It is only when the child sates himself, becomes bored, that he is

---

[1]"But paradoxically, the art experience cannot be effectively *used* for this purpose or any other. It must be a purposeless activity, as far as we understand 'purpose'. It can only be an experience in *being*—being a human organism doing what it must and what it is privileged to do—experiencing life keenly and wholly, expending energy and creating beauty in its own style—and the increased sensitivity, integrity, efficiency, and feeling of well-being are by-products."

From *Merrill-Palmer Quarterly* 3:36–47, 1956, by permission of the publisher and the author.

ready to turn to other, perhaps "higher," delights.

Then arise the inevitable questions. What holds him back? What prevents growth? Wherein lies the conflict? What is the alternative to growth forward? Why is it so hard and painful for some to grow forward? Here we must become more fully aware of the fixative and regressive power of ungratified deficiency-needs, of the attractions of safety and security, of the functions of defense and protection against pain, fear, loss, and threat, of the need for courage in order to grow ahead.

Every human being has *both* sets of forces within him. One set clings to safety and defensiveness out of fear, tending to regress backward, hanging on to the past, *afraid* to grow away from the primitive communion with the mother's uterus and breast, *afraid* to take chances, afraid to jeopardize what he already has, *afraid* of independence, freedom and separateness. The other set of forces impels him forward toward wholeness of Self and uniqueness of Self, toward full functioning of all his capacities, toward confidence in the face of the external world at the same time that he can accept his deepest, real, unconscious Self.

I can put all this together in a schema, which though very simple, is also very powerful, both heuristically and theoretically. This basic dilemma or conflict between the defensive forces and the growth trends I conceive to be existential, imbedded in the deepest nature of the human being, now and forever into the future. If it is diagrammed like this:

Safety←<PERSON>→Growth

then we can very easily classify the various mechanisms of growth in an uncomplicated way as

a. Enhancing the growthward vectors, e.g., making it more attractive and delight producing.
b. Minimizing the fears of growth,
c. Minimizing the safetyward vectors, i.e., making it less attractive,
d. Maximizing the fears of safety, defensiveness, pathology and regression.

We can then add to our basic schema these four sets of valences:

Enhance the dangers Enhance the attractions
Safety←<PERSON>→Growth
Minimize the attractions Minimize the dangers

Therefore we can consider the process of healthy growth to be a never ending series of free choice situations, confronting each individual at every point throughout his life, in which he must choose between the delights of safety and growth, dependence and independence, regression and progression, immaturity and maturity. Safety has both anxieties and delights; growth has both anxieties and delights. We grow forward when the delights of growth and anxieties of safety are greater than the anxieties of growth and the delights of safety.

So far it sounds like a truism. But it isn't to psychologists who are mostly trying to be objective, public, behavioristic. And it has taken many experiments with animals and much theorizing to convince the students of animal motivation that they must invoke what P. T. Young called a hedonic factor, over and above need-reduction, in order to explain the results so far obtained in free-choice experimentation. For example, saccharin is not need-reducing in any way and yet white rats will choose it over plain water. Its (useless) taste *must* have something to do with it.

Furthermore, observe that subjective delight in the experience is something that we can attribute to *any* organism, e.g., it applies to the infant as well as the adult, to the animal as well as to the human.

The possibility that then opens for us is very enticing for the theorist. Perhaps all these high-level concepts of Self, Growth, Self-realization, and Psychological Health can fall into the same system of explanation with appetite experiments in animals, free choice observations in infant feeding and in occupational choice, and the rich studies of homeostasis.

Of course this formulation of growth-through-delight also commits us to the necessary postulation that what tastes good is also, in the growth sense, "better" for us. We rest here on the faith that if free choice is *really* free and if the chooser is not too sick or frightened to choose, he will choose wisely, in a healthy and growthward direction, more often than not.

For this postulation there is already much experimental support, but it is mostly at the animal level, and much more detailed research is necessary with free choice in humans. We must know much more than we do about the reasons for bad and unwise choices, at the constitutional level and at the level of psychodynamics.

There is another reason why my systematizing side likes this notion of growth-through-delight. It is that then I find it possible to tie it in nicely with dynamic theory, with *all* the dynamic theories of Freud, Adler, Jung, Schachtel, Horney, Fromm and Rank, as well as The Self theories of Rogers, Buhler, Combs, Angyal, Allport, Goldstein and of the Growth-and-Being school, Dewey, Rasey, Kelley, Moustakas, Wilson, Perls, Lee, Mearns, etc.

I criticize the classical Freudians for tending (in the extreme instance) to pathologize everything and for not seeing clearly enough the healthward possibilities in the human being, for seeing everything through brown-colored glasses. But the growth school (in the extreme instance) is equally vulnerable, for they tend to see through rose-colored glasses and generally slide over the problems of pathology, of weakness, of *failure* to grow. One is like a theology of evil and sin exclusively; the other is like a theology without any evil at all, and is therefore equally incorrect and unrealistic.

One additional relationship between safety and growth must be specially mentioned. Apparently growth forward customarily takes place in little steps, and each step forward is made possible by the feeling of being safe, of operating out into the unknown from a safe home port, of daring because retreat is possible. We may use as a paradigm the toddler venturing away from his mother's knee into strange surroundings. Characteristically, he first clings to his mother as he explores the room with his eyes. Then he dares a little excursion, continually reassuring himself that the mother-security is intact. These excursions get more and more extensive. In this way, the child can explore a dangerous and unknown world. If suddenly the mother were to disappear, he would be thrown into anxiety, would cease to be interested in exploring the world, would wish only the return of safety, and might even lose his abilities, e.g., instead of daring to walk, he might creep.

I think we may safely generalize this example. Assured safety permits higher needs and impulses to emerge and to grow towards mastery. To endanger safety, means regression backward to the more basic foundation. What this means is that in the choice between giving up safety or giving up growth, safety will ordinarily win out. Safety needs are prepotent over growth needs. This means an expansion of our basic formula. In general, only a child who feels safe dares to grow forward

healthily. His safety needs must be gratified. He can't be *pushed* ahead, because the ungratified safety needs will remain forever underground, always calling for satisfaction. The more safety needs are gratified, the less valence they have for the child, the less they will beckon, and lower his courage.

Now, how can we know when the child feels safe enough to dare to choose the new step ahead? Ultimately, the only way in which we can know is by *his* choices, which is to say only *he* can ever really know the right moment when the beckoning forces ahead overbalance the beckoning forces behind, and courage outweighs fear.

Ultimately the person, even the child, must choose for himself. Nobody can choose for him too often, for this itself enfeebles him, cutting his self-trust, and confusing his *ability* to perceive his own internal delight in the experience, his *own* impulses, judgments, and feelings, and to differentiate them from the interiorized standards of others.[2]

If this is all so, if the child himself must finally make the choice by which he grows forward, since only he can know his subjective delight experience, then how can we reconcile this ultimate necessity for trust in the inner individual

---

[2]"From the moment the package is in his hands, he feels free to do what he wants with it. He opens it, speculates on what it is, recognizes what it is, expresses happiness or disappointment, notices the arrangement of the contents, finds a book of directions, feels the touch of the steel, the different weights of the parts, and their number, and so on. He does all this before he has attempted to do a thing with the set. Then comes the thrill of doing something with it. It may be only matching one single part with another. Thereby alone he gets a feeling of having done something, that he can do something, and that he is not helpless with that particular article. Whatever pattern is subsequently followed, whether his interest extends to the full utilization of the set and therefore toward further gaining a feeling of greater and greater accomplishment, or whether he completely discards it, his initial contact with the erector set has been meaningful.

"The results of active experiencing can be summarized approximately in the following way. There is physical, emotional, and intellectual self-involvement; there is a recognition and further exploration of one's abilities; there is initiation of activity or creativeness; there is finding out one's own pace and rhythm and the assumption of enough of a task for one's abilities at that particular time, which would include the avoidance of taking on too much; there is gain in skill which one can apply to other enterprises, and there is an opportunity each time that one has an active part in something, no matter how small, to find out more and more what one is interested in.

with the necessity for help from the environment? For he does need help. Without help he will be too frightened to dare. How can we help him to grow? Equally important, how can we endanger his growth?

The opposite of the subjective experience of delight (trusting himself), so far as the child is concerned, is the opinion of other people (love, respect, approval, admiration, reward from others, trusting others rather than himself). Since others are so important and vital for the helpless baby and child, fear of losing them (as providers of safety, food, love, respect, etc.) is a primal, terrifying danger. Therefore, the child, faced with a difficult choice between his own delight experiences and the experience of approval from others, must generally choose approval from others, and then handle his delight by repression or letting it die, or not noticing it or controlling it by will-power. In general, along with this will develop a disapproval of the delight experience, or shame and embarrassment and secretiveness about it, with finally, the inability even to experience it.[3]

The primal choice, the fork in the road, then, is between others' and one's own self. If the only way to maintain the self is to lose others, then the ordinary child will give up the self. This is true for the reason already mentioned, that safety is a most basic and prepotent need for children, more primarily necessary by far than independence and self-actualization. If adults force this choice upon him, of choosing between the loss of one (lower) vital necessity or another (higher) vital necessity, the child must choose safety even at the cost of giving up self and growth.

(In principle there is no need for forcing the child to make such a choice. People just *do* it often, out of their own sicknesses and out of ignorance. We know that it is not necessary because we have examples enough of children who are offered all these goods simultaneously, at no vital cost, who can have safety and love *and* respect too.)

"The above situation may be contrasted with another in which the person who brings home the erector set says to the child, 'Here is an erector set, let me open it for you.' He does so, and then points out all the things in the box, the various parts, etc., and, to top it off, he sets about building one of the complicated models, let us say, a crane. The child may be much interested in what he has seen being done, but let us focus on one aspect of what has really been happening. The child has had no opportunity to get himself involved with the erector set, with his body, his intelligence, or his feelings, he has had no opportunity to match himself up with something that is new for him, to find out what he is capable of or to gain further direction for his interests. The building of the crane for him may have brought in another factor. It may have left the child with an implied demand that he do likewise without his having had an opportunity to prepare himself for any such complicated task. The end becomes the object instead of the experience involved in the process of attaining the objective. Also, whatever he may subsequently do by himself will look small and mean compared to what had been made for him by someone else. He has not added to his total experience for coming up against something new for the next time. In other words, he has not grown from within but has had something superimposed from the outside. . . . Each bit of active experiencing is an opportunity toward finding out what he likes or dislikes, and more and more what he wants to make out of himself. It is an essential part of his progress toward the stage of maturity and self-direction."

[3]"How is it possible to lose a self? The treachery, unknown and unthinkable, begins with our secret psychic death in childhood—if and when we are not loved and are cut off from our spontaneous wishes. (Think: what is left?) But wait—victim might even 'outgrow' it—but it is a perfect double crime in which he him-it is not just this simple murder of a psyche. That might be written off, the tiny self also gradually and unwittingly takes part. He has not been accepted for himself, *as he is.* Oh they 'love' him, but they want him or force him or expect him to be different! Therefore he *must be unacceptable*. He himself learns to believe it and at last even takes it for granted. He has truly given himself up. No matter now whether he obeys them, whether he clings, rebels or withdraws—his behavior, his performance is all that matters. His center of gravity is in 'them,' not in himself—yet if he so much as noticed it he'd think it natural enough. And the whole thing is entirely plausible; all invisible, automatic, and anonymous!

"This is the perfect paradox. Everything looks normal; no crime was intended; there is no corpse, no guilt. All we can see is the sun rising and setting as usual. But what has happened? He has been rejected, not only by them, but by himself. (He is actually without a self.) What has he lost? Just the one true and vital part of himself: his own yes-feeling, which is his very capacity for growth, his root system. But alas, he is not dead. 'Life' goes on, and so must he. From the moment he gives himself up, and to the extent that he does so, all unknowingly he sets about to create and maintain a pseudo-self. But this is an expediency—a 'self' without wishes. This one shall be loved (or feared) where he is despised, strong where he is weak; it shall go through the motions (oh, but they are caricatures!) not for fun or joy but for survival; not simply because it wants to move but because it has to obey. This necessity is not life—not his life—it is a defense mechanism against death. It is also the machine of death. From now on he will be torn apart by compulsive (unconscious) *needs* or ground by (unconscious) conflicts into paralysis, every motion and every instant canceling out his being, his integrity; and all the while he is disguised as a normal person and expected to behave like one!

"In a word, I saw that we *become* neurotic seeking or defending a pseudo-self, a self-system; and we *are* neurotic to the extent that we are self-less."

Here we can learn important lessons from the therapy situation, the creative educative situation, creative art education and I believe also creative dance education. Here where the situation is set up variously as permissive, admiring, praising, accepting, safe, gratifying, reassuring, supporting, unthreatening, non-valuing, non-comparing, that is, where the person can feel completely safe and unthreatened, then it becomes possible for him to work out and express all sorts of lesser delights, e.g., hostility, neurotic dependency. Once these are sufficiently catharted, he then tends spontaneously to go to other delights which outsiders perceive to be "higher" or growthward, e.g., love, creativeness, and which he himself will prefer to the previous delights, once he has experienced them both. (It often makes little difference what kind of explicit theory is held by the therapist, teacher, helper, etc. The really good therapist who may espouse a pessimistic Freudian theory, *acts* as if growth were possible. The really good teacher who espouses verbally a completely rosy and optimistic picture of human nature, will *imply* in actual teaching, a complete understanding and respect for regressive and defensive forces. It is also possible to have a wonderfully realistic and comprehensive philosophy and belie it in practice, in therapy, or teaching or parenthood. Only the one who respects fear and defense can teach; only the one who respects health can do therapy.)

Part of the paradox in this situation is that in a very real way, even the "bad" choice is "good for" the neurotic chooser, or at least understandable and even necessary in terms of his own dynamics. We know that tearing away a functional neurotic symptom by force, or by too direct a confrontation or interpretation, or by a stress situation which cracks the person's defenses against too painful an insight, can shatter the person altogether. This involves us in the question of *pace* of growth. And again the good parent, or therapist or educator *practices* as if he understood that gentleness, sweetness, respect for fear, understanding of the naturalness of defensive and regressive forces, are necessary if growth is not to look like an overwhelming danger instead of a delightful prospect. He implies that he understands that growth can

emerge only from safety. He *feels* that if a person's defenses are very rigid this is for a good reason and he is willing to be patient and understanding even though knowing the path in which the child "should" go.

Seen from the dynamic point of view, ultimately *all* choices are in fact wise, if only we grant two kinds of wisdom, defensive-wisdom and growth-wisdom. Defensiveness can be as wise as daring; it depends on the particular person, his particular status and the particular situation in which he has to choose. The choice of safety is wise when it avoids pain that may be more than the person can bear at the moment. If we wish to help him grow (because we know that consistent safety-choices will bring him to catastrophe in the long run, and will cut him off from possibilities that he himself would enjoy if only he could savor them), then all we can do is help him if he asks for help out of suffering, or else simultaneously allow him to feel safe and beckon him onward to *try* the new experience like the mother whose open arms invite the baby to try to walk. We can't *force* him to grow, we can only *coax* him to, make it more possible for him, in the trust that simply experiencing the new experience will make him prefer it. *Only* he can prefer it; no one can prefer it for him. If it is to become part of him, *he* must like it. If he doesn't, we must gracefully concede that it is not for him at this moment.

This means that the sick child must be respected as much as the healthy one, so far as the growth process is concerned. Only when his fears are accepted respectfully, can he dare to be bold. We must understand that the dark forces are as "normal" as the growth forces.

This is a ticklish task, for it implies simultaneously that we know what is best for him (since we *do* beckon him on in a direction we choose), and also that only he knows what is best for himself in the long run. This means that we must *offer* only, and rarely force. We must be quite ready, not only to beckon forward, but to respect retreat to lick wounds, to recover strength, to look over the situation from a safe vantage point, or even to regress to a previous mastery or a "lower" delight, so that courage for growth can be regained.

And this again is where the helper comes in. He is needed, not only for making possible growth forward in the healthy child (by being "available" as the child desires) and getting out of his way at other times, but much more urgently, by the person who is "stuck" in fixation, in rigid defenses, in safety measures which cut off the possibilities of growth. Neurosis is self-perpetuating; so is character structure. We can either wait for life to prove to such a person that his system doesn't work, i.e., by letting him eventually collapse into neurotic suffering, or else by understanding him and helping him to grow by respecting and understanding both his deficiency needs and his growth needs.

This amounts to a revision of Taoistic "let-be," which often hasn't worked because the growing child needs help. It can be formulated as "helpful let-be." It is a *loving* and *respecting* Taoism. It recognizes not only growth and the specific mechanism which makes it move in the right direction, but it also recognizes and respects the fear of growth, the slow pace of growth, the blocks, the pathology, the reasons for not growing. It recognizes the place, the necessity and the helpfulness of the outer environment without yet giving it control. It implements inner growth by knowing its mechanisms and by being willing to help *it* instead of merely being hopeful or passively optimistic about it.

All the foregoing may now be related to the general motivation theory, set forth in my *Motivation and Personality,* particularly the theory of need gratification, which seems to me to be the most important single principle underlying all healthy human development. The single holistic principle that binds together the multiplicity of human motives is the tendency for a new and higher need to emerge as the lower need fulfills itself by being sufficiently gratified. The child who is fortunate enough to grow normally and well gets satiated and *bored* with the delights that he has savored sufficiently, and *eagerly* (without pushing) goes on to higher, more complex, delights as they become available to him without danger or threat.

This principle can be seen exemplified not only in the deeper motivational dynamics of the child but also in microcosm in the development of any of his more modest activities, e.g., in learning to read, or skate, or paint, or dance. The child who masters simple words en-

joys them intensely but doesn't stay there. In the proper atmosphere he spontaneously shows eagerness to go on to more and more new words, longer words, more complex sentences, etc. If he is forced to stay at the simple level he gets bored and restless with what formerly delighted him. He *wants* to go on, to move, to grow. Only if frustration, failure, disapproval, ridicule come at the next step does he fixate or regress and we are then faced with the intricacies of pathological dynamics and of neurotic compromises, in which the impulses remain alive but unfulfilled, or even of loss of impulse and of capacity.[4]

What we wind up with then is a subjective device to add to the principle of the hierarchical arrangement of our various needs, a device which guides and directs the individual in the direction of "healthy" growth. The principle holds true at any age. Recovering the ability to perceive one's own delights is the best way of rediscovering the sacrificed self even in adulthood. The process of therapy helps the adult to discover that the

---

[4] I think it is possible to apply this general principle to Freudian theory of the progression of libidinal stages. The infant in the oral stage, gets most of his delights through the mouth. And one in particular which has been neglected is that of mastery. We should remember that the *only* thing an infant can do well and efficiently is to suckle. In all else he is inefficient, incapable and if, as I think, this is the earliest precursor of self esteem (feeling of mastery), then this is the *only* way in which the infant can experience the delight of mastery (efficiency, control, self expression, volition.)

But soon he develops other capacities for mastery and control. I mean here not only anal control which though correct, has, in my opinion, been overplayed. Motility and sensory capacities also develop enough during the so-called "anal" stage to give feelings of delight and mastery. But what is important for us here is that the oral infant tends to play out his oral mastery and to become bored with it, just as he becomes bored with milk alone. In a free choice situation, he tends to give up the breast milk in favor of the more complex activities and tastes, or anyway, to add to the breast these other "higher" developments. Given sufficient gratification, free choice and lack of threat, he "grows" out of the oral stage and renounces it himself. He doesn't have to be "kicked upstairs," or forced on to maturity as is so often implied. He *chooses* to grow on to higher delights, to become bored with older ones. Only under the impact of danger, threat, failure, frustration, or stress does he tend to regress or fixate; only then does he prefer safety to growth. Certainly renunciation, delay in gratification and the ability to withstand frustration are also necessary for strength, and we know that unbridled gratification is dangerous. And yet it remains true that these qualifications are *subsidiary* to the principle that sufficient gratification of basic needs is *sine qua non.*

childish (repressed) necessity for the approval of others no longer need exist in the childish form and degree, and that the terror of losing these others with the accompanying fear of being weak, helpless and abandoned is no longer realistic and justified as it was for the child. For the adult, others can be and should be less important than for the child.

Our final formula then has the following elements:

1. The healthily spontaneous child, in his spontaneity, from within out, in response to his own inner Being, reaches out to the environment in wonder and interest, and expresses whatever skills he has.

2. To the extent that he is not crippled by fear, to the extent that he feels safe enough to dare.

3. In this process, that which gives him delight-experience is fortuitously encountered, or is offered to him by helpers.

4. He must be safe and self-accepting enough to be able to choose and prefer these delights, instead of being frightened by them.

5. If he *can* choose these experiences which are validated by the experience of delight, then he can return to the experience, repeat it, savor it to the point of repletion, satiation or boredom.

6. At this point, he shows the tendency to go on to more complex, richer experiences and accomplishments in the same sector (again, if he feels safe enough to dare).

7. Such experiences not only mean moving on, but have a feedback effect on the Self, in the feeling of certainty ("This I like; that I don't, for *sure*"); of capability, mastery, self-trust, self-esteem.

8. In this never ending series of choices of which life consists, the choice may generally be schematized as between safety (or, more broadly, defensiveness) and growth, and since only that child doesn't need safety who already has it, we may expect the growth choice to be made by the safety-need gratified child. Only he can afford to be bold.

9. In order to be able to choose in accord with his own nature and to develop it, the child must be permitted to retain the subjective experiences of delight and boredom, as *the* criteria of the correct choice for him. The alternative criterion is making the choice in terms of the wish of another person. The Self is lost when this happens. Also this constitutes restricting the choice to safety alone, since the child will give up trust in his own delight-criterion out of fear (of losing protection, love, etc.).

10. If the choice is really a free one, and if the child is not crippled, then we may expect him ordinarily to choose progression forward.[5]

11. The evidence indicates that what delights the healthy child, what tastes good for him, is also, more frequently than not, "best" for him in terms of far goals as perceivable by the spectator.

12. In this process the environment (parents, therapists, teachers) is important in various ways, even though the ultimate choice must be made by the child:

a. it can gratify his basic needs for safety, belongingness, love and respect, so that he can feel unthreatened, autonomous, interested and spontaneous and thus dare to choose the unknown;

b. it can help by making the growth choice positively attractive and less dangerous, and by making the regressive choice less attractive and more costly.

13. In this way the psychology of Being and the psychology of Becoming can be reconciled, and the child, simply being himself, can yet move forward and grow.

---

[5]A kind of pseudo-growth takes place very commonly when the person tries (by repression, denial, reaction-formation, etc.) to convince himself that an ungratified basic need has really been gratified, or doesn't exist. He then *permits* himself to grow on to higher-need-levels, which of course, forever after, rest on a very shaky foundation. I call this "pseudo-growth by bypassing the ungratified need." Such a need perseverates forever as an unconscious force (repetition compulsion).

PATHOLOGICAL PATTERNS

Phenomenological theorists express particular concern that contemporary man is trapped in a mechanistic mass society. Exposure to such an impersonal atmosphere results in feelings of social isolation and a sense of alienation from one's "true" self. Without a sure grasp of self, the individual lacks an identity, and cannot experience what is termed "being in the world." Unable to sense his own inner world, he cannot sense the inner world of others, and without meaningful social relationships, cannot break the vicious circle to expand experience and develop a sense of identity. Eventually, he may succumb to "nothingness" and disorder. Viktor Frankl has been a leading European exponent of the phenomenological approach to the study of psychopathology and society. Associated with the existential school, he believes that it is more fruitful to understand and treat patients in terms of the personal character of their experience than in terms of abstract theoretical concepts and diagnostic categories. The paper by R. D. Laing, a British existential psychiatrist, illuminates the nature of these personal experiences of isolation and anxiety. Beneath the sense of social loneliness lies a deep and profound alienation from one's self.

25. Meaninglessness: A Challenge to Psychologists[1]

VIKTOR E. FRANKL

Contemporary psychiatrists are more and more confronted with patients who complain of an abysmal feeling of meaninglessness, of a sense that their lives are completely futile, of what might be called an abyss experience in contradistinction to those peak experiences that have been investigated and so beautifully described by Abraham Maslow. These patients also speak of a feeling of emptiness, of an inner void, a condition which I have described and termed "the existential vacuum"[2].

If I were asked for a short explanation of the origins of the existential vacuum, I would refer to two facts: first, that man, unlike an animal, is not told by his drives and instincts what he must do; and second, that, unlike man in former times, he is no longer told by his traditions and values what he should do. Not knowing what he must do, not knowing what he should do, he often does not even know what he basically wishes to do. The danger in this is that either he will wish to do simply what other people do, and this makes for conformism, or he will simply do what other people wish him to do, and this makes for totalitarianism.

From *Psychologia Africana*, 1970, *13*, 87–95. Reprinted by permission.

[1]Parts of this article are reproduced from Frankl, V. E. (1968). *The task of education in an age of meaninglessness*. Letter, S. S. ed., Institute of Higher Education. New York, Columbia University, Teachers College Press. Professor Frankl's English language publications include *Man's Search for Meaning, Psychotherapy and Existentialism, The Will of Meaning*, and *The Doctor and the Soul*.

[2]Frankl, V. E. (1962) *Man's Search for Meaning, an Introduction to Logotherapy*, Boston, Beacon Press.

In other words, two outstanding phenomena observable in the Western and Eastern parts of the world respectively may well be explained, to some extent at least, by these effects of the existential vacuum. Recent literature available from behind the Iron Curtain reveals that, according to Stanislav Kratochvil, a Czechoslovakian psychologist, this existential frustration is by no means restricted to the capitalist states, but may be observed in communist countries, particularly among the youth.

A similar statement was made by the late Dr. Vymetal, psychiatrist of Olomouc University. He said, at a meeting of psychiatrists held behind the Iron Curtain, that we can no longer be content with psychotherapy that is based solely on Pavlovian concepts. "I am an old Pavlovian", he stated, "but I declare: sticking to the concepts of conditioned and/or unconditioned reflexes we can no longer cope with those patients who now complain of a sense of meaninglessness."

The existential vacuum is, of course, not the only origin and cause of totalitarianism and/or conformism, but it might well be a component within the etiology, within the pathogenesis. In addition to totalitarianism and conformism, there is a third result of the existential vacuum; this is neuroticism. There is a certain new kind of neurotic illness, a new syndrome, that I have termed the noögenic neurosis[3]. It is a neurosis deriving from existential frustration, from despair over the apparent meaninglessness of life. It is a neurosis that is not to be traced back to complexes or to conflicts between the ego and the superego, etc., but to spiritual and existential problems, and last but not least to the existential vacuum—to the sense of meaninglessness that is overwhelming so many people today.

James C. Crumbaugh[4], the research director of an American hospital, has worked out a special test that he calls the PIL (Purpose in Life) test in order to differentiate diagnostically the neuroses in the traditional or conventional sense—that is to say, psychogenic neuroses—from the

new, the noögenic neuroses. He has now obtained results from nearly twelve hundred subjects and the results show that the noögenic neurosis may well be differentiated from the conventional type. It is a new syndrome and it is by no means completely identical with the human condition. Based on similar results obtained in Europe and America, it would appear that about 20 per cent of neurotic cases should properly be diagnosed as noögenic.

As a kind of first aid in such cases, it seems to me to be necessary to show young people that their despair over the apparent meaninglessness of life is nothing to be ashamed of, but rather it is something of which to be proud. It is a human achievement because it is a prerogative of man not to take for granted that there is a meaning to life, but rather to venture to question this meaning. It is his prerogative not only to quest for meaning, but even to question it and to challenge the meaning of life. It is right if young people have the courage to do this. However, they should also have patience enough to wait until, sooner or later, meaning becomes clear to them, rather than commit suicide immediately out of this existential despair. In the first place, they should recognize that the fact that they venture to question the meaning of life is, after all, the manifestation of intellectual sincerity and honesty. Therefore it is truly something of which to be proud. However, they must first objectify; they must gain perspective by viewing this overwhelming problem from a distance. This in itself is beneficial in terms of mental hygiene. And they must realize the positive aspect, the fact that their questioning is something to be proud of.

The existential vacuum might also be understood and explained and interpreted as the frustration of what I personally regard to be the primary motivational force operant in man. As a deliberate oversimplification, I have called this the will to meaning[5]. Heuristically and for didactic purposes, it is opposed to the will to power (the concept that plays such an important rôle in the neurosis theory offered by Alfred Adler's individual psychology) and to the pleasure principle on which the whole psychoanalytic system developed by Freud is still based. Freud also rec-

[3]Frankl, V. E. (1965) The Doctor and the Soul. New York, Alfred A. Knopf.

[4]Crumbaugh, J. C. and L. T. Maholick (1967) An experimental study in existentialism: The psychometric approach to Frankl's concept of noögenic neurosis. In: Frankl, V. E. Psychotherapy and Existentialism. New York, Simon and Schuster.

[5]Frankl, V. E. (1969) The Will to Meaning. New York, The World Publishing Company.

ognized a reality principle counteracting, in a way, the operations and the strivings of the pleasure principle, but this does not alter this state of affairs because, according to Freud's own explicit statement, the reality principle is a servant and also seeks pleasure, delayed but secure pleasure. Nevertheless, psychoanalysis is still based on the validity of that concept called the pleasure principle.

You might conceive of the pleasure principle as a will to pleasure. There is, as I have mentioned, the will to power, and I have introduced the concept of a will to meaning by which I really mean the intrinsic self-transcendent quality of human existence. It is my contention that being human always points or is directed toward something other than itself, or to someone other than oneself. I deny that man really, basically, is striving to obtain, establish, or restore any state within himself. Such a concept is a monadologistic concept of man. It is a concept of man along the lines of a closed system. Man, on the contrary, is primarily reaching out for a meaning to fulfil out there in the world, reaching out to encounter another human being out there in the world, but he is never primarily concerned with anything within himself.

This is the basic feature of human existence, this self-transcendence as I call it, and it is only after man has once renounced his primary strivings that he comes back, he returns, and reflects upon himself. I would venture to say that whenever we observe in human beings the prevalence of a will to power and/or a will to pleasure rather than a will to meaning, it indicates that we are dealing with substitutes. The frustrated will to meaning makes a man long for pleasure and/or power, but primarily man is concerned with finding and fulfilling a meaning out there in the world, with encountering other beings. Man is never concerned primarily with himself but, by virtue of his self-transcendent quality, he endeavours to serve a cause higher than himself, or to love another person. Loving and serving a cause on the command of one's conscience are the principal manifestations of this self-transcendent quality of human existence that has been totally neglected by closed-system concepts such as the homeostasis principle. This principle is based on the presupposition that an organism, and also the human psyche, are primarily concerned with and striving to maintain or restore an inner equilibrium, a state without tension, regardless of whether these tensions are aroused by inner drives and instincts, by still unsatisfied needs, or by the clashes between ego and superego or between the interests of the societal environment and those of one's own psyche. This homeostasis principle has already been abandoned for many years, even in biology, as Ludwig von Bertalanffy in Canada could show. In neurology it was disproved and abandoned by the late Kurt Goldstein, the brain pathologist, and in psychology by the late Gordon Allport, by Charlotte Buhler and by Abraham Maslow. In education, however, it is still presupposed as a valid tenet.

This self-transcendent quality of human existence gives rise to a fact which a clinician can observe day by day, namely that the pleasure principle is actually self-defeating. In other words the "pursuit of happiness"[6] is self-defeating; it is a contradiction in itself. I daresay that precisely to the extent to which an individual sets out to pursue or to strive directly for happiness, to this same extent he cannot attain it. The more he strives to attain it, the further he misses it. How can this be understood?

Once a man has a reason to be happy, whether he has fulfilled a meaning or has lovingly encountered another human being, this makes him happy. Happiness ensues, happiness happens, and one must let happiness happen. What happens when a man strives directly for happiness? As illustrated by Figure 1, the more he pays attention to happiness or the more he embarks on a direct quest for happiness, precisely to this extent he loses sight of the reason to be happy and, consequently, happiness fades away because for him there is no longer any reason to be happy. He has shut out the reason for happiness. He no longer cares for meaning, for other beings; he cares for happiness by way of a direct intention. This we observe in sexual neuroses. I venture to say, based on decades of practice, that more than 95 per cent of the cases of impotence or frigidity may well be traced back to the fact that the male patient is directly striving to demonstrate his potency and the fe-

---

[6]Fabry, J. E. (1968) *The Pursuit of Meaning: Logotherapy Applied to Life.* Boston, Beacon Press.

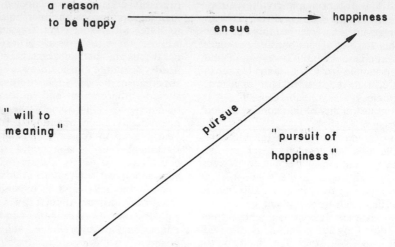

Figure 1.

male patient is directly striving to demonstrate to herself that she is capable of experiencing full orgasm. They are striving for happiness instead of letting happiness happen. They are "pursuing" happiness instead of letting happiness occur as a side effect. Pleasure is a side effect, not the goal, of human strivings; it is the side effect of fulfilling meaning, the side effect of a loving encounter with another human being. The moment one strives directly to attain pleasure, the goal is missed, because primarily man is concerned with a reason to become happy rather than with being happy. He is concerned with other human beings, with meanings; he is transcending himself rather than being a closed system that simply cares about reinstating in his brain or psyche a certain condition called pleasure, or homeostasis, or whatever concepts have been developed in the setting of those monadologistic concepts that treat man as if he were a closed system. In other words, happiness ensues as a side effect of fulfilling a meaning, of encountering another human being, of living out this self-transcendent quality of a human being, but it fades away to the extent that it is pursued or directly sought.

The two outstanding classical schools of psychotherapy developed the will to pleasure concept and the will to power concept when *both had to deal with neurotic individuals*. Only those neurotic people who have been frustrated in their primary and original striving for the fulfill-

ment of meaning, only those frustrated personalities are either intent on pleasure or content with power. They are intent on the effect rather than on the primary goal, or content with the means to the end because they have been frustrated in their strivings for the end itself, which is meaning.

The self-defeating quality of a direct striving for a side effect rather than a concern with the primary goal of human existence that is dictated by its self-transcendent quality, recurs in matters that are widely discussed. I am referring to the slogan of self-actualization. Self-transcendence implies that man is not capable of directly striving for self-actualization. One can actualize oneself only to the extent to which one is fulfilling a meaning out there in the world. Then self-actualization occurs, again as a side effect. It is a gift that falls into one's lap, but if one directly strives for self-actualization, one cannot obtain it, because there are no longer any grounds for self-actualization. If he has not fulfilled the task at hand, how can he actualize himself?

Self-actualization cannot be made the target of human strivings but must result from other sources, among which is self-transcendence through the fulfilment of meaning, or dedication and devotion to another human being through love. I could put it in one sentence by saying that Pindar was right when giving the admonition, "You should become what you are", but this is valid only when you add another statement once made by Karl Jaspers: "What a man is he only becomes through that cause which he has made his own."

We started with the proposition that the traditional values are on the wane, so let us ask ourselves whether it is not justifiable to contend that life is meaningless. This is not true because there is a distinction between values and meanings. Only values are affected by the wane of traditions, while meanings are spared. Values, I would say, are universal meanings. But meanings themselves are unique insofar as they refer to a unique person engaged in a unique situation. Meanings change from moment to moment, from situation to situation, and from person to person.

Meanings are unique and in this sense it might well be said that meanings are relative. They relate to a situation and to a person involved in this situation. The question is now raised whether they are also subjective, as is generally contended. Max Wertheimer, the founder of Gestalt psychology, once said explicitly that the requirement of a situation, that is to say what the situation means to the individual, is an objective quality. My great teacher, the late Rudolf Allers of Georgetown University (a philosopher rather than an experimental psychologist), was more cautious in just saying that it is a trans-subjective quality. Meanings, I would say, are objective in that they must be responsibly discovered rather than arbitrarily invented. (This, of course, is opposed to a view such as that developed by Jean-Paul Sartre.)

Incidentally, there are also subjective meanings. The person who is in the intoxicated state induced by LSD attributes meanings to the world. He finds subjective meanings, but they are not the objective meanings in wait for him, to be fulfilled by him. This reminds me of an experiment by Olds and Milner in California. They inserted electrodes into certain spots in the hypothalamus of rats and whenever they closed an electric circuit what the rats evidently experienced was sexual orgasm or the satisfaction of having ingested food. The rats learned to activate the lever by which the circuit was closed and they pressed this lever up to fifty thousand times a day, each time experiencing orgasm or the satisfaction of nutrition. After they obtained this subjective feeling, they neglected the real sexual partners and the real food offered to them. It is the same with those who take LSD. They may neglect the objective meanings waiting for them (the unique meanings they have to find) because they have restricted themselves merely to attributing meanings—profoundly subjective meanings—and they bypass their actual, their true, meanings and assignments (out there in the world) by only caring for subjective meanings.

In an age like ours, an age of the existential vacuum, man must be equipped with the capacity to discover meaning, to find for himself the individual meanings of the singular situations that together form a string called human life. He must be equipped with the means to find meaning in an age of meaninglessness. It is the particular task and assignment of education not only to content itself with transmitting traditions and values and knowledge, but also to see as one of its principal assignments the development and refining of that capacity always to find out, to smell out, the unique meanings of a given situation. This capacity is called conscience. In an age in which the Ten Commandments apparently are losing their unconditional validity for so many people, more than ever man must be equipped with the capacity to listen to the ten thousand commandments involved in the ten thousand of his life situations and mediated by his conscience. In other words, education must refine and sharpen the capacity of man to hear the voice of his conscience. Only when man has this capacity is he capable of counteracting those two effects which result from the existential vacuum—conformism and totalitarianism. Only a man with a vivid and alert conscience is capable of resisting totalitarianism and conformism.

We often see that, instead of embarking on this business of refining man's conscience, education is rather reinforcing the existential vacuum in the young people. This occurs as a result of that reductionism along the lines of which science is so often taught on campuses. I remember when I was thirteen years of age, in junior high school, our science teacher walked up and down the rows and taught or offered us the definition of what life ultimately is. "In the final analysis," he said, "life is nothing but a combustion, an oxidation process." Without asking permission, I sprang to my feet and threw the question into his face, "If this is true, then, Dr. Fritz, what meaning does life have?" It is a typical reductionist theory that life is nothing but an oxidation process. Actually, it is an example of oxidationism rather than reductionism.

In the United States the trend toward reductionist indoctrination is even more observable than it is elsewhere. At the University of Vienna, I found, for example, that 40 per cent of the German, Swiss, and Austrian students attending my lectures confessed that they had experienced this existential despair over the apparent meaninglessness of their own lives. In comparison, in a similar sample of American students attending my lectures, fully 81 per cent reported that they had experienced despair of this kind. I would say that the high incidence of existential despair among American students stems largely from the prevalence in the United States of the reductionist way of presenting facts and scientific data.

What is reductionism? I would define it thus: Reductionism is a pseudo-scientific procedure according to which a human phenomenon (such as love or conscience) is made into a mere epiphenomenon. It is thereby deprived of its very humanness. More specifically, human phenomena are deprived of their very humanness by being dynamically reduced to, or genetically deduced from, essentially subhuman phenomena. In other words, reductionism is a subhumanism.

Let me give an example. If love is defined as the sublimation of sex, it is reduced from a human phenomenon to a subhuman phenomenon, sexual instinct. Actually, love is not and never can be the mere sublimation of sex, simply because whenever sublimation is to take place the capacity to love is presupposed. In the final analysis, a person is capable of integrating his sexuality into the whole makeup of his personality only for the sake of another person whom he loves. Stated somewhat differently, the ego is capable of integrating its id only to the extent that it is lovingly directed toward a thou. Therefore, if sublimation of sex is only possible on the basis of the capacity to love, love can never be the result of sublimation.

As to conscience, something similar must be said by way of criticism. In the same way as love has been reduced to the id (sexuality) conscience is often reduced to or even identified with the superego, but there is an essential difference. Conscience can never be identical with or reduced to the superego simply because it is not the last and certainly not the least assignment of true conscience to contradict and oppose precisely those conventions and ideals and traditions that are channelled and transmitted through the superego. Thus if the superego must sometimes be contradicted and opposed by the conscience, the conscience cannot be identical with the superego.

Time and again it is said that conscience is the result of conditioning processes. This might be correct when it is applied, for example, to a dog that has wet the floor and then slinks under the couch with its tail between its legs. The animal undoubtedly displays something that resembles conscience, but it is not true conscience. I would say it is anticipatory anxiety, the fearful expectation of punishment, and this might well be the result of certain conditioning processes. When a man "hears the voice of his conscience," however, this has nothing to do with fear of punishment. This is something different, and it is only when this difference comes to the fore that the human dimension has been entered and the human quality of this phenomenon called conscience has been envisaged at all.

There are many persons who presuppose that, if there is anything such as conscience, it must be explainable in terms of the conditioning processes observable in animals. They reduce conscience to a conditioning process by their *a priori* assumption that what is human can be explained along the lines of animal psychology and animal behaviour. In this connection I am reminded of a Viennese joke about two neighbours who were quarrelling because one said that the other's cat had eaten two pounds of butter. The other neighbour denied that the cat ever ate butter and they went to the rabbi, asking him for a Solomonic judgment.

The rabbi pondered and said, "So you contend that two pounds of butter have been eaten by this cat?"

"Yes, two pounds of butter."

"Bring me the cat."

They brought him the cat. "Bring me scales," he said.

They brought him the scales and the rabbi put the cat on the scales and, believe it or not, the weight was exactly two pounds.

"Now I have the butter," said the rabbi, "but where is the cat?"

There was the *a priori* conviction on the part of the rabbi that if there is something which weighs two pounds it must be butter. Then he was searching in vain for the cat. The same is true of the animal behaviourists; they say that if there is anything in man it must be explainable by way of animal behaviour—reflexes, conditioning processes—and they have their conditioning processes, but where then is man? The *a priorism* which contradicts any true empiricism rests with the scientists who are reductionists rather than with the man who envisages the full scope of what is going on in man, who experiences conscience not as a conditioning process, but as something he has to follow because of his humanness—unless he just does away with his own humanness, and this would be contradicting his own self.

Why are we more and more confronted with reductionistically oriented scientists? This is because we are living in an age of specialists. I would say that a specialist is a man who no longer sees the forest of truth for the trees of facts. In other words, he is concerned with the scattered facts and data furnished by a compartmentalized science and is no longer capable of arriving at a unified concept of man[7].

The problem is whether disparate visions of man, or of a particular phenomenon in man, necessarily preclude our arriving at a unified concept of man. They do not. Consider the problem of stereoscopic vision. In stereoscopic vision two different pictures are given to the viewer. The pictures are disparate, but it is precisely this fact that opens up a new dimension—the dimension of space. In other words, the fact that the pictures obtained from scientific research are disparate need not necessarily make for confusion; all that is needed is what in physiology is called the fusion of the pictures at the retina. In other words, the

fact that the pictures provided by science are disparate need not result in loss of knowledge, but may produce a gain in knowledge, provided that we arrive at a fusion of the pictures which leads us to a unified *Weltanschauung,* or concept of man.

We cannot reverse the wheel of history; society cannot do without the specialist today. The style of modern research is profoundly characterized by what is called teamwork, that is by co-operative effort by teams of specialists. As I see it, the ultimate threat and danger do not lie in the fact that scientists more and more are specializing. The loss and consequent lack of universality are not what makes for reductionism. It is rather the totality of knowledge pretended by those specialists that makes for reductionism. In other words, we do not deplore the fact that more and more scientists are specializing, but rather that more and more specialists are generalizing. Specialists are making overgeneralized statements. For example, a biologist who contends that man's human life and existence can be explained entirely on the grounds of his biology, in merely biological terms, is making biology into biologism. Likewise, a specialist may make sociology into sociologism, psychology into psychologism, and so forth. At the very moment when we make such an overgeneralized statement on man, at the same moment we have turned our science into a mere ideology. In other words, what has been called the *terrible simplificateur* may well be complemented by a notion of the *terrible généralisateur.*

For instance "Man is nothing but a computer" is an overgeneralized statement. As a neurologist, I can vouch for the legitimacy of using the model of a computer as an analogy to explain the mode of functioning of the human central nervous system. But the error is in the phrase, "nothing but" which is not true because man is infinitely more than a computer.

Formerly, nihilism was masked behind the term "nothingness." Today nihilism unmasks itself by the use of the phrase "nothing but." This is the "nothing-butness" that characterizes nihilism today and it should not be confounded with existentialism. The true message delivered by existentialism is by no means the nothingness of man. I would say the true message of existentialism is the "no-

---

[7]Frankl, V. E. (1965) The concept of man in logotherapy. *In:* Dreyer, P. S. *and* S. J. Schoeman, *eds. Homo Viator: Fecsbundel Oberholzer.* Cape Town, Hollandsch Afrikaansche Uitgevers Maatschappij.

thingness" of man, the idea that a human being is not a thing, that a human being must never be reified, never totally objectified.

Let me return to reductionism. The devastating impact of an indoctrination along the lines of reductionism must not be underrated. Here I confine myself to quoting from a study by R. N. Gray and associates on 64 physicians, 11 of them psychiatrists. The study showed that during medical school, cynicism as a rule increases while humanitarianism decreases. Only after completion of medical studies is this trend reversed but unfortunately not in all subjects. Ironically, the author of the paper which reports these results, himself defines man as nothing but "an adaptive control system" and defines values as "homeostatic restraints in a stimulus-response process." According to another reductionist definition of values, they are nothing but reaction formations and defence mechanisms. My reaction to this theory was that I am not prepared to live for the sake of my reaction formations, even less to die for the sake of my defence mechanisms. Such reductionist interpretations are likely to undermine and erode the appreciation of values. As an example, let me report the following observation. A young American couple re-turned from Africa where they had served as Peace Corps volunteers, completely fed up and disgusted. At the outset, they had had to participate in mandatory group sessions led by a psychologist who played a game somewhat as follows: "Why did you join the Peace Corps?" "We wanted to help people less privileged." "So you must be superior to them." "In a way." "So there must be in you, in your unconscious, a need to prove to yourself that you are superior." "Well, I never thought of it that way but you are a psychologist, you certainly know better." And so it went on. The group was indoctrinated in interpreting their idealism and altruism as hang-ups. Even worse, the volunteers "were constantly on each other's backs, playing the 'what's *your* hidden motive' game", according to the report of a Fulbright fellow who studied in Vienna at my hospital last year. Here we are dealing with an instance of what I would call hyper-interpretation. Unmasking is perfectly legitimate but it must stop as soon as one is confronted with what is genuine, genuinely human, in man. If it does not, the only thing that is unmasked is the unmasking psychologist's own "hidden motive", namely, his unconscious need to belittle the greatness of man.

26.   Ontological Insecurity

R. D. LAING

A man may have a sense of his presence in the world as a real, alive, whole, and, in a temporal sense, continuous person. As such, he can live out into the world and meet others: a world and others experienced as equally real, alive, whole, and continuous.

Such a basically *ontologically*[1] se-cure person will encounter all the hazards of life, social, ethical, spiritual, biological, from a centrally firm sense of his own and other people's reality and identity. It is often difficult for a person with such a sense of his integral selfhood and personal identity, of the permanency of things, of the reliability of natural processes, of the substantiality of natural processes, of the substantiality of others, to transpose himself into the world of an individual whose experiences may be utterly lacking in any unquestionable self-validating certainties.

This study is concerned with the issues involved where there is the partial

---

From *The Divided Self*, chapter 3, copyright 1960, by permission of the author, Penguin Books and Tavistock Publications, Limited.

[1]Despite the philosophical use of "ontology" (by Heidegger, Sartre, Tillich, especially), I have used the term in its present empirical sense because it appears to be the best adverbial or adjectival derivative of "being."

or almost complete absence of the assurances derived from an existential position of what I shall call *primary ontological security:* with anxieties and dangers that I shall suggest arise *only* in terms of *primary ontological insecurity;* and with the consequent attempts to deal with such anxieties and dangers.

The literary critic, Lionel Trilling (1955), points up the contrast that I wish to make between a *basic existential position of ontological security* and one of *ontological insecurity* very clearly in comparing the worlds of Shakespeare and Keats on the one hand, and of Kafka on the other:

. . . for Keats the awareness of evil exists side by side with a very strong sense of personal identity and is for that reason the less immediately apparent. To some contemporary readers, it will seem for the same reason the less intense. In the same way it may seem to a contemporary reader that, if we compare Shakespeare and Kafka, leaving aside the degree of genius each has, and considering both only as expositors of man's suffering and cosmic alienation, it is Kafka who makes the more intense and complete exposition. And, indeed, the judgment may be correct, exactly because for Kafka the sense of evil is not contradicted by the sense of personal identity. Shakespeare's world, quite as much as Kafka's, is that prison cell which Pascal says the world is, from which daily the inmates are led forth to die; Shakespeare no less than Kafka forces upon us the cruel irrationality of the conditions of human life, the tale told by an idiot, the puerile gods who torture us not for punishment but for sport; and no less than Kafka, Shakespeare is revolted by the fetor of the prison of this world, nothing is more characteristic of him than his imagery of disgust. But in Shakespeare's cell the company is so much better than in Kafka's, the captains and kings and lovers and clowns of Shakespeare are alive and complete before they die. In Kafka, long before the sentence is executed, even long before the malign legal process is even instituted, something terrible has been done to the accused. We all know what that is—he has been stripped of all that is becoming to a man except his abstract humanity, which, like his skeleton, never is quite becoming to a man. He is without parents, home, wife, child, commitment, or appetite; he has no connection with power, beauty, love, wit, courage, loyalty, or fame, and the pride that may be taken in these. So that we may say that Kafka's knowledge of evil exists without the extradictory knowledge of the self in its health and validity, that Shakespeare's knowledge of evil exists with that contradiction in its fullest possible force (pp. 38–9).

We find, as Trilling points out, that Shakespeare does depict characters who evidently experience themselves as real and alive and complete however riddled by doubts or torn by conflicts they may be. With Kafka this is not so. Indeed, the effort to communicate what being alive is like in the absence of such assurances seems to characterize the work of a number of writers and artists of our time. Life, without feeling alive.

With Samuel Beckett, for instance, one enters a world in which there is no contradictory sense of the self in its "health and validity" to mitigate the despair, terror, and boredom of existence. In such a way, the two tramps who wait for Godot are condemned to live:

ESTRAGON: We always find something, eh, Didi, to give us the impression that we exist?
VLADIMIR (impatiently): Yes, yes, we're magicians. But let us persevere in what we have resolved, before we forget.

In painting, Francis Bacon, among others, seems to be dealing with similar issues. Generally, it is evident that what we shall discuss here clinically is but a small sample of something in which human nature is deeply implicated and to which we can contribute only a very partial understanding.

To begin at the beginning:

Biological birth is a definitive act whereby the infant organism is precipitated into the world. There it is, a new baby, a new biological entity, already with its own ways, real and alive, from *our* point of view. But what of the baby's point of view? Under usual circumstances, the physical birth of a new living organism into the world inaugurates rapidly ongoing processes whereby within an amazingly short time the infant *feels* real and alive and has a *sense* of being an entity, with continuity in time and a location in space. In short, physical birth and biological aliveness are followed by the baby becoming existentially born as real and alive. Usually this development is taken for granted and affords the certainty upon which all other certainties depend. This is to say, not only do adults see children to be real biologically visible entities but they experience themselves as whole persons who are real and alive, and conjunctively experience other human beings as real and alive. These are self-validating data of experience.

The individual, then, may experience his own being as real, alive, whole; as differentiated from the rest of the world in ordinary circumstances so clearly that his identity and autonomy are never in question; as a continuum in time; as having an inner consistency, substantiality, genuineness, and worth; as spatially coextensive with the body; and, usually, as having begun in or around birth and liable to extinction with death. He thus has a firm core of ontological security.

This, however, may not be the case. The individual in the ordinary circumstances of living may feel more unreal than real; in a literal sense, more dead than alive; precariously differentiated from the rest of the world, so that his identity and autonomy are always in question. He may lack the experience of his own temporal continuity. He may not possess an over-riding sense of personal consistency or cohesiveness. He may feel more insubstantial than substantial, and unable to assume that the stuff he is made of is genuine, good, valuable. And he may feel his self as partially divorced from his body.

It is, of course, inevitable that an individual whose experience of himself is of this order can no more live in a "secure" world than he can be secure "in himself." The whole "physiognomy" of his world will be correspondingly different from that of the individual whose sense of self is securely established in its health and validity. Relatedness to other persons will be seen to have a radically different significance and function. To anticipate, we can say that in the individual whose own being is secure in this primary experiential sense, relatedness with others is potentially gratifying; whereas the ontologically preserving rather than gratifying insecure person is preoccupied with himself: the ordinary circumstances of living threaten his *low threshold* of security.[2]

If a position of primary ontological security has been reached, the ordinary circumstances of life do not afford a

perpetual threat to one's own existence. If such a basis for living has not been reached, the ordinary circumstances of everyday life constitute a continual and deadly threat.

Only if this is realized is it possible to understand how certain psychoses can develop.

If the individual cannot take the realness, aliveness, autonomy, and identity of himself and others for granted, then he has to become absorbed in contriving ways of trying to be real, of keeping himself or others alive, of preserving his identity, in efforts, as he will often put it, to prevent himself losing his self. What are to most people everyday happenings, which are hardly noticed because they have no special significance, may become deeply significant in so far as they either contribute to the sustenance of the individual's being or threaten him with nonbeing. Such an individual, for whom the elements of the world are coming to have, or have come to have, a different hierarchy of significance from that of the ordinary person, is beginning, as we say, to "live in a world of his own," or has already come to do so. It is not true to say, however, without careful qualification that he is losing "contact with" reality, and withdrawing into himself. External events no longer affect him in the same way as they do others: it is not that they affect him less; on the contrary, frequently they affect him more. It is frequently not the case that he is becoming "indifferent" and "withdrawn." It may, however, be that the world of his experience comes to be one he can no longer share with other people.

But before these developments are explored, it will be valuable to characterize under three headings three forms of anxiety encountered by the ontologically insecure person: engulfment, implosion, petrification.

ENGULFMENT

An argument occurred between two patients in the course of a session in an analytic group. Suddenly, one of the protagonists broke off the argument to say, "I can't go on. You are arguing in order to have the pleasure of triumphing over me. At best you win an argument. At

---

[2]This formulation is very similar to those of H. S. Sullivan, Hill, F. Fromm-Reichmann, and Arieti in particular. Federn, although expressing himself very differently, seems to have advanced a closely allied view.

worst you lose an argument. *I am arguing in order to preserve my existence.*"

This patient was a young man who I would say was sane, but, as he stated, his activity in the argument, as in the rest of his life, was not designed to gain gratification but to "preserve his existence." Now, one might say that if he did, in fact, really imagine the loss of an argument would jeopardize his existence, then he was "grossly out of touch with reality" and was virtually psychotic. But this is simply to beg the question without making any contribution towards understanding the patient. It is, however, important to know that if you were to subject this patient to a type of psychiatric interrogation recommended in many psychiatric textbooks, within ten minutes his behaviour and speech would be revealing "signs" of psychosis. It is quite easy to evoke such "signs" from such a person whose threshold of basic security is so low that practically any relationship with another person, however tenuous or however apparently "harmless," threatens to overwhelm him.

A firm sense of one's own autonomous identity is required in order that one may be related as one human being to another. Otherwise, any and every relationship threatens the individual with loss of identity. One form this takes can be called engulfment. In this the individual dreads relatedness as such, with anyone or anything or, indeed, even with himself, because his uncertainty about the stability of his autonomy lays him open to the dread lest in any relationship he will lose his autonomy and identity. Engulfment is not simply envisaged as something that is liable to happen willy-nilly despite the individual's most active efforts to avoid it. The individual experiences himself as a man who is only saving himself from drowning by the most constant, strenuous, desperate activity. Engulfment is felt as a risk in being understood (thus grasped, comprehended), in being loved, or even simply in being seen. To be hated may be feared for other reasons, but to be hated as such is often less disturbing than to be destroyed, as it is felt, through being engulfed by love.

The main manoeuvre used to preserve identity under pressure from the dread of engulfment is isolation. Thus, instead of the polarities of separateness and relatedness based on individual autonomy, there is the antithesis between complete loss of being by absorption into the other person (engulfment), and complete aloneness (isolation). There is no safe third possibility of a dialectical relationship between two persons, both sure of their own ground and, on this very basis, able to "lose themselves" in each other. Such merging of being can occur in an "authentic" way only when the individuals are sure of themselves. If a man hates himself, he may wish to lose himself in the other: then being engulfed by the other is an escape from himself. In the present case it is an ever-present possibility to be dreaded. It will be shown later, however, that what at one "moment" is most dreaded and strenuously avoided can change to what is most sought.

This anxiety accounts for one form of a so-called "negative therapeutic reaction" to apparently correct interpretation in psychotherapy. To be understood correctly is to be engulfed, to be enclosed, swallowed up, drowned, eaten up, smothered, stifled in or by another person's supposed all-embracing comprehension. It is lonely and painful to be always misunderstood, but there is at least from this point of view a measure of safety in isolation.

The other's love is, therefore, feared more than his hatred, or rather all love is sensed as a version of hatred. By being loved one is placed under an unsolicited obligation. In therapy with such a person, the last thing there is any point in is to pretend to more "love" or "concern" than one has. The more the therapist's own necessarily very complex motives for trying to "help" a person of this kind genuinely converge on a concern for him which is prepared to "let him be" and is not *in fact* engulfing or merely indifference, the more hope there will be in the horizon.

There are many images used to describe related ways in which identity is threatened which may be mentioned here, as closely related to the dread of engulfment, e.g., being buried, being drowned, being caught and dragged down into quicksand. The image of fire recurs repeatedly. Fire may be the uncertain flickering of the individual's own inner aliveness. It may be a destructive alien power which will devastate him. Some psychotics say in the acute phase that they are on fire, that their bodies are being burned up. A patient describes himself as cold and dry. Yet he dreads any warmth or wet. He will be engulfed by the fire or the water, and either way be destroyed.

IMPLOSION

This is the strongest word I can find for the extreme form of what Winnicott terms the *impingement* of reality. Impingement does not convey, however, the full terror of the experience of the world as liable at any moment to crash in and obliterate all identity, as a gas will rush in and obliterate a vacuum. The individual feels that, like the vacuum, he is empty. But this emptiness is him. Although in other ways he longs for the emptiness to be filled, he dreads the possibility of this happening because he has come to feel that all he can be is the awful nothingness of just this very vacuum. Any "contact" with reality is then in itself experienced as a dreadful threat because reality, as experienced from this position, is necessarily *implosive* and thus, as was relatedness in engulfment, *in itself* a threat to what identity the individual is able to suppose himself to have.

Reality, as such, threatening engulfment or implosion, is the persecutor.

In fact, we are all only two or three degrees Fahrenheit from experiences of this order. Even a slight fever, and the whole world can begin to take on a persecutory, impinging aspect.

PETRIFICATION AND DEPERSONALIZATION

In using the term "petrification," one can exploit a number of the meanings embedded in this word:

1. A particular form of terror, whereby one is petrified, i.e., turned to stone.
2. The dread of this happening: the dread, that is, of the possibility of turning, or being turned, from a live person into a dead thing, into a stone, into a robot, an automaton, without personal autonomy of action, an *it* without subjectivity.
3. The "magical" act whereby one may attempt to turn someone else into stone, by "petrifying" him; and, by extension, the act whereby one negates the other person's autonomy, ignores his feelings, regards him as a thing, kills the life in him. In this sense one may perhaps better say that one depersonalizes him, or reifies him. One treats him not as a person, as a free agent, but as an *it*.

Depersonalization is a technique that is universally used as a means of dealing with the other when he becomes too tiresome or disturbing. One no longer allows oneself to be responsive to his feelings and may be prepared to regard him and treat him as though he had no feelings. The people in focus here both tend to feel themselves as more or less depersonalized and tend to depersonalize others; they are constantly afraid of being depersonalized by others. The act of turning him into a thing is, *for him*, actually petrifying. In the face of being treated as an *it*, his own subjectivity drains away from him like blood from the face. Basically he requires constant confirmation from others of his own existence as a person.

A partial depersonalization of others is extensively practised in everyday life and is regarded as normal if not highly desirable. Most relationships are based on some partial depersonalizing tendency in so far as one treats the other not in terms of any awareness of who or what he might be in himself but as virtually an android robot playing a role or part in a large machine in which one too may be acting yet another part.

It is usual to cherish if not the reality, at least the illusion that there is a limited sphere of living free from this dehumanization. Yet it may be in just this sphere that the greater risk is felt, and the ontologically insecure person experiences this risk in highly potentiated form.

The risk consists in this: if one experiences the other as a free agent, one is open to the possibility of experiencing oneself as an *object* of his experience and thereby of feeling one's own subjectivity drained away. One is threatened with the possibility of becoming no more than a thing in the world of the other, without any life for oneself, without any being for oneself. In terms of such anxiety, the very act of experiencing the other as a person is felt as virtually suicidal. Sartre discusses this experience brilliantly in Part 3 of *Being and Nothingness*.

The issue is in principle straightforward. One may find oneself enlivened and the sense of one's own being enhanced by the other, or one may experience the other as deadening and impoverishing. A person may have come to anticipate that any possible relationship with another will have the latter consequences. Any other is then a threat to his "self" (his capacity to act autonomously) not by reason of anything he or she may do or not do specifically, but by reason of his or her very existence.

Some of the above points are illustrated in the life of James, a chemist, aged twenty-eight.

The complaint he made all along was that he could not become a "person." He had "no self." "I am only a response to other people, I have no identity of my own." He felt he was becoming more and more "a mythical person." He felt he had no weight, no substance of his own. "I am only a cork floating on the ocean."

This man was very concerned about not having become a person: he reproached his mother for this failure. "I was merely her emblem. She never recognized my identity." In contrast to his own belittlement of and uncertainty about himself, he was always on the brink of being over-awed and crushed by the formidable reality that other people contained. In contrast to his own light weight, uncertainty, and insubstantiality, *they* were solid, decisive, emphatic, and substantial. He felt that in every way that mattered others were more "large scale" than he was.

At the same time, in practice he was not easily overawed. He used two chief manoeuvres to preserve security. One was an outward compliance with the other. The second was an inner intellectual Medusa's head he turned on the other. Both manoeuvres taken together safeguarded his own subjectivity which he had never to betray openly and which thus could never find direct and immediate expression for itself. Being secret, it

was safe. Both techniques together were designed to avoid the dangers of being engulfed or depersonalized.

With his outer behaviour he forestalled the danger to which he was perpetually subject, namely that of becoming someone else's *thing,* by pretending to be no more than a cork. (After all, what safer thing to be in an ocean?) At the same time, however, he turned the other person into a thing in his own eyes, thus magically nullifying any danger to himself by secretly totally disarming the enemy. By destroying, in his own eyes, the other person as a person, he robbed the other of his power to crush him. By depleting him of his personal aliveness, that is, by seeing him as a piece of machinery rather than as a human being, he undercut the risk to himself of this aliveness either swamping him, imploding into his own emptiness, or turning him into a mere appendage.

This man was married to a very lively and vivacious woman, highly spirited, with a forceful personality and a mind of her own. He maintained a paradoxical relationship with her in which, in one sense, he was entirely alone and isolated and, in another sense, he was almost a parasite. He dreamt, for instance, that he was a clam stuck to his wife's body.

Just because he could dream thus, he had the more need to keep her at bay by contriving to see her as no more than a machine. He described her laughter, her anger, her sadness, with "clinical" precision, even going so far as to refer to her as "it," a practice that was rather chilling in its effect. "It then started to laugh." She was an "it" because everything she did was a predictable, determined response. He would, for instance, tell her (it) an ordinary funny joke and when she (it) laughed this indicated her (its) entirely "conditioned," robot-like nature, which he saw indeed in much the same terms as certain psychiatric theories would use to account for all human actions.

I was at first agreeably surprised by his apparent ability to reject and disagree with what I said as well as to agree with me. This seemed to indicate that he had more of a mind of his own than he perhaps realized and that he was not too frightened to display some measure of autonomy. However, it became evident that his apparent capacity to act as an autonomous person with me was due to his secret manoeuvre of regarding me not as a live human being, a person in my own right with my own selfhood, but as a sort of robot interpreting device to which he fed input and which after a quick commutation came out with a verbal message to him. With this secret outlook on me as a thing he could appear to be a "person." What he could not sustain was a person-to-person relationship, experienced as such.

Dreams in which one or other of the above forms of dread is expressed are common in such persons. These dreams are not variations on the fears of being eaten which occur in ontologically secure persons. To be eaten does not necessarily mean to lose one's identity. Jonah was very much himself even within the belly of the whale. Few nightmares go so far as to call up anxieties about actual loss of identity, usually because most people, even in their dreams, still meet whatever dangers are to be encountered as persons who may perhaps be attacked or mutilated but whose basic existential core is not itself in jeopardy. In the classical nightmare the dreamer wakes up in terror. But this terror is not the dread of losing the "self." Thus a patient dreams of a fat pig which sits on his chest and threatens to suffocate him. He wakes in terror. At worst, in this nightmare, he is threatened with suffocation, but not with the dissolution of his very being.

The defensive method of turning the threatening mother- or breast-figure into a *thing* occurs in patients' dreams. One patient dreamt recurrently of a small black triangle which originated in a corner of his room and grew larger and larger until it seemed about to engulf him—whereupon he always awoke in great terror. This was a psychotic young man who stayed with my family for several months, and whom I was thus able to get to know rather well. There was only one situation as far as I could judge in which he could let himself "go" without anxiety at not recovering himself again, and that was in listening to jazz.

The fact that even in a dream the breast-figure has to be so depersonalized is a measure of its potential danger to the self, presumably on the basis of its frightening original personalizations and

the failure of *a normal process of depersonalization.*

Medard Boss (1957a) gives examples of several dreams heralding psychosis. In one, the dreamer is engulfed by fire:

A woman of hardly thirty years dreamt, at a time when she still felt completely healthy, that she was afire in the stables. Around her, the fire, an ever larger crust of lava was forming. Half from the outside and half from the inside her own body she could see how the fire was slowly becoming choked by this crust. Suddenly she was entirely outside this fire and, as if possessed, she beat the fire with a club to break the crust and to let some air in. But the dreamer soon got tired and slowly she (the fire) became extinguished. Four days after this dream she began to suffer from acute schizophrenia. In the details of the dream the dreamer had exactly predicted the special course of her psychosis. She became rigid at first and, in effect, encysted. Six weeks afterwards she defended herself once more with all her might against the choking of her life's fire, until finally she became completely extinguished both spiritually and mentally. Now, for some years, she has been like a burnt-out crater.

In another example, petrification of others occurs, anticipating the dreamer's own petrification:

. . . a girl of twenty-five years dreamt that she had cooked dinner for her family of five. She had just served it and she now called her parents and her brothers and sisters to dinner. Nobody replied. Only her voice returned as if it were an echo from a deep cave. She found the sudden emptiness of the house uncanny. She rushed upstairs to look for her family. In the first bedroom, she could see her two sisters sitting on two beds. In spite of her impatient calls they remained in an unnaturally rigid position and did not even answer her. She went up to her sisters and wanted to shake them. Suddenly she noticed that they were stone statues. She escaped in horror and rushed into her mother's room. Her mother too had turned into stone and was sitting inertly in her armchair staring into the air with glazed eyes. The dreamer escaped into the room of her father. He stood in the middle of it. In her despair she rushed up to him and, desiring his protection, she threw her arms round his neck. But he too was made of stone and, to her utter horror, he turned into sand when she embraced him. She awoke in absolute terror, and was so stunned by the dream experience that she could not move for some minutes. This same horrible dream was dreamt by the patient on four successive occasions within a few days. At that time she was apparently the picture of mental and physical health. Her parents used to call her the sunshine of the whole family. Ten days after the fourth repetition of the dream, the patient was taken ill with an acute form of schizophrenia displaying severe catatonic symptoms. She fell into a state which was remarkably similar to the physical petrification of her family that she had dreamt about. She was now overpowered in waking life by behaviour patterns that in her dreams she had merely observed in other persons.

It seems to be a general law that at some point those very dangers most dreaded can themselves be encompassed to forestall their actual occurrence. Thus, to forgo one's autonomy becomes the means of secretly safeguarding it; to play possum, to feign death, becomes a means of preserving one's aliveness (see Oberndorf, 1950). To turn oneself into a stone becomes a way of not being turned into a stone by someone else. "Be thou hard," exhorts Nietzsche. In a sense that Nietzsche did not, I believe, himself intend, to be stony hard and thus far dead forestalls the danger of being turned into a dead thing by another person. Thoroughly to understand oneself (engulf oneself) is a defense against the risk involved in being sucked into the whirlpool of another person's way of comprehending oneself. To consume oneself by one's own love prevents the possibility of being consumed by another.

It seems also that the preferred method of attack on the other is based on the same principle as the attack felt to be implicit in the other's relationship to oneself. Thus, the man who is frightened of his own subjectivity being swamped, impinged upon, or congealed by the other is frequently to be found attempting to swamp, to impinge upon, or to kill the other person's subjectivity. The process involves a vicious circle. The more one attempts to preserve one's autonomy and identity by nullifying the specific human individuality of the other, the more it is felt to be necessary to continue to do so, because with each denial of the other person's ontological status, one's own ontological security is decreased, the threat to the self from the other is potentiated and hence has to be even more desperately negated.

In this lesion in the sense of personal autonomy there is both a failure to sustain the sense of oneself as a person with the other, and a failure to sustain it alone. There is a failure to sustain a sense of one's own being without the presence of other people. It is a failure *to be* by oneself, a failure to exist alone. As James put it, "Other people supply me with my existence." This appears to be in direct contradiction to the aforementioned dread that other people will deprive him of his existence. But contradictory or absurd as it may be, these two attitudes existed in him side by side, and are indeed entirely characteristic of this type of person.

The capacity to experience oneself as autonomous means that one has really come to realize that one is a separate person from everyone else. No matter how deeply I am committed in joy or suffering to someone else, he is not me, and I am not him. However lonely or sad one may be, one can exist alone. The fact that the other person in his own actuality is not me, is set against the equally real fact that my attachment to him is a part of me. If he dies or goes away, he has gone, but my attachment to him persists. But in the last resort I cannot die another person's death. For that matter, as Sartre comments on this thought of Heidegger's, he cannot love for me or make my decisions, and I likewise cannot do this for him. In short, he cannot be me, and I cannot be him.

If the individual does not feel himself to be autonomous this means that he can experience neither his separateness from, nor his relatedness to, the other in the usual way. A lack of sense of autonomy implies that one feels one's being to be bound up in the other, or that the other is bound up in oneself, in a sense that transgresses the actual possibilities within the structure of human relatedness. It means that a feeling that one is in a position of ontological dependency on the other (i.e., dependent on the other for one's very being), is substituted for a sense of relatedness and attachment to him based on genuine mutuality. Utter detachment and isolation are regarded as the only alternatives to a clam- or vampire-like attachment in which the other person's life-blood is necessary for one's own survival, and yet is a threat to one's survival. Therefore, the polarity is between complete isolation or complete merging of identity rather than between separateness and relatedness. The individual oscillates perpetually between the two extremes, each equally unfeasible. He comes to live rather like those mechanical toys which have a positive tropism that impels them towards a stimulus until they reach a specific point, whereupon a built-in negative tropism directs them away until the positive tropism takes over again, this oscillation being repeated *ad infinitum*.

Other people were necessary for his existence, said James. Another patient, in the same basic dilemma, behaved in the following way: he maintained himself in isolated detachment from the world for months, living alone in a single room, existing frugally on a few savings, daydreaming. But in doing this, he began to feel he was dying inside; he was becoming more and more empty, and observed "a progressive impoverishment of my life mode." A great deal of his pride and self-esteem was implicated in thus existing on his own, but as his state of depersonalization progressed he would emerge into social life for a brief foray in order to get a "dose" of other people, but "not an overdose." He was like an alcoholic who goes on sudden drinking orgies between dry spells, except that in his case his addiction, of which he was as frightened and ashamed as any repentant alcoholic or drug-addict, was to other people. Within a short while, he would come to feel that he was in danger of being caught up or trapped in the circle he had entered and he would withdraw again into his own isolation in a confusion of frightened hopelessness, suspicion, and shame.

Some of the points discussed above are illustrated in the following two cases:

CASE 1. ANXIETY AT FEELING ALONE

Mrs. R.'s presenting difficulty was a dread of being in the street (agoraphobia). On closer inspection, it became clear that her anxiety arose when she began to feel on her own in the street or elsewhere. She could *be* on her own, as long as she did not feel that she was really alone.

Briefly, her story was as follows: she was an only and a lonely child. There was no open neglect or hostility in her family. She felt, however, that her parents were always too engrossed in each other for either of them ever to take notice of her. She grew up wanting to fill this hole in her life but never succeeded in becoming self-sufficient, or absorbed in her own world. Her longing was always to be important and significant *to someone* else. There always had to be someone else. Preferably she wanted to be loved and admired, but, if not, then to be hated was much to be preferred to being unnoticed. She wanted to be *significant* to someone else in whatever capacity, in contrast to her abiding memory of herself as a child that she did not really matter to her parents, that they neither loved nor hated, admired nor were ashamed of her very much.

In consequence, she tried looking at herself in her mirror but never managed to convince herself that she was *somebody*. She never got over being frightened if there was no one there.

She grew into a very attractive girl and was married at seventeen to the first man who really noticed this. Characteristically, it seemed to her, her parents had not noticed that any turmoil had been going on in their daughter until she announced that she was engaged. She was triumphant and self-confident under the warmth of her husband's attentions. But he was an army officer and shortly posted abroad. She was not able to go with him. At this separation she experienced severe panic.

We should note that her reaction to her husband's absence was not depression or sadness in which she pined or yearned for him. It was panic (as I would suggest) because of the dissolution of something in her, which owed its existence to the presence of her husband and his continued attentions. She was a flower that withered in the absence of one day's rain. However, help came to her through a sudden illness of her mother. She received an urgent plea for help from her father, asking her to come to nurse her mother. For the next year, during her mother's illness, she had never been, as she put it, so much herself. She was the pivot of the household. There was not a trace of panic until after her mother's death when the prospect of leaving the place where she had at last come to mean so much, to join her husband, was very much in her mind. Her experience of the last year had made her feel for the first time that she was now her parents' child. Against this, being her husband's wife was now somehow superfluous.

Again, one notes the absence of grief at her mother's death. At this time she began to reckon up the chances of her being alone in the world. Her mother had died; then there would be her father; possibly her husband: "beyond that— nothing." This did not depress her, it frightened her.

She then joined her husband abroad and led a gay life for a few years. She craved for all the attention he could give her but this became less and less. She was restless and unsatisfied. Their marriage broke up and she returned to live in a flat in London with her father. While continuing to stay with her father she became the mistress and model of a sculptor. In this way she had lived for several years before I saw her when she was twenty-eight.

This is the way she talked of the street: "In the street people come and go about their business. You seldom meet anyone who recognizes you; even if they do, it is just a nod and they pass on or at most you have a few minutes' chat. Nobody knows who you are. Everyone's engrossed in themselves. No one cares about you." She gave examples of people fainting and everyone's casualness about it. "No one gives a damn." It was in this setting and with these considerations in mind that she felt anxiety.

This anxiety was at being in the street alone or rather at feeling on her own. If she went out with or met someone who really knew her, she felt no anxiety.

In her father's flat she was often alone but there it was different. There she never felt *really* on her own. She made his breakfast. Tidying up the beds, washing up, was protracted as long as possible. The middle of the day was a drag. But she didn't mind too much. "Everything was familiar." There was her father's chair and his pipe rack. There was a picture of her mother on the wall looking down at her. It was as though all these familiar objects somehow illumined the house with the presence of the people who possessed and used them or had done so as a part of their lives. Thus, although she was by herself at home, she was always able to have someone with her in a magical way. But this magic was dispelled in the noise and anonymity of the busy street.

An intensive application of what is often supposed to be the classical psychoanalytic theory of hysteria to this patient might attempt to show this woman as unconsciously libidinally bound to her father; with, consequently, unconscious guilt and unconscious need and/or fear of punishment. Her failure to develop lasting libidinal relationships away from her father would seem to support the first view, along with her decision to live with him, to take her mother's place, as it were, and the fact that she spent most of her day, as a woman of twenty-eight, actually thinking about him. Her devotion to her mother in her last illness would be partly the consequences of unconscious guilt at her unconscious ambivalence to her mother; and her anxiety at her mother's death would be anxiety at her unconscious wish for her mother's death coming true. And so on.[3]

However, the central or pivotal issue in this patient's life is not to be discovered in her "unconscious"; it is lying quite open for her to see, as well as for us (although this is not to say that there are not many things about herself that this patient does not realize).

The pivotal point around which all her life is centered is her *lack of ontological autonomy*. If she is not in the actual presence of another person who knows her, or if she cannot succeed in evoking this person's presence in his absence, her sense of her own identity drains away from her. Her panic is at the fading away of her being. She is like Tinker Bell. In order to exist she needs someone else to believe in her existence. How necessary that her lover should be a sculptor and that she should be his model! How inevitable, given this basic premise of her existence, that when her existence was not recognized she should be suffused with anxiety. For her, *esse* is *percipi;* to be seen, that is, not as an anonymous passer-by or casual acquaintance. It was just that form of seeing which *petrified* her. If she was seen *as* an anonymity, *as* no one who especially mattered or as a *thing*, then she *was* no one in particular. She was as she was seen to be. If there was no one to see her, at the moment, she had to try to conjure up someone (father, mother, hus-

---

[3] For extremely valuable psychoanalytic contributions to apparently "hysterical" symptom-formation, see Segal (1954).

band, lover, at different times in her life) to whom she felt she mattered, for whom she was a *person,* and to imagine herself in his or her presence. If this person on whom her being depended went away or died, it was not a matter for grief, it was a matter for panic.

One cannot transpose her central problem into "the unconscious." If one discovers that she has an unconscious phantasy of being a prostitute, this does not explain her anxiety about street-walking, or her preoccupation with women who fall in the street and are not helped to get on their feet again. The conscious phantasy is, on the contrary, to be explained by and understood in terms of the central issue implicating her self-being, her being-for-herself. Her fear of being alone is not a "defense" against incestuous phantasies or masturbation. She had incestuous phantasies. *These phantasies were a defense against the dread of being alone,* as was her whole "fixation" on being a daughter. They were a means of overcoming her anxiety at being by herself. The unconscious phantasies of this patient would have an entirely different meaning if her basic existential position were such that she had a starting-point in herself that she could leave behind, as it were, in pursuit of gratification. As it was, *her sexual life and phantasies were efforts, not primarily to gain gratification, but to seek first ontological security.* In love-making an illusion of this security was achieved, and on the basis of this illusion gratification was possible.

It would be a profound mistake to call this woman narcissistic in any proper application of the term. She was unable to fall in love with her own reflection. It would be a mistake to translate her problem into phases of psychosexual development, oral, anal, genital. She grasped at sexuality as at a straw as soon as she was "of age." She was not frigid. Orgasm could be physically gratifying if she was temporarily secure in the prior ontological sense. In intercourse with someone who loved her (and she was capable of believing in being loved by another), she achieved perhaps her best moments. But they were short-lived. She could not be alone or let her lover be alone with her.

Her need to be taken notice of might facilitate the application of a further cliché to her, that she was an exhibitionist. Once more, such a term is only valid if it is understood existentially. Thus, and this will be discussed in greater detail subsequently, she "showed herself off" while never "giving herself away." That is, she exhibited herself while always holding herself in (inhibited). She was, therefore, always alone and lonely although superficially her difficulty was not in being together with other people; her difficulty was *least in evidence* when she was most together with another person. But it is clear that her realization of the autonomous existence of other people was really quite as tenuous as her belief in her own autonomy. If they were not there, they ceased to exist for her. Orgasm was a means of possessing herself, by holding in her arms the man who possessed her. But she could not be herself, by herself, and so could not really be herself at all.

CASE 2

A most curious phenomenon of the personality, one which has been observed for centuries, but which has not yet received its full explanation, is that in which the individual seems to be the vehicle of a personality that is not his own. Someone else's personality seems to "possess" him and to be finding expression through his words and action, whereas the individual's own personality is temporarily "lost" or "gone." This happens with all degrees of malignancy. There seem to be all degrees of the same basic process from the simple, benign observation that so-and-so "takes after his father," or "That's her mother's temper coming out in her," to the extreme distress of the person who finds himself under a compulsion to take on the characteristics of a personality he may hate and/or feel to be entirely alien to his own.

This phenomenon is one of the most important in occasioning disruption in the sense of one's own identity when it occurs unwanted and compulsively. The dread of this occurring is one factor in the fear of engulfment and implosion. The individual may be afraid to like anyone, for he finds that he is under a compulsion to become like anyone he likes.

The way in which the individual's self and personality are profoundly modified even to the point of threatened loss of his or her own identity and sense of reality by engulfment by such an alien sub-identity, is illustrated in the following case:

Mrs. D., a woman of forty, presented the initial complaint of vague but intense fear. She said she was frightened of everything, "even of the sky." She complained of an abiding sense of dissatisfaction, of unaccountable accesses of anger towards her husband, in particular of a "lack of a sense of responsibility." Her fear was "as though somebody was trying to rise up inside and was trying to get out of me." She was very afraid that she was like her mother, whom she hated. What she called "unreliability" was a feeling of bafflement and bewilderment which she related to the fact that nothing she did had ever seemed to please her parents. If she did one thing and was told it was wrong, she would do another thing and would find that they still said that was wrong. She was unable to discover, as she put it, "what they wanted me to be." She reproached her parents for this above all, that they hadn't given her any way of knowing who or what she really was or had to become. She could be neither bad nor good with any "reliability" because her parents were, or she felt they were, completely unpredictable and unreliable in their expressions of love or hatred, approval or disapproval. In retrospect, she concluded that they hated her; but at the time, she said, she was too baffled by them and too anxious to discover what she was expected to be to have been able to hate them, let alone love them. She now said that she was looking for "comfort." She was looking for a line from me that would give her an indication of the path she was to follow. She found my non-directive attitude particularly hard to tolerate since it seemed to her to be so clearly a repetition of her father's attitude: "Ask no questions and you'll be told no lies." For a spell, she became subject to compulsive thinking, in which she was under a necessity to ask such questions as, "What is this for?" or "Why is this?" and to provide herself with the answers. She interpreted this to herself as her effort to get comfort from her own thoughts since she could derive comfort from no one. She began to be intensely depressed and to make numerous complaints about her feelings, saying how childish they were. She spoke a great deal about how sorry she was for herself.

Now it seemed to me "she" was not really sorry for her own true self. She sounded to me much more like a querulous mother complaining about a difficult child. Her mother, indeed, seemed to be "coming out of her" all the time, complaining about "her" childishness. Not only was this so as regards the complaints which "she" was making about herself, but in other respects as well. For instance, like her mother, she kept screaming at her husband and child; like her mother,[4] she hated everyone; and like her mother she was forever crying. In fact, life was a misery to her by the fact that she could never be herself but was always being her mother. She knew, however, that when she felt lonely, lost, frightened, and bewildered she was more her true self. She knew also that she gave her complicity to becoming angry, hating, screaming, crying, or querulous, for if she worked herself up into being like that (i.e., being her mother), she did not feel frightened any more (at the expense, it was true, of being no longer herself). However, the backwash of this manoeuvre was that she was oppressed, when the storm had passed, by a sense of futility (at not having been herself) and a hatred of the person she had been (her mother) and of herself for her self-duplicity. To some extent this patient, once she had become aware of this false way of overcoming the anxiety she was exposed to when she was herself, had to decide whether avoiding experiencing such anxiety, by avoiding being herself, was a cure worse than her disease. The frustration she experienced with me, which called out intense hatred of me, was not fully to be explained by the frustration of libidinal or aggressive drives in the transference, but rather it was what one could term the existential frustration that arose out of the fact that I, by withholding from her the "comfort" she sought to derive from me, in that *I did not tell her what she was to be,* was imposing upon her the necessity to make her own decision about

---

[4] That is, like her notion of what her mother was. I never met her mother and have no idea whether her phantasies of her mother bore any resemblance to her mother as a real person.

the person she was to become. Her feeling that she had been denied her birthright because her parents had not discharged their responsibility towards her by giving her a definition of herself that could act as her starting-point in life was intensified by my refusal to offer this "comfort." But only by withholding it was it possible to provide a setting in which she could take this responsibility into herself.

In this sense, therefore, the task in psychotherapy was to make, using Jasper's expression, an appeal to the freedom of the patient. A good deal of the skill in psychotherapy lies in the ability to do this effectively.

References

Boss, M. *Analysis of Dreams*, London, Rider & Co., 1957.

Oberndorf, C. P., "The Role of Anxiety in Depersonalization," *International Journal of Psychoanalysis*, 1950, Vol. 31.

Segal, H., "Schizoid Mechanisms Underlying Phobia Formation," *International Journal of Psychoanalysis*, 1954, Vol. 35.

Trilling, Lionel, *The Opposing Self*, London, 1955, Secker & Warburg.

Phenomenological Theories

THERAPY

The goal of therapy, according to phenomenological theorists, should not be to understand the causes or to remove the symptoms of pathological behavior, but rather to free the patient to develop a constructive and confident image of his self-worth. Patients should be led to appreciate their "true identity" and encouraged to venture forth to test their personal tastes and values. The Swiss psychiatrists Ludwig Binswanger and Medard Boss have modified Freudian psychoanalytic therapy in line with this philosophy. In this recent essay, Binswanger summarized his position on Daseins-analysis and compares it with traditional intrapsychic therapy. The development of Boss' ideas are remarkably similar to those of Binswanger. In the present paper, he argues for a new basis for psychotherapy, one founded on the therapist's appreciation of the patient's total personality. Only by assuming a phenomenological attitude, according to Boss, can the therapist grasp the full nature of the patient's dilemmas and anxieties. Albert Ellis, though taking a more directive approach in his rational therapy, argues strongly for the view that the patient must judge his behavior not in terms of what others may believe, but in terms of what he senses is right for him. The goal of therapy is to enable the patient to commit himself to actions that correspond to his true value system.

27. Existential Analysis and Daseinsanalysis

LUDWIG BINSWANGER and MEDARD BOSS

PART I

Zürich is the birthplace of existential analysis *(Daseinsanalyse)* as a psychiatric-phenomenologic research method. I emphasize the term *research method*, for if the psychoanalytic theory of Freud or the teaching of Jung arose out of a dissatisfaction with preceding psychotherapy, thus owing their origin and development predominantly to psychotherapeutic impulses and aims, the existential research orientation in psychiatry arose from dissatisfaction with the prevailing efforts to gain scientific understanding in psychiatry; so that existential analysis owes its origin and de-velopment to an attempt to gain a new scientific understanding of the concerns of psychiatry, psychopathology and psychotherapy, on the basis of the analysis of existence *(Daseinsanalytik)* as it was developed in the remarkable work of Martin Heidegger: "Being and time" *(Sein und Zeit)*, in the year 1927. Psychology and psychotherapy, as sciences, are admittedly concerned with "man," but not at all primarily with mentally *ill* man, but with *man as such*. The new understanding of man, which we owe to Heidegger's analysis of existence, has its basis in the new conception that man is no longer understood in terms of some theory—be it a mechanistic, a biologic or a psychological one—but in terms of a purely phenomenologic elucidation of the total structure or total articula-

From *Progress in Psychotherapy* edited by F. Fromm-Reichmann and J. L. Moreno, 1956, 1957, Grune and Stratton, Inc., Vol. I and Vol. II, by permission of the publisher.

tion of existence as BEING-IN-THE-WORLD (*In-der-Welt-sein*). What this expression, fundamental for existential analysis, means, I unfortunately cannot develop here; be it only emphasized that it encompasses alike the individual's own world and the simultaneous and coextensive relationships with and to other people and things. Nor can I go into the difference between an ontologic-phenomenologic analysis of existence, an empiric-phenomenologic existential analysis, and an empiric discursive description, classification and explanation.

Once, in his interpretation of dreams, Freud said that psychiatrists had "forsaken the stability of the psychic structure too early." Existential analysis could say the same thing, albeit with an altogether different meaning. Freud, as is well known, had in mind the stability of the articulation of the life-history with the psychic structure, in contrast to the psychiatrists of his day who, at the very first opportunity, considered the psychic structure to be disrupted, and who resorted instead to physiologic processes in the cerebral cortex. Existential analysis, on the other hand, does not have in mind the solidity of the structure of the inner life-history, but rather the solidity of the transcendental structure preceding or underlying, a priori, all psychic structures as the very condition of this possibility. I regret that I cannot explain in fuller detail these philosophic expressions, already employed by Kant but here used in a much wider sense; those among you conversant with philosophy will readily understand me. I want to emphasize only that philosophy is not here in any way being introduced into psychiatry or psychotherapy, but rather that the philosophic bases of these sciences are being laid bare. Obviously, this in turn has an effect upon one's understanding of what constitutes their scientific object or field. This effect reveals itself in the fact that we have learned to understand and to describe the various psychoses and neuroses as specific *deviations* of the a priori, or the transcendental, structure of man's humanity, of the *condition humaine,* as the French say.

Be it noted in passing that the existential-analytic research method in psychiatry had to investigate the structure of existence as being-in-the-world, as Heidegger had outlined and delineated it

still further and along various new paths. Such, for instance, are its studies of various existential "dimensions," i.e., height, depth and width, thingness and resistance *(Materialität),* lighting and coloring of the world, fullness or emptiness of existence, etc. The investigation of psychotic or neurotic world-projects and existential structures such as, for example, those which we designate as manic, depressive, schizophrenic, or compulsive, have so occupied all of us who are engaged upon this work that only suggestions are at hand with regard to the significance of existential-analytic research for psychotherapy. I should like now very cursorily to indicate a few of the main trends of this relationship.

(1) A psychotherapy on existential-analytic bases investigates the life-history of the patient to be treated, just as any other psychotherapeutic method, albeit in its own fashion. It does not explain this life-history and its pathologic idiosyncrasies according to the teachings of any school of psychotherapy, or by means of its preferred categories. Instead, it *understands* this life-history as modifications of the total structure of the patient's being-in-the-world, as I have shown in my studies "On Flight of Ideas" (*Uber Ideenflucht*), in my studies of schizophrenia, and most recently in the case of "Suzanne Urban."

(2) A psychotherapy on existential-analytic bases thus proceeds *not* merely by showing the patient where, when and to what extent he has failed to realize the fullness of his humanity, but it tries to make him *experience* this as radically as possible—how, like Ibsen's master-builder, Solness, he has lost his way and footing in "airy heights" or "ethereal worlds of fantasy." In this case the psychotherapist could be compared to someone who is informed, e.g., a mountain guide, familiar with the particular terrain, who attempts the trip back to the valley with the unpracticed tourist who no longer dares either to proceed or to return. And inversely, the existential-analytically-oriented therapist seeks to enable the depressed patient to get out of his cavernous subterranean world, and to gain footing "upon the ground" once more, by revealing it to him as being the only mode of existence in which the fullness of human possibilities can be realized. And further, the existential-

analytically-oriented therapist will lead the twisted schizophrenic out of the autistic world of distortion and askewness in which he lives and acts, into the shared worlds, the *koinos kosmos* of Heraclitus; or he will strive to help a patient who, in her own words, lives "in two speeds" to "synchronize" these (again using her own expression). Yet, another time the therapist will see (as happened in one of Roland Kuhn's cases of anorexia mentalis) that the goal may be reached much more rapidly if one explores not the temporal but the spatial structures of a particular patient's world. It came as a surprise to us to find how easily some otherwise not particularly intelligent or educated patients proved accessible to an existential-analytic kind of exploration, and how thoroughly they felt understood by it in their singularity. This is, after all, an altogether indispensable prerequisite for any kind of psychotherapeutic success.

(3) Regardless of whether the existential analyst is predominantly psychoanalytic or predominantly jungian in orientation, he will always stand on the same plane with his patients—the plane of common existence. He will therefore not degrade the patient to an object toward which he is subject, but he will see in him an existential partner. He will therefore not consider the bond between the two partners to be as that of two electric batteries—a "psychic contact"—but as an *encounter* on what Martin Buber calls the "sharp edge of existence," an existence which *essentially* "is in the world," not merely as a self but also as a being-together with one another—relatedness and love. Also what has, since *Freud,* been called transference is, in the existential-analytic sense, a kind of encounter. For encounter is a being-with-others in *genuine presence,* that is to say, in the present which is altogether continuous with the *past* and bears within it the possibilities of a *future.*

(4) Perhaps you will also be interested in hearing what is the position of existential analysis toward the *dream,* and this again particularly with regard to psychotherapy. Here again it is removed from any theoretic "explanation" of the dream, especially from the purely sexual exegesis of dream contents in psychoanalysis; rather, it understands the dream, as I emphasized a long time ago, as a specific way of being-in-the-world, in other words, as a specific world and a specific way of existing. This amounts to saying that in the dream we see the whole man, the *entirety* of his problems, in a different existential modality than in waking, but against the background and with the structure of the a priori articulation of existence, and therefore the dream is also of paramount therapeutic importance for the existential analyst. For precisely by means of the structure of dreams he is enabled first of all to show the patient the structure of his being-in-the-world in an over-all manner, and secondly, he can, on the basis of this, free him for the *totality* of existential possibilities of being, in other words, for open resoluteness (*Entschlossenheit*); he can, to use Heidegger's expression, "retrieve" (*zurückholen*) existence from a dream existence to a genuine capacity for being itself. For the time being, I will refer you to Roland Kuhn's paper, "On the Existential Structure of a Neurosis" in Gebsattel's *Jahrbuch fur Psychologie und Psychotherapie.* I only ask of you not to imagine existential structure as something static, but as something undergoing constant change. Similarly, what we call neurosis represents a changed existential *process,* as compared with the healthy. Thus, existential analysis understands the task of psychotherapy to be the opening up of new structural possibilities to such altered existential processes.

As you see, existential analysis, instead of speaking in theoretic concepts, such as "pleasure principle" and "reality principle," investigates and treats the mentally-ill person with regard to the structures, structural articulations and structural alterations of his existence. Hence, it has not, by any means, consciousness as its sole object, as has been erroneously stated, but rather the whole man, prior to any distinction between conscious and unconscious, or even between body and soul; for the existential structures and their alterations permeate man's entire being. Obviously, the existential analyst, insofar as he is a therapist, will not, at least in the beginning of his treatment, be able to dispense with the distinction between conscious and unconscious, deriving from the psychology of consciousness and bound up with its merits and its drawbacks.

(5) Taking stock of the relationship between existential analysis and psycho-

therapy, it can be said that existential analysis cannot, over long stretches, dispense with the traditional psychotherapeutic methods; that, however, it can, as such, be therapeutically effective only insofar as it succeeds in opening up to the sick fellow man an understanding of the structure of human existence, and allows him to find his way back from his neurotic or psychotic, lost, erring, per-

forated or twisted mode of existence and world into the freedom of being able to utilize his own capacities for existence. This presupposes that the existential analyst, insofar as he is a psychotherapist, not only is in possession of existential-analytic and psychotherapeutic competence, but that he must dare to risk committing his own existence in the struggle for the freedom of his partner's.

PART II

MODERN PSYCHOTHERAPY IN NEED OF A BASIS

All problems, answers and resulting actions are invariably guided by the pre-scientific notions about the general nature and goal of man which each investigator carries within himself. No matter whether he is explicitly aware of his "philosophical" assumptions or whether he rejects all "philosophy" and attempts to be a "pure empiricist," the fact remains that such more or less hidden philosophical presuppositions, which are at the root of all science, are of fundamental importance. Up to now modern psychologists believed that their therapeutic approaches had found a sound basis in terms of their various psychodynamic theories about the human psyche. Freud thought of the human being as a telescope-like psychic apparatus; Reich, Alexander and Horney on the other hand attempt to explain all instinctual reactions in terms of a Total I or a Total Personality; for Jung the "psyche" is a self-regulating libidinal system controlled by the archetypes of the "Collective Unconscious"; Sullivan conceives of man as the product of interactions between him and his fellowmen; Fromm and others speak of man as a Self molded by society. Yet all these modern anthropologic theories can't possibly warrant an adequate understanding of the psychotherapeutic processes. For none of them answers what ought to be the first and foremost questions: what would have to be the nature of such a "Psyche," such a psychic apparatus, such a human I or Self or total personality in order that something like a mere perception of an object and of a human being, or even something like object relations and interpersonal and social relations, be at

all possible? How should a telescope-like psychic apparatus or a self-regulating libidinal system be able to perceive or understand the meaning of anything, or to love or to hate somebody? Even less can such anonymous psychic structures or forces develop a transference or a resistance in the course of psychotherapy. Yet all these phenomena are central factors for a true healing.

MARTIN HEIDEGGER'S "DASEINSANALYSIS" REVEALING MAN'S BASIC NATURE

The eminent importance of the "Daseinsanalysis" in the sense of Martin Heidegger's fundamental ontology for psychology and psychotherapy lies in the fact that it helps overcome just these shortcomings of the basic anthropologic concepts of our psychological thinking, shortcomings which until now actually kept us groping in the dark. The "Daseinsanalysis" is able to do so because its concept of man's basic nature is nothing more or less than an explicit articulation of that understanding of man which has always guided our therapeutic actions, independent of all secondary theories, although secretly only and without our awareness. Therefore, the daseinsanalytic understanding of man helps us comprehend directly and fundamentally why therapists *can* demand of their patients what they have in fact been asking all along, and why they even *must* demand it if they want to cure at all. In all their endeavors psychotherapists rely on the peculiar ability of man to exist in a variety of instinctual, feeling, thinking and acting relationships to the things and in social and interpersonal patterns of behavior towards the fellowmen of his world. The therapist tacitly counts on this human ability when he asks of his patient—and tries to help him achieve it by this or that psychotherapeutic method—that he knowingly and responsibly seize and adopt all his potentialities of relationships so that they no longer remain frozen in unconscious neurotic mental or physical symptoms because of early childhood inhibitions and repressions.

In order to gain real insight into these preconditions and this goal of all practical psychotherapeutic approaches, the daseinsanalytic thinking had to guard against approaching man dogmatically with preconceived notions about his reality, no matter how self-evident they might seem. It also had to avoid forcing man blindly, by means of such preconceived ideas, into categories whereby he would be nothing but a "Psyche," a "Person" or "Consciousness." On the contrary, the daseinsanalysis had to learn again to see man unbiased, in the manner in which he directly reveals himself, and, in so doing, it made a very simple but all the more significant discovery about the fundamental nature of man. It found that man exists only *in* his relations and *as* his relations to the objects and fellowmen of his world. In order to exist in such manner, however, man must intrinsically possess a fundamental understanding of the fact that something *is* and can *be* at all. Man's special manner of being-in-the-world can therefore only be compared to the shining of a light, in the brightness of which the presence of all that is can occur, in which all things can appear and reveal themselves in their own, proper nature. Man is fundamentally an essentially spiritual brightness and as such he genuinely exists in the world. As this world-revealing brightness he is claimed by the ultimate be-ness. If a primordial understanding of be-ness were not the very essence of man, where would he suddenly find the ability to acquire any special knowledge and insight? In fact, each single comprehension of the meaning of all the different encountering objects and all actual dealing with them is possible only because man is intrinsically "brightness" in the sense of being a primordial understanding of be-ness. This holds true in an all-embracing way: it is the prerequisite for the possibility to be concretely touched and affected by something as well as for all emotional experience and all conscious or unconscious instinctual behavior toward something: without it there can be no handling and grasping of mechanical tools, nor can there be conceptual grasping of scientific matters. This also refutes the widely heard objection that the daseinsanalysis is relevant only for the psychology of the conscious mind. The intrinsic ability of the human "dasein" to be open to the world in this way does not just discover things which can be located somewhere in space and time. It also opens up ways for the direct and immediate understanding of beings, who, as human beings, not only are altogether different from the things, but who, according to their manner of being as "dasein," are in the world in the same way as I am. These other human beings are likewise there and together with me. Humanity, as a whole, therefore, is best comparable to the full brightness of the day which also consists of the shining-together of all individual sun rays. Because of this being-together-in-the-world the world is always that which I share with others, the world of "dasein" is world-of-togetherness ("Mitwelt").[1]

Just as the objects cannot reveal themselves without such brightness of man, man cannot exist as that which he is without the presence of all he encounters. For if he did not find his proper place in the encounter with the objects, plants, animals and fellowmen, in his ability to be with them, in his relationship to them, how else could men be in this world as such brightening understanding of be-ness? Even physical light cannot appear as light unless it encounters an object and can make it shine.

THE DASEINSANALYTICALLY ORIENTED PSYCHOTHERAPIST

This then, is the anthropological essence of Martin Heidegger's Existential Analysis (Daseinsanalysis). Meanwhile, the term "existential analysis" has come to include a variety of philosophical, scientific, psychopathologic and psychotherapeutic schools of thought. Although they differ in their methods and goals, they are all derivatives of Heidegger's Daseinsanalysis. At least they re-

---

[1]M. Heidegger: *Sein und Zeit*. Halle, 1927. p. 118.

ceived from it their initial impetus even if, as in the case of J.-P. Sartre's philosophy, they have turned the real substance of the "Daseinsanalysis" into its complete opposite, namely, an extreme, subjectivistic Cartesianism.

The psychotherapist who lets himself be thoroughly pervaded by Heidegger's ontologic insight will not be able to derive new words or phrases from the daseinsanalysis for his psychopathologic descriptions. But he will win by it a tacit, but all the more reliable and all-embracing attitude toward his patient and the therapeutic process. If the therapist really understands that man is intrinsically a world-unfolding and world-opening being in the sense that in him, as the bright sphere of be-ness, comparable to a glade in a forest, all things, plants, animals and fellowmen can show and reveal themselves directly and immediately in all their significance and correlations, then he will have an unceasing reverence for the proper value of each phenomenon he encounters. At the same time he will have become aware that this way of being is the prerequisite that our destiny could claim man as a being who should care for the things and his fellowmen in the manner that all that is and may be can best unfold and develop. To exist in this sense is man's intrinsic task in life. How else could it be that his conscience tells him so relentlessly whenever he falls short of fulfilling it? This call from the conscience and this guilt feeling will not abate until man has taken over and responsibly accepted all those possibilities which constitute him, and has borne and carried them out in taking care of the things and fellowmen of his world. Thus, he has completed his full dasein and hence can consummate his individual, intrinsic temporality in a good death. The daseinsanalytic understanding of man makes the analyst gain so deep a respect for all phenomena he encounters that it bids him to abide even more fully and more firmly by the chief rule of psychoanalysis than Freud himself could, handicapped as he still was by theoretical prejudices. The therapist will now, according to Freud's technical prescriptions, really be able to accept as equally genuine all the new possibilities for communication which grow "on the playground of transference," without mutilating them through his own in-

tellectual and theoretical prejudices and his personal affective censure. The daseinsanalytically oriented psychoanalyst will have a clear conscience if he remains unpartial to all unproved scientific theories and abstractions and therefore refrains from attributing sole and only reality to one kind of behavior—the instinctual reactions, for instance—and does not consider them more "real" than all other potentialities. Thus, the danger of a so-called unresolved transference can often be avoided. This therapeutic difficulty usually develops only because the analyst has attempted to interpret and thereby reduce a new possibility of communication which unfolded for the first time in the therapeutic situation to a mere repetition of a relationship which existed earlier in life, considering this one primary and causal. Therefore, this new possibility can never properly unfold and mature and thus must inevitably remain in its embryonic state, i.e., the "transference fixation." How different, though, if one respects for instance the divine, which also reveals itself during psychoanalysis, in its divineness, just as one is ready to concede to the earthly its earthliness, and does not degrade the divine to a mere product of sublimation of an infantile-libidinal fixation, nor to a mere subjectivistic "psychic reality" produced by some supposed archetypal structure in the psyche of a human subject.

Of equally decisive influence on the attitude of the analyst is a thorough daseinsanalytic understanding of the fact that man is intrinsically and essentially always together with others. Heidegger's fundamental ontology helps us understand this in terms of a primary participation of all men in being the same open sphere of the be-ness. This insight teaches us that there is a being-together which is of such intrinsic and essential nature that no man can in fact perceive another even in the distance, without being already—through the mere art of perceiving—involved in the other's particular world-relatedness in some specific way. Thus, from the very first encounter between the therapist and patient the therapist is already together with his patient in the patient's way of existing, just as the patient already partakes in the therapist's manner of living, no matter whether, either on the part of the therapist or the patient, their being-together manifests itself for some time only in aloof observation, indifference or even intense resistance.

Already the knowledge of just this one essential trait of man provides an enormous impetus and a firm basis even for psychotherapeutic endeavors which formerly were a venture requiring an almost blind courage. For, only in the primordial being-together as it was brought to light by Heidegger's "Daseinsanalysis" we are able now to recognize the very foundation of all psychotherapeutic possibilities. Owing to this basic structure of man's existence, the most seriously ill schizophrenic patient, for instance, partakes in some way or other as human being in the wholesome mode of living of his psychotherapist; hence, such a patient's fundamental possibility of being cured by the adequate being-together of a psychotherapeutic situation through which he may recollect his true self again.[2]

Apart from the confidence which we derive from the daseinsanalytic insights for our practical dealings with such difficult patients, the daseinsanalytic way of thinking affords us also some important "theoretical" gain. For example, it helps us understand such central phenomena as "psychic projection" and "transference."

---

[2]M. Boss: *Psychoanalyse und Daseinsanalytik.* Bern, Hans Huber, 1957.

Until now modern psychology could conceive of them only in terms of a tossing-out and carrying-over of psychic contents from within a "psyche" into something in the external world. Those concepts, however, are entirely unexplainable and can only be maintained on the basis of abstract intellectual constructions. The daseinsanalytic thinking allows us to understand these phenomena simply and with full justice to reality out of the primary, intrinsic being-together of all men in the same world.[3]

---

[3]M. Boss: *The Dream and Its Interpretation.* London, 1957.

References

Binswanger, L.: Freud's Auffassung vom Menschen im Lichte der Anthropologie. Bern, A. Francke, 1947.

Boss, M.: The Dream and Its Interpretation. London, Rider, 1957.

———: Einfuhrung in die psychosomatische Medizin. Bern, Huber, 1957.

———: Psychoanalyse und Daseinsanalytik. Bern, Huber, 1957.

Heidegger, M.: Sein und Zeit, Tübingen, Niemeyer. 1927.

———: Ueber den Humanismus. Frankfurt a.M, Klostermann, 1953.

———: Einfuhrung in die Metaphysik, Tübingen, Niemeyer, 1933.

———: Was heisst Denken? Tübingen, Niemeyer, 1947.

28.   Rational Psychotherapy

ALBERT ELLIS

The central theme of this paper is that psychotherapists can help their clients to live the most self-fulfilling, creative, and emotionally satisfying lives by teaching these clients to organize and discipline their thinking. Does this mean that *all* human emotion and creativity can or should be controlled by reason and intellect? Not exactly.

The human being may be said to possess four basic processes—perception,

---

From *The Journal of General Psychology,* 1958, 59, 35–49. Reprinted by permission.

movement, thinking, and emotion—all of which are integrally inter-related. Thus, thinking, aside from consisting of bioelectric changes in the brain cells, and in addition to comprising remembering, learning, problem-solving, and similar psychological processes, also is, and to some extent has to be, sensory, motor, and emotional behavior (1, 4). Instead, then, of saying, "Jones thinks about this puzzle," we should more accurately say, "Jones perceives-moves-feels-THINKS about this puzzle." Because, however, Jones' activity in relation to the puzzle may be *largely* focussed upon solving it, and only *incidentally* on seeing, manipulating, and emoting about it, we may perhaps justifiably emphasize only his thinking.

Emotion, like thinking and the sensori-motor processes, we may define as an exceptionally complex state of human reaction which is integrally related to all the other perception and response processes. It is not *one* think, but a combination and holistic integration of several seemingly diverse, yet actually closely related, phenomena (1).

Normally, emotion arises from direct stimulation of the cells in the hypothalamus and autonomic nervous system (e.g., by electrical or chemical stimulation) or from indirect excitation via sensori-motor, cognitive, and other conative processes. It may theoretically be controlled, therefore, in four major ways. If one is highly excitable and wishes to calm down, one may (a) take electroshock or drug treatments; (b) use soothing baths or relaxation techniques; (c) seek someone one loves and quiet down for his sake; or (d) reason oneself into a state of calmness by showing oneself how silly it is for one to remain excited.

Although biophysical, sensori-motor, and emotive techniques are all legitimate methods of controlling emotional disturbances, they will not be considered in this paper, and only the rational technique will be emphasized. Rational psychotherapy is based on the assumption that thought and emotion are not two entirely different processes, but that they significantly overlap in many respects and that therefore disordered emotions can often (though not always) be ameliorated by changing one's thinking.

A large part of what we call emotion, in other words, is nothing more or less than a certain kind—a biased, prejudiced, or strongly evaluative kind—of thinking. What we usually label as thinking is a relatively calm and dispassionate appraisal (or organized perception) of a given situation, an objective comparison of many of the elements in this situation, and a coming to some conclusion as a result of this comparing or discriminating process (4). Thus, a thinking person may observe a piece of bread, see that one part of it is mouldy, remember that eating this kind of mould previously made him ill, and therefore cut off the mouldy part and eat the non-mouldy section of the bread.

An emoting individual, on the other hand, will tend to observe the same piece of bread, and remember so violently or prejudicedly his previous experience with the mouldy part, that he will quickly throw away the whole piece of bread and therefore go hungry. Because the thinking person is relatively calm, he uses the maximum information available to him —namely, that mouldy bread is bad but non-mouldy bread is good. Because the emotional person is relatively excited, he may use only part of the available information—namely, that mouldy bread is bad.

It is hypothesized, then, that thinking and emoting are closely interrelated and at times differ mainly in that thinking is a more tranquil, less somatically involved (or, at least, perceived), and less activity-directed mode of discrimination than is emotion. It is also hypothesized that among adult humans raised in a social culture thinking and emoting are so closely interrelated that they usually accompany each other, act in a circular cause-and-effect relationship, and in certain (though hardly all) respects are essentially the *same thing,* so that one's thinking *becomes* one's emotion and emotion *becomes* one's thought. It is finally hypothesized that since man is a uniquely sign-, symbol-, and language-creating animal, both thinking and emoting tend to take the form of self-talk or internalized sentences; and that, for all practical purposes, the sentences that human beings keep telling themselves *are* or *become* their thoughts and emotions.

This is not to say that emotion can under *no* circumstances exist without thought. It probably can; but it then tends to exist momentarily, and not to be sustained. An individual, for instance, steps on your toe, and you spontaneously, immediately become angry. Or you hear a piece of music and you instantly begin to feel warm and excited. Or you learn that a close friend has died and you quickly begin to feel sad. Under these circumstances, you may feel emotional without doing any concomitant thinking. Perhaps, however, you do, with split-second rapidity, start thinking "This person who stepped on my toe is a blackguard!" or "This music is wonderful!" or "Oh, how awful it is that my friend died!"

In any event, assuming that you don't, at the very beginning, have any conscious or unconscious thought accompanying your emotion, it appears to be difficult to *sustain* an emotional outburst without bolstering it by repeated ideas. For unless you keep telling yourself on the order of "This person who stepped on my toe is a blackguard!" or "How could he do a horrible thing like that to me!" the pain of having your toe stepped on will soon die, and your immediate reaction will die with the pain. Of course, you can keep getting your toe stepped on, and the continuing pain may sustain your anger. But assuming that your physical sensation stops, your emotional feeling, in order to last, normally has to be bolstered by some kind of thinking.

We say "normally" because it is theoretically possible for your emotional circuits, once they have been made to reverberate by some physical or psychological stimulus, to keep reverberating under their own power. It is also theoretically possible for drugs or electrical impulses to keep acting directly on your hypothalamus and autonomic nervous system and thereby to keep you emotionally aroused. Usually, however, these types of continued direct stimulation of the emotion-producing centers do not seem to be important and are limited largely to pathological conditions.

It would appear, then, that positive human emotions, such as feelings of love or elation, are often associated with or result from thoughts, or internalized sentences, stated in some form or variation of the phrase "This is good!" and that negative human emotions, such as feelings of anger or depression, are frequently associated with or result from thoughts or sentences which are stated in some form of variation of the phrase "This is bad!" Without an adult human being's employing, on some conscious or unconscious level, such thoughts and sentences, much of his emoting would simply not exist.

If the hypothesis that sustained human emotion often results from or is directly associated with human thinking and self-verbalization is true, then important corollaries about the origin and perpetuation of states of emotional disturbance, or neurosis, may be drawn. For neurosis would appear to be disordered, over- or under-intensified, uncontrollable emotion; and this would seem to be the result of (and, in a sense, the very same thing as)

illogical, unrealistic, irrational, inflexible, and childish thinking.

That neurotic or emotionally disturbed behavior is illogical and irrational would seem to be almost definitional. For if we define it otherwise, and label as neurotic *all* incompetent and ineffectual behavior, we will be including actions of *truly* stupid and incompetent individuals—for example, those who are mentally deficient or brain injured. The concept of neurosis only becomes meaningful, therefore, when we assume that the disturbed individual is *not* deficient or impaired but that he is theoretically capable of behaving in a more mature, more controlled, more flexible manner than he actually behaves. If, however, a neurotic is essentially an individual who acts significantly below his own potential level of behaving, or who defeats his own ends though he is theoretically capable of achieving them, it would appear that he behaves in an illogical, irrational, unrealistic way. Neurosis, in other words, consists of stupid behavior by a non-stupid person.

Assuming that emotionally disturbed individuals act in irrational, illogical ways, the questions which are therapeutically relevant are: (*a*) How do they originally get to be illogical? (*b*) How do they keep perpetuating their irrational thinking? (*c*) How can they be helped to be less illogical, less neurotic?

Unfortunately, most of the good thinking that has been done in regard to therapy during the past 60 years, especially by Sigmund Freud and his chief followers (5, 6, 7), has concerned itself with the first of these questions rather than the second and the third. The assumption has often been made that if psychotherapists discover and effectively communicate to their clients the main reasons why these clients originally became disturbed, they will thereby also discover how their neuroses are being perpetuated and how they can be helped to overcome them. This is a dubious assumption.

Knowing exactly how an individual originally learned to behave illogically by no means necessarily informs us precisely how he *maintains* his illogical behavior, nor what he should do to change it. This is particularly true because people are often, perhaps usually, afflicted with *secondary* as well as *primary* neuroses, and the two may significantly differ. Thus, an individual may originally become disturbed because he discovers that he has strong death wishes against his father and (quite illogically) thinks he should be blamed and punished for having these wishes. Consequently, he may develop some neurotic symptom, such as a phobia against dogs because, let us say, dogs remind him of his father, who is an ardent hunter.

Later on, this individual may grow to love or be indifferent to his father; or his father may die and be no more of a problem to him. His fear of dogs, however, may remain: not because, as some theorists would insist, they still remind him of his old death wishes against his father, but because he now hates himself so violently for *having* the original neurotic symptom—for behaving, to his mind, so stupidly and illogically in relation to dogs—that every time he thinks of dogs his self-hatred and fear of failure so severely upset him that he cannot reason clearly and cannot combat his illogical fear.

In terms of self-verbalization, this neurotic individual is first saying to himself: "I hate my father—and this is awful!" But he ends up by saying: "I have an irrational fear of dogs—and this is awful!" Even though both sets of self-verbalizations are neuroticizing, and his secondary neurosis may be as bad as or worse than his primary one, the two can hardly be said to be the same. Consequently, exploring and explaining to this individual—or helping him gain insight into—the origins of his primary neurosis will not necessarily help him to understand and overcome his perpetuating or secondary neurotic reactions.

If the hypotheses so far stated have some validity, the psychotherapist's main goals should be those of demonstrating to clients that their self-verbalizations have been and still are the prime source of their emotional disturbances. Clients must be shown that their internalized sentences are illogical and unrealistic at certain critical points and that they now have the ability to control their emotions by telling themselves more rational and less self-defeating sentences.

More precisely: the effective therapist should continually keep unmasking his client's past and, especially, his present illogical thinking or self-defeating verbalizations by (a) bringing them to his attention or consciousness; (b) showing the client how they are causing and maintaining his disturbance and unhappiness; (c) demonstrating exactly what the illogical links in his internalized sentences are; and (d) teaching him how to re-think and re-verbalize these (and other similar) sentences in a more logical, self-helping way. Moreover, before the end of the therapeutic relationship, the therapist should not only deal concretely with the client's specific illogical thinking, but should demonstrate to this client what, *in general,* are the main irrational ideas that human beings are prone to follow and what more rational philosophies of living may usually be substituted for them. Otherwise, the client who is released from one specific set of illogical notions may well wind up by falling victim to another set.

It is hypothesized, in other words, that human beings are the kind of animals who, when raised in any society similar to our own, tend to fall victim to several major fallacious ideas; to keep reindoctrinating themselves over and over again with these ideas in an unthinking, autosuggestive manner; and consequently to keep actualizing them in overt behavior. Most of these irrational ideas are, as the Freudians have very adequately pointed out, instilled by the individual's parents during his childhood, and are tenaciously clung to because of his attachment to these parents and because the ideas were ingrained, or imprinted, or conditioned before later and more rational modes of thinking were given a chance to gain a foothold. Most of them, however, as the Freudians have not always been careful to note, are also instilled by the individual's general culture, and particularly by the media of mass communication in this culture.

What are some of the major illogical ideas or philosophies which, when originally held and later perpetuated by men and women in our civilization, inevitably lead to self-defeat and neurosis? Limitations of space preclude our examining all these major ideas, including their more significant corollaries; therefore, only a few of them will be listed. The illogicality of some of these ideas will also, for the present, have to be taken somewhere on faith, since there again is no space to outline the many reasons *why* they are irrational. Anyway, here, where angels fear to tread, goes the psychological theoretician!

1. The idea that it is a dire necessity for an adult to be loved or approved by everyone for everything he does—instead of his concentrating on his own self-respect, on winning approval for necessary purposes (such as job advancement), and on loving rather than being loved.

2. The idea that certain acts are wrong, or wicked, or villainous, and that people who perform such acts should be severely punished—instead of the idea that certain acts are inappropriate or antisocial, and that people who perform such acts are invariably stupid, ignorant, or emotionally disturbed.

3. The idea that it is terrible, horrible, and catastrophic when things are not the way one would like them to be—instead of the idea that it is too bad when things are not the way one would like them to be, and one should certainly try to change or control conditions so that they become more satisfactory, but that if changing or controlling uncomfortable situations is impossible, one had better become resigned to their existence and stop telling oneself how awful they are.

4. The idea that much human unhappiness is externally caused and is forced on one by outside people and events—instead of the idea that virtually all human unhappiness is caused or sustained by the view one takes of things rather than the things themselves.

5. The idea that if something is or may be dangerous or fearsome one should be terribly concerned about it—instead of the idea that if something is or may be dangerous or fearsome one should frankly face it and try to render it non-dangerous and, when that is impossible, think of other things and stop telling oneself what a terrible situation one is or may be in.

6. The idea that it is easier to avoid than to face life difficulties and self-responsibilities—instead of the idea that the so-called easy way is invariably the much harder way in the long run and that the only way to solve difficult problems is to face them squarely.

7. The idea that one needs something other or stronger or greater than oneself on which to rely—instead of the idea that it is usually far better to stand on one's own feet and gain faith in oneself and

one's ability to meet difficult circumstances of living.

8. The idea that one should be thoroughly competent, adequate, intelligent, and achieving in all possible respects—instead of the idea that one should *do* rather than always try to do *well* and that one should accept oneself as a quite imperfect creature, who has general human limitations and specific fallibilities.

9. The idea that because something once strongly affected one's life, it should indefinitely affect it—instead of the idea that one should learn from one's past experiences but not be overly-attached to or prejudiced by them.

10. The idea that it is vitally important to our existence what other people do, and that we should make great efforts to change them in the direction we would like them to be—instead of the idea that other people's deficiencies are largely *their* problems and that putting pressure on them to change is usually least likely to help them do so.

11. The idea that human happiness can be achieved by inertia and inaction—instead of the idea that humans tend to be happiest when they are actively and vitally absorbed in creative pursuits, or when they are devoting themselves to people or projects outside themselves.

12. The idea that one has virtually no control over one's emotions and that one cannot help feeling certain things—instead of the idea that one has enormous control over one's emotions if one chooses to work at controlling them and to practice saying the right kinds of sentences to oneself.

It is the central theme of this paper that it is the foregoing kinds of illogical ideas, and many corollaries which we have no space to delineate, which are the basic causes of most emotional disturbances or neuroses. For once one believes the kind of nonsense included in these notions, one will inevitably tend to become inhibited, hostile, defensive, guilty, anxious, ineffective, inert, uncontrolled, or unhappy. If, on the other hand, one could become thoroughly released from all these fundamental kinds of illogical thinking, it would be exceptionally difficult for one to become too emotionally upset, or at least to sustain one's disturbance for very long.

Does this mean that all the other so-called basic causes of neurosis, such as the Oedipus complex or severe maternal rejection in childhood, are invalid, and that the Freudian and other psychodynamic thinkers of the last 60 years have been barking up the wrong tree? Not at all. It only means, if the main hypotheses of this paper are correct, that these psychodynamic thinkers have been emphasizing secondary causes or results of emotional disturbances rather than truly prime causes.

Let us take, for example, an individual who acquires, when he is young, a full-blown Oedipus complex: that is to say, he lusts after his mother, hates his father, is guilty about his sex desires for his mother, and is afraid that his father is going to castrate him. This person, when he is a child, will presumably be disturbed. But, if he is raised so that he acquires none of the basic illogical ideas we have been discussing, it will be virtually impossible for him to *remain* disturbed.

For, as an adult, this individual will not be too concerned if his parents or others do not approve of his actions, since he will be more interested in his *own* self-respect than in *their* approval. He will not believe that his lust for his mother is wicked or villainous, but will accept it as a normal part of being a limited human whose sex desires may easily be indiscriminate. He will realize that the actual danger of his father castrating him is exceptionally slight. He will not feel that because he was once afraid of his Oedipal feelings he should forever remain so. If he still feels it would be improper for him to have sex relations with his mother, instead of castigating himself for even thinking of having such relations he will merely resolve not to carry his desires into practice and will stick determinedly to his resolve. If, by any chance, he weakens and actually has incestuous relations, he will again refuse to castigate himself mercilessly for being weak but will keep showing himself how self-defeating his behavior is and will actively work and practice at changing it.

Under these circumstances, if this individual has a truly logical and rational approach to life in general, and to the problem of Oedipal feelings, in particular, how can he possibly *remain* disturbed about his Oedipal attachment?

Take, by way of further illustration, the case of an individual who, as a child,

is continually criticized by his parents, who consequently feels himself loathesome and inadequate, who refuses to take chances at failing at difficult tasks, and who therefore comes to hate himself more. Such a person will be, of course, seriously neurotic. But how would it be possible for him to *sustain* his neurosis if he began to think in a truly logical manner about himself and his behavior?

For, if this individual does use a consistent rational approach to his own behavior, he will stop caring particularly what others think of him and will start primarily caring what he thinks of himself. Consequently, he will stop avoiding difficult tasks and, instead of punishing himself for being incompetent when he makes a mistake, will say to himself something like: "Now this is not the right way to do things; let me stop and figure out a better way." Or: "There's no doubt that I made a mistake this time; now let me see how I can benefit from making it."

This individual, furthermore, will if he is thinking straight, not blame his defeats on external events, but will realize that he himself is causing them by his illogical or impractical behavior. He will not believe that it is easier to avoid facing difficult things, but will realize that the so-called easy way is always, actually, the harder and more idiotic one. He will not think that he needs something greater or stronger than himself to help him, but will independently buckle down to difficult tasks himself. He will not feel that because he once defeated himself by avoiding doing things the hard way that he must always do so.

How, with this kind of logical thinking, could an originally disturbed person possibly maintain and continually revivify his neurosis? He just couldn't. Similarly, the spoiled brat, the worrywart, the egomaniac, the autistic stay-at-home—all of these disturbed individuals would have the devil of a time indefinitely prolonging their neuroses if they did not continue to believe utter nonsense: namely, the kinds of basic irrational postulates previously listed.

Neurosis, then, usually seems to originate in and be perpetuated by some fundamentally unsound, irrational ideas. The individual comes to believe in some unrealistic, impossible, often perfectionistic goals—especially the goals that he should always be approved by everyone, should do everything perfectly well, and should never be frustrated in any of his desires—and then, in spite of considerable contradictory evidence, refuses to give up his original illogical beliefs.

Some of the neurotic's philosophies, such as the idea that he should be loved and approved by everyone, are not entirely inappropriate to his childhood state; but all of them are quite inappropriate to average adulthood. Most of his irrational ideas are specifically taught him by his parents and his culture; and most of them also seem to be held by the great majority of adults in our society—who theoretically should have been but actually never were weaned from them as they chronologically matured. It must consequently be admitted that the neurotic individual we are considering is often statistically normal; or that ours is a generally neuroticizing culture, in which most people are more or less emotionally disturbed because they are raised to believe, and then to internalize and to keep reinfecting themselves with, arrant nonsense which must inevitably lead them to become ineffective, self-defeating, and unhappy. Nonetheless: it is not absolutely *necessary* that human beings believe the irrational notions which, in point of fact, most of them seem to believe today; and the task of psychotherapy is to get them to disbelieve their illogical ideas, to change their self-sabotaging attitudes.

This, precisely, is the task which the rational psychotherapist sets himself. Like other therapists, he frequently resorts to the usual techniques of therapy which the present author has outlined elsewhere (2, 3), including the techniques of relationship, expressive-emotive, supportive, and insight-interpretive therapy. But he views these techniques, as they are commonly employed, as kinds of preliminary strategies whose main functions are to gain rapport with the client, to let him express himself fully, to show him that he is a worthwhile human being who has the ability to change, and to demonstrate how he originally became disturbed.

The rational therapist, in other words, believes that most of the usual therapeutic techniques wittingly or unwittingly show the client *that* he is illogical and how he *originally* became so. They often fail to show him, however, how he is presently *maintaining* his illogical think-ing, and precisely what he must do to change it by building general rational philosophies of living and by applying these to practical problems of everyday life. Where most therapists directly or indirectly show the client that he is behaving illogically, the rational therapist goes beyond this point to make a forthright, unequivocal *attack* on the client's general and specific irrational ideas and to try to *induce* him to adopt more rational ones in their place.

Rational psychotherapy makes a concerted attack on the disturbed individual's irrational positions in two main ways: (*a*) the therapist serves as a frank counter-propagandist who directly contradicts and denies the self-defeating propaganda and superstitions which the client has originally learned and which he is now self-propagandistically perpetuating. (*b*) The therapist encourages, persuades, cajoles, and at times commands the client to partake of some kind of activity which itself will act as a forceful counter-propagandist agency against the nonsense he believes. Both these main therapeutic activities are consciously performed with one main goal in mind: namely, that of finally getting the client to internalize a rational philosophy of living just as he originally learned and internalized the illogical propaganda and superstitions of his parents and his culture.

The rational therapist, then, assumes that the client somehow imbibed illogical ideas or irrational modes of thinking and that, without so doing, he could hardly be as disturbed as he is. It is the therapist's function not merely to show the client that he has these ideas or thinking processes but to persuade him to change and substitute for them more rational ideas and thought processes. If, because the client is exceptionally disturbed when he first comes to therapy, he must first be approached in a rather cautious, supportive, permissive, and warm manner, and must sometimes be allowed to ventilate his feeling in free association, abreaction, role playing, and other expressive techniques, that may be all to the good. But the therapist does not delude himself that these relationship-building and expressive-emotive techniques in most instances really get to the core of the client's illogical thinking and induce him to think in a more rational manner. Occasionally, this is true: since the client may come to see, through relationship and emotive-expressive methods, that he *is* acting illogically, and he may therefore resolve to change and actually do so. More often than not, however, his illogical thinking will be so ingrained from constant self-repetitions, and will be so inculcated in motor pathways (or habit patterns) by the time he comes for therapy, that simply showing him, even by direct interpretation, *that* he is illogical will not greatly help. He will often say to the therapist: "All right, now I understand that I have castration fears and that they are illogical. But I *still* feel afraid of my father."

The therapist, therefore, must keep pounding away, time and again, at the illogical ideas which underlie the client's fears. He must show the client that he is afraid, really, not of his father, but of being blamed, of being disapproved, of being unloved, of being imperfect, of being a failure. And such fears are thoroughly irrational because (*a*) being disapproved is not half so terrible as one *thinks* it is; because (*b*) no one can be thoroughly blameless or perfect; because (*c*) people who worry about being blamed or disapproved essentially are putting themselves at the mercy of the opinion of *others,* over whom they have no real control; because (*d*) being blamed or disapproved has nothing essentially to do with one's *own* opinion of oneself; etc.

If the therapist, moreover, merely tackles the individual's castration fears, and shows how ridiculous *they* are, what is to prevent this individual's showing up, a year or two later, with some *other* illogical fear—such as the fear that he is sexually impotent? But if the therapist tackles the client's *basic* irrational thinking, which underlies *all* kinds of fear he may have, it is going to be most difficult for this client to turn up with a new neurotic symptom some months or years hence. For once an individual truly surrenders ideas of perfectionism, of the horror of failing at something, of the dire need to be approved by others, of the opinion that the world owes him a living, and so on, what else is there for him to be fearful of or disturbed about?

To give some idea of precisely how the rational therapist works, a case summary will now be presented. A client came in one day and said he was depressed but did not know why. A little questioning showed that he had been putting off the inventory-keeping he was required to do as part of his job as an apprentice glass-staining artist. The therapist immediately began showing him that his depression was related to his resenting having to keep inventory and that this resentment was illogical for several reasons:

(*a*) The client very much wanted to learn the art of glass-staining and could only learn it by having the kind of job he had. His sole logical choice, therefore, was between graciously accepting this job, in spite of the inventory-keeping, or giving up trying to be a glass-stainer. By resenting the clerical work and avoiding it, he was choosing neither of these two logical alternatives, and was only getting himself into difficulty.

(*b*) By blaming the inventory-keeping, and his boss for making him perform it, the client was being irrational since, assuming that the boss was wrong about making him do this clerical work, the boss would have to be wrong out of some combination of stupidity, ignorance, or emotional disturbance; and it is silly and pointless blaming people for being stupid, ignorant, or disturbed. Besides, maybe the boss was quite right, from his own standpoint, about making the client keep the inventory.

(*c*) Whether the boss was right or wrong, resenting him for his stand was hardly going to make him change it; and the resentment felt by the client was hardly going to do him, the client, any good or make him feel better. The saner attitude for him to take, then, was that it was too bad that inventory-keeping was part of his job, but that's the way it was, and there was no point in resenting the way things were when they could not, for the moment, be changed.

(*d*) Assuming that the inventory-keeping was irksome, there was no sense in making it still *more* annoying by the client's continually telling himself how awful it was. Nor was there any point in shirking this clerical work, since he eventually would have to do it anyway and he might as well get this unpleasant task out of the way quickly. Even more important: by shirking a task that he knew that, eventually, he just had to do, he would lose respect for himself and his loss of self-respect would be far worse than the slight, rather childish satisfaction he might receive from trying to sabotage his boss's desires.

While showing this client how illogical was his thinking and consequent behavior, the therapist specifically made him aware that he must be telling himself sentences like these: "My boss makes me do inventory-keeping. I do not like this. . . . There is no reason why I have to do it. . . . He is therefore a blackguard for making me do it. . . . So I'll fool him and avoid doing it. . . . And then I'll be happier." But these sentences were so palpably foolish that the client could not really believe them, and began to finish them off with sentences like: "I'm not really fooling my boss, because he sees what I'm doing. . . . So I'm not solving my problem this way. . . . So I really should stop this nonsense and get the inventory-keeping done. . . . But I'll be damned if I'll do it for him!" . . . . However, if I don't do it, I'll be fired. . . . But I still don't want to do it for him! . . . . I guess I've got to, though. . . . Oh, why must I always be persecuted like this? . . . And must I keep getting myself into such a mess? . . . I guess I'm just no good. . . . And people are against me. . . . Oh, what's the use?"

Whereupon, employing these illogical kinds of sentences, the client was becoming depressed, avoiding doing the inventory-keeping, and then becoming more resentful and depressed. Instead, the therapist pointed out, he could tell himself quite different sentences, on this order: "Keeping inventory is a bore. . . . But it is presently an essential part of my job. . . . And I also may learn something useful by it. . . . Therefore, I had better go about this task as best I may and thereby get what *I* want out of this job."

The therapist also emphasized that whenever the client found himself intensely angry, guilty, or depressed, there was little doubt that he was then thinking illogically, and that he should immediately question himself as to what was the irrational element in his thinking, and set about replacing it with a more logical element or chain of sentences.

The therapist then used the client's current dilemma—that of avoiding inventory-keeping—as an illustration of his general neurosis, which in his case largely took the form of severe alcoholic tendencies. He was shown that his alcoholic trends, too, were a resultant of his trying to do things the easy way, and of poor thinking preluding his avoidance of self-responsibilities. He was impressed with the fact that, as long as he kept thinking illogically about relatively small things, such as the inventory-keeping, he would also tend to think equally illogically about more important aspects, such as the alcoholism.

Several previous incidents of illogical thinking leading to emotional upheaval in the client's life were then reviewed, and some general principles of irrational thought discussed. Thus, the general principle of blamelessness was raised and the client was shown precisely why it is illogical to blame anyone for anything. The general principle of inevitability was brought up and he was shown that when a frustrating or unpleasant event is inevitable, it is only logical to accept it uncomplainingly instead of dwelling on its unpleasant aspects. The general principle of self-respect was discussed, with the therapist demonstrating that liking oneself is far more important than resentfully trying to harm others.

In this matter, by attempting to show or teach the client some of the general rules of logical living, the therapist tried to go beyond his immediate problem and mode of thinking or problem solving that would enable him to deal effectively with almost any future similar situation that might arise.

The rational therapist, then, is a frank propagandist who believes wholeheartedly in a most rigorous application of the rules of logic, of straight thinking, and of scientific method to everyday life, and who ruthlessly uncovers every vestige of irrational thinking in the client's experience and energetically urges him into more rational channels. In so doing, the rational therapist does not ignore or eradicate the client's emotions; on the contrary, he considers them most seriously, and helps change them, when they are disordered and self-defeating, through the same means by which they commonly arise in the first place—that is, by thinking and acting. Through exerting consistent interpretive and philosophic pressure on the client to change his thinking or his self-verbalizations and to change his experiences or his actions, the rational therapist gives a specific impetus to the client's movement toward mental health without which it is not impossible, but quite unlikely, that he will move very far.

Can therapy be effectively done, then, with *all* clients mainly through logical analysis and reconstruction? Alas, no. For one thing, many clients are not bright enough to follow a rigorously rational analysis. For another thing, some individuals are so emotionally aberrated by the time they come for help that they are, at least temporarily, in no position to comprehend and follow logical procedures. Still other clients are too old and inflexible; too young and impressionable; too philosophically prejudiced against logic and reason; too organically or biophysically deficient; or too something else to accept, at least at the start of therapy, rational analysis.

In consequence, the therapist who *only* employs logical reconstruction in his therapeutic armamentarium is not likely to get too far with many of those who seek his help. It is vitally important, therefore, that any therapist who has a basically rational approach to the problem of helping his clients overcome their neuroses also be quite eclectic in his use of supplementary, less direct, and somewhat less rational techniques.

Admitting, then, that rational psychotherapy is not effective with all types of clients, and that it is most helpful when used in conjunction with, or sub-sequent to, other widely employed therapeutic techniques, I would like to conclude with two challenging hypotheses: *(a)* that psychotherapy which includes a high dosage of rational analysis and reconstruction, as briefly outlined in this paper, will prove to be more effective with more types of clients than any of the non-rational or semi-rational therapies now being widely employed; and *(b)* that a considerable amount of—or, at least, proportion of—rational psychotherapy will prove to be virtually the only type of treatment that helps to undermine the basic neuroses (as distinguished from the superficial neurotic symptoms) of many clients, and particularly of many with whom other types of therapy have always been shown to be ineffective.

References

1. Cobb, S. *Emotions and clinical medicine.* New York: Norton, 1950.
2. Ellis, A. New approaches to psychotherapy techniques. *Journal of Clinical Psychology, Monograph Supplement,* No. 11. Brandon, Vermont: *Journal of Clinical Psychology,* 1955.
3. Ellis, A. Psychotherapy techniques for use with psychotics. *American Journal of Psychotherapy,* 1955, *9,* 452–476.
4. Ellis, A. An operational reformation of some of the basic principles of psychoanalysis. *Psychoanalytic Review,* 1956, *43,* 163–180.
5. Fenichel, O. *The psychoanalytic theory of neurosis.* New York: Norton, 1945.
6. Freud, S. *Basic Writings.* New York: Modern Library, 1938.
7. Freud, S. *Collected Papers.* London: Hogarth Press, 1924–1950.

Phenomenological Theories

CRITICAL EVALUATION

The *phenomenologist's portrayal of the dilemmas of man is striking, but we must distinguish between skillful literary depiction and effective theorizing. No matter how compelling and vivid a theory may be, the crucial test does not lie in elegant persuasion, but in explicit hypothesis. Although phenomenologists are among the most acute observers of the human condition, their formulation of these observations into a theory is sporadic and casual. Perhaps these formulations should not be thought of as theory, but as a set of loosely connected observations and notions. So discursive a body of work, little concerned with problems of integration, structure, and continuity, lacking in tautness of systematic argument, cannot be viewed as a scientific theory at all. At best, it represents a consistent point of view; at worst, it is an ill-constructed social commentary.*

Other critics object not to the loose structure of phenomenological theory but to what these theories propose. Particular exception is taken to their idealistic conception of man's inherent nature. The notion that man would be a constructive, rational, and socially conscious being, were he free of the malevolent distortions of society, seems not only sentimental but invalid. There is something grossly naïve in exhorting man to live life to the fullest and then expecting socially beneficial consequences to follow. What evidence is there that one's inherent self-interest would not clash with the self-interests of others? There is something as banal as the proverbialism of a fortune cookie in the suggestion "be thyself." Conceiving man's emotional disorders as a failure to "be thyself" seems equally naïve and banal.

The critiques of M. Brewster Smith and Robert Holt presented here are not entirely unfriendly to the phenomenological position. Rather they argue against a number of naïve and romantic assumptions common among phenomenologists which would preclude the development of an adequate science of personality and psychopathology.

29. The Phenomenological Approach in Personality Theory: Some Critical Remarks

M. BREWSTER SMITH

The "phenomenological approach" has recently come to be something of a rallying cry to a number of psychologists who share the "tender-minded" bias that

From *J. Abnormal & Social Psychol. 45:* 516–522, 1950, by permission of the American Psychological Association and the author.

psychology must, after all, come to terms with human experience, and who go so far as to believe that careful attention to this experience will leave the science of psychology not merely more satisfying to like-minded people, but also better science. Sharing this point of view and agreeing heartily with the program recommended by MacLeod (1947) in his article on "The Phenomenological Approach in Social Psychology," the present writer has been dismayed by some recent publications which, it seems to him, misconstrue the appropriate role of a phenomenological approach in a way that invites the critical to reject a humanized psychology lock, stock, and barrel. Since the writer would regard such an outcome as highly unfortunate, he feels that a clarification of the issues is badly needed, and herewith makes an attempt in this direction.

The position with which he would take particular issue is that of Snygg and Combs (1949; Combs, 1949) whose point of view has also been espoused by Rogers (1947). These authors contrast the objective or external frame of reference in psychology with the phenomenological, or internal frame of reference, and, declaring their stand firmly with phenomenology, proceed to muster on their side the names of Lewin, Lecky, Allport, Murphy, and Angyal, among others, even including the seemingly less tractable father-figure of Freud. In essence, their contention is that the locus of psychological causation lies entirely within the phenomenal field of conscious experience, and that it therefore behooves the psychological theorist—and therapist—to formulate his problems and concepts accordingly. Snygg and Combs give much attention to the individual's perceptual-cognitive field, particularly to the *self*, as its most salient feature. Written from this standpoint, psychology comes close to a rapprochement with common sense.

While applauding their emphasis on perception and the self, the present writer proposes that they are confusing phenomenology with what may be termed the subjective frame of reference. Sharply maintained, this distinction further helps to clarify certain persistent ambiguities in the theory of ego and self.

PHENOMENOLOGY AND COMMON SENSE

One of the genuine merits of the phenomenological approach is that it brings psychology somewhat closer to the world of common sense. There is always the danger that psychology, in its concern for rigor and neatness, may divorce itself too completely from this source of problems and partial insights. Focussing scientific attention on the phenomenal world as it is presented to us, the world from which common sense also takes its start, the phenomenological approach can bring into the ken of the psychologist data and problems too often left to common sense by default. Like common sense, and unlike some current varieties of psychological theory, it does deal with experience, and thus presents itself as an attractive alternative to those who find a behavioristic psychology uncongenial.

But phenomenology is not common sense, nor can it rightly be called upon to justify a common-sense psychology. In MacLeod's phrase, the phenomenological approach "involves the adoption of what might be called an attitude of disciplined naïveté" (1947, p. 194). In many respects, its result may run exactly counter to common-sense conclusions. Common sense, with its preconceived categories and stock explanations, neither disciplined nor naïve, is full of pseudo-scientific theory, while phenomenology limits its concern to the unprejudiced *description* of the world of phenomena. To take the phenomenal world presented in conscious experience as completely explanatory of behavior is closer to common sense than to phenomenology or adequate science.

Yet this is essentially what Snygg and Combs have done in their attempt to rewrite psychology in a "phenomenological frame of reference." *"All behavior, without exception,"* they say, *"is completely determined by and pertinent to the phenomenal field of the behaving organism"* (1949, p. 15, italics theirs). And they go on to explain that

by the phenomenal field we mean the entire universe, including himself, as it is experienced by the individual at the instant of action. . . . Unlike the "objective" physical field, the phenomenal field is not an abstraction or an artificial construction. It is simply the universe of naive experience in which each individual lives, the everyday situation of self and surroundings which each person takes to be reality (1949, p. 15).

While they bow unnecessarily to current prejudice in avoiding the word *consciousness*, their meaning is clear, and their index spells it out: "Consciousness, *see* Phenomenal field."

It is one variant of common sense

that consciousness completely explains behavior, but at this juncture, it is hard to see how such a view can be regarded as an acceptable scientific postulate. Quite apart from the metaphysical controversy about the status of consciousness as "real" or respectable, we have behind us Würzburg and we have behind us Freud, to mention but two major sources of evidence that a psychology of experience or consciousness has distinct explanatory limits. Where is the determining tendency represented in the phenomenal field? What of the inacceptable strivings that warp our behavior, what of our defensive techniques of adjustment that so often prove most effective precisely when we are least aware of them? It is no satisfactory solution to speak, as Snygg and Combs do, of a "unified field of figure-ground phenomena of which the individual is more or less conscious . . . [in which] the vague and fuzzy aspects of behavior correspond to and are parts of the vague and incompletely differentiated aspects of the field" (1949, p. 17). The clinical literature abounds with instances of unconsciously determined behavior which, far from being "vague and fuzzy," is on the contrary highly differentiated.

One suspects that such a psychology of consciousness has an element of common-sense appeal not unlike the attraction of allied forms of psychotherapy. It does make sense to the layman: it accords with what he is ready and able to recognize in himself. And it has distinct value within limits that it refuses to recognize. Because it over-states its claims, however, it may tend to promote the state of affairs away from which we have been striving—every man his own psychologist.

But McLeod has already made the relevant point succinctly: "The phenomenological method, in social psychology as in the psychology of perception [and we would add, psychology generally] can never be more than an approach to a scientific inquiry" (1947, p. 207). It provides certain kinds of data, not *all* the data. It furnishes the basis for certain valuable theoretical constructs; it does not give birth to them in full concreteness. It sets some problems and provides some clues; the psychologist, theorist or clinician, must *infer* the answers.

SUBJECTIVE CONSTRUCTS AND THE OBSERVER'S FRAME OF REFERENCE

Here we reach the crux of the matter. If a psychology of consciousness is necessarily incomplete yet we do not abandon our hope for a psychology that comes to terms with human experience, what is the solution? A discussion of two lesser questions may indicate the nature of the answer. In the first place, does the decision to frame our psychological concepts and theories in terms appropriate to the "private world" of the behaving person commit us to the exclusive use of phenomenal concepts? Secondly, what is the appropriate role of the phenomenological approach in the service of this kind of theory-building?

Lewin, whose psychological life space Snygg and Combs equate to their phenomenal field (1949, p. 15), was entirely clear in maintaining a sharp distinction between the two concepts. He said:

It is likewise doubtful whether one can use consciousness as the sole criterion of what belongs to the psychological life space at a given moment in regard to social facts and relationships. The mother, the father, and brothers and sisters are not to be included as real facts in the psychological situation of the child only when they are immediately present. For example, the little child playing in the garden behaves differently when he knows his mother is at home than when he knows she is out. One cannot assume that this fact is continually in the child's consciousness. Also a prohibition or a goal can play an essential role in the psychological situation without being clearly present in consciousness. . . . Here, as in many other cases it is clear that one must distinguish between "appearance" and the "underlying reality" in a dynamic sense. In other words, the phenomenal properties are to be distinguished from the conditional-genetic characteristics of objects and events, that is, from the properties which determine their casual relationships. . . . As far as the conceptual derivation is concerned, one may use effectiveness as the criterion for existence: *"What is real is what has effects"* (1936, p. 19).

Lewin's life space, then, is *not* merely the phenomenal field. And he adds to our previous considerations cogent reasons for thinking that a psychology of the phenomenal field cannot be adequately explanatory. His life space is not immediately given in the concreteness of experience; it is an abstract, hypothetical construct, inferred by the psychologist-observer to account for the individual's behavior.

It is, however, a construct of a type that differs from constructs of behavioristic psychology. It is formulated in terms of what is behaviorally real to the acting individual, not primarily in terms of what is physically observable to the scientist. Hence it is legitimate to speak of theories like Lewin's as anchored in a *subjective* (not phenomenological) *frame of reference*. Lewin's concepts and many of Freud's are in this sense *subjective constructs,* not because they are built of the stuff of conscious experience, but because they attempt to deal with what is effectively real to the individual, even when it is real to the scientific observer only in this secondary, indirect way.

The subjective frame of reference in theory construction is to be contrasted with the *objective frame of reference*, wherein concepts are chosen so as to be rooted as closely as possible in effective realities shared by any qualified observer. This is the distinction that Snygg and Combs seek, which makes them see both Freud and Lewin as precursors. There is no absolute difference between the two frames of reference; it is rather a question of which criteria are weighted most strongly in the selection of constructs.

Both the subjective and objective frames of reference pertain to the choice of constructs and the theoretical context in which they are embedded. They in no sense conflict with what has been called the *observer's frame of reference*, which, indeed, lies at the foundation of all science. The problem of establishing a bridge between the point of view of the observer and *either* subjective or objective inferential constructs is the familiar one of operational definition. It cannot, in the last analysis, be avoided unless one chooses the alternative of claiming *direct* access to the point of view of the observed. This is the position of intuitionism, which asserts that the observer's and subject's points of view can be merged. But is this science? Not in the sense of a systematic search for understanding that can withstand the equally systematic doubt of the man from Missouri.

Subjective constructs framed in terms of the "private world" of the behaving in-

dividual remain constructs, and as such must ultimately be rooted in data accessible to the observer's frame of reference. There is no reason at all why their source should be restricted to the data of communicated conscious experience, in answer to our first question. But the phenomenological approach, or, more generally, any means of access to the experience of the subject, is of course crucial to the formulation of subjective constructs and the investigation of their relationships. Perhaps the point has been labored, but it is an essential one: the phenomenological approach, the clinical interview, the projective protocol, the behavioral observation—none of these yield direct knowledge of psychological constructs, subjective or objective, while all of them can provide the basis for inferring explanatory constructs and their relationships. If the canons of inference can be made sufficiently explicit, they provide the operational definitions that secure the constructs in the scientific home base of the observer's frame of reference.

Methods that get the subject to reveal his private world as he sees it need to be supplemented by others which permit the observer to infer effective factors that are distorted or disguised in the subject's awareness. But the broadly phenomenological methods remain a signally important source of data. Certain important subjective constructs such as the *self,* moreover, are anchored fairly directly in the data of phenomenological report.

EGO, SELF, AND PHENOMENOLOGY

Although there is still considerable confusion in usage, a degree of consensus seems to be emerging to employ the term *self* for the phenomenal content of the experience of personal identity. A salient feature of the phenomenal field that has figured largely in personality theory, the self in this sense has the conceptual properties of a phenomenal object. Murphy (1947) and Chein (1944) use it with this meaning. Snygg and Combs agree, writing with somewhat franker circularity:

Of particular importance in the motivation of behavior will be those parts of the phenomenal field perceived by him to be part or characteristic of himself. To refer to this important aspect of the total field we have used the term *phenomenal self* (1949, p. 111).

Within the phenomenal self, they distinguish as a stable core the *self-concept:* "Those parts of the phenomenal field which the individual has differentiated as definite and fairly stable characteristics of himself" (1949, p. 112).

Sharing with Murphy a strong emphasis on responses to the self as fundamental to motivational theory, Snygg and Combs go so far as to state that the basic human need is "the preservation and enhancement of the phenomenal self" (1949, p. 58). Changes in the perception of the self play a major role in the theory of the therapeutic process that they share with Rogers (1947).

Let us look more closely, however, at how these writers actually use the term. Passages like the following can readily be found:

. . . when the self is free from any threat of attack or likelihood of attack, then it is possible for the self to consider these hitherto rejected perceptions, to make new differentiations, and to reintegrate the self in such a way as to include them (Rogers, 1947, p. 365).

A self threatened by its perceptions may deny the perception by simply refusing to enter the situation where such a perception is forced upon him (Snygg and Combs, 1949, p. 148).

Can a phenomenal self consider perceptions and reintegrate itself; can a threatened phenomenal self deny perceptions; or is this rather double-talk resulting from the attempt to make one good concept do the work of two? If, as this writer suspects, the latter is the case, what is the nature of the hidden second concept, which evidently is not merely a percept or phenomenal entity? To give it a name he would suggest the conventional term *ego*, realizing that usage in this respect is even more ambiguous than with the term *self*. The important point is that the concept, implicit in the writings of Rogers and of Snygg and Combs, is a subjective construct but does not refer to a phenomenal entity, whereas the self, on the other hand, is a coordinate subjective construct that does. The relation between the two will bear closer examination.

It is not necessary, at this juncture, to propose a definitive theory of the ego, nor to enter into an involved discussion of alternative views about its nature. What is relevant is that starting from an attempt to write a psychology in phenomenal terms, our authors in spite of themselves give implicit recognition to organizing, selective processes in the personality which are somehow guided by the nature and status of the self (among other things) and somehow, in turn, have an influence in its nature and status. So conceived, the relation of ego and self is highly interdependent[1] but by no means an identity. The distinction is that between a dynamic configuration of on-going processes, inferred from many facts of biography and behavior, and a phenomenal entity resulting from these processes and affecting them in turn, inferred primarily (but not exclusively) from phenomenological report.

Approaching the problem on a slightly different tack, we may find it rewarding to consider three of the eight conceptions of the ego listed by Allport (1943, p. 459) in the light of the distinction just made: the ego "as one segregated behavioral system among others," "as knower," and "as object of knowledge." The fundamental conception advanced here is not unlike the first of these senses, if one reads into it a dynamic quality not expressed in Allport's formulation. As an on-going system of organizing and selective processes mediating the individual's intercourse with reality, it includes a variety of processes without being coterminous with the total personality.[2] Among these processes or functions is that of the ego as "knower," which the writer would take in a less metaphysical sense than Allport's to embrace the cognitive-perceptual functions of personality. These have been described with reason in psychoanalytic theory (Freud, 1933, pp. 105-106) as an integral aspect of the ego system. Among the phenomena that the ego "knows" is the *self*, Allport's "ego as object of knowledge." Like any cognitive-perceptual object, the self only imperfectly mirrors the physical, psychological, and social facts that underlie the perception. And also like similar phenomenal objects it serves as a guide to appropriate behavior. But the relation of self to ego-processes is no more and no less obscure than the relation of cognitive structures to behavior generally.

---

[1] The writer doubts that it is advisable to construct the ego as narrowly around the self as do Chein (1944) and Murphy (1947).

[2] How to distinguish within the personality between *ego* and *non-ego* is, of course, an important problem, though it will not be attempted here. The distinction, however, is not the same as the phenomenal one between the *self* and *notself* (often described, confusingly, as *ego-alien*).

"EGO-INVOLVEMENTS" AND "EGO DEFENSE"

We have sought to reinstate the ego as a subjective but non-phenomenal construct mainly through an examination of the pitfalls encountered by the attempt to avoid such a concept. If the ego-self distinction as outlined above is worth making, however, it should make a difference in the formulation of other knotty problems. Does it? Two such problems—the nature of "ego-involvements" and of the "mechanisms of defense"—will be examined briefly as test cases.

As it emerges in the work of Sherif and Cantril (1947), the concept of ego-involvement lacks clarity and focus. Widely divergent sorts of psychological facts turn out to be embraced by the term, which, like so many in popular psychological currency, rather identifies a disparate group of problems than clarifies them. More often than not, ego-involvement means the involvement of a person's pride and self-esteem in a task; he feels put to the test and ready to be ashamed of a poor performance. In other instances, the term is invoked to cover immersion in a cause, or falling in love—cases in which the person, to be sure, cares as deeply about outcomes as in the first type, but may be engrossed to the point of losing self-awareness.

Now the present self-ego distinction makes excellent sense when applied here. Since the distinctive character of the first sort of examples lies in the fact that the individual's conception of his self and its worth is at stake, these can aptly be described as *self-involvement*. The second type of case can often still be called ego-involvement without inconsistency. The situation in the latter instances touches on the person's central system of on-going psychological processes so closely that he may lose himself in it. Similar engrossment can, to be sure, result from the involvement of equally imperative non-ego processes: who is to say, without intimate acquaintance with the principals, whether being in love should be called ego-involvement or "id-involvement"! However that may be, note that self-involvement and ego-involvement thus conceived may vary independently. A person may care about a task both because of its intrinsic meaning for him

and with after-thought for its bearing on his prestige and self-esteem. Or either or neither may be the case. The behavioral conditions and consequences of ego- and self-involvement should furthermore be quite distinct.

The situation is somewhat different in regard to the theoretical status of the mechanisms of defense. Here the classical formulation by Anna Freud (1946) regards the defense mechanisms as employed by the ego (the term is used essentially in our sense) to protect itself, primarily from disruption by strong unassimilated urges, but also from threats from the external world. As a more or less precariously balanced system mediating between inner strivings and outer reality, the ego, in this view, has recourse to these sometimes drastic techniques in order to preserve its balance, and maintain the course of behavior at a lower level of adjustment if need be rather than run the risk of its catastrophic disruption. Murphy (1947), and later Snygg and Combs (1949), on the other hand, say in effect that it is rather the self that is defended. Under conditions of threat, enhancement and preservation of the self may be achieved by the classical defense mechanisms. Is it necessary to choose between these divergent formulations, or can the conflict be resolved?

The present writer would maintain that the mechanisms of defense can ultimately all be conceived as defenses of the ego, since they serve to bolster up the ego's adjustive compromise. As contributors to this compromise, they can also best be regarded as a part of the activity included in the ego system. But in a more immediate sense, any particular one of an individual's defenses may or may *not* be a *self*-defense mechanism. Since the maintenance of a favorable self-image is important to sound ego functioning, though not its only requisite, the end of ego defense can often be served most efficiently by self-defense mechanisms. Certain mechanisms, like identification, may, indeed, always take effect through the defense of the self. There are, however, instances of ego-defense mechanisms which involve the self only indirectly if at all. In regression, for example, one can hardly suppose that the self is enhanced in any way. What is more likely is that by retreating to an earlier, more deeply established, or simpler level of ego organization, the person seeks, perhaps ineptly, to cope with disturbing experiences that, by reason of circumstance, constitution, or previous learning, he has not the strength to meet maturely. In most cases, the relative significance of the self in the defensive process probably cannot be assessed in any simple way, since changes in the self for better or worse may be the *consequence* of the fortunes of the ego and its defenses, as well as the focus of defensive techniques.

A formulation of this sort, which seems to agree with present clinical experience, again suggests the usefulness of a distinction between phenomenal and non-phenomenal (shall we say *functional?*) subjective constructs, with both employed in proper coordination. A purely phenomenological psychology, on the other hand, cannot adequately describe *all* the defensive processes, since neither all the effective threats to the ego nor all the defenses against them are registered accurately in conscious awareness. Indeed, it is largely the consequence of "silent" defensive processes that phenomenological reports must be viewed with so much circumspection in personality research.

CONCLUSIONS

Starting from a discussion of Snygg and Combs' proposal of a phenomenological frame of reference for psychology (1949) the writer has sought to establish the following major points:

1. While common sense may favor an explanatory psychology framed entirely in terms of conscious experience, such a psychological system does violence to currently available knowledge.

2. Phenomenology, as distinct from common sense, is descriptive, not explanatory. It is an approach or method ancillary to the formulation of problems and derivation of constructs, and does not give birth to these constructs full blown.

3. The subjective and objective frames of reference, which denote relatively different alternative contexts within which constructs may be selected, are both entirely compatible with the observer's frame of reference. Subjective

constructs to be scientifically admissible must ultimately be anchored in the data of observation.

4. The phenomenological approach provides one method of deriving subjective constructs. But not all subjective constructs need represent phenomenal entities. They may, thus, denote functional entities that are either absent from the phenomenal field or inaccurately presented in it.

5. The coordinate use of phenomenal and non-phenomenal subjective constructs, maintained in clear distinction from one another, serves to clarify the theory of the ego and the self. It is proposed that an adequate theory of personality must distinguish, among other constructs,

a. the *ego*, a *non-phenomenal* subjective construct representing a configuration of ongoing processes, among which is the cognitive-perceptual function. Through exercise of this function, the ego "knows," among other things,

b. the *self*, a *phenomenal* subjective construct.

6. When carried into current problems concerning the nature of "ego-involvement" and of the "mechanisms of defense," the above distinction seems productive.

References

Allport, G. W. The ego in contemporary psychology. *Psychol. Rev.*, 1943, *50*, 451–478.
Chein, I. The awareness of self and the structure of the ego. *Psychol. Rev.*, 1944, *51*, 304–314.
Combs, A. W. A phenomenological approach to adjustment. *J. abnorm. soc. Psychol.*, 1949, *44*, 29–35.
Freud, A. *The ego and the mechanisms of defense.* New York: International Universities Press, 1946.
Freud, S. *New introductory lectures on psychoanalysis.* New York: Norton, 1933.
Lewin, K. *Principles of topological psychology.* New York: McGraw-Hill, 1936.
MacLeod, R. B. The phenomenological approach to social psychology. *Psychol. Rev.*, 1947, *54*, 193–210.
Murphy, G. *Personality: A biosocial approach to origins and structure.* New York: Harper, 1947.
Rogers, C. R. Some observations on the organization of personality. *Amer. Psychologist*, 1947, *2*, 358–368.
Sherif, M., and Cantril, H. *The psychology of ego-involvements.* New York: Wiley, 1947.
Snygg, D., and Combs, A. W. *Individual behavior: A new frame of reference for psychology.* New York: Harper, 1949.

30. The Logic of the Romantic Point of View in Personology

ROBERT R. HOLT

Let us now consider each of the main propositions that make up the romantic point of view, and state the logical objections to them systematically.

1. *The goal of personology must be understanding, not prediction and control.* The goal of those who profess an idiographic point of view is not anything so antiseptic and inhuman as a family of curves; it is *understanding*. In one sense, it is proper to say that we understand poliomyelitis when we have isolated the responsible viruses and have identified the conditions under which they attack and cripple a person, but this is not *Verstehen*. That conception is an empathic, intuitive *feeling* of knowing a phenomenon from the inside, as it were. To take a more congenial example, we do not understand why a particular boy becomes delinquent from knowing that he comes from a neighborhood that an ecological survey has determined to be economically deprived and socially disorganized; whereas after we have read Farrell's *Studs Lonigan* and have seen such conditions and the embeddedness of delinquency in them portrayed with artistic power and vividness, then we understand (in the sense of *Verstehen*) the relation between these phenomena.

From this example, it should be clear that the feeling of understanding is a subjective effect aimed at by artists, not scientists. In science, when we say we understand something, we mean that we can predict and control it, but such aims are foreign to the romantic viewpoint. When Allport says (as of course Freud and many others have said also) that novelists and poets have been great intuitive psychologists, in some ways the greatest psychologists, the statement has two (not necessarily coexistent) meanings: that literary men have known many significant variables of and propositions about personality (e.g., the role of unconscious incestuous wishes

in determining many kinds of behavior), or, that they have been able to create the most vivid, compelling portraits of people, which give us the sense of knowing and understanding them. The latter effect is achieved by judicious selection and artful distortion, not by exhaustive cataloguing and measurement of traits, motives, or structural relations. Indeed, the idea of a catalogue is the very antithesis of art, just as a painful realism that tries to copy nature slavishly is the death of an artistic endeavor.

Here we see the issues drawn clearly. Is personology to be an art, devoted to word portraits that seek to evoke in the reader the thrill of recognition, the gratifying (if perhaps illusory) feeling of understanding unique individuals? Or is it to be a science, which enables us to study these same persons in all their uniqueness and to derive from such study general propositions about the structure, development, and other significant aspects of personality? If we elect for a science, we must abandon art whenever it takes us in a different direction than the one demanded by the scientific method, and we must recognize that the ideal of an idiographic science is a will-o'-the-wisp, an artistic and not a scientific goal. Science may be supplemented by art, but not combined with it.

There is a legitimate art of personality, literary biography. An artist like André Maurois is not hindered by not being a scientist of any kind. We should recognize that an artist's quest for "truth" differs from a scientist's in being a striving not for strict verisimilitude but for allusive illumination; its criterion is the effect on some audience—something to which science must remain indifferent.

Since some personologists (notably Freud, Murphy, Allport, and Murray) have had much of the artist in them as well as the scientist and have been masters of prose writing, it is no wonder that at times the artistic side of their identities has come uppermost. If Allport had been less aesthetically sensitive, he might not have failed to distinguish between artistic and

Abridged from "Individuality and Generalization in the Psychology of Personality," *J. Personality 30*:377–402, 1962, by permission of the publisher and the author.

scientific goals. Often, too, poor scientists are at the same time poor writers, and an inferior case study may be poor either because its facts are wrong and its interpretations undiscerning, or because it is poorly put together and lacks the literary touch that can put the breath of life into even a routine case report. The more art a scientist possesses—so long as he does not let it run away with him—the more effective a scientist he can be, because he can use his aesthetic sense in constructing theory as well as in communicating his findings and ideas to others.

2. *The proper methods of personology are intuition and empathy, which have no place in natural science.* As has been indicated above, intuition and empathy were used by the romantics as ways of gaining direct and definitive understanding, and were considered to be complete scientific methods. The contemporary personologist has no quarrel with their use in the practical arts of clinical psychology and psychoanalysis, nor as ways of making discoveries and formulating hypotheses. Indeed, the more secure scientists are in their methodological position, the more respect they usually have for intuition (and in psychology for the closely related methods of empathy and recipathy). Thus, the claim that these operations have no place in natural science is false; they are used by all scientists in the most exciting and creative phase of scientific work: when they decide what to study, what variables to control, what empirical strategies to use, and when they make discoveries within the structure of empirical data. As to their sufficiency, I need only remind the reader that the methodology of verification, the hypothesis-testing phase of scientific work, involves well-developed rules and consensually established procedures, and that intuition and empathy have no place in it.

3. *Personology is a subjective discipline as contrasted to objective branches of psychology, being concerned with values and meanings, which cannot be subjected to quantification.* Elsewhere (Holt, 1961), I have dealt with the contention that there is a fundamental methodological difference between disciplines that deal with verbal meanings and values, and those that deal with objective facts. Briefly, the argument is the

familiar one that objectivity is only intersubjectivity, and that meanings (including values) may be perceived and dealt with in essentially the same ways as the data of natural science, which must be discriminated and recognized also. Moreover, a logical analysis of the operations carried out in disciplines such as literature, concerned with the understanding of individual works and little (if at all) with generalization, shows that these workers outside of science use many of the *same* methods of analyzing texts as the quantitative content-analysis of social psychology, with their exclusive concern with generalization. Their work has shown that meanings may be quantified and in other ways treated as objectively as any other facts of nature. Other objections to quantification grow out of antipathy to abstract variables of analysis, and will be considered in the following section.

4. *The concepts of personology must be individualized, not generalized as are the concepts of natural science.* The belief that the concern of personology with unique individuals (see below) contrasts fundamentally with the exclusive concern of nomothetic science with generalities logically implies that the two types of discipline must have different types of concepts. As the chief spokesman for the romantic point of view in psychology, Allport calls for the use of individual traits, which are specific to the person being studied, not common traits, which are assumed to be present to some degree in all persons. But to describe an individual trait, we have to take one of two courses: either we create a unique word (a neologism) for each unique trait, or we use a unique configuration of existing words. The first approach is clearly impossible for communication, let alone science; personology would be a complete Babel. The second solution, however, turns out to be a concealed form of nomothesis, for what is a unique configuration of existing words but a "fallacious attempt to capture something ineffably individual by a complex net of general concepts"? Allport himself has explicitly ruled out this possibility:

. . . each psychologist tends to think of individuals as combinations of whatever abstractions he favors for psychological analysis. This procedure, common as it is, is wholly unsuitable for the psychology of personality.

For one thing, such abstract units are not distinctively *personal* (1937a, p. 239).*

An idiographic discipline thus must be a dumb or an incomprehensible one, for intelligible words—even some of Allport's favorite, literary ones, like *Falstaffian,* which he does consider "personal" —abstract and generalize, proclaiming a general pattern of resemblance between at least two unique individuals, Falstaff and the case being described. Any such trait thus becomes common, not individual.

One of the great methodologists of social science, Max Weber (1949) developed an apposite analysis of scientific concepts and their development in reaction against the romantic movement in his country at the turn of the century (cf. Parsons, 1957). He had the insight to see that the exponents of *Geisteswissenschaft* were trying to do the impossible: to capture the full richness of reality. There are three identifiable stages in the scientific study of anything, Weber said. To begin with, one selects from nature the historical individual (or class thereof) one wishes to focus on; for example, the Boston Massacre, the personality of Einstein, the cathedral at Chartres. Even though limited, each of these is infinitely rich in potentially specifiable aspects and configurations. One could study one of these, or even a tiny "flower in a crannied wall," until doomsday and not exhaust everything that could be known about it. Without doing any more abstracting than focusing on a particular topic, one can only contemplate it; and this is where the idiographic approach logically must stop. The method of intuition or *Verstehen* is essentially a wordless act of identification with the object, or some other attempt to "live in it" without analyzing its Gestalt.

The second stage, that of the ideal type, is a rudimentary attempt to see similarities between historical individuals, while staying as close as possible to their concrete particularity. Ideal types are much used in psychology, especially in diagnosis, for any syndrome such as

schizophrenia is a complex of identifiably separate but loosely covarying elements, never encountered in exact textbook form. The lure of ideal types is that they give the brief illusion of getting you close to the individual while still allowing a degree of generality. But this advantage is illusory, the apparent advantage of a compromise that denies satisfaction to either party. Concrete reality (fidelity to the unique individual) *is* forsworn, and the advantages of truly general concepts are not attained. An ideal type does not fit any particular case exactly, and the failure of fit is different in kind as well as degree from one case to another. For an ideal type "is a conceptual construct which is neither historical reality nor even the 'true' reality. It is even less fitted to serve as a schema under which a real situation or action is to be subsumed as one *instance.* It has the significance of a purely ideal *limiting* concept with which the real situation or action is compared and surveyed for the explication of certain of its significant components" (Weber, 1949, p. 93).

The final stage of scientific development, therefore, is the fractionation of ideal types into their constituent dimensions and elements, which Weber called abstract analytical variables. Paradoxically, only a truly abstract concept can give an exact fit to any particular individual! I cannot say exactly how Falstaffian or how schizophrenic or how big any particular subject may be, but I can name a particular value of an abstract analytical variable, height, that fits him as closely as his skin. The example would be less convincing if chosen from psychology because we do not have as well-established, unitary dimensions as the physical ones, and not as simple and unarguable operations for measuring them as the use of the meter stick; the principle, however, is the same.

The fit is exact, of course, only because an abstract analytical concept does not purport to do more than one thing. If I try to measure the breadth of a person's interests, I make no pretensions to have "captured the essence of his personality." Not having tried, I cannot properly be accused of failing. But I have chosen a variable that can be measured, and thus potentially its relations to other aspects of personality can be discovered and precisely stated.

---

*Allport wrote these words in the context of rejecting Murray's system of needs (1937a); yet elsewhere (Allport, 1937b) he praises as "strikingly personal" such concepts (or dimensions) of W. Stern (1938) as depth-surface, embeddedness-salience, nearness-remoteness, and expectancy-retrospect!

Curiously, Allport attacks general variables on the ground that they "merely *approximate* the unique cleavages which close scrutiny shows are characteristic of each separate personality" (Allport, 1946; his emphasis). His preferred *ad hoc* approach may seem less approximate because many of the general variables used in personology are ideal types, lacking true abstract generality. The solution, however, lies in a direction diametrically opposed to the one toward which Allport beckons. And it does not consist in escaping from approximation. Scientific models of reality can *never* fit perfectly; the attempt to force such identity between concept and referent sacrifices the flexibility and power of abstract concepts in a chimerical quest for the direct grasp of noumena.

Parenthetically, the recent vogue of existentialism and Zen Buddhism in psychology may be partly attributed to the promise they extend of providing a way of grasping the total richness of reality. Part of the lure of *satori* or any other mystical ecstasy of a direct contact with the world, unmediated by concepts, may stem from the necessary distance imposed by the scientific necessity to abstract. But despite their confusing jargons, which make them seem superficially quite different from the late nineteenth-century romantic movement we have been considering, both of these fashionable doctrines suffer from the same fallacies. Mystical experience, like aesthetic experience, offers nothing to the scientist qua scientist except an interesting phenomenon that may be subjected to scientific study.

5. *The only kind of analysis allowable in personology is structural, not abstract, while natural science is not concerned with structure.* It is true that the scientific psychology of Dilthey's heyday had no place for structural analysis in the sense introduced by the romantics. Psychology dealt with a number of functions, which were treated implicitly or explicitly as quite independent of one another. It had no methods parallel to those of exegetic Biblical scholarship or literary criticism, which seek out the internal organization of ideas in a specific text. And the reductionistic enthusiasts for analyzing things were not interested in putting the pieces back together again, nor very clear themselves that analysis need not mean

dismemberment. This state of affairs made it easy to think that analysis could be destructive, and that structural relations between the parts of the personality could be studied only in concrete, unique individuals, so that structure* seemed to be an exclusive concern of idiographic disciplines.

There are really two points here: the distrust of analysis, and the emphasis on structure. The first of these has been partly dealt with in the preceding section; it was based on a misunderstanding of the nature of abstract concepts.

On the second point, structural concepts and structural analyses are commonplace in science at large today. Such structural disciplines as stereochemistry and circuit design were (at best) in their infancy at the time of the idiographic manifestoes. Today, natural science uses abstract, structural, and dispositional concepts simultaneously with a minimum of confusion. Presumably, the same may be true of personology someday, too.

One merit of the romantic tradition in personology is that it has consistently highlighted the problem of structure. At the time Allport was taking his position on these matters (in the late 1920's and early 1930's), the predominant American conceptions of personality were "and-summative" (the sum total of a person's habits, traits, etc.), and the problem of structure was ignored. The early academic personologists who concentrated their efforts on personality inventories, single variables, or factor analyses, all tended to disregard entirely the structuring of these elements or to assume simple, universal answers (e.g., orthogonal factor-structure).

At the same time, however, Freud (1947) was developing the structural point of view in psychoanalysis, and today psychoanalytic psychology is increasingly concerned with the problem and has developed a variety of variables to deal with it (cf. Rapaport and Gill, 1959; Holt, 1960;

---

*Ironically, in psychology the adherents of structuralism were among those who carried atomistic, reductionistic analysis to its most absurd extreme: the Titchenerian introspectionists. The Gestalt psychologists, though appalled by the equally atomistic behaviorism and structuralism alike, concentrated their efforts on perceptual patterning, leaving untouched most of the structural problems that concern personology, particularly the enduring invariances of molar behavior.

and see the recent work of G. S. Klein and his associates on cognitive controls as structural variables: Gardner *et al.*, 1959). Drawing on this tradition and that of psychopathology generally, psychodiagnosis concerns itself with structural variables and their constellation into a limited number of ideal types (e.g., the obsessive-compulsive type of ego-structure) which, in the best practice, are used not as pigeonholes but as reference-points in terms of which the clinician creates individualized analyses of personality structure.

6. *There can be no general laws of personality because of the role of chance and free will in human affairs.* There are hardly any contemporary personologists who openly espouse this argument. It played an important part in the development of the romantic point of view, as we have seen, and persists in Catholic psychology. It is generally admitted, however, that scientific work requires the basic assumption of strict determinism throughout. Closely examined, chance becomes ignorance; when we discover systematic effects where "error" existed before, the chance (at least in part) disappears. Theoretically, the exact path of a bolt of lightning and the exact events of a human life could be predicted rigorously, if we only had all of the necessary data at hand.

7. *General laws are not possible in personology because its subject matter is unique individuals, which have no place in natural science.* It is not difficult to dispose of this last, supposedly critical point of difference between *Naturwissenschaft* and *Geisteswissenschaft.*

The mechanistic, pre-field theoretical science of Windelband's day contained a curious dictum that has been one of the principal sources of confusion on this whole issue: *Scientia non est individuorum* — science does not deal with individual cases. This hoary slogan dates back to the days when Aristotle was the last word on matters scientific, and the whole point of view it expresses is outdated in the physical sciences. According to this philosophy, the individual case was not lawful, since laws were conceived of as empirical regularities. This is the point of view (Plato's idealism or what Popper calls *essentialism*) that considers an average to be the only fact, and all deviation from it mere error.

Freud and Lewin have taught us that psychic determinism is thoroughgoing (see above), and the individual case is completely lawful. It is just difficult to know what the laws *are* from a study of one case, no matter how thorough. We can surmise (or, if you will, intuit) general laws from a single case in the hypothesis-forming phase of scientific endeavor, but we can verify them only by resorting to experimental or statistical inquiry or both.

There is truth in the old adage only in one sense, then: We cannot carry out the complete scientific process by the study of an individual. It is true that in certain of the disciplines concerned with man, from anatomy to sensory psychology, it has usually been assumed that the phenomena being studied are so universal that they can be located for study in any single person, and so autonomous from entanglement in idiosyncratically variable aspects of individuals that the findings of intensive investigation will have general applicability to people at large. Every so often, however, these assumptions turn out not to be tenable. For example, when Boring repeated Head's study (in one case, himself) of the return of sensation after the experimental section of a sensory nerve in his arm, he did not find the protopathic-epicritic sequential recovery, which had been so uncritically accepted as to be firmly embedded in the literature. No matter how intensively prolonged, objective, and well-controlled the study of a single case, one can never be sure to what extent the lawful regularities found can be generalized to other persons, or in what ways the findings will turn out to be contingent on some fortuitously present characteristic of the subject—until the investigation is repeated on an adequate sample of persons. As excellent a way as it is to make discoveries, the study of an individual cannot be used to establish laws; bills of attainder (that is, laws concerned with single individuals) are as unconstitutional in science as in jurisprudence. Note, however, that law of either kind, when promulgated, is still conceived as holding quite rigorously for the single individual.

Science is defined by its methods, not its subject matter; to maintain the opposite, as Skaggs (1945) did in an attack on Allport, is to perpetuate the confusion, not resolve it, and Allport (1946) was an easy victor in the exchange. There can be and is scientific study of all sorts of individuals. Particular hurricanes are individualized to the extent of being given personal names and are studied by all the scientific means at the meteorologist's command. A great part of the science of astronomy is given over to the study of a number of unique individuals: the sun, moon, and planets, and even individual stars and nebulae. There may not be another Saturn, with its strange sets of rings, in all of creation,* yet it is studied by the most exact, quantitative and—if you must—nomothetic methods, and no one has ever considered suggesting that astronomy is for these reasons not a science nor that there should be two entirely different astronomical sciences, one to study individual heavenly bodies and the other to seek general laws. Further examples are easily available from geology, physics, and biology. Once we realize that individuals are easily within the realm of orthodox scientific study, and that science does not strive for artistic illusions of complete understanding, the issue is easily seen as a pseudo-problem. Psychology as a science remains methodologically the same, whether its focus be on individual cases or on general laws.

Granted, then, that individual personalities may and must be studied by the scientific method in personology, with the use of general concepts, what is the role of general laws in such a science? Where does it get us to make scientific studies of personalities, if each is unique, and if that uniqueness is the heart of the matter?

Personalities *are* in many ways unique, but as Kluckhohn and Murray (1953) point out, every man is also like all men in some ways and like a limited number of others in still other ways, making generalization possible. If every personality structure were as much a law unto itself as Allport implies, it would be impossible to gain useful information in this field; there would be no transfer from one case study to another. As anyone knows who has tried it, there is a great deal.

It is a mistake to focus personology on just those aspects of a person that are unique, as Weber (1949) saw clearly half a century ago. "The attempt to understand 'Bismarck,' " he said for example, "by leaving out of account everything which he has in common with other men and keeping what is 'particular' to him would be an instructive and amusing exercise for beginners. One would in that case . . . preserve, for example, as one of those 'finest flowers' [of such an analysis of uniqueness] his 'thumbprint,' that most specific indication of 'individuality.' " And some of the most critical points about him for predicting his behavior would have to be excluded because he shared them with other persons. Indeed, in contemporary psychodiagnosis, it is considered most useful to treat as a quantitative variable the degree to which a person's responses resemble those of the group as a whole.

The only kind of law that Allport could conceive for personology was one (like his principle of functional autonomy) that describes how uniqueness comes about. Personology has not been much restrained from seeking general relationships among its variables by this narrow view, however; the journals are full of investigations in which aspects of personality are studied genetically (that is, are related to the abstract variable of age) or are correlated, one with another. Once one treats uniqueness not with awe but with the casual familiarity due any other truistic fact of life, it ceases to pose any difficulty for personology.

Writing intensive case studies (on the genesis and structure of individual personalities) turns out not to be a particularly fruitful method, except for the generation of hypotheses. This is a very important exception, but the point is that personology does not proceed mainly by adding one exhaustive scientific biography to another, looking for generalizations afterwards. The Gestaltist taboo on studying any variable out of its context in the individual life is an overstatement. There is, of course, such a phenomenon as the interaction of variables, but it is not so far-reachingly prevalent as to make impossible any study of two variables at a time. As Falk (1956) has shown, this condition of interactive nonsummativeness is

---

*After these words had been written, I was amused to find that Cournot used this same example, and even similar wording, in supporting his position that "it is no longer necessary to accept to the letter the aphorism of the ancients to the effect that the individual and particular have no place in science" (1956, p. 443).

found in many other kinds of subject matter besides personality and creates no major difficulties of method or procedure.

In summary, in this section we have looked at the major propositions of the romantic point of view as applied to personology, and have found that the "basic differences" between this field and natural science are completely illusory. No basis for a separate methodology exists, and the objections to applying the general methodology of science to personalities turn out to be based on misunderstandings or on a narrow conception of natural science that is an anachronism today.

References

Allport, G. W. *Personality, a psychological interpretation*. New York: Holt, 1937a.

Allport, G. W. The personalistic psychology of William Stern. *Char. & Pers.*, 1937b, *5*, 231–246.

Allport, G. W. Personalistic psychology as science: A reply. *Psychol. Rev.*, 1946, *53*, 132–135.

Cournot, A. A. *An essay on the foundations of our knowledge*. (Trans. by M. H. Moore.) New York: Liberal Arts Press, 1956.

Falk, J. L. Issues distinguishing nomothetic from idiographic approaches to personality theory. *Psychol. Rev.*, 1956, *63*, 53–62.

Freud, S. *The ego and the id*. London: Hogarth, 1947.

Gardner, R., Holzman, P. S., Klein, G. S., Linton, Harriet B., and Spence, D. P. Cognitive control: A study of individual consistencies in cognitive behavior. *Psychol. Issues*, 1959, *1*, No. 4.

Holt, R. R. Recent developments in psychoanalytic ego psychology and their implications for diagnostic testing. *J. proj. Tech.*, 1960, *24*, 254–266.

Holt, R. R. Clinical judgment as a disciplined inquiry. *J. nerv. ment. Dis.*, 1961, *133*, 369–382.

Kluckhohn, C., and Murray, H. A. Personality formation: The determinants. In C. Kluckhohn and H. A. Murray (Eds.), *Personality in nature, society, and culture*. New York: Knopf, 1953.

Parsons, T. *The structure of social action*. Glencoe, Ill.: Free Press, 1957.

Rapaport, D., and Gill, M. M. The points of view and assumptions of metapsychology. *Int. J. Psychoanal.*, 1959, *40*, 153–162.

Skaggs, E. B. Personalistic psychology as science. *Psychol. Rev.*, 1945, *52*, 234–238.

Stern, W. *General psychology from a personalistic standpoint*. (Trans. by H. D. Spoerl.) New York: Macmillan, 1938.

Weber, M. *The methodology of the social sciences*. (Trans. and ed. by E. A. Shils and H. A. Finch.) Glencoe, Ill.: Free Press, 1949. (The material collected here was originally published from 1904 to 1917.)

Part IV

Behavioral Theories

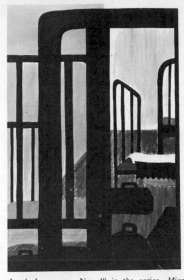

Jacob Lawrence—No. 48 in the series, *Migration of the Negro*.

INTRODUCTION

Taken in its strictest form, the behavioral approach requires that all concepts and propositions be anchored precisely to measurable properties in the empirical world. That behavioral concepts are, in fact, not always formulated as operational concepts is a concession to the limits of practicality. Nevertheless, empirically unanchored speculation is anathema to behaviorists; hypothetical constructs, which abound in intrapsychic and phenomenological theories, are rarely found in behavioral theories.

Behaviorism originated with the view that subjective introspection was "unscientific" and that it should be replaced by the use of objectively observable behavior. Further, all environmental influences upon behavior were likewise to be defined objectively. If unobservable processes were thought to exist within the individual, they were to be defined strictly in terms of observables which indicate their existence.

Recent theories of behavioral pathology have included concepts generated originally in experimental learning research. They are not simple translations of psychoanalytic concepts into behavioral terminology, as were earlier theories of behavioral pathology, but are based on the ostensible "empirical" laws of learning. Theorists using these concepts lay claim to the virtues of science since their heritage lies with the objective studies of systematic learning research and not with the dubious methods of clinical speculation.

That learning concepts are helpful in understanding pathology cannot be denied, but behavioral theorists take a stronger position. They state that pathological behavior is learned behavior that develops according to the same laws as those governing the development of normal behavior. Disturbed behavior differs from normal behavior only in magnitude, frequency, and social adaptiveness. Were these behavior patterns more adaptive, or less frequent and extreme, they would possess no other distinguishing features.

Behavioral Theories

ORIENTATION

The first theory to restrict its conception of pathology entirely to objective behavioral processes, eschewing all reference to internal phenomena such as the unconscious or innate anxiety dispositions, was formulated by the eminent learning theorist B. F. Skinner and his disciples. According to strict behaviorism, as presented in the paper reprinted here, it is unnecessary and misleading to posit the existence of unobservable emotional states to account for pathological behavior. The excerpt from the paper by Leonard Ullmann and Leonard Krasner elaborates what they refer to as the "psychological model" of psychopathology. They discard all reference to hypothetical inner states and offer a formulation based solely in terms of stimulation and reinforcement. Reinforcements shape the behavioral repertoire of the individual, and differences between adaptive and maladaptive behavior results from differences in the reinforcement pattern to which individuals were exposed.

31.   What Is Psychotic Behavior?

B. F. SKINNER

Since my field of specialization lies some distance from psychiatry, it may be well to begin with credentials. The first will be negative. In the sense in which my title is most likely to be understood, I am wholly unqualified to discuss the question before us. The number of hours I have spent in the presence of psychotic people (assuming that I am myself sane) is negligible compared with what many of you might claim, and the time I have spent in relevant reading and discussion would suffer equally from the same comparison. I am currently interested in some research on psychotic subjects, to which I shall refer again later, but my association with that program in no way qualifies me as a specialist.

Fortunately, I am not here to answer the question in that sense at all. A more accurate title would have been "What is *behavior?*—with an occasional reference

to psychiatry." Here I will list such positive credentials as seem appropriate. I have spent a good share of my professional life in the experimental analysis of the behavior of organisms. Almost all my subjects have been below the human level (most of them rats or pigeons) and all, so far as I know, have been sane. My research has not been designed to test any theory of behavior, and the results cannot be evaluated in terms of the statistical significance of such proofs. The object has been to discover the functional relations which prevail between measurable aspects of behavior and various conditions and events in the life of the organism. The success of such a venture is gauged by the extent to which behavior can, as a result of the relationships discovered, actually be predicted and controlled. Here we have, I think, been fortunate. Within a limited experimental arrangement, my colleagues and I have been able to demonstrate a lawfulness in behavior which seems to us quite remarkable. In more recent research it has been possible to maintain—actually, to sharpen—this degree of

From *Theory and Treatment of the Psychoses,* pages 77–99, 1956, Washington University Studies, by permission of the Washington University Press and the author.

lawfulness while slowly increasing the complexity of the behavior studied. The extent of the prediction and control which has been achieved is evident not only in "smoothness of curves" and uniformity of results from individual to individual or even species to species, but in the practical uses which are already being made of the techniques—for example, in providing baselines for the study of pharmacological and neurological variables, or in converting a lower organism into a sensitive psychophysical observer.

Although research designed in this way has an immediate practical usefulness, it is not independent of one sort of theory. A primary concern has been to isolate a useful and expedient measure. Of all the myriad aspects of behavior which present themselves to observation, which are worth watching? Which will prove most useful in establishing functional relations? From time to time many different characteristics of behavior have seemed important. Students of the subject have asked how well organized behavior is, how well adapted it is to the environment, how sensitively it maintains a homeostatic equilibrium, how purposeful it is, or how successfully it solves practical problems or adjusts to daily life. Many have been especially interested in how an individual compares with others of the same species or with members of other species in some arbitrary measure of the scope, complexity, speed, consistency, or other property of behavior. All these aspects may be quantified, at least in a rough way, and any one may serve as a dependent variable in a scientific analysis. But they are not all equally productive. In research which emphasizes prediction and control, the topography of behavior must be carefully specified. Precisely what is the organism doing? The most important aspect of behavior so described is its probability of emission. How likely is it that an organism will engage in behavior of a given sort, and what conditions or events change this likelihood? Although probability of action has only recently been explicitly recognized in behavior theory, it is a key concept to which many classical notions, from reaction tendencies to the Freudian wish, may be reduced. Experimentally we deal with it as the *frequency* with which an organism behaves in a given way under specified circumstances, and our methods

are designed to satisfy this requirement. Frequency of response has proved to be a remarkably sensitive variable, and with its aid the exploration of causal factors has been gratifyingly profitable.

One does not engage in work of this sort for the sheer love of rats or pigeons. As the medical sciences illustrate, the study of animals below the level of man is dictated mainly by convenience and safety. But the primary object of interest is always man. Such qualifications as I have to offer in approaching the present question spring about equally from the experimental work just mentioned and from a parallel preoccupation with human behavior, in which the principles emerging from the experimental analysis have been tested and put to work in the interpretation of empirical facts. The formal disciplines of government, education, economics, religion, and psychotherapy, among others, together with our everyday experience with men, overwhelm us with a flood of facts. To interpret these facts with the formulation which emerges from an experimental analysis has proved to be strenuous but healthful exercise. In particular, the nature and function of *verbal* behavior have taken on surprisingly fresh and promising aspects when reformulated under the strictures of such a framework.

In the long run, of course, mere interpretation is not enough. If we have achieved a true scientific understanding of man, we should be able to prove this in the actual prediction and control of his behavior. The experimental practices and the concepts emerging from our research on lower organisms have already been extended in this direction, not only in the experiments on psychotic subjects already mentioned, but in other promising areas. The details would take us too far afield, but perhaps I can indicate my faith in the possibilities in a single instance by hazarding the prediction that we are on the threshold of a revolutionary change in methods of education, based not only upon a better understanding of learning processes, but upon a workable conception of knowledge itself.

Whether or not this brief personal history seems to you to qualify me to discuss the question before us, there is no doubt that it has created a high probability that I will do so, as shown by the fact that I am here. What I have to say is admittedly methodological. I can understand a certain impatience with such discussion particularly when, as in the field of psychiatry, many pressing problems call for action. The scientist who takes time out to consider human nature when so many practical things need to be done for human welfare is likely to be cast in the role of a Nero, fiddling while Rome burns. (It is quite possible that the fiddling referred to in this archetypal myth was a later invention of the historians, and that in actual fact Nero had called in his philosophers and scientists and was discussing "the fundamental nature of combustion" or "the epidemiology of conflagration.") But I should not be here if I believed that what I have to say is remote from practical consequences. If we are now entering an era of research in psychiatry which is to be as extensive and as productive as other types of medical research, then a certain detachment from immediate problems, a fresh look at human behavior in general, a survey of applicable formulations, and a consideration of relevant methods may prove to be effective practical steps with surprisingly immediate consequences.

The study of human behavior is, of course, still in its infancy, and it would be rash to suppose that anyone can foresee the structure of a well-developed and successful science. Certainly no current formulation will seem right fifty years hence. But although we cannot foresee the future clearly, it is not impossible to discover in what direction we are likely to change. There are obviously great deficiencies in our present ways of thinking about men; otherwise we should be more successful. What are they, and how are they to be remedied? What I have to say rests upon the assumption that the behavior of the psychotic is simply part and parcel of human behavior, and that certain considerations which have been emphasized by the experimental and theoretical analysis of behavior in general are worth discussing in this special application.

It is important to remember that I am speaking as an experimental scientist. A conception of human behavior based primarily on clinical information and practice will undoubtedly differ from a conception emanating from the laboratory. This does not mean that either is superior to the other, or that eventually a common formulation will not prove useful to both. It is possible that questions which have been suggested by the exigencies of an experimental analysis may not seem of first importance to those of you who are primarily concerned with human behavior under therapy. But as psychiatry moves more rapidly into experimental research and as laboratory results take on a greater clinical significance, certain problems in the analysis of behavior should become common to researcher and therapist alike, and should eventually be given common and cooperative solutions.

———

The study of behavior, psychotic or otherwise, remains securely in the company of the natural sciences so long as we take as our subject matter the observable activity of the organism, as it moves about, stands still, seizes objects, pushes and pulls, makes sounds, gestures, and so on. Suitable instruments will permit us to amplify small-scale activities as part of the same subject matter. Watching a person behave in this way is like watching any physical or biological system. We also remain within the framework of the natural sciences in explaining these observations in terms of external forces and events which act upon the organism. Some of these are to be found in the hereditary history of the individual, including his membership in a given species as well as his personal endowment. Others arise from the physical environment, past or present. We may represent the situation as in Figure 1. Our organism emits the behavior we are to account for, as our dependent variable, at the right. To explain this, we appeal to certain external, generally observable, and possibly controllable hereditary and environmental conditions, as indicated at the left. These are the independent variables of which behavior is to be expressed as a function. Both input and output of such a system may be treated within the accepted dimensional systems of physics and biology. A complete set of such relations would permit us to predict and, insofar as the independent variables are under our control, to modify or generate behavior at will. It would also permit us to *interpret* given instances of behavior by inferring plausible variables of which we lack direct information. Admittedly the data are subtle and complex, and many relevant conditions are hard to get at, but the pro-

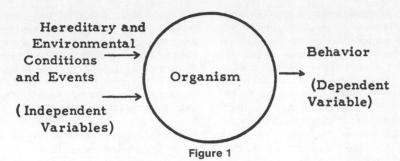

Figure 1

gram as such is an acceptable one from the point of view of scientific method. We have no reason to suppose in advance that a complete account cannot be so given. We have only to try and see.

It is not, however, the subtlety or complexity of this subject matter which is responsible for the relatively undeveloped state of such a science. Behavior has seldom been analyzed in this manner. Instead, attention has been diverted to activities which are said to take place within the organism. All sciences tend to fill in causal relationships, especially when the related events are separated by time and space. If a magnet affects a compass needle some distance away, the scientist attributes this to a "field" set up by the magnet and reaching to the compass needle. If a brick falls from a chimney, releasing energy which was stored there, say, a hundred years ago when the chimney was built, the result is explained by saying that the brick has all this time possessed a certain amount of "potential energy." In order to fill such spatial and temporal gaps between cause and effect, nature has from time to time been endowed with many weird properties, spirits, and essences. Some have proved helpful and have become part of the sub-

ject matter of science, especially when identified with events observed in other ways. Others have proved dangerous and damaging to scientific progress. Sophisticated scientists have usually been aware of the practice and alert to its dangers. Such inner forces were, indeed, the hypotheses which Newton refused to make.

Among the conditions which affect behavior, hereditary factors occupy a primary position, at least chronologically. Differences between members of different species are seldom, if ever, disputed, but differences between members of the same species, possibly due to similar hereditary factors, are so closely tied up with social and ethical problems that they have been the subject of seemingly endless debate. In any event, the newly conceived organism begins at once to be influenced by its environment; and when it comes into full contact with the external world, environmental forces assume a major role. They are the only conditions which can be changed so far as the individual is concerned. Among these are the events we call "stimuli," the various interchanges between organism and environment such as occur in breathing or eating, the events which generate the changes in behavior

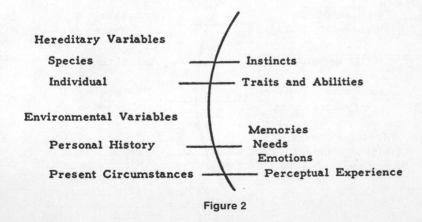

Figure 2

we call emotional, and the coincidences between stimuli or between stimuli and behavior responsible for the changes we call learning. The effects may be felt immediately or only after the passage of time—perhaps of many years. Such are the "causes"—the independent variables—in terms of which we may hope to explain behavior within the framework of a natural science.

In many discussions of human behavior, however, these variables are seldom explicitly mentioned. Their place is taken by events or conditions within the organism for which they are said to be responsible (see Figure 2). Thus, the species status of the individual is dealt with as a set of instincts, not simply as patterns of behavior characteristic of the species, but as biological drives. As one text puts it, "instincts are innate biological forces, urges, or impulsions driving the organism to a certain end." The individual genetic endowment, if not carried by body-type or other observable physical characteristic, is represented in the form of inherited traits or abilities, such as temperament or intelligence. As to the environmental variables, episodes in the past history of the individual are dealt with as memories and habits, while certain conditions of interchange between organism and environment are represented as needs or wants. Certain inciting episodes are dealt with as emotions, again in the sense not of patterns but of active causes of behavior. Even the present environment as it affects the organism is transmuted into "experience," as we turn from what is the case to what "seems to be" the case to the individual.

The same centripetal movement may be observed on the other side of the diagram (see Figure 3). It is rare to find behavior dealt with as a subject matter in its own right. Instead it is regarded as evidence for a mental life, which is then taken as the primary object of inquiry. What the individual does—the topography of his behavior—is treated as the functioning of one or more personalities. It is clear, especially when personalities are multiple, that they cannot be identified with the biological organism as such, but are conceived of, rather, as inner behavers of doubtful status and dimensions. The act of behaving in a given instance is neglected in favor of an impulse or wish, while the probability of such an act is represented as an excitatory tendency or in terms of psychic energy. Most important of all, the changes in behavior which represent the fundamental behavioral processes are characterized as mental activities—such as thinking, learning, discriminating, reasoning, symbolizing, projecting, identifying, and repressing.

The relatively simple scheme shown in the first figure does not, therefore, represent the conception of human behavior characteristic of most current theory. The great majority of students of human behavior assume that they are concerned with a series of events indicated in the expanded diagram of Figure 4. Here the hereditary and environmental conditions are assumed to generate instincts, needs, emotions, memories, habits, and so on, which in turn lead the personality to engage in various activities characteristic of the mental apparatus, and these in turn generate the observable behavior of the

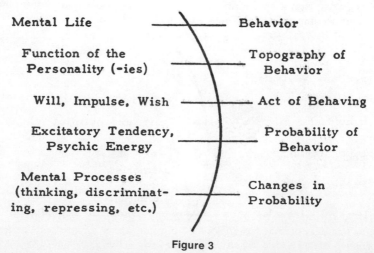

Figure 3

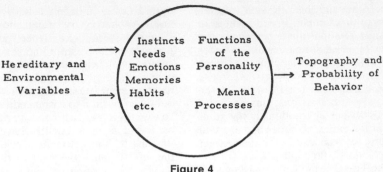

Figure 4

organism. All four stages in the diagram are accepted as proper objects of inquiry. Indeed, far from leaving the inner events to other specialists while confining themselves to the end terms, many psychologists and psychiatrists take the mental apparatus as their primary subject matter.

Perhaps the point of my title is now becoming clearer. Is the scientific study of behavior—whether normal or psychotic—concerned with the behavior of the observable organism under the control of hereditary and environmental factors, or with the functioning of one or more personalities engaged in a variety of mental processes under the promptings of instincts, needs, emotions, memories, and habits? I do not want to raise the question of the supposed *nature* of these inner entities. A certain kinship between such an explanatory system and primitive animism can scarcely be missed, but whatever the historical sources of these concepts, we may assume that they have been purged of dualistic connotations. If this is not the case, if there are those who feel that psychiatry is concerned with a world beyond that of the psychobiological or biophysical organism, that conscious or unconscious mind lacks physical extent, and that mental processes do not affect the world according to the laws of physics, then the following arguments should be all the more cogent. But the issue is not one of the nature of these events, but of their usefulness and experience in a scientific description.

It can scarcely be denied that the expansion of subject matter represented by Figure 4 has the unfortunate effect of a loss of physical status. This is more than a question of prestige or "face." A subject matter which is unquestionably part of the field of physics and biology has been relinquished for one of doubtful characteristics. This cannot be corrected merely by asserting our faith in the ultimately physical nature of inner processes. To protest that the activities of the conscious and unconscious mind are only in some sense an aspect of the biological functioning of the organism will not answer the practical question. In abandoning the dimensional systems of physics and biology, we abandon the techniques of measurement which would otherwise be a natural heritage from earlier achievements in other sciences. This is possibly an irreparable loss. If we come out flatly for the existence of instincts, needs, memories, and so on, on the one hand, and the mental processes and functions of the personality on the other, then we must accept the responsibility of devising methods of observing these inner events and of discovering dimensional systems according to which they can be measured. The loss of the opportunity to measure and manipulate in the manner characteristic of the physical sciences would be offset only by some extraordinary advantage gained by turning to inner states or conditions.

It is possible, however, to argue that these inner events are merely ways of representing the outer. Many theorists will contend that a habit is only a sort of notation useful in reporting a bit of the history of the individual, just as so-called "mental processes" are ways of talking about changes in behavior. This is a tempting position, for we may then insist that the only dimensional systems required are those appropriate to the terminal events. But if we are to take that line, a great deal still needs to be done to put our house in scientific order. The concepts which one encounters in current behavior theory represent the observable events in an extremely confusing way. Most of them have arisen from theoretical or practical considerations which have little reference to their validity or usefulness as scientific constructs, and they bear the scars of such a history. For example, Freud pointed to important relationships between the behavior of an adult and certain episodes in early childhood, but he chose to bridge the very considerable gap between cause and effect with activities or states of the mental apparatus. Conscious or unconscious wishes or emotions in the adult represent the earlier episodes and are said to be directly responsible for their effect upon behavior. The adult is said, for example, to be suffering from conscious or unconscious anxiety generated when as a child he was punished for aggressive behavior toward a sibling. But many details of the early episode are glossed over (and may, as a result, be neglected) in attributing the disturbances in his behavior to a current anxiety rather than to the earlier punishment. The number of references to anxiety in treatises on behavior must greatly exceed the number of references to punishing episodes, yet we must turn to the latter for full details. If the details are not available, nothing can take their place.

Other kinds of independent variables provide similar examples. Everyone is familiar with the fact that, in general, organisms eat or do not eat depending upon a recent history of deprivation or ingestion. If we can establish that a child does not eat his dinner because he has recently eaten other food, there may seem to be no harm in expressing this by saying that "he is not hungry," provided we explain this in turn by pointing to the history of ingestion. But the concept of hunger represents quite inadequately the many features of schedules of deprivation and other conditions and events which alter the behavior of eating. In the same way the inner surrogates of hereditary variables function beyond the line of duty. We often have no other explanation of a given bit of behavior than that, like other features of anatomy and physiology, it is characteristic of a species; but when we choose instead to attribute this behavior to a set of instincts, we obscure the negative nature of our knowledge and suggest more active causes than mere species status warrants. Similarly, we accept the fact that individuals differ in their behavior, and we may, in some instances, show a relation between aspects of the behavior of successive generations, but these differences and relationships are optimistically misrepresented when we speak of hereditary traits and abilities. Again, the term "experience" incorrectly represents our information about a stimulating field. It has often been observed, for example, that some trivial incident generates a reaction altogether out of proportion to its magnitude. A person seems to be reacting, not to the physical world as such, but to what the world "means to him." Eventually, of course, the effect must be explained—for example, by pointing to some earlier connection with more important events. But whatever the explanation, it is almost certainly not adequately expressed by the notion of a momentary experience. There are obvious difficulties involved in representing a physical environment *plus a personal history* as a current psychological environment alone.

So far as our independent variables are concerned, then, the practice we are examining tends to gloss over many important details and complexities. The conceptual structure conceals from us the inadequacy of our present knowledge. Much the same difficulty is encountered with respect to the dependent variable, when observable behavior takes second place to mental functionings of a personality. Just as the physical environment is transmuted into experience, so physical behavior comes to be described in terms of its purpose or meaning. A man may walk down the street in precisely the same way upon two occasions, although in one instance he is out for exercise and in another he is going to mail a letter. And so it is thought necessary to consider, not the behavior itself, but "what it means" to the behaving individual. But the additional information we are trying to convey is not a property of behavior but of an independent variable. The behavior we observe in the two cases *is* the same. In reading meaning or intention into it, we are speculating about some of its causes. To take another example, it is commonly said that we can "see" aggression. But we "see" it in two steps: (1) we observe the behavior of an organism, and (2) we relate it to observed or inferred variables having to do with injurious consequences and with the kinds of circumstances which make such behavior probable. No behavior is itself aggressive by nature, although some forms of behavior are so often a function of variables which make them aggressive that we are inclined to overlook the inferences involved. Similarly, when we observe two or more behavioral systems in the same individual and attribute them to different personalities, we gain a considerable advantage for certain descriptive purposes. For example, we can then describe oppositions between such systems as we would between different persons. But we have almost certainly suggested a unity which is not justified by the observed systems of behavior, and we have probably made it more difficult to represent the actual extent of any conflict as well as to explain its origins. And when we observe that the behavior of a person is characterized by a certain responsiveness or probability of responding and speak instead of a given amount of psychic energy, we neglect many details of the actual facts and dodge the responsibility of finding a dimensional system. Lastly, mental processes are almost always conceived of as simpler and more orderly than the rather chaotic material from which they are inferred and which they are used to explain. The "learning process" in experimental psychology, for example, does not give us an accurate account of measured changes in behavior.

We look inside the organism for a *simpler* system, in which the causes of behavior are less complex than the actual hereditary and environmental events and in which the behavior of a personality is more meaningful and orderly than the day-to-day activity of the organism. All the variety and complexity of the input in our diagram seems to be reduced to a few relatively amorphous states, which in turn generate relatively amorphous functions of the personality, which then suddenly explode into the extraordinary variety and complexity of behavior. But the simplification achieved by such a practice is, of course, illusory, for it follows only from the fact that a one-to-one correspondence between inner and outer events has not been demanded. It is just this lack of correspondence which makes such an inner system unsuitable in the experimental analysis of behavior. If "hunger" is something which is produced by certain schedules of deprivation, certain drugs, certain states of health, and so on, and if in turn it produces changes in the probability of a great variety of re-

sponses, then it must have very complex properties. It cannot be any simpler than its causes or its effects. If the behavior we observe simply expresses the functioning of a personality, the personality cannot be any simpler than the behavior. If some common learning process is responsible for the changes observed in a number of different situations, then it cannot be any simpler than these changes. The apparent simplicity of the inner system explains the eagerness with which we turn to it, but from the point of view of scientific method it must be regarded as a spurious simplicity, which foreshadows ultimate failure of such an explanatory scheme.

There is another objection. Although speculation about what goes on within the organism seems to show a concern for completing a causal chain, in practice it tends to have the opposite effect. Chains are left incomplete. The layman commonly feels that he has explained behavior when he has attributed it to something in the organism—as in saying "He went *because* he wanted to go," or "He could not work *because* he was worried about his health." Such statements may have value in suggesting the relevance of one set of causes as against another, but they do not give a full explanation until it is explained *why* the person wanted to go, or *why* he was worried. Frequently this additional step is taken, but perhaps just as often these incomplete explanations bring inquiry to a dead stop.

No matter how we may wish to represent such a sequence of causal events, we cannot satisfy the requirements of interpretation, prediction, or control unless we go back to events acting upon the organism from without— events, moreover, which are observed as any event is observed in the physical and biological sciences. It is only common sense, therefore, as well as good scientific practice, to make sure that the concepts which enter into a theory of behavior are explicitly and carefully related to such events. What is needed is an operational definition of terms. This means more than simple translation. The operational method is commonly misused to patch up and preserve concepts which are cherished for extraneous and irrelevant reasons. Thus it might be possible to set up acceptable definitions of instincts, needs, emotions, memories, psychic energy, and so on, in which each term would be carefully related to certain behavioral and environmental facts. But we have no guarantee that these concepts will be the most useful when the actual functional relationships are better understood. A more reasonable program at this stage is to attempt to account for behavior without appeal to inner explanatory entities. We can do this within the accepted framework of biology, gaining thereby not only a certain personal reassurance from the prestige of a well-developed science, but an extensive set of experimental practices and dimensional systems. We shall be prevented from oversimplifying and misrepresenting the available facts because we shall not transmute our descriptions into other terms. The practical criteria of prediction and control will force us to take into account the complete causal chain in every instance. Such a program is not concerned with establishing the existence of inferred events, but with assessing the state of our knowledge.

This does not mean, of course, that the organism is conceived of as actually empty, or that continuity between input and output will not eventually be established. The genetic development of the organism and the complex interchanges between organism and environment are the subject matters of appropriate disciplines. Some day we shall know, for example, what happens when a stimulus impinges upon the surface of an organism, and what happens inside the organism after that, in a series of stages the last of which is the point at which the organism acts upon the environment and possibly changes it. At that point we lose interest in this causal chain. Some day, too, we shall know how the ingestion of food sets up a series of events, the last of which to engage our attention is a reduction in the probability of all behavior previously reinforced with similar food. Some day we may even know how to bridge the gap between the behavioral characteristics common to parents and offspring. But all these inner events will be accounted for with techniques of observation and measurement appropriate to the physiology of the various parts of the organism, and the account will be expressed in terms appropriate to that subject matter. It would be a remarkable coincidence if the concepts now used to

refer inferentially to inner events were to find a place in that account. The task of physiology is not to find hungers, fears, habits, instincts, personalities, psychic energy, or acts of willing, attending, repressing, and so on. Nor is that task to find entities or processes of which all these could be said to be other "aspects." Its task is to account for the causal relations between input and output which are the special concern of a science of behavior. Physiology should be left free to do this in its own way. Just to the extent that current conceptual systems fail to represent the relationships between terminal events correctly, they misrepresent the task of these other disciplines. A comprehensive set of causal relations stated with the greatest possible precision is the best contribution that we, as students of behavior, can make in the co-operative venture of giving a full account of the organism as a biological system.

But are we not overlooking one important source of knowledge? What about the direct observation of mental activity? The belief that the mental apparatus is available to direct inspection anticipated the scientific analysis of human behavior by many hundreds of years. It was refined by the introspective psychologists at the end of the nineteenth century into a special theory of knowledge which seemed to place the newly created science of consciousness on a par with natural science by arguing that all scientists necessarily begin and end with their own sensations and that the psychologist merely deals with these in a different way for different purposes. The notion has been revived in recent theories of perception, in which it has been suggested that the study of what used to be called "optical illusions," for example, will supply principles which help in understanding the limits of scientific knowledge. It has also been argued that the especially intimate empathic understanding which frequently occurs in psychotherapy supplies a kind of direct knowledge of the mental processes of other people. Franz Alexander and Lawrence Kubie have argued in this manner in defense of psychoanalytic practices. Among clinical psychologists Carl Rogers has actively defended a similar view. Something of the same notion may underlie the belief that the psychiatrist may better understand the psychotic if, through the use of lysergic acid, for example, he may temporarily experience similar mental conditions.

Whether the approach to human behavior which I have just outlined ignores some basic fact, whether it is unable to take into account the "stubborn fact of consciousness," is part of a venerable dispute which will not be settled here. Two points may be made, however, in evaluating the evidence from direct "introspection" of the mental apparatus. Knowledge is not to be identified with how things look to us, but rather with what we do about them. Knowledge is power because it is action. How the surrounding world soaks into the surface of our body is merely the first chapter of the story and would be meaningless were it not for the parts which follow. These are concerned with behavior. Astronomy is not how the heavens look to an astronomer. Atomic physics is not the physicist's perception of events within the atom, or even of the macroscopic events from which the atomic world is inferred. Scientific knowledge is what people *do* in predicting and controlling nature.

The second point is that knowledge depends upon a personal history. Philosophers have often insisted that we are not aware of a difference until it makes a difference, and experimental evidence is beginning to accumulate in support of the view that we should probably not know anything at all if we were not forced to do so. The discriminative behavior called knowledge arises only in the presence of certain reinforcing contingencies among the things known. Thus, we should probably remain blind if visual stimuli were never of any importance to us, just as we do not hear all the separate instruments in a symphony or see all the colors in a painting until it is worth while for us to do so.

Some interesting consequences follow when these two points are made with respect to our knowledge of events within ourselves. That a small part of the universe is enclosed within the skin of each of us, and that this constitutes a private world to which each of us has a special kind of access can scarcely be denied. But the world with which we are in contact does not for that reason have any special physical or metaphysical status. Now, it is presumably necessary to learn to observe or "know" external events, and our knowledge will consist of doing something about them. But the society from which we acquire such behavior is at a special disadvantage. It is easy to teach a child to distinguish between colors by presenting different colors and reinforcing his responses as right or wrong accordingly, but it is much more difficult to teach him to distinguish between different aches or pains, since the information as to whether his responses are right or wrong is much less reliable. It is this limited accessibility of the world within the skin, rather than its nature, which has been responsible for so much metaphysical speculation.

Terms which refer to private events tend to be used inexactly. Most of them are borrowed in the first place from descriptions of external events. (Almost all the vocabulary of emotion, for example, has been shown to be metaphorical in origin.) The consequences are well known. The testimony of the individual regarding his mental processes, feeling, needs, and so on, is, as the psychiatrist above all others has insisted, unreliable. Technical systems of terms referring to private events seldom resemble each other. Different schools of introspective psychology have emphasized different features of experience, and the vocabulary of one may occasionally be unintelligible to another. This is also true of different dynamic theories of mental life. The exponent of a "system" may show extraordinary conviction in his use of terms and in his defense of a given set of explanatory entities, but it is usually easy to find someone else showing the same conviction and defending a different and possibly incompatible system. Just as experimental psychology once found it expedient to train observers in the use of terms referring to mental events, so the education of experimental psychologists, educators, applied psychologists, psychotherapists, and many others concerned with human behavior is not always free from a certain element of indoctrination. Only in this way has it been possible to make sure that mental processes will be described by two or more people with any consistency.

Psychiatry itself is responsible for the notion that one need not be aware of the feelings, thoughts, and so on, which are said to affect behavior. The individual often behaves *as if* he were thinking or feeling in a given way although he cannot himself say that he is doing so. Mental processes which do not have the support of the testimony supplied by introspection are necessarily defined in terms of, and measured as, the behavioral facts from which they are inferred. Unfortunately, the notion of mental activity was preserved in the face of such evidence with the help of the notion of an unconscious mind. It might have been better to dismiss the concept of mind altogether as an explanatory fiction which had not survived a crucial test. The modes of inference with which we arrive at knowledge of the unconscious need to be examined with respect to the conscious mind as well. Both are conceptual entities, the relations of which to observed data need to be carefully re-examined.

In the long run the point will not be established by argument, but by the effectiveness of a given formulation in the design of productive research. An example of research on psychotic subjects which emphasizes the end terms in our diagram is the project already mentioned. This is not the place for technical details, but the rationale of this research may be relevant.* In these experiments a patient spends one or more hours daily, alone, in a small pleasant room. He is never coerced into going there, and is free to leave at any time. The room is furnished with a chair, and contains a device similar to a vending machine, which can be operated by pushing a button or pulling a plunger. The machine delivers candies, cigarettes, or substantial food, or projects colored pictures on a translucent screen. Most patients eventually operate the machine, are "reinforced" by what it delivers, and then continue to operate it daily for long periods of time—possibly a

*Dr. Harry Solomon of the Boston Psychopathic Hospital has served as co-director of the project, although the preceding arguments do not necessarily represent his views. Ogden R. Lindsley is in immediate charge and responsible for much of the overall experimental design as well as for the actual day-to-day conduct of the experiments. Support has been provided by the Office of Naval Research and by the National Institute of Mental Health. The work is being carried out at the Metropolitan State Hospital in Waltham, Massachusetts, with the co-operation of Dr. William McLaughlin, Superintendent, and Dr. Meyer Asakoff, Director of Research.

year or more. During this time the behavior is reinforced on various "schedules"—for example, once every minute or once for every thirty responses—in relation to various stimuli. The behavior is recorded in another room in a continuous curve which is read somewhat in the manner of an electrocardiogram and which permits a ready inspection and measurement of the rate of responding.

The isolation of this small living space is, of course, not complete. The patient does not leave his personal history behind as he enters the room, and to some extent what he does there resembles what he does or has done elsewhere. Nevertheless, as time goes on, the conditions arranged by the experiment begin to compose, so to speak, a special personal history, the important details of which are known. Within this small and admittedly artificial life space, we can watch the patient's behavior change as we change conditions of reinforcement, motivation, and to some extent emotion. With respect to these variables the behavior becomes more and more predictable and controllable or—as characteristic of the psychotic subject—fails to do so in specific ways.

The behavior of the patient may resemble that of a normal human or infrahuman subject in response to similar experimental conditions, or it may differ in a simple quantitative way—for example, the record may be normal except for a lower over-all rate. On the other hand, a performance may be broken by brief psychotic episodes. The experimental control is interrupted momentarily by the intrusion of extraneous behavior. In some cases it has been possible to reduce or increase the time taken by these interruptions, and to determine where during the session they will occur. As in similar work with other organisms, this quantitative and continuous account of the behavior of the individual under experimental control provides a highly sensitive base line for the observation of the effects of drugs and of various forms of therapy. For our present purposes, however, the important thing is that it permits us to apply to the psychotic a fairly rigorous formulation of behavior based upon much more extensive work under the much more propitious control of conditions obtained with other species.

This formulation is expressed in terms of input and output without reference to inner states.

The objection is sometimes raised that research of this sort reduces the human subject to the status of a research animal. Increasing evidence of the lawfulness of human behavior only seems to make the objection all the more cogent. Medical research has met this problem before and has found an answer which is available here. Thanks to the parallel work on animals, it has been possible, in some cases at least, to generate healthier behavior in men, even though at this stage we are not directly concerned with such a result.

Another common objection is that we obtain our results only through an over-simplification of conditions, and that they are therefore not applicable to daily life. But one always simplifies at the start of an experiment. We have already begun to make our conditions more complex and will proceed to do so as rapidly as the uniformity of results permits. It is possible to complicate the task of the patient without limit, and to construct not only complex intellectual tasks but such interactions between systems of behavior as are seen in the Freudian dynamisms.

One simplification sometimes complained of is the absence of other human beings in this small life space. This was, of course, a deliberate preliminary measure, for it is much more difficult to control social than mechanical stimulation and reinforcement. But we are now moving on to situations in which one patient observes the behavior of another working on a similar device, or observes that the other patient receives a reinforcement whenever he achieves one himself, and so on. In another case the patient is reinforced only when his behavior corresponds in some way to the behavior of another. Techniques for achieving extraordinarily precise competition and co-operation between two or more individuals have already been worked out with lower organisms, and are applicable to the present circumstances.

This project has, of course, barely scratched the surface of the subject of psychotic behavior. But so far as it has gone, it seems to us to have demonstrated the value of holding to the observable data. Whether or not you will all find them significant, the data we report have a special kind of simple objectivity. At least we can say: this is what a psychotic subject did under these circumstances, and this is what he failed to do under circumstances which would have had a different effect had he not been psychotic.

Although we have been able to describe and interpret the behavior observed in these experiments without reference to inner events, such references are, of course, not interdicted. Others may prefer to say that what we are actually doing is manipulating habits, needs, and so on, and observing changes in the structure of the personality, in the strength of the ego, in the amount of psychic energy available, and so on. But the advantage of this over a more parsimonious description becomes more difficult to demonstrate, as evidence of the effectiveness of an objective formulation accumulates. In that bright future to which research in psychiatry is now pointing, we must be prepared for the possibility that increasing emphasis will be placed on immediately observable data and that theories of human behavior will have to adjust themselves accordingly. It is not inconceivable that the mental apparatus and all that it implies will be forgotten. It will then be more than a mere working hypothesis to say—to return at long last to my title—that psychotic behavior, like all behavior, is part of the world of observable events to which the powerful methods of natural science apply and to the understanding of which they will prove adequate.

32.   The Psychological Model

LEONARD P. ULLMANN and LEONARD KRASNER

In the following parts of this section, we shall discuss the psychological model, starting with a brief review of elementary learning concepts. This review will be at a level that the student who used an elementary text such as Kendler (1962), Munn (1961), Hilgard (1962), or Morgan (1961) should have no difficulty. Next, we shall take up the major topics we have discussed in terms of the medical model: formulation of maladaptive behavior and the alteration of maladaptive behavior. Specifically, the parts of this section will deal with learning concepts, the formulation of maladaptive behavior, methods of behavior modification, and characteristics of the behavior therapist. The burden of the argument throughout will be that maladaptive behavior is both learned and unlearned in the same manner as all other behavior.

LEARNING THEORY CONCEPTS

At present, only the broadest, most thoroughly established concepts, those common to all learning theories, are used in a clinical setting. This may be supported by two examples of authors writing about the clinical application of learning theory. Dollard and Miller (1950) state: "All that is needed for the present purpose is a reinforcement theory in the broadest sense of those words," and Eysenck (1959): "Those points about which argument rages are usually of academic interest rather than of practical importance . . . there would be general agreement in any particular case about the optimum methods of achieving a quick rate of conditioning, or extinction. . . ."

In this book, more of those authors dealing with hospitalized subjects or children are likely to use terms derived from the work of B. F. Skinner, while authors of articles dealing with adult neurotic or sexual problems are more likely to use the language and concepts of Hull's system. One of the authors in giving the rationale on which he based his treatment, makes use of concepts drawn from Guthrie. The point is that psychologists engaged in behavior modification make use of a variety of learning theories, but their actual operations can be described with ease by any one of a number of learning theories, the fine points that differentiate the theories being relatively minute and not at present reflected in psychologists' behavior in clinical settings.

Basic to concepts of learning is the acquisition of a functional connection between an environmental stimulus and some subject response. Two major, albeit parallel, forms of learning may be noted: classical, or Pavlovian, or respondent conditioning, in which the stimulus elicits the response, and operant conditioning in which the subject must emit the response to the situation prior to the environmental event that becomes associated with and alters its frequency of occurrence in the future either by contiguity or reinforcement.*

In the Pavlovian or respondent conditioning situation, a stimulus that initially has no power to elicit a respondent behavior may come to have such power if it is associated with a stimulus that does have the power to elicit the respondent. In this situation, the pairing of the conditioned and the unconditioned stimuli is called *reinforcement* because any tendency for the response to the conditioned stimulus is facilitated by the presence of the unconditioned stimulus and the response to it. Once formed, the conditioned response undergoes systematic changes in strength depending upon the

---

---

*Guthrie's concept of contiguity avoids a theoretical difficulty involved in a strict reinforcement theory: we will say that a reinforcing stimulus is one which alters the frequency of an emitted behavior, and then at times imply that a reinforcing stimulus is defined by its effect on the frequency of behavior. This can easily lead to an embarrassing circular definition situation, which, as Dr. Lloyd Humphreys has pointed out to the authors, makes the contiguity theory preferable. While the authors agree, the preponderance of reinforcement theorists among authors in this volume led to the selection of the easier didactic procedure of a reinforcement rather than contiguity frame of reference.

arrangement of the environment. If the unconditioned stimulus is repeatedly omitted, the conditioned response gradually diminishes, and the repetition of the conditioned stimulus without reinforcement is called *extinction*. This is not a passive disappearance, but rather there is learned an inhibition or tendency not to respond. When a conditioned response to one stimulus has been acquired, other similar stimuli will also evoke the response. This observed behavior leads to the concept of *generalization,* a reaction to novel situations in accordance with their degree of similarity to familiar ones. The amount of generalization decreases as the second stimulus becomes less similar to the original conditioned stimulus. A process complementary to *generalization* is *discrimination*. Conditioned discrimination is brought about through selective reinforcement and extinction so that of two stimuli similar to each other, the one reinforced (followed by the unconditioned stimulus) will elicit the respondent while the one extinguished will not elicit the respondent.

In general, respondent behavior is associated with involuntary musculature and operant behavior is associated with voluntary musculature. From birth, the individual makes massive, random responses, both verbal and motoric. He literally "operates" on his environment, hence the Skinnerian term "operant." An operant behavior that is closely followed by a reinforcing stimulus is likely to be changed in frequency of emission. If the reinforcing stimulus is a pleasant one, for example, one that reduces some current deprivation, it is a positive reinforcement, one that increases the likelihood, when the environmental setting is repeated, of the emission of the act with which it was associated. If the reinforcing stimulus is unpleasant or aversive, the emitted behavior is less likely to occur on repetition of the circumstances. Withdrawal of an aversive stimulus is a positive reinforcing event. It is crucial to state explicitly that frequency of emitted behavior is the prime operational definition of reinforcing stimuli (although latency and amplitude may, at times, be used also). Where positive reinforcement increases emission, and negative reinforcement decreases emission, repeated absence of reinforcement leads to extinction and a return of the rate of response emission to the level observed prior to reinforcement.

We may talk of discriminative stimuli: any stimulus that marks a time or place of reinforcement, positive or negative, being presented or removed, is a discriminative stimulus. A discriminative stimulus marks the time or place when an operant will have reinforcing consequences. A discriminative stimulus does not elicit a response. Elicitation is a characteristic that holds only for respondents, that is, the green traffic light, a discriminative stimulus, does not set people going across the street in the same way that a bright light flashed in their eyes constricts their pupils. A discriminated operant is one controlled by a preceding discriminative stimulus. A person who typically responds under the control of discriminative stimuli is said to be discriminating, and the procedure of bringing an operant under such control is called discrimination. Whenever some particular stimulus, through association with reinforcement, takes on discriminative stimulus properties, then other stimuli (although not directly associated with reinforcement) will also take on discriminative stimulus properties to the extent they are similar to the original discriminative stimulus. This phenomenon is called *operant stimulus generalization*.

Discriminative stimuli may become reinforcing. On highways in California pedestrians are able to press a traffic button that will change the light for them. In order to obtain the discriminative stimulus, the green light, they perform operants, that is, push buttons. Discriminative stimuli become reinforcers with adults and comprise the major environmental stimuli that are systematically associated with reinforcement, for example, money. Reinforcers that have achieved their reinforcing powers through their prior service as discriminative stimuli are called *acquired or secondary reinforcers.*

As will be seen in this volume, particularly in Ayllon's work with hospitalized psychiatric patients and in the Harris, *et al.* work with nursery school children, attention is a very strong acquired or secondary reinforcer. For the child, it is usually necessary to obtain an adult's attention before satisfaction of other needs can be obtained. Once established, a secondary reinforcer can strengthen responses other than those used during its original establishment, and can do so with motives other than the motive prevailing during the original training.

The rate at which reinforcements are delivered may follow different patterns, and these patterns are called *schedules of reinforcement.* Reinforcement can be presented upon completion of acts or at the completion of time intervals. A ratio of reinforcement (one reinforcement for one act, one every two acts, and so forth) or an interval of reinforcement (one every ten seconds, one every minute) may be talked about. Further, these programs may be "fixed" every *n*th act (a fixed ratio) or "variable" (randomly on a one-third or one-tenth ratio). Similarly, there may be fixed interval or variable interval schedules. In general, learning is more resistant to extinction if the reinforcement is intermittent and/or variable.

An important aspect of work applying operant conditioning techniques is the method of *approximations or shaping.* Isaacs, Thomas, and Goldiamond's article in this volume describes and makes use of shaping. The experimenter reinforces only those responses that move in the direction of the final performance, which is the goal, and he extinguishes or does not reinforce all other responses. In shaping the responses, he may, in many instances, only approximate the final desired behaviors. Such selective reinforcement is a powerful tool in bringing about a "new" behavior.

A final note should be made of another technique, that of *response chaining,* in which an increasingly long set of responses is gradually built up prior to the reinforcement. It should be explicit that a schedule of reinforcement, as well as the behavior reinforced, may gradually be changed during the course of time. These procedures, all of which depend eventually upon response contingent reinforcement, both help explain the development of maladaptive behavior and provide tools for its change.

The range of acquired reinforcers, discriminative stimuli, and complex performances is great indeed. Perhaps the most important, and certainly the one given the greatest attention in traditional therapy, is language. While research reports and experimental (as distinct from theoretical) foundations do not fall within the scope of the present work, it is worth while to note that the vocal behavior c chickens (Lane, 1961), cats (Molliver 1963), and dogs (Salzinger and Waller 1962) have been brought under control c reinforcing stimuli, and that infants' smi ing (Brackbill, 1958) and vocalization (Rheingold, Gewirtz, and Ross, 1959 have been increased through respons contingent social reinforcement.

Simple performances, once estab lished, may become parts of more com plex ones. Both the increasing demand of the person's society, and his increase range due to language and communi cated experience (lectures, readings lead to increasingly complex perfor mances which become techniques fo solving further problems. Skinner (1963 talks of plans and logical analyses a discriminative stimuli, Miller and Dol lard (1941) demonstrate the learning of a relationship, imitation in animals, an Berger (1961), Kanfer and Marston (1963 and particularly Bandura and Walter (1963) have investigated, within socia reinforcement terms, vicarious reinforce ment and modeling.

The learning concepts we have jus reviewed are those of Skinner. The mos frequent alternative formulation is that o Hull. While for the present purposes, a we have mentioned, the differences be tween the two schools are of relatively lit tle importance, we will now turn to Hull' formulations. Where Skinner's concept are based on the frequency of emission o overt behaviors, Hull distinguishes be tween performance, the overt behavior and habit, the modification of the centra nervous system, which mediates learning and which is not directly measurable. A performance is the product of habi strength and drives such as hunger o thirst. Important concepts for behavio therapy, particularly of tics, are those of reactive inhibition and conditioned in hibition. All activity produces some fatigue and this fatigue produces a drive (reactive inhibition which decreases with rest) and a negative habit (conditioned in hibition). The Hullian system with its con cept of drive and mediation through habit is perhaps a stronger explanatory tool than Skinner's system and certainly lends itself more readily (compare Dollard and Miller, 1950) to the translation of psy choanalytic concepts. The Skinnerian system with its orientation to what Boring called "an empty organism" is more likely to focus on the stimulus environment rather than the internal state of the organism. With a concept of mediation and autonomic responses associated with meanings, the Hullian system may rely more heavily on Pavlovian or respondent conditioning than Skinnerian formulations. Hull's system certainly facilitates the comprehension of Wolpe's systematic desensitization procedure in which a conditioned drive, anxiety, may be inhibited by associating the appropriate stimulus with an image or other cue mediating the response to the anxiety provoking stimulus.

In closing this brief section we must add a few related points. The first is that while we have discussed operant and respondent behavior as though they were separate, in reality the two are usually intertwined and operant behaviors have respondent consequences. Especially for the behavior change techniques reported in this book, the concepts of operant and respondent conditioning, role learning and modeling, serve to complement each other. A behavior such as acting pleasantly may have genuine conditioned respondent consequences through prior association with the effects of such behavior, for example, an increase in the positive reinforcing stimuli emitted by other people (Ullmann, Krasner, and Gelfand, 1963). This leads to the concept that an important aspect of the individual's simulus environment is composed of his own behavior. Performing an appropriate behavior, studying for an exam, may, because of prior experience, lead to an increase in reinforcing stimuli. The operant behavior, studying, may reduce the autonomic consequences of being unprepared. In discussing appropriate behavior of such a molar nature we arrive at a concept of role, a group of behaviors that have been shaped by the environment to meet the expectation of others (that is, to be reinforced) as appropriate for an individual in a given situation. Just as in typing, telegraphy, or piano playing increasing skill leads to larger functional units in which particular enactments may serve as stimuli for subsequent actions, so a complex social response may be developed from fine discriminations of the stimulus situation and generalization from previous situations. The person may learn to identify situations and use his own verbal responses as stimuli, which indicate the similarity or difference of a present situation to ones which were previously punishing or rewarding. This formulation may also include the labeling of patterns of behaviors that have previously been useful such as "Do what the other person is doing" or "It is likely that what happens to him will happen to me" or "This situation—exam—is likely to be painful." The subject responds to the situation with a vocal behavior that in turn is a discriminative stimulus. Finally, just as we noted the complex association of operant and respondent behaviors at the beginning of this paragraph, we should note that the human stimulus situation is considerably more uncontrolled, complex, changeable, and filled with more useful and more irrelevant stimuli than a Skinner box. A small and selected sample of these cues is probably used to match current situations with past ones and provide the self-stimulus of a label. Responses based on self-stimulation are necessary for reasonably prompt social responses, but they may well be inaccurate, superstitious, and self-validating. However, these responses, or the stimuli that control them, may be identified and reconditioned. It is this line of reasoning, the individual's own behavior as a source of stimuli and the patterning of social behavior into roles as units of behavior that we think may offer a fruitful extension of reinforcement theory into increasingly complex areas of social behavior.

MALADAPTIVE BEHAVIOR: A PSYCHOLOGICAL FORMULATION

Maladaptive behaviors are learned behaviors, and the development and maintenance of a maladaptive behavior is no different from the development and maintenance of any other behavior. There is no discontinuity between desirable and undesirable modes of adjustment or between "healthy" and "sick" behavior. The first major implication of this view is the question of how a behavior is to be identified as desirable or undesirable, adaptive or maladaptive. The general answer we propose is that because there are no disease entities involved in the majority of subjects displaying maladaptive behavior, the designation of a behavior as pathological or not is dependent upon the individual's society. Specifically, while there are no single behaviors that would be said to be adaptive in all cultures, there are in all cultures definite expectations or roles for functioning adults in terms of familial and social responsibility. Along with role enactments, there are a full range of expected potential reinforcements. The person whose behavior is maladaptive does not fully live up to the expectations for one in his role, does not respond to all the stimuli actually present, and does not obtain the typical or maximum forms of reinforcement available to one of his status. The difference between the types of reinforcement that maintain adaptive and maladaptive behavior is that the latter is maintained by more direct and immediate forms of reinforcement than the former. Behavior that one culture might consider maladaptive, be it that of the Shaman or the paranoid, is adaptive in another culture if the person so behaving is responding to all the cues present in the situation in a manner likely to lead to his obtaining reinforcement appropriate to his status in that society. Maladaptive behavior is behavior that is considered inappropriate by those key people in a person's life who control reinforcers. Such maladaptive behavior leads to a reduction in the range or the value of positive reinforcement given to the person displaying it.

In a major article, Scott (1958) reviewed definitions of mental health in order to determine if there was available an operational definition of mental health or illness that could be used for purposes of research. His conclusion was that the current definitions were unworkable and at variance with each other. Such findings are not surprising in view of the questionable model on which a concept of "mental health" is based. Definitions of adjustment must be situation specific. In particular, by definition, a person comes to the therapist or to a hospital because someone wants to change him. That someone may be the person himself, his relatives, friends, employer, or authorities empowered to make the judgment that his behavior is a danger to himself or others so that he or his society would benefit from his treatment. This set of circumstances means that the definition of adjustment is not absolute but shifts from time to time and place to place. Further

as the number of mental health professionals increases, it is likely that the number of people specified as requiring treatment will also increase. Jerome Frank (1961, pp.6-7) summarizes this concept as follows:

An interesting, if somewhat unfortunate, consequence of the fact that social attitudes play such a big role in the definition of mental illness is that mental health education may be a two-edged sword. By teaching people to regard certain types of distress or behavioral oddities as illnesses rather than as normal reactions to life's stresses, harmless eccentricities, or moral weaknesses, it may cause alarm and increase the demand for psychotherapy. This may explain the curious fact that the use of psychotherapy tends to keep pace with its availability. The greater the number of treatment facilities and the more widely they are known, the larger the number of persons seeking their help. Psychotherapy is the only form of treatment which, at least to some extent, appear to create the illness it treats.

The next question becomes one of how we can account for the regularities of behavior seen in the "mentally ill" that compose the body of descriptive psychiatry. At a first level, as we have previously implied, these regularities may be far less frequent than is generally supposed. The grouping of people as exemplars of underlying causes or illness is a matter leading to a great deal of argument and constant revision, and expansion under sociological pressures. Textbook cases are hard to find in the psychiatric hospital because most cases manifest only a few of the specific symptoms that compose a syndrome, while many hospitalized people show specific behaviors that belong to more than one syndrome. A factor analytic approach to the question of the covariation of symptomatic behaviors is likely to indicate that classic syndromes are infrequent and may even be labels that do not reflect the behavior actually present. Another instance of this is the increasing use of the concept of premorbid adjustment (Phillips, 1953) or the process-reactive continuum (Ullmann and Giovannoni, 1964) to predict differential responses to stimulus situations either within or across major diagnostic categories. In short, the regularities presupposed by a medical model may not exist.

At a second level there is a matter of role learning. Any behavior that increases positive reinforcement or helps reduce aversive stimuli is likely to be increased. A person who is "sick" is considered unlucky, excused from responsibility, and a proper object of pity and forebearance. In our society, the patient is one who bears or endures suffering without complaint, who is long-suffering, and who is acted upon and receives treatment. At the present time, the person who is a mental patient is frequently considered incompetent legally and yet is in a position to demand attention and forgiveness from his peers. Just as the manifestations of the hypnotic role have changed over time, so have the manifestations of the mentally ill role changed over time and, during the same period, from one social class to another. Illustrations of this are the greater frequency of psychosomatic ills among officers than enlisted men during World War II, the decrease of hysterical symptoms, and the different patterns of maladaptive behavior in different social classes. Kelly (1955, p. 366) notes: "It seemed to the writer, in comparing the complaints of psychologically sophisticated people with those of the psychologically naive, that there was a definite tendency, once a person had chosen a psychological name for his discomfort, to display all of the symptoms in whatever book he had read, even if he had to practice them diligently. It suggested that psychological symptoms may frequently be interpreted as the rationale by which one's chaotic experiences are given a measure of structure and meaning."

The psychiatrist or other mental health professional may do much to foster the regularities supposedly seen in mental illness. During the diagnostic interview, the psychiatrist will focus on, and thereby reinforce with attention, the material that is meaningful to him. Hollingworth (1930, pp. 233-236) makes this point very clearly in his discussion of symptoms rendered vivid by attention. He describes how a medical examination may emphasize complaints: ". . . it is astonishing to find how many bodily sensations have hitherto escaped attention and now clamor for report. Fixation upon them, prolonged attention to them, minute scrutiny of them, increases their vividness, and they now stand out with distinctness. This is the characteristic effect of attention everywhere." (p. 234). If there is pressure to

admit a person to the hospital, the psychiatrist will look for behaviors that are symptomatic and permit the statement that a particular syndrome exists. Once this has been accomplished, he can make a medical decision, a diagnosis, and hospitalize the individual. The patient is shaped into giving the physician what is wanted and expected.

Once within the hospital, there are strong pressures on the individual to assume the proper passive, non-troublesome "good patient" role. In particular, the nursing assistants or attendants have the responsibility to keep large groups of patients safe, clean, quiet, and cooperative. The aide culture (Belknap, 1956; Dunham and Weinberg, 1960; Goffman, 1961; Lehrman, 1961) can impose a strong set of explicit reinforcements to obtain expected behavior. Among these are the granting of privileges such as freedom of movement, passes, better accommodations, and the threat of punishment such as electroconvulsive therapy and transfer to a ward peopled by more disturbed patients. The apathy and withdrawal that are the most difficult and prognostically unfavorable symptoms of schizophrenia may well arise from the training given the patient not to be assertive or insistent upon his legitimate human rights. In the typical hospital setting, there is also a marked decrease in normal social contact and sensory stimulation. A number of authors have hypothesized that the social and sensory deficits involved in this situation parallel the production of behaviors similar to psychoses observed in sensory deprivation experiments (McReynolds, Acker, and Daily, 1959). The psychological correlates of playing a particular role and the physical conditions of diet, exercise, and living accommodations may lead to biochemical similarities that are the results and not the cause of hospitalization (Kety, 1960).

While perhaps less severe, there is definite role training observed in outpatient treatment. We shall return to this matter, particularly in the work of Goldstein (1962), when we discuss traditional therapy as behavior therapy. At this point we merely wish to indicate that it is possible to build a case for patients learning the regularities expected of them.

Let us turn to a more intensive analysis of the development of specific symptoms within a learning theory context. Again, for purposes of exposition, we will make distinctions between operant and respondent behavior when in fact the two are intertwined.

In terms of respondent or "surplus conditioned reactions" (Eysenck, 1959), we shall describe the concepts and terminology of Wolpe (1954). However, we have reservations about the usefulness of a drive concept; and the concept of "anxiety" currently has so many extraneous and poorly defined uses as to be a hindrance at times rather than an aid in communication (English and English, 1958, p. 35; Sarbin, 1963). To quote Wolpe (1954): "By 'anxiety' is meant the autonomic response pattern or patterns that are characteristically part of the organism's response to noxious stimulation. . . . An anxiety response is unadaptive when it is evoked in circumstances in which there is objectively no threat." Such responses occur within the paradigm of classic or Pavlovian conditioning. A noxious stimulus is paired with a previously indifferent stimulus, and at a later time the previously neutral stimulus alone elicits the response appropriate to the prior situation (when the noxious stimulus was present), but which is no longer adaptive or appropriate. Watson and Rayner (1920) present the experimental development of a phobia, complete with generalization, by this technique. Moss (1924) used a similar procedure to establish food aversion in two children and anecdotal material illustrative of this point abounds (Burnham, 1924). On a more general level, we may quote Eysenck (1959):

Many conditioned responses are unadaptive, and consequently may embarrass the individual and even drive him into a mental hospital if sufficiently intense. Yet other conditioned responses are obviously necessary and desirable; indeed, many of them are indispensable for survival. It has been argued very strongly that the whole process of socialization is built up on the principle of conditioning; the overt display of aggressive and sexual tendencies is severely punished in the child, thus producing conditioned fear and pain responses (anxiety) to situations in which the individual is likely to display such tendencies. He consequently refrains from acting in the forbidden manner . . . because only by not indulging, and physically removing himself can he relieve the very painful conditioned anxiety responses to the whole situation. Anxiety thus acts as a mediating drive. . . .

Another way in which this might be put is that the behaviors that reduce the likelihood of aversive stimuli are positively reinforcing and likely to recur. A result is the avoidance of objects, situations, acts, and so forth, that have been associated with noxious stimuli. However, there is likely to be generalization, and in the very nature of withdrawal, a failure to differentiate between those elements of a situation from which it is adaptive to withdraw and those from which it is maladaptive to withdraw. Similarly, a behavior that has been associated with termination of aversive stimuli is likely to be repeated, even if such a behavior had no association with the reinforcement other than contiguity. Other responses may be continued because they were once appropriate to situations that were similar in some aspect irrelevant to the realities of the current situation. The reader's attention is called to our previous comment that the human stimulus situation is uncontrolled, complex, changeable, and filled with cues that are both relevant and irrelevant. This situation leads to responses to situations based on a limited sample of the available cues. Hollingworth's formulation of maladaptive behavior as redintegrated reactions (Hollingworth, 1930, pp. 249–255) is particularly germane. A major difference between physical and mental reactions is the response to symbols of the situation rather than reinstitution of all the original stimuli. "Mental processes . . . are those in which a partial stimulus serves adequately or approximately to provoke responses formerly occasioned only by more elaborate situations." (Hollingworth, 1930, p. 249). The eliciting of a response by a partial detail of its former antecedent is what Hollingworth means by redintegration. Hollingworth (1930, p. 250) writes:

. . . the response may be overdetermined by the detail, without due regard to other features now occurring with it. The response is thus determined by past contexts rather than by present contexts. It is therefore likely to be bizarre, inutile, maladjusted, and hence neurotic. Prepotency of special cues or fragments of a situation may thus result in ineffective adjustment to that situation. Effective adjustment demands that all present facts be allowed to constellate, to *determine jointly* the nature of the response. Individuals in whom this synergy or adequate cooperation of all the details of a situation does not effectively take place are lacking in a characteristic which we may for convenience call *scope* or *sagacity*.

For purposes of exposition, we may distinguish between an adaptive response that has not been learned and a maladaptive response that now must be changed.

In terms of deficient prior learning, we may conceive of a person who was isolated and socially withdrawn as a child. Such a person is less likely to have practiced, been reinforced for, and learned effective social skills. This deficit in training may make future social situations less rewarding and lead to the development of a vicious cycle. The development of attention and interest is exemplified by Birnbrauer *et al.* in the present volume. Another example of this area is the treatment of enuresis. The association between bladder tension and wakefulness may be taught within a simple conditioning paradigm. In terms of symptom substitution, it is interesting that Mowrer and Mowrer (1938) who made the major breakthrough in this area write: "Personality changes, when any have occurred as a result of the application of the present method of treating enuresis, have uniformly been in a favorable direction. In no case has there been any evidence of 'symptom substitution.' " Morgan and Witmer (1939), Davidson and Douglass (1950), and Geppert (1953) are among authors who also remark on the general personality improvement associated with overcoming enuresis by conditioning techniques. In short, there may have been a simple failure to learn a particular behavior that can be taught easily.

A second group of maladaptive behaviors may be learned through operant conditioning. The behavior is associated with positive reinforcement of some sort. In the present volume, the child in the report by Wolf, *et al.* found that the maladaptive behavior, vomiting, through misguided kindness, led to release from a potentially uncomfortable situation. When the reinforcement maintaining the behavior, release from the situation, ceased, the maladaptive response to the situation decreased and finally ceased. Mees (1964) summarizes the general principle: "If you want an explanation for this behavior—this monster behavior—I believe we can account for all of it with one general principle: *it pays off*. It pays

off for the individual who can't seem to find other, nonmonstrous behaviors to get him what he wants."

Patterns of behaviors are increased, shaped, and maintained through reinforcement. If a person emits a behavior and reinforcement follows soon after, the frequency with which that behavior will be emitted in the future is altered. In terms of the development of maladaptive behavior, we have mentioned the work of Watson and Rayner (1920) and Moss (1924). To this, we may add the Haughton and Ayllon work on the production and elimination of symptomatic behavior printed in this book. In this work, a person for whom cigarettes were reinforcing was handed a broom and given a cigarette. Broom holding became a stimulus associated with being given cigarettes, and the person developed the "bizarre, maladaptive" behavior of holding a broom and refusing to let it go. In another article, Ayllon and Haughton (1964) systematically manipulated the symptomatic verbal behavior of three patients. When the staff responded with interest and attention to bizarre talk, these verbalizations increased in frequency. Withholding social reinforcement (extinction) resulted in a decrease in the frequency of symptomatic verbal responses. The articles in the first section of this book illustrate operant techniques to promote adjustive responses, but, by implication, if adjustive responses are under stimulus control, we may hypothesize that so are maladjustive ones. In studies in which either control groups or periods of no reinforcement (extinction) have been used, Salzinger and Pisoni (1958, 1961) and Weiss, Krasner, and Ullmann (1963) have illustrated that affect self-references and use of emotional words by hospitalized patients may be altered by reinforcement. Many people have posited that a crucial symptom in schizophrenia is disorganization of thinking. Sommer, Witney, and Osmond (1962) have increased, through selective reinforcement of desirable responses, the frequency of common associations of hospitalized patients in a word association situation. Ullmann, Krasner, and Edinger (1964) replicated this result, and perhaps as noteworthy, found that even with long-term schizophrenic patients, the non-reinforced control group decreased in their rate of emission of common associations. Work on nursery school behavior, Allen *et al.* with social isolation, Harris *et al.* with regressed crawling, and Hart *et al.* with operant crying, illustrate with the same paradigm used by Ayllon and Haughton (1964) that these behaviors may be increased or decreased contingent upon adult attention. These three studies of nursery school behavior indicate clearly how a behavior "paying off" may lead to its increase. Finally, avoidance of aversive stimuli is reinforcing: stuttering was instigated in three normally fluent subjects when a persistent shock was introduced and its cessation for a brief period was made contingent upon nonfluent verbal behavior (Flanagan, Goldiamond, and Azrin, 1959). In our introductions to specific groups of case histories, we shall offer additional material, but at the present, we may point to the instigation and manipulation (both increase and decrease) of maladaptive behavior through procedures of reinforcement. While there are relatively few studies that set out to develop maladaptive responses to stimuli, every article that utilizes a psychological technique for the direct alteration of adaptive behavior buttresses by implication this formulation of the development of maladaptive behavior.

A question that follows the development of maladaptive responses is why, or more accurately how, these behavior patterns are maintained. The answer is by the same manner, reinforcement, as they were developed. Some of the evidence for this may be found in the articles cited in the previous paragraph. Further evidence comes from the effect of removing reinforcement (such as attention) in articles such as those of Ayllon and Ayllon and Michael. Additional material appears in the Isaacs, Thomas, and Goldiamond article in which a previously mute patient verbalized his wishes with those people who did not respond to his gestures, but continued to be mute with those people with whom the nonverbal behavior was effective. Williams' article on temper tantrums provides an instance of a relapse, a naturalistic experiment similar to the systematic instances reported in the group of nursery school papers previously cited. In Ayllon, "emotional responses" which, if reinforced, might have become highly frequent behaviors, did not become so due to being ignored. The current reinforce-

ment obtained for maladaptive behavior need not be the same as the reinforcement that led to the development of the behavior: *all* that is argued is that the maladaptive behavior is maintained by some reinforcement. An example may make this point clear. A person known to the authors once had a roommate who snored. To drown out the snoring he started using a second pillow to cover his ear. A pillow over the ear was associated with reinforcement, going to sleep, and became a discriminative stimulus for sleeping. Ten years after the original situation he continued to have difficulty going to sleep without a second, covering pillow. Although the original stimulus, the snoring roommate, was no longer present, the behavior continued because it was still associated with a pleasant stimulus, that is, going to sleep. Reinforcing stimuli can, particularly in humans, be different from the stimuli in the original situation. It is neither parsimonious nor necessary to explain behavior by either functional autonomy or underlying causes. It goes without saying that we doubt whether analyzing the dynamics of the comfort pattern of clinging to a soft, white object, such as a pillow, first observed when the subject was separated from his home and mother, would be particularly useful in changing the behavior.

We have noted that because there is no distinction between the development and maintenance of adaptive and maladaptive behavior, what we say of one applies to the other. For this reason, in line with our discussion of the maintenance of maladaptive behavior, we would now like to turn to the generalization of gains made in the professional behavior modification setting to the extra-therapy environment. The explicit techniques for the alteration of maladaptive behavior and fostering of new, more adaptive behavior, will be discussed in the next part of this introduction. But if we assume that the new behavior has developed, we may offer a number of means by which it is maintained.

First and foremost, the new behavior pays off. It is more likely to lead to reinforcement. Lazarus' case (1959) of a boy treated with Wolpe's (1958, pp. 184-185) anxiety-relief technique for sleeping with his mother is an example. The new behavior was welcomed by both parents and the siblings, and the entire family situation was changed. In short, because the subject's behavior leads to responses from other people, a new pattern of behavior by the subject puts him in a new environment. This point is important because evocative therapists typically argue that the person must be "basically" changed (for example, his ego strengthened) before he can withstand the stress of returning to the environment in which he had previously developed a pattern of maladaptive behavior. Using this concept as a solution, alternative, or supplement, expressive therapists are likely to press for the treatment of parents so that they will solve *their* problems.

People who are likely to be important in regard to the maintenance of new adaptive behavior can be taught and literally programed as alternate therapists. In the present volume there are many examples of this. In Ayllon and Michael's and Bachrach, Erwin, and Mohr's articles we will see the nurse being given instructions as to her behavior toward hospitalized patients. In Wolf, Risley, and Mees' article, an aide who worked with the child in the hospital went home with him to teach the parents. Davison discusses the training of college undergraduates for work with severely disturbed children. Parents play a key role in selecting and reinforcing behavior in papers by Rickard and Mundy (stuttering), Patterson (school phobia), Williams (temper tantrums), Bentler (phobia), Peterson and London, and Madsen (toilet training). School teachers play a key role in the majority of the work with children in social situations, and retardates. Finally, in Sulzer's paper we will see the subject's friends making their reinforcing behavior contingent on his not drinking. It is important to note that this approach is readily understandable to parents and other significant people in the child's environment and thus may lead to a rapid and hearty adoption by them. For example, Jersild and Holmes (1935) discuss the techniques that parents devised to overcome children's fears, and the most effective of these closely parallel the reconditioning techniques that are presented in this book. A second point is that these techniques are more likely to be accepted and utilized by those members of the lower social classes who are likely to have difficulty in utilizing more traditional forms of psychotherapy (Hollingshead and Red-

lich, 1958). There are many parents who do not value self-insight and neither understand nor believe in the efficacy of working on their basic problems to alleviate their child's maladaptive behavior. For those people, who may well expect prescription and direction, withdrawal from therapy follows a rigid approach which assumes that the focus of difficulty lies in them. By accepting whatever the parent has been doing as evidence of good faith, the person interested in behavior modification can reduce the parents' feelings of inadequacy and pave the way for the development of more effective parental responses to the child's behavior. The therapist's goal is to program the parents to respond to and nurture the desired changes toward adaptive behavior. Behavior therapy may extend the number of cases the therapist is likely to undertake. For example, Phillips notes that with his assertion-structured therapy 53 of 59 patients entered therapy and 51 of these 53 obtained benefit in an average of less than eight sessions. In contrast, at the same clinic, and with no noticeable bias of assignment, of 190 cases initially interviewed 103 were judged unsuitable for treatment by psychoanalytically oriented therapists, 42 refused therapy themselves, and the remaining 45 completed a course of therapy averaging 17 sessions. For approximately 75 per cent of these 45 cases, benefit was reported. Aside from the difference in the rate of benefit of those actually undergoing treatment, the assertion-structured approach was found serviceable in a far greater proportion of the population that came for help. Thus behavior therapy may have an additional value in terms of the scope of the population served. Finally, behavior may be maintained by subject feedback. An obvious aspect of this is the increase of positive environmental reinforcement. Another aspect is that certain new behaviors are inconsistent with other maladaptive behaviors. An example may be found in the Ayllon and Michael article in which, with self-feeding and a considerable weight gain, an "untreated" delusion of poisoned food ceased. It seems reasonable to hypothesize that hearty self-feeding is a behavior incompatible with the claim of poisoned food. There is also a matter of generalization: as Eysenck (1959) has noted, removal of one symptom, rather than exacerbating or leading to development of new symptoms, facilitates removal of other maladaptive behaviors. On one level, the person observes that he can be different and can change. On a different level of abstraction, it seems reasonable that if maladaptive responses can generalize, a technique that has been adaptive in one situation will also be tried out as a response to other situations. Finally, as we noted in our discussion of learning concepts, operant and respondent behaviors are intertwined and a considerable portion of the subject's environment is composed of his own behavior. We may hypothesize that this part of the environment is appreciably changed for the better as he emits more adaptive responses. In short, there are many ways in which behavior, whether adaptive or maladaptive, can be maintained without reference to an underlying, historical cause.

References

Ayllon, T., and Haughton, E. Control of the behavior of schizophrenic patients by food. *J. exp. Anal. Behav.*, 1962, *5*, 343–352.

Bandura, A., and Walters, R. H. *Social learning and personality development*. New York: Holt, Rinehart and Winston, Inc., 1963.

Belknap, I. *Human problems of a state mental hospital*. New York: McGraw-Hill, 1956.

Berger, S. M. Incidental learning through vicarious reinforcement. *Psychol. Rep.*, 1961, *9*, 477–491.

Brackbill, Yvonne. Extinction of the smiling response in infants as a function of reinforcement schedule. *Child Develpm.*, 1958, *29*, 115–124.

Burnham, W. H. *The normal mind*. New York: Appleton, 1924.

Davidson, J. R., and Douglass, E. Nocturnal enuresis: a special approach to treatment. *Brit. Med. J.*, 1950, *1*, 1345–1347.

Dollard, J., and Miller, N. E. *Personality and psychotherapy*. New York: McGraw-Hill, 1950.

Dunham, H. W., and Weinberg, S. K. *The culture of the state mental hospital*. Detroit: Wayne State University Press, 1960.

English, H. B., and English, Ava C. *A comprehensive dictionary of psychological and psychoanalytical terms: a guide to usage*. New York: Longmans, 1958.

Eysenck, H. J. Learning theory and behaviour therapy. *J. ment. Sci.*, 1959, *105*, 61–75. (In Eysenck, 1960a)

Flanagan, B., Goldiamond, I., and Azrin, N. H. Instatement of stuttering in normally fluent individuals through operant procedures. *Science*, 1959, *130*, 979–981.

Frank, J. D. *Persuasion and healing*. Baltimore: Johns Hopkins Press, 1961.

Geppert, T. V. Management of nocturnal enuresis by conditioned response. *J. Amer. med. Ass.*, 1953, *152*, 381–383.

Goffman, E. *Asylums*. New York: Anchor Books, 1961.

Goldstein, A. P. *Therapist-patient expectancies in psychotherapy*. New York: Pergamon, 1962.

Hilgard, E. R. *Introduction to psychology* (3rd ed.). New York: Harcourt, 1962.

Hollingshead, A. B. and Redlich, F. C. *Social class and mental illness*. New York: Wiley, 1958.

Hollingworth, H. L. *Abnormal psychology*. New York: Ronald, 1930.

Jersild, A. T., and Holmes, Frances B. Methods of overcoming children's fears. *J. Psychol.*, 1935, *1*, 75–104.

Kanfer, F. H., and Marston, A. R. Human reinforcement: vicarious and direct. *J. exp. Psychol.*, 1963, *65*, 292–296.

Kelly, G. A. *The psychology of personal constructs*. New York: Norton, 1955. 2 vols.

Kendler, H. K. *Basic psychology*. New York: Appleton, 1962.

Kety, S. S. Recent biochemical theories of schizophrenia. In D. D. Jackson (Ed.), *The etiology of schizophrenia*. New York: Basic Books, 1960.

Lane, H. Operant control of vocalizing in the chicken. *J. exp. Anal. Behav.*, 1961, *4*, 171–177.

Lazarus, A. A. The elimination of children's phobias by deconditioning. *Med. Proc. S. Afr.*, 1959, *5*, 261–265. (In Eysenck, 1960a)

Lehrman, N. S. Do our hospitals help make acute schizophrenia chronic? *Dis. nerv. Syst.*, 1961, *22*, 489–493.

McReynolds, P., Acker, Mary, and Daily, J. On the effects of perceptual enhancement on certain schizophrenic symptoms. *Res. Rept. V A Palo Alto*, 1959, No. 1.

Mees, H. How to create a monster. Unpublished manuscript, 1964.

Miller, N. E., and Dollard, J. *Social learning and imitation*. New Haven: Yale University Press, 1941.

Molliver, M. E. Operant control of vocal behavior in the cat. *J. exp. Anal. Behav.*, 1963, *6*, 197–202.

Morgan, C. T. *Introduction to psychology*. (2nd ed.) New York: McGraw-Hill, 1961.

Morgan, J. J. B., and Witmer, Frances J. The treatment of enuresis by the conditioned reaction technique. *J. genet. Psychol.*, 1939, *55*, 59–65.

Moss, F. A. Note on building likes and dislikes in children. *J. exp. Psychol.*, 1924, *7*, 475–478.

Mowrer, O. H., and Mowrer, Willie M. Enuresis: a method for its study and treatment. *Amer. J. Orthopsychiat.*, 1938, *8*, 436–459.

Munn, N. L. *Psychology*. (4th ed.) New York: Houghton Mifflin, 1961.

Phillips, E. L. *Psychotherapy: a modern theory and practice*. Englewood Cliffs, N.J.: Prentice-Hall, 1956.

Phillips, L. Case history data and prognosis in schizophrenia. *J. nerv. ment. Dis.*, 1953, *117*, 515–525.

Rheingold, Harriet L., Gerwitz, J. L., and Ross, Helen W. Social conditioning of vocalizations in the infant. *J. comp. physiol. Psychol.*, 1959, *52*, 68–73.

Salzinger, K., and Pisoni, Stephanie. Reinforcement of affect responses of schizophrenics during the clinical interview. *J. abnorm. soc. Psychol.*, 1958, *57*, 84–90.

Salzinger, K., and Pisoni, Stephanie. Some parameters of the conditioning of verbal affect responses in schizophrenic subjects. *J. abnorm. soc. Psychol.*, 1961, *63*, 511–516.

Salzinger, K., and Waller, M. B. The operant control of vocalization in the dog. *J. exp. Anal. Behav.*, 1962, *5*, 383–389.

Sarbin, T. R. Anxiety: the reification of a metaphor. Paper presented to West. Psychiat. Assoc., San Francisco, Sept. 1963.

Scott, W. A. Research definitions of mental health and mental illness. *Psychol. Bull.*, 1958, *55*, 29–45.

Skinner, B. F. Operant behavior. *Amer. Psychologist*, 1963, *18*, 503–515.

Sommer, R., Witney, Gwynneth, and Osmond, H. Teaching common associations to schizophrenics. *J. abnorm. soc. Psychol.*, 1962, *65*, 58–61.

Ullmann, L. P., and Giovannoni, Jeanne M. The development of a self-report measure of the process-reactive continuum. *J. nerv. ment. Dis.*, 1964, *138*, 38–42.

Ullmann, L. P., Krasner, L., and Edinger, R. L. Verbal conditioning of common associations in long-term schizophrenic patients. *Behav. Res. Ther.*, 1964, *2*, 15–18.

Ullmann, L. P., Krasner, L., and Gelfand, Donna M. Changed content within a reinforced response class. *Psychol. Rep.*, 1963, *12*, 819–829.

Watson, J. B., and Rayner, Rosalie. Conditioned emotional reactions. *J. exp. Psychol.*, 1920, *3*, 1–14. (In Eysenck, 1960a)

Weiss, R., Krasner, L., and Ullmann, L. P. Responsivity of psychiatric patients to verbal conditioning: "success" and "failure" conditions and patterns of reinforced trials. *Psychol. Rep.*, 1963, *12*, 423–426.

Wolpe, J. Reciprocal inhibition as the main basis of psychotherapeutic effects. *AMA Arch. Neurol. Psychiat.*, 1954, *72*, 205–226. (In Eysenck, 1960a)

Wolpe, J. *Psychotherapy by reciprocal inhibition.* Stanford, Calif.: Stanford University Press, 1958.

ETIOLOGY AND DEVELOPMENT

Behaviorists are concerned minimally with when and what is learned. The specific events which may be associated with the development of pathological behavior interest them little; what they have to say on this score usually is a rewording of the speculations of the intrapsychic theorists. Their distinction lies in proposing a limited number of rigorously derived principles which can account for a wide variety of learned pathological behavior patterns. Behaviorists are wary of the excessive number of empirically unanchored concepts included in intrapsychic theory, and propose that all behavior—normal or pathological—can be reduced to a few objective principles and concepts. Their focus on the process of learning in behavioral pathology, rather than on the content of what is learned, has added a precision and clarity to the study of psychopathology that has been sorely lacking.

The excerpts reprinted here from papers by John Dollard and Neal Miller and by Albert Bandura and Richard Walters illustrate how these basic learning principles can be applied in the analysis of pathological behavior.

33. How Symptoms Are Learned

JOHN DOLLARD and NEAL E. MILLER

PHOBIAS

In a phobia acquired under traumatic conditions of combat the relevant events are recent and well known. Such cases provide one of the simplest and most convincing illustrations of the learning of a symptom.

The essential points are illustrated by the case of a pilot who was interviewed by one of the authors. This officer had not shown any abnormal fear of airplanes before being sent on a particularly difficult mission to bomb distant and well-defended oil refineries. His squadron was under heavy attack on the way to the target. In the confusion of flying exceedingly low over the target against strong defensive fire, a few of the pre-

ceding planes made a wrong turn and dropped their bombs on the section that had been assigned to the pilot's formation. Since not enough bombs were dropped to destroy the installations, the pilot's formation had to follow them to complete the job. As they came in above the rooftops, bombs and oil tanks were exploding. The pilot's plane was tossed violently about and damaged while nearby planes disappeared in a wall of fire. Since this pilot's damaged plane could not regain altitude, he had to fly back alone at reduced speed and was subject to repeated violent fighter attack which killed several crew members and repeatedly threatened to destroy them all. When they finally reached the Mediterranean, they were low on gas and had to ditch the airplane in the open sea. The survivors drifted on a life raft and eventually were rescued.

Many times during this mission the pilot was exposed to intensely fear-

From *Personality and Psychotherapy* by John Dollard and Neal E. Miller, copyright 1950, used by permission of McGraw-Hill Book Company and the authors.

provoking stimuli such as violent explosions and the sight of other planes going down and comrades being killed. It is known that intense fear-provoking stimuli of this kind act to reinforce fear as a response to other cues present at the same time.* In this case the other cues were those from the airplane, its sight and sound, and thoughts about flying. We would therefore expect the strong drive of intense fear to be learned as a response to all of these cues.

When a strong fear has been learned as a response to a given set of cues, it tends to generalize to other similar ones (Miller, 1950). Thus one would expect the fear of this airplane and of thoughts about flying it to generalize to the similar sight and sound of other airplanes and thoughts about flying in them. This is exactly what happened; the pilot felt strongly frightened whenever he approached, looked at, or even thought about flying in any airplane.

Because he had already learned to avoid objects that he feared, he had a strong tendency to look away and walk away from all airplanes. Whenever he did this, he removed the cues eliciting the fear and hence felt much less frightened. A reduction in any strong drive such as fear serves to reinforce the immediately preceding responses. Therefore we would expect any response that produced successful avoidance to be learned as a strong habit. This is what occurred; the pilot developed a strong phobia of airplanes and everything connected with them.

Similarly, he felt anxious when thinking or talking about airplanes and less anxious when he stopped thinking or talking about them. The reduction in anxiety reinforced the stopping of thinking or of talking about airplanes; he became reluctant to think about or discuss his experience.

To summarize, under traumatic conditions of combat the intense drive of fear was learned as a response to the airplane and everything connected with it. The fear generalized from the cues of this airplane to the similar ones of other airplanes. This intense fear motivated responses of avoiding airplanes, and whenever any one of these responses was successful, it was reinforced by a reduction in the strength of the fear.

When all of the circumstances are understood, as in this case, there is no mystery about the phobia. In fact, such things as the avoidance of touching hot stoves or stepping in front of speeding cars usually are not called "phobias" because the conditions reinforcing the avoidance are understood. Our contention is that the laws of learning are exactly the same, although the conditions are often different and much more obscure, especially when the fear is elicited by the internal cues of thoughts or drives.

Fear Aroused by Drive to Perform a Punished Response. The way fear can be elicited by the temptation to perform a forbidden act is illustrated in the case of a four-year-old boy who showed a sudden and prolonged flare-up of extreme resistance to going to bed. Previously the little boy had only shown the normal reluctance. Suddenly this became greatly intensified. He protested at having to leave his toys, asked for extra bedtime stories, came down repeatedly for drinks of water, was found sitting at the head of the stairs, expressed various fears of the bedroom that were hard for the parents to understand, and had to be put back to bed as many as fifteen or twenty times in a single night.

The parents realized that their child was seriously disturbed but could not figure out why; they were baffled and annoyed. At first they thought that the main interest of the child, who was an only child, was staying up with adults. As they took increasingly firm measures to keep him out of the living room so that they could lead a semblance of a normal social life, they found him sleeping in strange and uncomfortable places such as the threshold of the entrance to the bedroom, in the hall, and even on the stairs. It began to appear that his real motivation was to avoid his bed. Occasionally he would go to sleep wearing two pairs of pants in spite of the fact that it was the middle of the summer in a hot Midwestern city.

The parents tried everything they could think of but nothing seemed to help. Finally they took him to a clinic. There the following facts were gradually pieced together. The mother had had a much younger brother who was severely punished for masturbation during his infancy and so she had resolved that she was never going to treat her own children like that. She began by giving this child com-

---

*For a similar analysis of other combat cases, see Dollard (1945).

plete freedom in this respect and then gradually made him understand that he could masturbate only when he was alone or in his own house without strangers being present. The trouble about going to bed began shortly after a new maid was hired. The mother remembered that the afternoon before the trouble started the little boy had reported to her that the maid had said he was nasty and had slapped him "like she slaps her own little boys." Because the maid seemed so gentle and affectionate the mother had doubted this, and in the face of these doubts the little boy had guessed that he had imagined it. Later the maid was observed to tell the little boy that he was nasty when she found him fingering his penis and was privately told to ignore this kind of behavior. The symptom had faded away somewhat during the week the maid was absent to take care of her sick mother and flared up again when the maid returned.

On the advice of the psychiatrist at the clinic, the mother made it perfectly clear to the child that the maid was not to punish him for masturbating; she dramatized this by making the maid apologize to him and say that she was wrong in calling him nasty. After this the extreme resistance to going to bed suddenly disappeared, with only a few minor recurrences that were easily met by further reassurance. There was also a marked improvement in the child's cooperativeness and happy, independent spontaneity.

In this case it seems fairly evident that punishment and disapproval from the maid had attached fear to the response of masturbation. The child seems to have been more strongly tempted to masturbate when he was alone in bed. Thus the fear was aroused in bed. (It is also possible that some of the punishments were administered in bed, but unfortunately we have no evidence on this point.) Whenever the child approached the bed or was told to go to bed, his fear was increased; any response that took him away from bed was reinforced by a reduction in the strength of this fear. He learned a variety of such responses. Putting on the two pairs on pants probably also tended to reduce the fear of masturbating in bed, not by physical escape but by covering up the penis. When the fear of masturbation was reduced, the motivation to perform all of these responses (*i.e.,* symptoms)

was removed. Freedom from this source of anxiety and conflict also improved the lad's general mood.

Origin of Response. When the fear-provoking stimulus is clearly circumscribed (like a hot radiator), the avoidance response that reduces the fear often occurs immediately with relatively little trial and error. Apparently it is either an innate response or is learned early in life and quickly generalized to new situations containing the similar element of a localized fear-provoking stimulus. In cases in which direct avoidance is physically or socially difficult (like dealing with the school bully), the individual may show considerable trial and error, reasoning and planning. Once the responses producing successful avoidance are elicited by any one of these means, they are reinforced by the reduction in the strength of fear and quickly learned as strong habits.

Origin of Fear. In phobias, the origin of the responses of avoidance and the way they produce the reinforcing reduction in fear is usually quite clear. The origin of the fear is often obscure, stemming from the childhood conflicts about sex and aggression that were described in the preceding chapter. Further research is needed to enable us to describe in terms of rigorous behavior principles and social conditions all the detailed steps intervening between infancy and adulthood.

How Fear is Transferred to New Cues. Theoretically one would expect the strong fears involved in phobias to transfer to new cues in a number of different ways:

1. PRIMARY STIMULUS GENERALIZATION. When a person learns to fear one situation, he should also tend to fear other similar ones. Stimuli more similar to the original traumatic ones should elicit stronger generalized fear. This is called a *gradient of generalization*.

2. HIGHER-ORDER CONDITIONING. After strong fear is learned as a response to certain cues, they will serve as learned (*i.e.,* secondary) reinforcing agents so that any cues that consistently precede them will acquire the ability to elicit fear (Pavlov, 1927).

3. SECONDARY, OR RESPONSE-MEDIATED, GENERALIZATION. When the fear is attached to response-produced cues, any new stimulus that becomes able to

elicit the response producing these cues will arouse the fear they elicit. For example, a young man may have fear attached to the cues produced by the first incipient responses of sexual excitement. Then if a previously indifferent girl is labeled "sexy," she may arouse incipient responses of sexual excitement which in turn elicit fear.

When a response produces the cues eliciting the fear, any increase in the drive motivating that response will be expected to cause it to generalize to a greater variety of stimulus situations. In other words, when the young man's sex urge increases, he will be expected to find a wider variety of situations sexually exciting and, hence, frightening. Conversely, when his sexual motivation is low, only the most provocative situations will be exciting and, hence, frightening. In short, the variety of situations feared will be expected to vary with the strength of the drive motivating the response mediating the fear.

Extinction of Phobias. If a response to a given cue continues to be repeated without reinforcement, it gets progressively weaker. This is called *extinction*. It will be remembered that such experimental evidence as we have seems to indicate that the internal "response" of fear follows the same laws in this respect also and is subject to extinction. In the case of a strong fear, however, this extinction may proceed so slowly that it is scarcely noticeable within 200 trials. In this case, if only a small sample of behavior were observed, one might easily be led to the false conclusion that no extinction was occurring.

In some cases the extinction of phobias can be noticed. For instance, the pilot in the first example was somewhat less afraid of airplanes several months after his traumatic experience. Similarly, a young man with a moderately strong fear of high places gradually lost his fear when he was strongly motivated to participate in mountain climbing and gradually exposed himself to a series of increasingly steep heights.

In other cases, the fears involved in phobias seem to be enormously resistant to extinction. It will be remembered that the following variables are known to increase resistance to extinction: a stronger drive of pain or fear involved in the original learning; a larger number of reinforced learning trials; intermittent, or so-called partial, reinforcement; the generalization of reinforcement from other similar situations; the similarity of the phobic situation to the original traumatic one; the variability of the cues in the stimulus situation; and, as will be seen, the subject's memory for the original circumstances under which the fear was learned. Phobias also tend to be preserved because subjects usually manage to avoid the phobic situation and so do not receive many extinction trials.

As long as the subject can avoid the cues that elicit fear or that evoke the internal cue-producing responses eliciting fear, he will be expected to experience no fear. Thus the pilot in the first example was not afraid as long as he could stay completely away from airplanes, and the little boy in the second example was reasonably unafraid when he was safely away from the bed. If the social conditions allow successful avoidance of the fear-provoking situations, all that will be noticed is a blank area in the person's life. But as soon as he is forced to go into the phobic situation, strong fear will appear.

To summarize, in phobias the responses of avoidance and their reinforcement by a reduction in the strength of the fear is almost always quite clear. The origin of the drive of fear may be obvious or obscure; it often traces back to childhood conflicts about sex and aggression. Fear can be exceedingly resistant to extinction. The more exact determination of the factors that affect this resistance is a problem with important therapeutic implications.

COMPULSIONS

It is well known that if a compulsive response, for example excessive hand washing, is interrupted by a command or physical restraint, the subject experiences a marked increase in anxiety; he reports that he just feels awful. As soon as the compulsion is resumed, the anxiety disappears (Fenichel, 1945, pp. 306–307; White, 1948, p. 277). Thus it seems clear that the compulsion is reinforced in exactly the same way as the avoidance response in the phobia and the responses of turning the wheel, pressing the bar, or pulling of the handle in the experiments described in an earlier chapter. In fact, a phobia of dirt, which leads the subject to remove visible dirt by washing, may shade over by imperceptible degrees into hand washing where the subject fears dirt even when the hands seem clean, or where he does not know what he fears.

While the existence of the fear, guilt, or other drive motivating compulsive responses usually becomes obvious if the patient is forced to stop performing the compulsive response, the source of this drive is often quite obscure. Frequently a hand-washing compulsion must be traced back to childhood conflicts in which cleanliness training produces an abnormal fear of dirt or sex training results in a strong fear of venereal disease.

The responses involved in compulsions may be the result of more or less random trial and error but often are ones that have already been learned in other more or less similar situations. For example, the mother who arouses anxiety in the child by criticising him for dirty hands teaches him to wash his hands when they are dirty.

Similarly, the anxiety-reducing effects of a particular act, such as hand washing, are often due to social training. Then the act of washing the hands may have a direct reassuring effect because it has been so frequently associated during childhood with escape from criticism for having dirty hands. Stated more exactly, the cues produced by the act may elicit responses that inhibit fear. In other cases the effect may be more indirect; the function of the act may be to elicit thoughts that are incompatible with the ones eliciting the fear. For example, the thought "I have washed my hands so they must be clean" will be incompatible with the one "Perhaps my hands are contaminated."

In other instances the compulsive act may have an anxiety-reducing effect because it serves as a distraction. Keeping the hands busy with an innocent response may help to keep them out of anxiety-provoking mischief.

Usually the compulsive act produces only a temporary reduction in the anxiety. After a relatively short time, the anxiety starts to increase again so that the patient is motivated to repeat the compulsive act.

In conclusion, the drive-increasing effect of interfering with compulsions and the drive-reducing effect of performing them is usually clear-cut. The origin of the fear (or other drive) and the reason why a particular compulsive act reduces it is often not obvious and must be tracked down or inferred.

HYSTERICAL SYMPTOMS

Our analysis of how hysterical symptoms are learned will start with a case of war neurosis where the causation is relatively recent and clear. This is case 12 reported by Grinker and Spiegel (1945b, pp. 28-29). The patient had been directing the firing of an artillery platoon under great danger and with heavy responsibilities. After the acute phase of battle, he was lying on the ground exhausted when three shells landed nearby and exploded, blowing him off the ground each time. He was somewhat shaken up but otherwise fit. Half an hour later he found that he could not remove his right hand from his trouser pocket, having almost complete paralysis. He did not report sick and stayed with his company regaining some strength in his arm but still suffering partial paralysis. Then he was sent to the hospital, where he was calm and cooperative and had no anxiety, tremor, or terror dreams.

His condition was not organic (*i.e.,* it must have been learned) because under pentothal narcosis he was able to move his arm in all directions with ease. With reeducation and a short series of therapeutic interviews the condition cleared up. When it became obvious, however, that he was fit to return to his unit, he developed frank anxiety and tremor in both arms. The anxiety now appeared directly in relation to his battle experience and had to be dealt with as a separate problem.

Reinforcement vs. Adaptiveness. In this case it is obvious that the symptom of a paralyzed arm served a certain adaptive function in that it kept the soldier out of combat. More general evidence that escape from combat is involved in reinforcing the symptoms of war neurosis is given by the fact that they vary with the requirements of the combat task. Thus aviators are likely to turn up with disturbances in depth perception or night vision, symptoms that are peculiarly suited to interfere with flying, while paratroopers are likely to have paralyzed legs (Grinker and Spiegel, 1945a, pp. 104).

For the more rigorous type of theory that we are trying to construct, however, merely pointing out the adaptiveness of the symptom is not enough; the reinforcement should be described more exactly. In the case of the soldier with the paralyzed arm, the eventual hospitalization and escape from combat could not have been the original reinforcement because it occurred only after the symptom was firmly established. The original reinforcement must have occurred while the symptom was being learned. Furthermore, we know that in order to be effective in strengthening a response, reinforcement must occur soon after it.

In this case the drive is fear and the origin of the fear in combat is quite clear. Since the fear was not experienced as long as the symptom persisted but reappeared as soon as the symptom was interrupted, it is apparent that the symptom reduced the fear. But a reduction in the strength of fear is known to act as a reinforcement. Therefore, the symptom of partial paralysis seems to have been reinforced by the immediate reduction that it produced in the strength of fear.

The symptom of paralysis produced this reduction in fear because the patient knew that it would prevent his return to combat. As soon as the patient noticed that it was difficult to move his hand, he probably said to himself something like "They won't let me fight with a paralyzed hand," and this thought produced an immediate reduction in fear. Though the fear reduction probably was mediated by a thought, its reinforcing effect on the symptoms was direct and automatic. In other words, the patient did not say to himself anything like "Since a paralyzed hand will keep me out of combat, I should try to have a paralyzed hand." In fact, when such a patient becomes convinced of the causal relationship between the escape from fear and the symptom, a strong increase in guilt counteracts any reduction in fear. The reinforcement is removed and there is strong motivation to abandon the symptom.

Malingering. Now we can see how the hysterical symptom differs from malingering. In malingering, the guilt attached to thoughts of performing a response in order to escape from a responsibility, such as combat, is not as strong as the fear of the responsibility. Therefore the subject is able to plan to perform a response in order to escape. In hysteria, the response is made directly to the drive, such as fear; in malingering, it is made to the verbal cues of the plan. Therefore we would expect hysterical symptoms to vary with the drive and malingered ones to vary with the plan. Perhaps this is why, as Grinker and Spiegel (1945b, pp. 47, 95) report, hysterical symptoms are relieved by drugs such as pentothal (which according to us operate by reducing the drive of fear) while malingered ones are unaffected. It can also be seen that only responses that are under verbal (*i.e.,* voluntary) control can be involved in malingering, while any response that can occur may be reinforced as an hysterical symptom. In fact, the more plausible the response seems as an involuntary organic defect, the less likely it is to arouse guilt.

Origin of Response. Phobias involve the exceedingly natural response of avoidance, and compulsions usually involve common responses. Often the responses involved in hysterical symptoms are much more unusual. Thus there is more of a problem concerning how the response occurs and is available for the initial reinforcement. Often symptoms have an organic basis at first and then persist after the organic basis has been cured (Grinker and Spiegel, 1945a, pp. 111-112). This seems to be a way of getting the response to occur so that it can be reinforced. Aviators' symptoms resemble diseases that often occur in fliers—pseudo air emboli, air sickness, and so forth (Grinker and Spiegel, 1945a, p. 57). Many symptoms appear to be responses that are relatively normal to the drive of strong fear. In spite of these suggestive facts, the factors determining exactly which symptoms will occur are still somewhat of a mystery. For example, does allowing children to escape from school for certain kinds of pains or mild illnesses predispose them to the use of pseudo illnesses to escape from difficulties in later life?

To summarize, in hysteria the reinforcement, or primary gain from the symptom, is often relatively clear; the drives involved may be unclear at first, and the factors determining the occurrence of a particular response may be quite obscure.

References

Dollard, John, March 9, 1945. Exploration on morale factors among combat air crewmen—memorandum to research branch, information and education division. *Psychol. Service Center J.*, 1950.

Fenichel, O., 1945. "The Psychoanalytic Theory of Neuroses." Norton, New York.

Grinker, R. R., and Spiegel, J. P., 1945a. "Men Under Stress." Blakiston, New York.

Grinker, R. R., and Spiegel, J. P., 1945b. "War Neurosis." Blakiston, New York.

Miller, N. E., 1950. Learnable drives and rewards. In S. Stevens (ed.), "Handbook of Experimental Psychology." Wiley, New York.

Pavlov, I. P., 1927. "Conditioned Reflexes," trans. by G. V. Anrep. Oxford, London.

White, R. W., 1948. "The Abnormal Personality." Ronald, New York.

34. Social Learning of Dependence Behavior

ALBERT BANDURA and RICHARD H. WALTERS

In the psychological literature such responses as seeking proximity and physical contact, help, attention, reassurance, and approval have been categorized as dependent (Beller, 1955). Since the human infant is almost totally helpless and remains relatively incapable of caring for himself for a number of years, dependent responses receive a considerable amount of positive reinforcement in most societies (Whiting and Child, 1953). Although independence training in North America is usually initiated in early childhood, this training is primarily focused on the mastery of developmental tasks. For example, the child is taught to clothe, feed, and occupy himself, and later on to master certain instrumental social and occupational skills that will permit him in adulthood to maintain an independent socio-vocational adjustment.

While there are very marked changes in *task-oriented* dependent responses from infancy to adulthood, *person-oriented* dependency is expected and reinforced throughout all stages of development. Some changes in the form of person-oriented dependency occur, but these are largely attributable to the acquisition of instrumental skills. On the other hand, there are major changes in the objects to which this kind of dependency is expressed. Seeking proximity and

physical contact, for example, is not merely permitted but actually expected at all stages of an individual's life, and particularly during adolescent and adult years as he increasingly engages in heterosexual behavior. Eventually, dependent responses of this kind become focused primarily on a single object, the marriage partner, although in attenuated forms they may still be expressed toward other persons. Indeed, it is culturally expected that within the marriage partnership husband and wife will engage in physical manifestations of dependency that do not differ greatly from those that occur in the parent-child relationship.

Other forms of person-oriented dependency—for example, the seeking of approval and help—are expected to be shown toward a wide variety of persons, such as friends, colleagues, and members of one's reference groups.

Failure to develop task-oriented independent responses is usually attributed to a lack of such factors as motivation, initiative, or achievement drive, to limitations of capacity, social resources, or opportunity, or to just plain laziness, but is rarely, in and of itself, regarded as indicative of psychopathology. Failure to develop and maintain appropriate person-oriented dependency is, in contrast, one of the main criteria for identifying certain forms of behavior disorder. It should be noted that overdeveloped person-oriented dependency does not usually constitute, nor become labeled as, a serious form of deviation. In fact, overdependent individuals are usually regarded as self-indulgent, egocentric, or "spoiled," but not as emotionally disturbed. This perhaps accounts for the paucity of studies of overdependency in the clinical literature. By contrast, deficits in person-oriented dependency have received a great deal of attention, for example, in studies of autism, of the effects of prolonged institutionalization, and of children who have been deprived of a normal family life.

Certain classes of patients, such as psychopaths, are usually regarded as incapable of forming person-oriented dependent relationships; on the other hand, they are also described as possessing highly developed manipulatory skills designed to secure person-oriented dependency gratifications. In fact, in most cases, their deviant behavior is characterized not by an absence of such dependency, but by the transience of the dependency relationships into which they enter. Such failures to maintain appropriate dependency attachments have been of considerable concern to workers in the mental health field.

DEFINITION OF DEPENDENCY

Dependency may be defined as a class of responses that are capable of eliciting positive attending and ministering responses from others. Since dependency responses are prosocial in nature, the presence of intent can perhaps be more readily established than in the case of aggression. These responses, however, do not inevitably elicit positive reactions from others, particularly when they are of high frequency or inappropriately timed. Under these circumstances, the agent may wittingly or unwittingly feign states of disability, lack of capacity, or illness in order to ensure positive rather than negative counter-responses. If the agent does not actively seek attention or care, but simply presents himself as relatively helpless or suffering, the object of dependency may appear not to be the initiator of the interaction sequence, and the problem of intent then arises.

The problem of intent also occurs in the case of high magnitude responses. For example, a young child kicks his mother's leg, when he has failed to obtain a desired toy that is placed beyond his reach, and the mother has not attended to his verbal requests for assistance. If the kick is mild, there is a good chance that the child's response will be regarded as dependent; if the kick is strongly administered, it is more likely that the response will be labeled "aggressive." The covert assumption, of course, is that a hard kick is *intended* to hurt. But in the case cited, it may be argued that the hard, as well as the mild, kick is intended to procure the mother's attention and so can be categorized as dependent. The intentionality criterion can thus lead to categorization of a single response sequence as both dependent and aggressive. Indeed, negative attention-seeking behavior provides a good example of a response pattern the categorization of which consistently baffles research workers (Bandura and Walters, 1959; Sears, Whiting, Nowlis, and Sears, 1953).

POSITIVE TRAINING IN DEPENDENCY

There have been relatively few observational and interview studies of direct training in dependency and still fewer experimental investigations; research into children's dependency has instead been focused on identifying changes in dependency objects and on the development of independence, on the assumption that independence emerges from dependency. Moreover, greater attention has been given to generalized parental variables such as acceptance, affection, child-centeredness, and indulgence, than to specific aspects of dependency training.

It has generally been assumed that adult nurturance is a critical factor in the establishing of dependency in children. Nurturance involves positive reinforcement of dependency, the active eliciting of dependency responses, and the conditioning of positive emotional responses to the nurturant adult. The occurrence of nurturant behavior, itself complex, has usually been inferred from such parent characteristics as affectional demonstrativeness and warmth that may, but need not, involve all three facets of nurturance and certainly involve many other facets of parent behavior.

Positive relationships between parental demonstrativeness and warmth and the dependency of children have emerged from a number of field studies. Sears, Maccoby, and Levin (1957) found that mothers who were affectionately demonstrative responded positively to the children's dependent behavior and described them as high in dependency. Bandura and Walters (1959) reported that mothers of nonaggressive adolescent boys who were relatively high in dependency showed more warmth than mothers of relatively nondependent aggressive boys; the fathers of the high-dependent boys were both warmer and more affectionately demonstrative than the fathers of the low-dependent group. Moreover, a correlational analysis of data from families of aggressive and inhibited children indicated that parents who were warm, affectionate, rewarded dependency, and had spent a good deal of time in caring for their sons had children who tended to display a high degree of dependency behavior (Bandura, 1960).

Rheingold (1956) carried out an experimental study of "mothering" in which she performed caretaking acts toward institutionalized children for a period of eight weeks. A control group of children remained in the usual hospital routine. An assessment of the children's social behavior at the end of the eight-week period indicated that the infants who had received the nurturant care of the experimenter were more socially responsive both to the experimenter and to an examiner than were the control children. Clinical case material suggests that an extreme degree of "mothering" may create very strong dependency habits in children. For example, Levy (1943) found that highly indulgent mothers who were extremely solicitous in caring for their children's needs and were constantly rewarding dependency responses had highly dependent children.

Additional indirect evidence that maternal permissiveness for, and reward of, dependency increases children's dependency behavior was obtained by Heathers (1953). Six- to twelve-year-old children were blindfolded and then requested to walk along a narrow unstable plank, which was balanced on springs and raised eight inches from the floor. As the child stood on the starting end of the plank, the experimenter touched the back of the child's hand and waited for him to accept or reject the implied offer of help.

Parent-training measures, in the form of ratings previously secured by means of the Fels Parent Behavior Scales (Baldwin, Kalhorn, and Breeze, 1945), were available to the experimenter and were related to the performance of the children. The analysis showed that children who accepted the experimenter's hand on the initial trial of the Walk-the-Plank Test tended to have child-centered parents who encouraged their children to lean on others rather than to take care of themselves and who held their children back from developing age-appropriate skills.

Unlike aggression and sex, dependency is generally regarded as a prosocial form of behavior. Consequently, parents are usually reluctant to acknowledge any failure to reward, or any punishment of, their children's dependency. It is therefore not surprising that field studies in which parental handling of dependency has been directly investigated have generally failed to reveal any strong relationships between the parent behavior and the dependency responses of children. In Bandura's (1960) study, however, thematic interview material secured from aggressive and inhibited boys revealed that the former group of boys, who displayed a great deal of dependency behavior, depicted parents as providing a considerable amount of intermittent reward for their son's dependency responses.

The reward of dependency responses has rarely been used as an antecedent variable within experimental studies. Nelsen (1960) investigated the effects of both reward and punishment of dependency on the incidence of children's dependent responses in a subsequent social-interaction situation. During training half the children were shown approval for dependency while the remaining children received mild verbal rebukes for acting in a dependent manner. Pretest-to-posttest changes indicated that reward for dependency resulted in an increase in dependency responses toward the rewarding agent, while punishment for dependency resulted in a decrease of such responses. The effects of reward were more marked for girls than for boys.

Cairns (1962) reported that prior reward for dependency facilitated children's learning when correct responses were reinforced by verbal approval. Grade-school children were first shown some toys in a cabinet and were told that they could play with a new toy each time a bell rang. For two groups of children the doors of the cabinet were closed, and the toys were therefore accessible only through the help of the experimenter. The children in one of these groups were rewarded, through the experimenter's compliance, for asking help or seeking attention in response to the signal that another toy might be taken from the cupboard; similar behavior from the children in the other group was consistently ignored. The children in a third group were given free access to the toys and experienced rewarding responses from the experimenter that were not contingent upon their exhibiting dependency behavior. Following the experimental treatments, all children were set a discrimination task by a second experimenter, who said "Good" each time a child made a correct response. Children who had been previously reinforced for dependent responses learned more rapidly than children in either of the other two groups. Cairns' results suggest that children in whom dependency habits are strongly developed are more responsive to social reinforcers. Support for this interpretation is provided by Ferguson (1961), who used Beller's (1955) scale to select high-dependent and low-dependent children and then compared their performance on a task similar to that used in Cairns' study. The results indicated that high-dependent children, when rewarded by approval, learned more rapidly than low-dependent children.

Parents who encourage and reward dependency also serve as nurturant models for their children. Consequently, parental reward of dependency should be one antecedent of strongly developed affiliative patterns in children. This joint reinforcement and modeling effect appears to be reflected in the finding of Hartup and Keller (1960) that nursery-school children who sought help and affection relatively often tended also to give frequent attentive, affectionate, protective, and reassuring responses in their interactions with their peers.

PUNISHMENT AND INHIBITION OF DEPENDENCY

Warmth, affectional demonstrativeness, and "mothering" have been selected for study as possible antecedents of the development of dependency habits; similarly, rejection, another nonspecific parent characteristic, has been made the focus of attention in studies of the negative conditioning of dependency. One important component of severe rejection is probably the punishment of dependency behavior; however, if rejection is not extreme, both reward and punishment may occur, and the effects of rejection will then depend on the extent to which one or other of these types of parental responses predominate.

The effects of punishment on dependency are inevitably modified by the effects of the rewards that are dispensed for dependency from time to time, particularly during the child's early years, in almost every family situation. Thus dependency training contrasts strongly with sex training, during which rewards are rarely, if ever, dispensed, and with aggression training, which in most homes involves only intermittent, highly selective, and relatively infrequent dispensing of rewards. Moreover, especially in early childhood, dependency behavior cannot be relinquished as readily as sexual or aggressive behavior, since a child's immediate needs must receive some attention from even reluctant adults. Consequently, initial discouragement of dependency is likely to intensify a child's efforts to obtain dependency rewards. Indeed, Sears, Maccoby, and Levin (1957) found rejection to have little relationship to dependency if there was, at other times, little reward for dependency, but to have a positive relationship to dependency if the mother had also rewarded this kind of behavior.

In the case of the more severe forms of rejection, one would expect inhibition of dependency behavior, an outcome that is reflected in the finding of Bandura and Walters (1959) that aggressive boys who had experienced a good deal of parental rejection showed much less dependent behavior than more accepted nonaggressive boys. In this study parents who expressed rejection of their children were found to have punished dependency to a greater extent than those who were more accepting; moreover, ratings of the boys' dependency made from interviews with the boys were negatively correlated with ratings of paternal rejection made from father interviews. Finally, boys who felt rejected by their parents showed a low incidence of dependency responses toward parents, teachers, and peers.

When rejection involves primarily the withholding of positive reinforcers, rather than the presentation of negative reinforcers, its effect may be to intensify the dependency toward the frustrating agent. Hartup (1958), in an experimental study of nurturance withdrawal, found that children who had experienced delay of reward for dependency exhibited more dependent behavior than children whose dependency had been consistently rewarded. Similarly, Gewirtz (1954) demonstrated that children displayed more attention-seeking behavior in the presence of a nonresponsive adult than in the presence of an adult who centered his attention on the child. Withholding of positive reinforcers appears to produce more sustained increases in dependency behavior in children whose past social-learning experiences have made them highly dependent than in children in whom dependency habits are weakly established (Baer, 1962; Beller and Haeberle, 1961a, 1961b). Thus, the occurrence of a dependent response to frustration is more likely if dependent responses are dominant in children's response hierarchies.

In the study by Nelsen (1960) children who were negatively reinforced for dependency showed a subsequent decrease in dependency responses; in this case the effect was more pronounced for boys. An analysis of patient-therapist interaction sequences by Winder, Ahmad, Bandura, and Rau (1962) indicated that whereas positive reinforcement of dependency responses greatly increased the extent to which these were emitted in therapy sessions, negative reinforcement resulted in a marked decrease in their frequency. Thus, even with adults, relatively consistent punishment of dependency appears to have an inhibitory effect.

When active punishment is combined with reward, its effects on dependency behavior may under some circumstances be the same as when rewards are intermittently withheld. Fisher (1955) compared the social responses of two groups of puppies. One of these was consistently petted and fondled by the experimenter for approach responses, while the second group of puppies was administered the same kind of reward treatment with the addition of training sessions in which the puppies were handled roughly and on occasions electrically shocked for approach responses. Tests of dependency behavior conducted toward the end of, and following, thirteen weeks' training indicated that the puppies which had received both reward and punishment exhibited greater dependency behavior in the form of remaining close to a human than did the puppies in the reward-only group.

While the withholding of rewards for dependency seems to produce an increase in dependency behavior, active punishment appears to reduce its incidence unless there is relatively frequent concurrent reward. Consequently, since withholding of reward is generally regarded as a less severe disciplinary technique than punishment, it is understandable that Sears, Whiting, Nowlis, and Sears (1953) found some support for the hypothesis that there is a curvilinear relationship between the complex variable of maternal frustration-and-punishment of dependency and the incidence of dependency in preschool children.

The correlational data from Bandura's (1960) investigation into the child-training antecedents of aggressive and inhibited behavior indicated that punishment for dependency behavior decreased its directness, but that significant relationships between punitiveness for dependency and its frequency were largely absent. The only exceptions were found in the case of the aggressive boys, for whom maternal punishment for dependency seemed to have the effect of *increasing* dependency responses to adults. This outcome was also reflected in the boys' thematic interview responses, which strongly suggested that differential reinforcement histories had led the aggressive and inhibited boys to respond to dependency frustration in quite different ways.

In the first place, the mothers of aggressive boys tended to ignore mild forms of dependency behavior, whereas more intense forms secured their attention. If more vigorous responses are thus differentially reinforced, one would expect these responses, which might well be labeled as aggressive, to become strongly established. Rewarding of responses of this kind in order temporarily to terminate their occurrence could be one means of establishing troublesome behavior. Indeed, teachers were beginning to complain that the dependency behavior of the aggressive boys had become burdensome.

In the case of the inhibited boys, nonaggressive withdrawal reactions occupied a dominant position in the hierarchy of responses elicited by situations in which dependency was frustrated. When the mother punished dependency, inhibited boys depicted the frustrated child as giving up the goal of gaining the mother's nurturance and attention and making dependency responses to other persons. In addition, they reported more withdrawal behavior following frustration of dependency by peers; since there was no indication that they had been greatly punished by peers for exhibiting dependency behavior, it is reasonable to conclude that the withdrawal response had generalized from the home situation to peer interactions.

There was one notable difference between the findings of Bandura's investigation and the authors' earlier study of aggressive adolescent boys (Bandura and Walters, 1959). In contrast to the adolescents, who showed relatively little dependency behavior and a marked inhibition of dependency responses, Bandura's aggressive preadolescent boys exhibited a great deal of dependency behavior toward their parents, teachers, and peers. This difference seems in part to reflect a developmental process, and in part the influence of differential reinforcement histories. In the first place, preadolescents are necessarily more dependent than adolescents; in fact, a number of the parents of the aggressive adolescents had commented on the strength of their sons' dependency behavior during preadolescent years. When the preadolescents expressed dependency, they tended to do so in forms that elicited mild punishment from others, and such forms of dependency had apparently also predominated in the earlier histories of the delinquent adolescents. With increasing age, the aggressive preadolescents would be expected to show a marked decrease in dependency behavior, assuming that their dependency responses continued to be ignored and to elicit punishment.

Moreover, once boys begin to exhibit serious anti-social behavior, as many of the delinquent adolescents had already done, they tend to be openly rejected by parents, teachers, and the majority of peers, and this consequence inevitably promotes dependency inhibition. In addition, there were some differences between the two groups of families, for example, a difference in socioeconomic status, which could have influenced parents' child-training practices and consequently further increased the difference between the two groups of boys in their readiness to express dependency behavior.

Investigations into the effects of maternal privation have shown that institutionalized and other mentally deprived children are socially nonresponsive and nondependent (Bowlby, 1952; Freud and Burlingham, 1944; Gewirtz, 1961; Goldfarb, 1943; Lowrey, 1940; Spitz, 1945; Yarrow, 1961). However, they have also incidentally noted the occurrence of frequent, direct, and intense dependency responses in some children presumably deprived of maternal care. This differential effect would be expected if the children under investigation had experienced differential amounts of reward, nonreward, and punishment for dependency behavior.

References

Baer, D. M. A technique of social reinforcement for the study of child behavior: Behavior avoiding reinforcement withdrawal. *Child Develpm.,* 1962, *33,* 847–858.

Baldwin, A. L., Kalhorn, Joan, and Breeze, Fay H. Patterns of parent behavior. *Psychol. Monogr.,* 1945, *58,* No. 3 (Whole No. 268).

Bandura, A. Relationship of family patterns to child behavior disorders. Progress Report, U.S.P.H. Research Grant M-1734. Stanford Univer., 1960.

Bandura, A., and Walters, R. H. *Adolescent aggression.* New York: Ronald, 1959.

Beller, E. K. Dependency and independence in young children, *J. genet. Psychol.,* 1955, *87,* 25–35.

Beller, E. K., and Haeberle, Ann W. Dependency and the frustration-aggression hypothesis. Unpublished manuscript, Child Develpm. Center, New York City, 1961 (a).

Beller, E. K., and Haeberle, Ann W. Dependency and the frustration-aggression hypothesis: II. Paper read at the Annual Meeting of the Eastern Psychol. Assoc., Philadelphia, 1961 (b).

Bowlby, J. *Maternal care and mental health.* Geneva: World Health Organization, 1952 (WHO Monogr. Series, No. 2).

Cairns, R. B. Antecedents of social reinforcer effectiveness. Unpublished manuscript, Indiana Univer., 1962.

Ferguson, P. E. The influence of isolation, anxiety, and dependency on reinforcer effectiveness. Unpublished M.A. thesis, Univ. of Toronto, 1961.

Fisher, A. E. The effects of differential early treatment on the social and exploratory behavior of puppies. Unpublished doctoral dissertation, Penn. State Univer., 1955.

Freud, Anna, and Burlingam, Dorothy T. *Infants without families.* New York: International Universities, 1944.

Gewirtz, J. L. Three determinants of attention seeking in young children. *Monogr. Soc. Res. Child Develpm.,* 1954, *19,* No. 2 (Serial No. 59).

Gewirtz, J. L. A learning analysis of the effects of normal stimulation, privation, and deprivation on the acquisition of social motivation and attachment. In B. M. Foss (Ed.). *Determinants of infant behavior.* New York: Wiley, 1961, pp. 213–283.

Goldfarb, W. Infant rearing and problem behavior. *Amer. J. Orthopsychiat.,* 1943, *13,* 249–265.

Hartup, W. W. Nurturance and nurturance-withdrawal in relation to the dependency behavior of preschool children. *Child Develpm.,* 1958, *29,* 191–201.

Hartup, W. W., and Keller, E. D. Nurturance in preschool children and its relation to dependency. *Child Develpm.,* 1960, *31,* 681–689.

Heathers, G. Emotional dependence and independence in a physical threat situation. *Child Develpm.,* 1953, *24,* 169–179.

Levy, D. M. *Maternal overprotection.* New York: Columbia Univer. Press, 1943.

Lowrey, L. G. Personality distortion and early institutional care. *Amer. J. Orthopsychiat.,* 1940, *10,* 576–586.

Nelsen, E. A. The effects of reward and punishment of dependency on subsequent dependency. Unpublished manuscript, Stanford Univer., 1960.

Rheingold, Harriet L. The modification of social responsiveness in institutional babies. *Monogr. Soc. Res. Child Develpm.,* 1956, *21,* No. 2 (Serial No. 63).

Sears, R. R., Maccoby, Eleanor E., and Levin, H. *Patterns of child rearing.* New York: Harper, 1957.

Sears, R. R. Whiting, J. W. M., Nowlis, V., and Sears, Pauline S. Some child-rearing antecedents of aggression and dependency in young children. *Genet. Psychol. Monagr.,* 1953, *47,* 135–234.

Spitz, R. A. Hospitalism: An inquiry into the genesis of psychiatric conditions in early childhood. *Psychoanal. Study Child,* 1945, *1,* 53–74.

Whiting, J. W. M., and Child, I. L. *Child training and personality.* New Haven: Yale Univer. Press, 1953.

Winder, C. L., Ahmad, Farrukh Z., Bandura, A., and Rau, Lucy C. Dependency of patients, psychotherapists' responses, and aspects of psychotherapy. *J. consult. Psychol.,* 1962, *26,* 129–134.

Yarrow, L. J. Maternal deprivation: Toward an empirical and conceptual reevaluation. *Psychol. Bull.,* 1961, *58,* 459–490.

Behavioral Theories

PATHOLOGICAL PATTERNS

Pathology is defined by most behaviorists as socially maladaptive or deficient behavior. Since the varieties of such behavior are infinite, these theorists feel that the traditional classification system adopted by the psychiatric profession is a figment of Kraepelin's imagination. As evidence for this view they point to the fact that classification schemes are constantly revised and rarely hold up under research analysis. To them, whatever regularities are found can be accounted for by similarities in cultural patterns of conditioning.

Joseph Wolpe, a major figure in behavioral therapy, describes his analysis of a number of traditional neurotic disorders in the excerpt printed here. Although he accepts the traditional schema of syndromes, it is evident that he reconstructs these disorders in terms consistent with behavioral theory. A more adventuresome and detailed reformulation of the traditional approach to classification is undertaken in the paper by Frederick Kanfer and George Saslow.

35. Etiology of Human Neuroses

JOSEPH WOLPE

THE CAUSAL RELATIONS OF PERVASIVE ("FREE-FLOATING") ANXIETY

Under certain circumstances it is not only to well-defined stimulus configurations that anxiety responses are conditioned, but also to more or less omnipresent properties of the environment, of which extreme examples would be light, light and shade contrasts, amorphous noise, spatiality, and the passage of time. Since each of these enters into most, if not all, possible experience, it is to be expected that if any of them becomes connected to anxiety responses the patient will be persistently, and apparently causelessly anxious. He will be suffering from what is erroneously called "free-

From *Psychotherapy by Reciprocal Inhibition* by Joseph Wolpe, pages 83–94, copyright 1958 by the Board of Trustees of the Leland Stanford Junior University. With the permission of the publishers, Stanford University Press.

floating" anxiety, and for which a more suitable label would be *pervasive anxiety*.

It must be unequivocally stated, in case it is not quite self-evident, that there is no sharp dividing line between specific anxiety-evoking stimuli and stimuli to pervasive anxiety. The pervasiveness of the latter is a function of the pervasiveness of the stimulus element conditioned; and there are degrees of pervasiveness ranging from the absolute omnipresence of time itself through very common elements like room walls to rarely encountered configurations like hunchbacks.

What reason is there for believing that pervasive anxiety has definable stimulus sources?

Questioning of patients with pervasive anxiety usually reveals that definable aspects of the environment are especially related to this anxiety. For example, one patient reported increased anxiety in the presence of any very large object; another an uncomfortable intrusiveness of all sharp contrasts in his visual field—even the printed words on a page, and particularly contrasts in the periphery of the field. A third felt overwhelmed by physical space. Frequently, patients with pervasive anxiety observe that noise causes a rise in the level of their anxiety. In some cases the noise need not be loud, and in some even music is disturbing.

Although pervasive anxiety is usually felt less when the patient lies down and closes his eyes, it does not disappear. To some extent this may be explained on the basis of perseveration due to prolonged reverberation of the effects of the stimulus in the nervous system. But this does not account for the fact that usually *some* anxiety is already felt at the moment of waking. An obvious explanation is that anxiety evocable by stimuli that enter into the very structure of experience is likely to be produced by the first contents of the awakening subject's imagination. Anxiety increases when the outside world makes its impact; and it is consonant with this that, very commonly, the level of pervasive anxiety gradually rises as the day goes on.

This diurnal rise in level is less likely to occur when the general level of pervasive anxiety is low; for then there is a greater likelihood of the arousal, during a normal day's experience, of other emotions which may be physiologically antagonistic to anxiety, so that the anxiety will be inhibited and its habit strength each time slightly diminished. On the other hand, invariably (in my experience) the patient with pervasive anxiety also has unadaptive anxiety reactions to specific stimuli, and if he should encounter and react to any one of the latter during that day, the level of pervasive anxiety will promptly rise. In the normal course of events it is to be expected that level of pervasive anxiety will fluctuate because of "chance" occurrences which strengthen or weaken its habit strength.

Sometimes, when a patient is fortunate enough not to meet with any specific disturbing stimuli over an extended period, his pervasive anxiety may practically cease, but subsequent response to a relevant specific anxiety-evoking stimulus will condition it lastingly again. This reconditioning was beautifully demonstrated in one of my patients, who, in addition to pervasive anxiety, had a number of severe phobias on the general theme of illness. The pervasive anxiety responded extremely well to La Verne's carbon dioxide-oxygen inhalation therapy. The patient stopped coming for treatment until several months later when the pervasive anxiety was reinduced after he had witnessed an epileptic fit in the street. The pervasive anxiety was again speedily removed by carbon dioxide-oxygen and the patient again stopped treatment after a few more interviews. The essence of this sequence was repeated about ten times before the patient finally allowed desensitization to the phobic stimuli to be completed.

The question naturally arises: What factors determine whether or not pervasive anxiety will be part of a patient's neurosis? At the moment two possible factors may be suggested on the basis of clinical impressions. One seems to be the intensity of anxiety evocation at the time of the induction of the neurosis. It is hypothesized that the more intense the anxiety the more stimulus aspects are likely to acquire *some* measure of anxiety conditioning. Indirect support for this hypothesis comes from the observation that, on the whole, it is the patient who reacts more severely to specific stimuli who is also likely to suffer from pervasive anxiety.

The second possible factor is a lack of clearly defined environmental stimuli at the time of neurosis induction. For example, one patient's pervasive anxiety began after a night in a hotel during which he had attempted intercourse with a woman to whom he felt both sexual attraction and strong revulsion. He had felt a powerful and strange, predominantly nonsexual excitation, and ejaculation had occurred very prematurely without pleasure. The light had been switched off, and *only the dark outlines of objects could be seen.* After this, so great was his feeling of revulsion to the woman that he spent the remainder of the night on the carpet. This experience left him, as he subsequently found, with an anxiety toward a wide range of sexual objects, along with much pervasive anxiety, characterized by a special intrusiveness of all heavy dark objects.

THE CAUSAL PROCESS IN HYSTERIA

Hysterical reactions are clearly distinguishable from the rather diffuse discharges of the autonomic nervous system that characterize anxiety reactions. In most instances hysterical reactions do not find expression in the autonomic nervous system at all, but in the sensory system, the motor system, or groups of functional units involved in the production of imagery or of consciousness in general. Thus, they may take the form of anesthesias, paresthesias, hyperesthesias, or disturbances of vision or hearing; of paralyses, pareses, tics, tremors, disturbances of balance, contractures or fits; of amnesias, fugues, or "multiple personality" phenomena. Occasionally, hysterical reactions do appear to involve functions within the domain of the autonomic nervous system—in the form of vomiting (or nausea) or enuresis, but it is noteworthy that each of the two functions involved is to some extent within voluntary control.

Anxiety frequently accompanies hysterical reactions and then they occur side by side as two distinct forms of *primary* neurotic response. This state of affairs must be sharply distinguished from that in which sensory or motor phenomena are secondary effects of the normal components of anxiety, and as such do not qualify as hysterical. For example, a headache due to tension of the temporal muscles, backache due to tension of the longitudinal spinal muscles, or paresthesia due to hyperventilation are not to be regarded as hysterical.

It is necessary also to differentiate hysterical from obsessional reactions. Hysterical reactions are at a relatively low level of organization, affecting well-defined sensory areas and specific motor units, and causing changes in the general character of consciousness or the exclusion from consciousness of "blocks" of experience limited in terms of a time span or some other broad category. The details of the reactions tend to be fixed and unchanging. Obsessional reactions consist by contrast of highly organized movements or of elaborate and complex thinking, in either of which there is a great variety in the individual instances of expression of a specific constant theme.

Like other neurotic reactions, hysterical reactions are acquired by learning. It is intriguing to note that Freud's very early observations on hysterical subjects could easily have led him to this conclusion had he not been sidetracked by a spurious deduction from observations on

therapeutic effects. In a paper published in 1893, speaking of the relation of the symptoms of hysteria to the patients' reactions at the time of the precipitating stress, he states:

The connection is often so clear that it is quite evident how the exciting event has happened to produce just this and no other manifestation; the phenomenon is determined in a perfectly clear manner by the cause; to take the most ordinary example, a painful effect, which was originally excited while eating, but was suppressed, produces nausea and vomiting, and this continues for months, as hysterical vomiting. A child who is very ill at last falls asleep, and its mother tries her utmost to keep quiet and not to wake it; but just in consequence of this resolution (hysterical counterwill) she makes a clucking noise with her tongue. On another occasion when she wishes to keep absolutely quiet this happens again, and so a tic in the form of tongue-clicking develops which for a number of years accompanies every excitement. . . . A highly intelligent man assists while his brother's ankylosed hip is straightened under an anesthetic. At the instant when the joint gives way with a crack, he feels a violent pain in his own hip joint which lasts almost a year. . . . (pp. 25-26)

The attack then arises spontaneously as memories commonly do; but they may also be provoked, just as any memory may be aroused according to the laws of association. Provocation of an attack occurs either by stimulation of a hysterogenic zone or by a new experience resembling the pathogenic experience. We hope to be able to show that no essential difference exists between the two conditions, apparently so distinct; and in both cases a hyperaesthetic memory has been stirred. (p. 40)

Apart from the reference to the possibility of attacks arising "spontaneously" (which Freud later explicitly repudiated) we have here an account of the formation by learning of stimulus-response connections. That Freud did not *see* this was mainly because, having observed patients cured when they recalled and narrated the story of the precipitating experience, he concluded that the symptoms were due to the imprisonment of emotionally disturbing memories. He states ". . . we are of opinion that the psychical trauma, or the memory of it acts as a kind of foreign body constituting an effective agent in the present, even long after it has penetrated. . . ." There can be little doubt that this statement would not have been made, and the mind-structure theory that is psychoanalytic theory would not have been born, if Freud could have known that memories do not exist in the form of thoughts or images in some kind of repository within us, but depend on the establishment, through the learning process, of specific neural interconnections that give *a potentiality* of evocation of particular thoughts and images when and only when certain stimulus conditions, external or internal, are present.

When a clear history of the onset of hysterical symptoms is obtained, it is usually found, as illustrated in Freud's cases quoted above, that the hysterical reaction displays a repetition of features that were present in response to the initiating disturbing experience. The stimulus to the reaction varies. Sometimes it is a fairly specific sensory stimulation. For example, a 33-year-old woman had as a hysterical reaction an intolerable sensation of "gooseflesh" in her calves in response to any rectal sensation such as a desire to defecate, ever since, three years previously, a surgeon had unceremoniously performed a rectal examination upon her, while, drowsy from premedication with morphia, she was awaiting the administration of an anesthetic for an abdominal operation.

In other cases it appears that the hysterical reaction is aroused by ubiquitous stimuli, being then the hysterical equivalent of pervasive ("free-floating") anxiety. An example of this is wryneck that is present throughout the working day and relaxes the moment the patient falls asleep. In yet others anxiety appears to *mediate* the hysterical reaction. The hysteria of one of my patients had both a pervasive component and an anxiety-mediated component. This was a 58-year-old woman who 18 months earlier had encountered a deadly snake in a copse. She had been terrified and momentarily paralyzed; her ears were filled with the sound of waves and she had been unable to speak for two hours. The sound of waves had never left her, and any considerable anxiety such as might arise from tension in her home would intensify this sound and then lead to vertigo, loss of balance, and a feeling of great weakness in all her limbs, so that she sometimes fell.

The central feature of hysterical reactions is the conditioning, in situations of stress, of neurotic reactions other than anxiety, although anxiety is often also conditioned as well. It is necessary to ask what determines this. There are two possible answers. One is that these reactions are conditioned when they happen to be evoked in addition to anxiety. The other is that although such reactions may be evoked by stress in all subjects, they become the neurotic responses conditioned only in those in whom some special factor is present that gives preference to nonanxiety conditioning. Since, in fact, the immediate response to neurotigenic stimulation always seems to implicate all response systems, the latter possibility is the more likely to be relevant. And there is evidence that it is people with distinct personality features who usually develop hysterical reactions.

Jung (1923) long ago observed that hysterics tend to exhibit extravert character traits while other neurotic subjects tend to be introverted. In this partition of personalities he was followed by other writers who, while differing in many ways, agreed, as Eysenck (1947, p. 58) concluded from a survey, in the following particulars: *(a)* the introvert has a more subjective, the extravert a more objective outlook; *(b)* the introvert shows a higher degree of cerebral activity, the extravert a higher degree of behavioral activity; *(c)* the introvert shows a tendency to self-control (inhibition), the extravert a tendency to lack of such control. Eysenck (1955b) has pointed out on the basis of experiments performed by Franks (1956) and himself (1955a) that extraverted subjects besides learning more poorly also generate reactive inhibition more readily than introverts do. He postulates (1955b, p. 35) that subjects in whom reactive inhibition is generated quickly and dissipated slowly "are predisposed thereby to develop extraverted patterns of behaviour and to develop hysterico-psychopathic disorders in cases of neurotic breakdown." Clearly what his facts actually demonstrate is that the hysterical type of breakdown is particularly likely in subjects in whom reactive inhibition has the feature stated. The *causal* role of reactive inhibition is not shown, nor is a possible mechanism suggested.

A possibility is this: that in addition to their easily generated and persistent reactive inhibition (and perhaps in some indirect way bound up with it) extraverted people have one or both of the following characteristics: *(a)* when exposed to anxiety-arousing stimuli they respond with relatively low degrees of anxiety so that other responses are unusually prominent; *(b)* when anxiety and other responses are simultaneously evoked in them, contiguous stimuli become conditioned to the other responses rather than to the anxiety—by contrast with introverts.

This hypothesis lends itself readily to direct experimentation. In the meantime a survey from my records of the 22 patients with hysterical symptoms has yielded some suggestive evidence. Nine of them (41 per cent) had initial Willoughby scores below 30. This is in striking contrast to 273 nonhysterical neurotic patients, in only 50 (18 per cent) of whom were the initial scores below this level. The Kolmogorov-Smirnov test shows the difference to be significant at the .05 level. It is interesting to note that insofar as this supports our hypothesis it accords with the time-worn conception of the hysterical patient with little or no anxiety—*la belle indifference.* It is relevant to the same point that the hysterical patients with low Willoughby scores all benefited by procedures that varied greatly but did not obviously affect anxious sensitivity. By contrast, in the 13 patients whose hysterical reactions were accompanied by much anxiety there was a direct correlation between diminution of anxious sensitivity and decreased strength of hysterical reactions except in two cases where this consisted purely of amnesia, which was unaffected. (In one of these the events of the forgotten period were later retrieved under hypnosis, in the other they remained forgotten. It seemed to make no difference either way to the patient's recovery.)

Summarizing the above facts, it may be said that hysterical reactions may either accompany anxiety or occur on their own. In the former case their treatment is the treatment of anxiety, in the latter it is different in a way that will be discussed in the chapter on treatment. It is supposed that anxiety is a feature when hysteria occurs in subjects relatively far from the extraverted extreme of Eysenck's introversion-extraversion dimension, just because the hypothetical preferential conditioning of responses other than anxiety to neurotigenic stimuli is less marked in these people. This supposition needs to be tested.

Meanwhile it may be noted that there is experimental evidence of a competitive relationship in certain contexts between autonomic and motor responses. Mowrer and Viek (1948), using two groups of rats, placed each animal after a period of starvation on the electrifiable floor of a rectangular cage and offered him food on a stick for ten seconds. Whether the animal ate or not, shock was applied ten seconds later. In the case of one group of ten rats, jumping into the air resulted in the experimenter switching off the shock (shock-controllable group). Each animal in this group had an experimental "twin" to which the shock was applied for the same length of time as it had taken its counterpart to jump into the air (shock-uncontrollable group). One trial a day was given to each animal. The animals in each group whose eating responses during the ten seconds were inhibited (by conditioned anxiety responses resulting from the shocks) were charted each day, and it was found that in the shock-controllable group the number of eating inhibitions was never high and declined to zero, whereas in the shock-uncontrollable group the number rose to a high level and remained there. Apparently, the constant evocation of jumping in the former group resulted in gradual development of conditioned inhibition of anxiety. By contrast with this, in the typical Cornell technique for producing experimental neuroses (p. 43) a very localized musculoskeletal conditioned response comes to be increasingly dominated by autonomic anxiety responses. This whole matter has been discussed in more detail elsewhere (Wolpe, 1953a).

OBSESSIONAL BEHAVIOR

Sometimes, besides the autonomic discharges characteristic of anxiety, ideational, motor, and sensory responses are prominent in a neurosis. If simple and invariate in character, they are labeled *hysterical.* The term *obsessional* is applied to behavior that is more complex and variable in detail, consisting of well-defined and often elaborate thought sequences or relatively intricate acts which, though they may differ in outward form from one occasion to the next, lead or tend to lead to the same kind of result. The term is applicable even to those cases characterized by an obstinate impulse to behavior that rarely or never becomes manifest. Examples of obsessions predominantly of thought are a woman's insistent idea that she might throw her child from the balcony of her apartment, or a man's need to have one of a restricted class of "pleasant" thoughts in his mind before he can make any well-defined movement such as entering a doorway or sitting down. Exhibitionism and compulsive handwashing are characteristic examples of predominantly motor obsessional behavior.

Sometimes the word *compulsive* has been preferred to obsessional for those cases in which motor activity predominates. However, as most cases display both elements, there is little practical value in the distinction. Furthermore, the term compulsive is open to the objection that *all* behavior is compulsive in a sense, for causal determinism implies that the response that occurs is always the only one that could have occurred in the circumstances. The feature of any example of obsessional behavior is not its inevitability but its *intrusiveness*. Its elicitation or the impulse toward it is an encumbrance and an embarrassment to the patient.

If hysterical and obsessional reactions involve similar elements, we may expect that borderline cases will be found. An example of this is a 47-year-old male nurse employed in an industrial first-aid room who for 17 years had an uncontrollable impulse to mimic any rhythmic movements performed before him, e.g., waving of arms or dancing, and to obey any command no matter from whom. In this was combined the basic simplicity of hysteria and the situationally determined variability of obsessional behavior.

It may be stated almost as dogma that the strength and frequency of evocation of obsessional behavior is directly related to the amount of anxiety being evoked in the patient. Pollitt (1957) in a study of 150 obsessional cases noted that obsessional symptoms became more severe and prominent "when anxiety and tension increased for whatever causes." However, it is not always that the source of the anxiety is irrelevant. Sometimes the obsessional behavior is evident only when anxiety arises from specific, usually neurotic sources. For example, an exhibitionist experienced impulses to expose himself when he felt inadequate and inferior among his friends but not when he was anxious about the results of a law examination.

Anxiety-Elevating Obsessions. Two types of obsessional behavior are clearly distinguishable in clinical practice. One type appears to be part and parcel of the immediate response to anxiety-evoking stimulation and has secondary effects entirely in the direction of increasing anxiety. When a motor mechanic of 45 had neurotic anxiety exceeding a certain fairly low level, he would have a terrifying though always controllable impulse to strike people. From the first moment of awareness of the impulse he would feel increased anxiety, and if at the time he was with an associate or even among strangers—for example, in a bus—he would thrust his hands firmly into his pockets "to keep them out of trouble." In the history of such patients one finds that behavior similar to that constituting the obsession was present during an earlier situation in which conditioning of anxiety took place. In 1942 this motor mechanic, on military service, had been sentenced to 30 days' imprisonment in circumstances which he had with some justice felt to be grossly unfair. Then, as he had resisted the military police rather violently in protest, he was taken to a psychiatrist who said there was nothing wrong with him and that the sentence should be carried out. At this his feeling of helpless rage had further increased and he was taken out by force. Then for the first time he had had "this queer feeling" in his abdomen and had struck a military policeman who tried to compel him to work. Horror at the implications of this act intensified his disturbed state. The obsession to strike people made its first appearance in 1953, eleven years later. He had been imprisoned overnight (for the first time since 1942) because, arriving home one night to find his house crowded with his wife's relatives, he had shouted and been violent until his wife had called the police. After emerging from jail, burning with a sense of injustice much like that experienced during his imprisonment in the army, he had felt the impulse to strike a stranger who was giving him a lift in an automobile, and then again, much more strongly, a few days later toward his wife at their first meeting since his night in jail. This time he had gone into a state of panic, and since then, for a period of five months, the obsession had recurred very frequently and in an increasing range of conditions, e.g., at work he would often have a fear-laden desire to hit fellow workmen with any tool he happened to be holding. (There was subsequently a secondary conditioning of anxiety to the *sight* of tools, including knives and forks.)

Anxiety-Reducing Obsessions. The second type of obsessional behavior occurs as a *reaction* to anxiety, and its performance *diminishes* anxiety to some extent, for at least a short time. It occurs in many forms—tidying, handwashing, eating, buying—activities which are of course "normal" when prompted by usual motivations and not by anxiety; rituals like touching poles, perversions like exhibitionism, and various thinking activities. In some of these cases secondary heightening of anxiety occurs as a response to some aspect of the obsessional behavior. For example, in a case of obsessional eating, the anxiety was at first reduced by the eating, and then its level would rise in response to the idea of getting fat.

Obsessional behavior of this kind owes its existence to the previous conditioning of anxiety-relieving responses. This has been strikingly demonstrated in a recent experiment by Fonberg (1956). This writer conditioned each of several dogs to perform a definite movement in response to several auditory and visual stimuli using food reinforcement. When these instrumental conditioned responses had been firmly established, she proceeded to elaborate defensive instrumental conditioned responses, employing stimuli and responses distinct from those of the alimentary training. The noxious stimulus used was either an electric shock to the right foreleg or a strong air puff to the ear. As a result of this conditioning, upon presentation of the conditioned stimulus an animal would be able to avert the noxious stimulus—for example, by lifting a particular foreleg. The dogs were then made neurotic by conditioning an excitatory alimentary response to a strong tone of 50 cycles and an inhibitory response to a very weak tone of the same frequency, and then bringing the two differentiated tones nearer and nearer to each other from session to session either by progressive strengthening of the inhibitory tone or by both strengthening the inhibitory and weakening the excitatory. In all animals, as soon as neurotic

behavior appeared it was accompanied by the previously elaborated defensive motor reaction. Besides this deliberately conditioned reaction, "shaking off" movements were observed in those dogs in whom the noxious stimulation had originally been air puffed into the ear. The more intense the general disturbance the more intense and frequent were the defensive movements. The alimentary conditioned reflexes disappeared completely. With the disappearance of general disturbed symptoms, the defensive move-outburst of behavioral disturbance.

It appears clear from these observations that in elaborating the conditioned defensive reaction to the auditory stimulus, anxiety-response-produced stimuli were also conditioned to evoke the defensive reaction, and this reaction was consequently evocable *whenever* the animal had anxiety responses, no matter what the origin of these may have been.

Similarly, in the history of patients displaying this kind of obsessional behavior, it is found that at an earlier period, some important real threat was consistently removed by a single well-defined type of behavior, and this behavior later appears as a response to *any* similar anxiety. The behavior must owe its strength to its association with exceptionally strong reinforcement-favoring conditions—either very massive or very numerous anxiety-drive reductions or both. Its development is also, no doubt, greatly favored when from the outset no other significant anxiety-relieving activity has occurred to compete with it. Its maintenance depends upon the reduction of anxiety it is able to effect at each performance.

One patient was the youngest daughter of a man who despised females and would not forgive his wife for failing to bear him a son. She was very clever at school, and found that intellectual achievement, and that alone, could for brief periods abate her father's blatant hostility and therefore her own anxiety. Consequently, "thinking things out" became her automatic response to *any* anxiety. Since there are many objective fears for which careful thought is useful, there were no serious consequences for years. But when a series of experiences in early adult life led to a severe anxiety state in her, she automatically resorted to her characteristic "problem-solving" behavior. Because the anxiety responses now arose from such sources as imaginary social disapproval, and could not be removed by the solution of a well-defined problem, she began to set herself complex problems in which she usually had to decide whether given behavior was morally "good" or "bad." Partial and brief alleviation of anxiety followed both the formulation of a "suitable" problem and the solution thereof, while prolonged failure to solve a problem increased anxiety sometimes to terror. Although the anxiety soon returned in full force, its temporary decrements at the most appropriate times for reinforcement maintained the problem-finding and problem-solving obsessions, and could well have continued to do so indefinitely.

In other cases obsessional behavior is less episodically determined because everyday circumstances contain aspects of the special situation in which the obsessional mode of behavior alone brought relief from severe anxiety. A history of more than 100 undetected thefts of money by a 17-year-old university student began at the age of 5 when his mother joined the army and left him in the care of an elder sister who beat him severely or tied him to a tree for a few hours if he was slightly dirty or did anything "wrong." He feared and hated her and retaliated by stealing money from her. He was never caught and the possession of the stolen gains gave him a feeling of "munificence and security." The kleptomania continued all through the early home life and school life and was clearly connected with the chronic presence of punishment-empowered authority in the shape of parents or teachers.

It is not surprising, if obsessional behavior is so consistently followed by reduction of anxiety drive, that it is apt to become conditioned to other stimuli too, especially any that happen to be present on repeated occasions. Thus, after therapy had rendered the young woman with the problem-solving obsession mentioned above practically free from neurotic anxieties, mild problem-solving activity was still occasionally aroused by a trifling question, such as "Is it cloudy enough to rain?" The conditioned stimulus was apparently the mere awareness of doubt. Similarly an exhibitionist whose exhibiting had almost entirely disappeared with the overcoming of his anxious sensitivities,

still had some measure of the impulse when he saw a girl dressed in a school ("gym") uniform, because he had in the past exhibited to schoolgirls particularly frequently and with special relish. Of course, in this instance sex-drive reduction may have played as important a role in the reinforcement as anxiety-drive reduction.

AMNESIA AND "REPRESSION"

The amnesias that are usually encountered in the course of neurotic states can be conveniently divided into two classes, according to the emotional importance of the incidents forgotten. Patients who are in a chronic state of emotional disturbance frequently fail to register many trifling events that go on around them. For example, a patient may go into a room and conduct a brief conversation with his wife and an hour later have no recollection whatever that he went into that room at all. Here we seem to have a simple case of deficient registration of impressions (retrograde amnesia). Apparently, the patient's attention is so much taken up by his unpleasant anxious feelings that very little is left to be devoted to what goes on around him.

The forgetting of the contents of highly emotionally charged experiences has been given foremost importance by Freud and his followers as the cause of neurosis. It seems, however, that forgetting of this character is rather unusual, and when it does occur it appears to be merely one more of the conditionable occurrences in the neurotigenic situation. It does not appear that the repression as such plays any part in the maintenance of neurosis. It is quite possible for the patient to recover emotionally although the forgotten incidents remain entirely forgotten.

References

Eysenck, H. J. (1947) Dimensions of Personality. London, Routledge.
———. (1955a) A dynamic theory of anxiety and hysteria. *J. Ment. Sci. 101*: 28.
———. (1955b) Cortical inhibition, figural after-effect and theory of personality. *J. Abnorm. Soc. Psychol. 51*: 94.
Fonberg, E. (1956) On the manifestation of condi-

tioned defensive reactions in stress. *Bull. Soc. Sci. Lettr. Lodz. Class III. Sci. Math. Natur.* 7: 1.

Franks, C. M. (1956) Conditioning and personality: A study of normal and neurotic subjects. *J. Abnorm. Soc. Psychol. 52*: 143.

Freud, S. (1893) On the psychical mechanism of hysterical phenomena. In Collected Works of Freud, Vol. I. London, Hogarth Press, 1949.

Jung, C. G. (1923) Psychological Types. New York, Harcourt, Brace.

Mowrer, O. H., and Viek, P. (1948) Experimental analogue of fear from a sense of helplessness. *J. Abnorm. Soc. Psychol. 43*: 193.

Pollitt, J. (1957) Natural history of obsessional states: A study of 150 cases. *Brit. Med. J. 1*: 194.

Wolpe, J. (1953a) Learning theory and "abnormal fixations." *Psychol. Rev. 60*: 111.

36. Behavioral Analysis: An Alternative to Diagnostic Classification

FREDERICK H. KANFER and GEORGE SASLOW

During the past decade attacks on conventional psychiatric diagnosis have been so widespread that many clinicians now use diagnostic labels sparingly and apologetically. The continued adherence to the nosological terms of the traditional classificatory scheme suggests some utility of the present categorization of behavior disorders, despite its apparently low reliability[1,21]; its limited prognostic value[7,26]; and its multiple feebly related assumptive supports. In a recent study of this problem, the symptom patterns of carefully diagnosed paranoid schizophrenics were compared. Katz et al[12] found considerable divergence among patients with the same diagnosis and concluded that "diagnostic systems which are more circumscribed in their intent, for example, based on manifest behavior alone, rather than systems which attempt to comprehend etiology, symptom patterns and prognosis, may be more directly applicable to current problems in psychiatric research" (p 202).

We propose here to examine some sources of dissatisfaction with the present approach to diagnosis, to describe a framework for a behavioral analysis of individual patients which implies both suggestions for treatment and outcome criteria for the single case, and to indicate the conditions for collecting the data for such an analysis.

PROBLEMS IN CURRENT DIAGNOSTIC SYSTEMS

Numerous criticisms deal with the internal consistency, the explicitness, the precision, and the reliability of psychiatric classifications. It seems to us that the more important fault lies in our lack of sufficient knowledge to categorize behavior along those pertinent dimensions which permit prediction of responses to social stresses, life crises, or psychiatric treatment. This limitation obviates anything but a crude and tentative approximation to a taxonomy of effective individual behaviors.

Zigler and Phillips,[28] in discussing the requirement for an adequate system of classification, suggest that an etiologically-oriented closed system of diagnosis is premature. Instead, they believe that an empirical attack is needed, using "symptoms broadly defined as meaningful and discernible behaviors, as the basis of the classificatory system" (p 616). But symptoms as a class of responses are defined after all only by their nuisance value to the patient's social environment or to himself as a social being. They are also notoriously unreliable in predicting the patient's particular etiological history or his response to treatment. An alternate approach lies in an attempt to identify classes of dependent variables in human behavior which would allow inferences about the particular controlling factors, the social stimuli, the physiological stimuli, and the reinforcing stimuli, of which they are a function. In

From the *Archives of General Psychiatry 12:* 529–538, June 1965, copyright 1965 by the American Medical Association, by permission of the publisher and the authors.

the present early stage of the art of psychological prognostication, it appears most reasonable to develop a program of analysis which is closely related to subsequent treatment. A classification scheme which implies a program of behavioral change is one which has not only utility but the potential for experimental validation.

The task of assessment and prognosis can therefore be reduced to efforts which answer the following three questions: *(a)* which specific behavior patterns require change in their frequency of occurrence, their intensity, their duration or in the conditions under which they occur, *(b)* what are the best practical means which can produce the desired changes in this individual (manipulation of the environment, of the behavior, or the self-attitudes of the patient), and *(c)* what factors are currently maintaining it and what are the conditions under which this behavior was acquired. The investigation of the history of the problematic behavior is mainly of academic interest, except as it contributes information about the probable efficacy of a specific treatment method.

Expectations of Current Diagnostic Systems. In traditional medicine, a diagnostic statement about a patient has often been viewed as an essential prerequisite to treatment because a diagnosis suggests that the physician has some knowledge of the origin and future course of the illness. Further, in medicine diagnosis frequently brings together the accumulated knowledge about the pathological process which leads to the manifestation of the symptoms, and the experiences which others have had in the past in treating patients with such a disease process. Modern medicine recognizes that any particular disease need not have a single cause or even a small number of antecedent conditions. Nevertheless, the diagnostic label attempts to define at least the necessary conditions which are most relevant in considering a treatment program. Some diagnostic classification system is also invaluable as a basis for many social decisions involving entire populations. For example, planning for treatment facilities, research efforts and educational programs take into account the distribution frequencies of specified syndromes in the general population.

Ledley and Lusted[14] give an excellent conception of the traditional model in medicine by their analysis of the reasoning underlying it. The authors differentiate between a disease complex and a symptom complex. While the former describes known pathological processes and their correlated signs, the latter represents particular signs present in a particular patient. The bridge between disease and symptom complexes is provided by available medical knowledge and the final diagnosis is tantamount to labeling the disease complex. However, the current gaps in medical knowledge necessitate the use of probability statements when relating disease to symptoms, admitting that there is some possibility for error in the diagnosis. Once the diagnosis is established, decisions about treatment still depend on many other factors including social, moral, and economic conditions. Ledley and Lusted[14] thus separate the clinical diagnosis into a two-step process. A statistical procedure is suggested to facilitate the primary or diagnostic labeling process. However, the choice of treatment depends not only on the diagnosis proper. Treatment decisions are also influenced by the moral, ethical, social, and economic conditions of the individual patient, his family and the society in which he lives. The proper assignment of the weight to be given to each of these values must in the last analysis be left to the physician's judgment (Ledley and Lusted[14]).

The Ledley and Lusted model presumes available methods for the observation of relevant behavior (the symptom complex), and some scientific knowledge relating it to known antecedents or correlates (the disease process). Contemporary theories of behavior pathology do not yet provide adequate guidelines for the observer to suggest what is to be observed. In fact, Szasz[25] has expressed the view that the medical model may be totally inadequate because psychiatry should be concerned with problems of living and not with diseases of the brain or other biological organs. Szasz[25] argues that "mental illness is a myth, whose function it is to disguise and thus render more potable the bitter pill of moral conflict in human relations" (p 118).

The attack against use of the medical model in psychiatry comes from many quarters. Scheflen[23] describes a model of somatic psychiatry which is very similar to the traditional medical model of disease. A pathological process results in onset of an illness; the symptoms are correlated with a pathological state and represent our evidence of "mental disease." Treatment consists of removal of the pathogen, and the state of health is restored. Scheflen suggests that this traditional medical model is used in psychiatry not on the basis of its adequacy but because of its emotional appeal.

The limitations of the somatic model have been discussed even in some areas of medicine for which the model seems most appropriate. For example, in the nomenclature for diagnosis of disease of the heart and blood vessels, the criteria committee of the New York Heart Association[17] suggests the use of multiple criteria for cardiovascular diseases, including a statement of the patient's functional capacity. The committee suggests that the functional capacity be ". . . estimated by appraising the patient's ability to perform physical activity" (p 80), and decided largely by inference from his history. Further,[17] ". . . (it) should not be influenced by the character of the structural lesion or by an opinion as to treatment or prognosis" (p 81). This approach makes it clear that a comprehensive assessment of a patient, regardless of the physical disease which he suffers, must also take into account his social effectiveness and the particular ways in which physiological, anatomical, and psychological factors interact to produce a particular behavior pattern in an individual patient.

Multiple Diagnosis. A widely used practical solution and circumvention of the difficulty inherent in the application of the medical model to psychiatric diagnosis is offered by Noyes and Kolb.[18] They suggest that the clinician construct a diagnostic formulation consisting of three parts: (1) A *genetic* diagnosis incorporating the constitutional, somatic, and historical-traumatic factors representing the primary sources or determinants of the mental illness; (2) A *dynamic* diagnosis which describes the mechanisms and techniques unconsciously used by the individual to manage anxiety, enhance self-esteem, ie, that traces the psychopathological processes;

and (3) A *clinical* diagnosis which conveys useful connotations concerning the reaction syndrome, the probable course of the disorder, and the methods of treatment which will most probably prove beneficial. Noyes' and Kolb's multiple criteria[18] can be arranged along three simpler dimensions of diagnosis which may have some practical value to the clinician: (1) etiological, (2) behavioral, and (3) predictive. The kind of information which is conveyed by each type of diagnostic label is somewhat different and specifically adapted to the purpose for which the diagnosis is used. The triple-label approach attempts to counter the criticism aimed at use of any single classificatory system. Confusion in a single system is due in part to the fact that a diagnostic formulation intended to describe current behavior, for example, may be found useless in an attempt to predict the response to specific treatment, or to postdict the patient's personal history and development, or to permit collection of frequency data on hospital populations.

Classification by Etiology. The Kraepelinian system and portions of the 1952 APA classification emphasize etiological factors. They share the assumption that common etiological factors lead to similar symptoms and respond to similar treatment. This dimension of diagnosis is considerably more fruitful when dealing with behavior disorders which are mainly under control of some biological condition. When a patient is known to suffer from excessive intake of alcohol his hallucinatory behavior, lack of motor coordination, poor judgment, and other behavioral evidence disorganization can often be related directly to some antecedent condition such as the toxic effect of alcohol on the central nervous system, liver, etc. For these cases, classification by etiology also has some implications for prognosis and treatment. Acute hallucinations and other disorganized behavior due to alcohol usually clear up when the alcohol level in the blood stream falls. Similar examples can be drawn from any class of behavior disorders in which a change in behavior is associated primarily or exclusively with a single, *particular* antecedent factor. Under these conditions this factor can be called a pathogen and the situation closely approximates the condition described by the traditional medical model.

Utilization of this dimension as a basis for psychiatric diagnosis, however, has many problems apart from the rarity with which a specified condition can be shown to have a direct "causal" relationship to a pathogen. Among the current areas of ignorance in the fields of psychology and psychiatry, the etiology of most common disturbances probably takes first place. No specific family environment, no dramatic traumatic experience, or known constitutional abnormality has yet been found which results in the same pattern of disordered behavior. While current research efforts have aimed at investigating family patterns of schizophrenic patients, and several studies suggest a relationship between the mother's behavior and a schizophrenic process in the child,[10] it is not at all clear why the presence of these same factors in other families fails to yield a similar incidence of schizophrenia. Further, patients may exhibit behavior diagnosed as schizophrenic when there is no evidence of the postulated mother-child relationship.

In a recent paper Meehl[16] postulates schizophrenia as a neurological disease, with learned content and a dispositional basis. With this array of interactive etiological factors, it is clear that the etiological dimension for classification would at best result in an extremely cumbersome system, at worst in a useless one.

Classification by Symptoms. A clinical diagnosis often is a summarizing statement about the way in which a person behaves. On the assumption that a variety of behaviors are correlated and consistent in any given individual, it becomes more economical to assign the individual to a class of persons than to list and categorize all of his behaviors. The utility of such a system rests heavily on the availability of empirical evidence concerning correlations among various behaviors (response-response relationships), and the further assumption that the frequency of occurrence of such behaviors is relatively independent of specific stimulus conditions and of specific reinforcement. There are two major limitations to such a system. The first is that diagnosis by symptoms, as we have indicated in an earlier section, is often misleading because it implies common etiological factors. Freedman[7] gives an excellent illustration of the differences both in probable antecedent factors and

subsequent treatment response among three cases diagnosed as schizophrenics. Freedman's patients were diagnosed by at least two psychiatrists, and one would expect that the traditional approach should result in whatever treatment of schizophrenia is practiced in the locale where the patients are seen. The first patient eventually gave increasing evidence of an endocrinopathy, and when this was recognized and treated, the psychotic episodes. Freedman[7] suggests The second case had a definite history of seizures and appropriate anticonvulsant medication was effective in relieving his symptoms. In the third case, treatment directed at an uncovering analysis of the patient's adaptive techniques resulted in considerable improvement in the patient's behavior and subsequent relief from psychotic episodes. Freedman[7] suggests that schizophrenia is not a disease entity in the sense that it has a unique etiology, pathogenesis, etc., but that it represents the evocation of a final common pathway in the same sense as do headache, epilepsy, sore throat, or indeed any other symptom complex. It is further suggested that the term "schizophrenia has outlived its usefulness and should be discarded" (p 5). Opler[19,20] has further shown the importance of cultural factors in the divergence of symptoms observed in patients collectively labeled as schizophrenic.

Descriptive classification is not always this deceptive, however. Assessment of intellectual performance sometimes results in a diagnostic statement which has predictive value for the patient's behavior in school or on a job. To date, there seem to be very few general statements about individual characteristics, which have as much predictive utility as the IQ.

A second limitation is that the current approach to diagnosis by symptoms tends to center on a group of behaviors which is often irrelevant with regard to the patient's total life pattern. These behaviors may be of interest only because they are popularly associated with deviancy and disorder. For example, occasional mild delusions interfere little or not at all with the social or occupational effectiveness of many ambulatory patients. Nevertheless, admission of their occurrence is often sufficient for a diagnosis of psychosis. Refinement of such an approach beyond current usage appears possible, as shown for example by Lorr et al[15] but this does not remove the above limitations.

Utilization of a symptom-descriptive approach frequently focuses attention on by-products of larger behavior patterns, and results in attempted treatment of behaviors (symptoms) which may be simple consequences of other important aspects of the patient's life. Emphasis on the patient's subjective complaints, moods and feelings tends to encourage use of a syndrome-oriented classification. It also results frequently in efforts to change the feelings, anxieties, and moods (or at least the patient's report about them), rather than to investigate the life conditions, interpersonal reactions, and environmental factors which produce and maintain these habitual response patterns.

Classification by Prognosis. To date, the least effort has been devoted to construction of a classification system which assigns patients to the same category on the basis of their similar response to specific treatments. The proper question raised for such a classification system consists of the manner in which a patient will react to treatments, regardless of his current behavior, or his past history. The numerous studies attempting to establish prognostic signs from projective personality tests or somatic tests represent efforts to categorize the patients on this dimension.

Windle[26] has called attention to the low degree of predictability afforded by personality (projective) test scores, and has pointed out the difficulties encountered in evaluating research in this area due to the inadequate description of the population sampled and of the improvement criteria. In a later review Fulkerson and Barry[8] came to the similar conclusion that psychological test performance is a poor predictor of outcome in mental illness. They suggest that demographic variables such as severity, duration, acuteness of onset, degree of precipitating stress, etc., appear to have stronger relationships to outcome than test data. The lack of reliable relationships between diagnostic categories, test data, demographic variables or other measures taken on the patient on the one hand, and duration of illness, response to specific treatment, or degree of recovery, on the other hand, precludes the construction of a simple empiric framework for a diagnostic-

prognostic classification system based only on an array of symptoms.

None of the currently used dimensions for diagnosis is directly related to methods of modification of a patient's behavior, attitudes, response patterns, and interpersonal actions. Since the etiological model clearly stresses causative factors, it is much more compatible with a personality theory which strongly emphasizes genetic-developmental factors. The classification by symptoms facilitates social-administrative decisions about patients by providing some basis for judging the degree of deviation from social and ethical norms. Such a classification is compatible with a personality theory founded on the normal curve hypothesis and concerned with characterization by comparison with a fictitious average. The prognostic-predictive approach appears to have the most direct practical applicability. If continued research were to support certain early findings, it would be indeed comforting to be able to predict outcome of mental illness from a patient's premorbid social competence score,[28] or from the patient's score on an egostrength scale,[4] or from many of the other signs and single variables which have been shown to have some predictive powers. It is unfortunate that these powers are frequently dissipated in cross validation. As Fulkerson and Barry[8] have indicated single predictors have not yet shown much success.

A FUNCTIONAL (BEHAVIORAL-ANALYTIC) APPROACH

The growing literature on behavior modification procedures derived from learning theory[3,6,11,13,27] suggests that an effective diagnostic procedure would be one in which the eventual therapeutic methods can be directly related to the information obtained from a continuing assessment of the patient's current behaviors and their controlling stimuli. Ferster[6] has said ". . . a functional analysis of behavior has the advantage that it specifies the causes of behavior in the form of explicit environmental events, which can be objectively identified and which are potentially manipulable" (p 3). Such a diagnostic undertaking makes the assumption that a description of the problematic behavior, its controlling factors, and the means by which it can be changed are the most appropriate "explanations." It further makes the assumption that a diagnostic evaluation is never complete. It implies that additional information about the circumstances of the patient's life pattern, relationships among his behaviors, and controlling stimuli in his social milieu and his private experience is obtained continuously until it proves sufficient to effect a noticeable change in the patient's behavior, thus resolving "the problem." In a functional approach it is necessary to continue evaluation of the patient's life pattern and its controlling factors, concurrent with attempted manipulation of these variables by reinforcement, direct intervention, or other means until the resultant change in the patient's behavior permits restoration of more efficient life experiences.

The present approach shares with some psychological theories the assumption that psychotherapy is *not* an effort aimed at removal of intrapsychic conflicts, nor at a change in the personality structure by therapeutic interactions of intense nonverbal nature, (eg, transference, self-actualization, etc.). We adopt the assumption instead that the job of psychological treatment involves the utilization of a variety of methods to devise a program which controls the patient's environment, his behavior, and the consequences of his behavior in such a way that the presenting problem is resolved. We hypothesize that the essential ingredients of a psychotherapeutic endeavor usually involve two separate stages: (1) a change in the perceptual discriminations of a patient, ie, in his approach to perceiving, classifying, and organizing sensory events, including perception of himself, and (2) changes in the response patterns which he has established in relation to social objects and to himself over the years.[11] In addition, the clinician's task may involve direct intervention in the patient's environmental circumstances, modification of the behavior of other people significant in his life, and control of reinforcing stimuli which are available either through self-administration, or by contingency upon the behavior of others. These latter procedures complement the verbal interactions of traditional psychotherapy. They require that the clinician, at the invitation of the patient or his family, participate more fully in planning

the total life pattern of the patient outside the clinician's office.

It is necessary to indicate what the theoretical view here presented does *not* espouse in order to understand the differences from other procedures. It does *not* rest upon the assumption that (a) insight is a sine qua non of psychotherapy, (b) changes in thoughts or ideas inevitably lead to ultimate changes in actions, (c) verbal therapeutic sessions serve as replications of and equivalents for actual life situations, and (d) a symptom can be removed only by uprooting its cause or origin. In the absence of these assumptions it becomes unnecessary to conceptualize behavior disorder in etiological terms, in psychodynamic terms, or in terms of a specifiable disease process. While psychotherapy by verbal means may be sufficient in some instances, the combination of behavior modification in life situations as well as in verbal interactions serves to extend the armamentarium of the therapist. Therefore verbal psychotherapy is seen as an *adjunct* in the implementation of therapeutic behavior changes in the patient's total life pattern, not as an end in itself, nor as the sole vehicle for increasing psychological effectiveness.

In embracing this view of behavior modification, there is a further commitment to a constant interplay between assessment and therapeutic strategies. An initial diagnostic formulation seeks to ascertain the major variables which can be directly controlled or modified during treatment. During successive treatment stages additional information is collected about the patient's behavior repertoire, his reinforcement history, the pertinent controlling stimuli in his social and physical environment, and the sociological limitations within which both patient and therapist have to operate. Therefore, the initial formulation will constantly be enlarged or changed, resulting either in confirmation of the previous therapeutic strategy or in its change.

A Guide to a Functional Analysis of Individual Behavior. In order to help the clinician in the collection and organization of information for a behavioral analysis, we have constructed an outline which aims to provide a working model of the patient's behavior at a relatively low level of abstraction. A series of questions are so organized as to yield immediate implications for treatment. This outline has been found useful both in clinical practice and in teaching. Following is a brief summary of the categories in the outline.

1. Analysis of a Problem Situation: *The patient's major complaints are categorized into classes of behavioral excesses and deficits. For each excess or deficit the dimensions of frequency, intensity, duration, appropriateness of form, and stimulus conditions are described. In content, the response classes represent the major targets of the therapeutic intervention. As an additional indispensable feature, the behavioral assets of the patient are listed for utilization in a therapy program.

2. Clarification of the Problem Situation: Here we consider the people and circumstances which tend to maintain the problem behaviors, and the consequences of these behaviors to the patient and to others in his environment. Attention is given also to the consequences of changes in these behaviors which may result from psychiatric intervention.

3. Motivational Analysis: Since reinforcing stimuli are idiosyncratic and depend for their effect on a number of unique parameters for each person, a hierarchy of particular persons, events, and objects which serve as reinforcers is established for each patient. Included in this hierarchy are those reinforcing events which facilitate approach behaviors as well as those which, because of their aversiveness, prompt avoidance responses. This information has as its purpose to lay plans for utilization of various reinforcers in prescription of a specific behavior therapy program for the patient, and to permit utilization of appropriate reinforcing behaviors by the therapist and significant others in the patient's social environment.

4. Developmental Analysis: Questions are asked about the patient's biological equipment, his sociocultural experiences, and his characteristic behavioral development. They are phrased in such a way as (a) to evoke descriptions of his habitual behavior at various chronological stages of his life, (b) to relate specific new stimulus conditions to noticeable

changes from his habitual behavior, and (c) to relate such altered behavior and other residuals of biological and sociocultural events to the present problem.

5. Analysis of Self-Control: This section examines both the methods and the degree of self-control exercised by the patient in his daily life. Persons, events, or institutions which have successfully reinforced self-controlling behaviors are considered. The deficits or excesses of self-control are evaluated in relation to their importance as therapeutic targets and to their utilization in a therapeutic program.

6. Analysis of Social Relationships: Examination of the patient's social network is carried out to evaluate the significance of people in the patient's environment who have some influence over the problematic behaviors, or who in turn are influenced by the patient for his own satisfactions. These interpersonal relationships are reviewed in order to plan the potential participation of significant others in a treatment program, based on the principles of behavior modification. The review also helps the therapist to consider the range of actual social relationships in which the patient needs to function.

7. Analysis of the Social-Cultural-Physical Environment: In this section we add to the preceding analysis of the patient's behavior as an individual, consideration of the norms in his natural environment. Agreements and discrepancies between the patient's idiosyncratic life patterns and the norms in his environment are defined so that the importance of these factors can be decided in formulating treatment goals which allow as explicitly for the patient's needs as for the pressures of his social environment.

The preceding outline has as its purpose to achieve definition of a patient's problem in a manner which suggests specific treatment operations, or that none are feasible, and specific behaviors as targets for modification. Therefore, the formulation is *action oriented*. It can be used as a guide for the initial collection of information, as a device for organizing available data, or as a design for treatment.

The formulation of a treatment plan follows from this type of analysis because knowledge of the reinforcing conditions suggests the motivational controls at the disposal of the clinician for the modification of the patient's behavior. The analysis of specific problem behaviors also provides a series of goals for psychotherapy or other treatment, and for the evaluation of treatment progress. Knowledge of the patient's biological, social, and cultural conditions should help to determine what resources can be used,

---

*For each patient a detailed analysis is required. For example, a list of behavioral excesses may include specific aggressive acts, hallucinatory behaviors, crying, submission to others in social situations, etc. It is recognized that some behaviors can be viewed as excesses or deficits depending on the vantage point from which the imbalance is observed. For instance, excessive withdrawal and deficient social responsiveness, or excessive social autonomy (nonconformity) and deficient self-inhibitory behavior may be complementary. The particular view taken is of consequence because of its impact on a treatment plan. Regarding certain behavior as excessively aggressive, to be reduced by constraints, clearly differs from regarding the same behavior as a deficit in self-control, subject to increase by training and treatment.

and what limitations must be considered in a treatment plan.

The various categories attempt to call attention to important variables affecting the patient's *current* behavior. Therefore, they aim to elicit descriptions of low-level abstraction. Answers to these specific questions are best phrased by describing classes of events reported by the patient, observed by others, or by critical incidents described by an informant. The analysis does not exclude description of the patient's habitual verbal-symbolic behaviors. However, in using verbal behaviors as the basis for this analysis, one should be cautious not to "explain" verbal processes in terms of postulated internal mechanisms without adequate supportive evidence, nor should inference be made about nonobserved processes or events without corroborative evidence. The analysis includes many items which are not known or not applicable for a given patient. Lack of information on some items does not necessarily indicate incompleteness of the analysis. These lacks must be noted nevertheless because they often contribute to the better understanding of what the patient needs to learn to become an autonomous person. Just as important is an inventory of his existing socially effective behavioral repertoire which can be put in the service of any treatment procedure.

This analysis is consistent with our earlier formulations of the principles of comprehensive medicine[9,22] which emphasized the joint operation of biological, social, and psychological factors in psychiatric disorders. The language and orientation of the proposed approach are rooted in contemporary learning theory. The conceptual framework is consonant with the view that the course of psychiatric disorders can be modified by systematic application of scientific principles from the fields of psychology and medicine to the patient's habitual mode of living.

This approach is not a substitute for assignment of the patient to traditional diagnostic categories. Such labeling may be desirable for statistical, administrative, or research purposes. But the current analysis is intended to replace other diagnostic formulations purporting to serve as a basis for making decisions about specific therapeutic interventions.

METHODS OF DATA COLLECTION FOR A FUNCTIONAL ANALYSIS

Traditional diagnostic approaches have utilized as the main sources of information the patient's verbal report, his nonverbal behavior during an interview, and his performance on psychological tests. These observations are sufficient if one regards behavior problems only as a property of the patient's particular pattern of associations or his personality structure. A mental disorder would be expected to reveal itself by stylistic characteristics in the patient's behavior repertoire. However, if one views behavior disorders as sets of response patterns which are learned under particular conditions and maintained by definable environmental and internal stimuli, an assessment of the patient's behavior output is insufficient unless it also describes the conditions under which it occurs. This view requires an expansion of the clinician's sources of observations to include the stimulation fields in which the patient lives, and the variations of patient behavior as a function of exposure to these various stimulational variables. Therefore, the resourceful clinician need not limit himself to test findings, interview observations in the clinician's office, or referral histories alone in the formulation of the specific case. Nor need he regard himself as hopelessly handicapped when the patient has little observational or communicative skill in verbally reconstructing his life experiences for the clinician. Regardless of the patient's communicative skills the data must consist of a description of the patient's behavior *in relationship* to varying environmental conditions.

A behavioral analysis excludes no data relating to a patient's past or present experiences as irrelevant. However, the relative merit of any information (as, eg, growing up in a broken home or having had homosexual experiences) lies in its relation to the independent variables which can be identified as controlling the current problematic behavior. The observation that a patient has hallucinated on occasions may be important only if it has bearing on his present problem. If looked upon in isolation, a report about hallucinations may be misleading, resulting in emphasis on classification rather than treatment.

In the *psychiatric interview* a behavioral-analytic approach opposes acceptance of the content of the verbal self-report as equivalent to actual events or experiences. However, verbal reports provide information concerning the patient's verbal construction of his environment and of his person, his recall of past experiences, and his fantasies about them. While these self-descriptions do not represent data about events which actually occur internally, they do represent current behaviors of the patient and indicate the verbal chains and repertoires which the patient has built up. Therefore, the verbal behavior may be useful for description of a patient's thinking processes. To make the most of such an approach, variations on traditional interview procedures may be obtained by such techniques as role playing, discussion, and interpretation of current life events, or controlled free association. Since there is little experimental evidence of specific relationships between the patient's verbal statements and his nonverbal behavioral acts, the verbal report alone remains insufficient for a complete analysis and for prediction of his daily behavior. Further, it is well known that a person responds to environmental conditions and to internal cues which he cannot describe adequately. Therefore, any verbal report may miss or mask the most important aspects of a behavioral analysis, ie, the description of the relationship between antecedent conditions and subsequent behavior.

In addition to the use of the clinician's own person as a controlled stimulus object in interview situations, *observations of interaction with significant others* can be used for the analysis of variations in frequency of various behaviors as a function of the person with whom the patient interacts. For example, use of prescribed standard roles for nurses and attendants, utilization of members of the patient's family or his friends, may be made to obtain data relevant to the patient's habitual interpersonal response pattern. Such observations are especially useful if in a later interview the patient is asked to describe and discuss the observed sessions. Confrontations with tape recordings for comparisons between the patient's report and the actual session as witnessed by the observer may provide information about the patient's perception of himself and others as well as his habitual behavior toward peers, authority figures, and other significant people in his life.

Except in working with children or family units, insufficient use has been made of material obtained from *other informants* in interviews about the patient. These reports can aid the observer to recognize behavioral domains in which the patient's report deviates from or agrees with the descriptions provided by others. Such information is also useful for contrasting the patient's reports about his presumptive effects on another person with the stated effects by that person. If a patient's interpersonal problems extend to areas in which social contacts are not clearly defined, contributions by informants other than the patient are essential.

It must be noted that verbal reports by other informants may be no more congruent with actual events than the patient's own reports and need to be equally related to the informant's own credibility. If such crucial figures as parents, spouses, employers can be so interviewed, they also provide the clinician with some information about those people with whom the patient must interact repeatedly and with whom interpersonal problems may have developed.

Some observation of the patient's daily *work behavior* represents an excellent source of information, if it can be made available. Observation of the patient by the clinician or his staff may be preferable to descriptions by peers or supervisors. Work observations are especially important for patients whose complaints include difficulties in their daily work activity or who describe work situations as contributing factors to their problem. While freer use of this technique may be hampered by cultural attitudes toward psychiatric treatment in the marginally adjusted, such observations may be freely accessible in hospital situations or in sheltered work situations. With use of behavior rating scales or other simple measurement devices, brief samples of patient behaviors in work situations can be obtained by minimally trained observers.

The patient himself may be asked to provide samples of his own behavior by using tape recorders for the recording of segments of interactions in his family, at work, or in other situations during his everyday life. A television monitoring system for the patient's behavior is an excellent technique from a theoretical viewpoint but it is extremely cumbersome and expensive. Use of recordings for diagnostic and therapeutic purposes has been reported by some investigators.[2,5,24] Playback of the recordings and a recording of the patient's reactions to the playback can be used further in interviews to clarify the patient's behavior toward others and his reaction to himself as a social stimulus.

Psychological tests represent problems to be solved under specified interactional conditions. Between the highly standardized intelligence tests and the unstructured and ambiguous projective tests lies a dimension of structure along which more and more responsibility for providing appropriate responses falls on the patient. By comparison with interview procedures, most psychological tests provide a relatively greater standardization of stimulus conditions. But, in addition to the specific answers given on intelligence tests or on projective tests these tests also provide a behavioral sample of the patient's reaction to a problem situation in a relatively stressful interpersonal setting. Therefore, psychological tests can provide not only quantitative scores but they can also be treated as a miniature life experience, yielding information about the patient's interpersonal behavior and variations in his behavior as a function of the nature of the stimulus conditions.

In this section we have mentioned only some of the numerous life situations which can be evaluated in order to provide information about the patient. Criteria for their use lies in economy, accessibility to the clinician, and relevance to the patient's problem. While it is more convenient to gather data from a patient in an office, it may be necessary for the clinician to have first-hand information about the actual conditions under which the patient lives and works. Such familiarity may be obtained either by utilization of informants or by the clinician's entry into the home, the job situation, or the social environment in which the patient lives. Under all these conditions the clinician is effective only if it is possible for him to maintain a nonparticipating, objective, and observational role with no untoward consequences for the patient or the treatment relationship.

The methods of data collecting for a functional analysis described here differ from traditional psychiatric approaches only in that they require inclusion of the physical and social stimulus field in which the patient actually operates. Only a full appraisal of the patient's living and working conditions and his way of life allow a description of the actual problems which the patient faces and the specification of steps to be taken for altering the problematic situation.

SUMMARY

Current psychiatric classification falls short of providing a satisfactory basis for the understanding and treatment of maladaptive behavior. Diagnostic schemas now in use are based on etiology, symptom description, or prognosis. While each of these approaches has a limited utility, no unified schema is available which permits prediction of response to treatment or future course of the disorder from the assignment of the patient to a specific category.

This paper suggests a behavior-analytic approach which is based on contemporary learning theory, as an alternative to assignment of the patient to a conventional diagnostic category. It includes the summary of an outline which can serve as a guide for the collection of information and formulation of the problem, including the biological, social, and behavioral conditions which are determining the patient's behavior. The outline aims toward integration of information about a patient for formulation of an action plan which would modify the patient's problematic behavior. Emphasis is given to the particular variables affecting the *individual* patient rather than determination of the similarity of the patient's history or his symptoms to known pathological groups.

The last section of the paper deals with methods useful for collection of information necessary to complete such a behavior analysis.

This paper was written in conjunction with Research grant MH 06921-03 from the National Institutes of Mental Health, United States Public Health Service.

References

1. Ash, P. Reliability of Psychiatric Diagnosis, J Abnorm Soc Psychol 44:272–277, 1949.
2. Bach, G. In Alexander, S. Fight Promoter for Battle of Sexes, Life 54:102–108 (May 17) 1963.
3. Bandura, A. Psychotherapy as Learning Process, Psychol Bull 58:143–159, 1961.
4. Barron, F.: Ego-Strength Scale Which Predicts Response to Psychotherapy, J Consult Psychol 17:235–241, 1953.
5. Cameron, D. E., et al. Automation of Psychotherapy, Compr Psychiat 5:1–14, 1964.
6. Ferster, C. B. Classification of Behavioral Pathology in Ullman, L. P. and Krasner, L. (eds.). Behavior Modification Research, New York: Holt, Rinehart & Winston, 1965.
7. Freedman, D. A. Various Etiologies of Schizophrenic Syndrome, Dis Nerv Syst 19:1–6, 1958.
8. Fulkerson, S. E., and Barry, J. R. Methodology and Research on Prognostic Use of Psychological Tests, Psychol Bull 58: 177–204, 1961.
9. Guze, S. B., Matarazzo, J. D., and Saslow, G. Formulation of Principles of Comprehensive Medicine With Special Reference to Learning Theory, J Clin Psychol 9:127–136, 1953.
10. Jackson, D. D. A. Etiology of Schizophrenia, New York: Basic Books Inc., 1960.
11. Kanfer, F. H. Comments on Learning in Psychotherapy, Psychol Rep 9:681–699, 1961.
12. Katz, M. M., Cole, J. O., and Lowery, H. A. Nonspecificity of Diagnosis of Paranoid Schizophrenia, Arch Gen Psychiat 11:197–202, 1964.
13. Krasner, L. "Therapist as Social Reinforcement Machine," in Strupp, H., and Luborsky, L. (eds.). Research in Psychotherapy. Washington, D.C. American Psychological Association, 1962.
14. Ledley, R. S., and Lusted, L. B. Reasoning Foundations of Medical Diagnosis, Science 130: 9–21, 1959.
15. Lorr, M., Klett, C. J., and McNair, D. M. Syndromes of Psychosis, New York: Macmillan Co., 1963.
16. Meehl, P. E. Schizotaxia, Schizotypy, Schizophrenia, Amer Psychol 17:827–838, 1962.
17. New York Heart Association. Nomenclature and Criteria for Diagnosis of Diseases of the Heart and Blood Vessels, New York: New York Heart Association, 1953.
18. Noyes, A. P., and Kolb, L. C. Modern Clinical Psychiatry, Philadelphia: W. B. Saunders & Co., 1963.
19. Opler, M. K. Schizophrenia and Culture, Sci Amer 197:103–112, 1957.
20. Opler, M. K. Need for New Diagnostic Categories in Psychiatry, J Nat Med Assoc 55:133–137, 1963.
21. Rotter, J. B. Social Learning and Clinical Psychology, New York: Prentice-Hall, 1954.
22. Saslow, G. On Concept of Comprehensive Medicine, Bull Menninger Clin 16:57–65, 1952.
23. Scheflen, A. E. Analysis of Thought Model Which Persists in Psychiatry, Psychosom Med 20: 235–241, 1958.
24. Slack, C. W. Experimenter-Subject Psychotherapy —A New Method of Introducing Intensive Office Treatment for Unreachable Cases, Ment Hyg 44:238–256, 1960.
25. Szasz, T. S. Myth of Mental Illness, Amer Psychol 15:113–118, 1960.
26. Windle, C. Psychological Tests in Psychopathological Prognosis, Psychol Bull 49: 451–482, 1952.
27. Wolpe, J. Psychotherapy in Reciprocal Inhibition, Stanford, Calif: Stanford University Press, 1958.
28. Zigler, E., and Phillips, L. Psychiatric Diagnosis: Critique, J Abnorm Soc Psychol 63:607–618, 1961.

Behavioral Theories

THERAPY

Behavioral therapy consists of the direct application of experimentally derived principles of learning to the treatment of pathological disorders. The therapist does not seek to remove the "underlying" causes of psychopathology, nor does he give the patient free rein to explore his attitudes and feelings. Instead, he arranges a program of conditioning and extinction in which the behavior patterns he wishes to alter are specified, the environmental elements which have reinforced the maladaptive behavior are eliminated, and a series of new reinforcements are instituted in order to condition new adaptive behaviors. The British psychologist Hans Eysenck has been in the forefront as an exponent of behavioral therapy. In the paper presented here, he offers an illuminating commentary on the logic and rationale of the entire behavioral movement. Julian Rotter, a major exponent of the social learning approach, provides the basic thesis of his views on therapy in the excerpt reprinted here. Central to his theory is the notion of altering the patient's reinforcement expectancies, thereby modifying the source which motivates his overt behavior.

37. Learning Theory and Behaviour Therapy*

H. J. EYSENCK

It would probably be true to say that the present position in the psychiatric treatment of neurotic disorders is characterized by the following features. (1) With the exception of electroshock, the only method of treatment at all widely used is psychotherapy. (2) In practically all its manifestations, psychotherapy is based on Freudian theories. (3) With the exception of intelligence testing, psychological contributions consist almost entirely in the administration and interpretation of projective tests, usually along psychoanalytic lines. I have argued in the past and quoted numerous experiments in support of these arguments, that there is little evidence for the practical efficacy of psychotherapy,† whether strictly Freudian or "eclectic"[7,8]; that Freudian theories are outside the realm of science because of their failure to be consistent, or to generate testable deductions[9]; and that projective tests

From *J. Mental Science 105*: 61–75, 1959, by permission of the Royal Medico-Psychological Association and the author.

*This paper was delivered on 3 July 1958 to a meeting of the R.M.P.A., and its style inevitably bears traces of the fact that it was originally prepared for verbal presentation. It was followed by another paper, delivered by Mr. Gwynne Jones, giving concrete examples of the application of behaviour therapy from our own experience. Some of these are discussed in his article published in this Journal,[1] and it is suggested that readers interested in the theories here advanced may like to consult this article in order to obtain some notion of the practical methods emanating from these theories. A more detailed discussion of many theoretical points that arise may be found in *Dynamics of Anxiety and Hysteria*,[2] as well as several of my previous books.[3,4,5]

†When I first suggested that the literature did not contain any kind of unequivocal proof of the efficacy of psychotherapeutic treatment, this conclusion was widely criticized. Since then however, Dr. Weinstock, Chairman of the Fact-Finding Committee of the Amer. Psychoanalyt. Assoc., has explicitly stated in a lecture delivered at the Maudsley Hospital that his Association made *no claims of therapeutic usefulness for psychoanalytic methods* and in this country Glover[6] has equally explicitly disavowed such claims. On this point, therefore, leading psychoanalysts appear to share my views to a considerable extent.

are so unreliable and lacking in validity that their use, except in research, cannot be defended.[10]* I shall not here argue these points again; the evidence on which these views are based is quite strong and is growing in strength every year. I shall, instead, try to make a somewhat more constructive contribution by discussing an alternative theory of neurosis, an alternative method of treatment and an alternative way of using the knowledge and competence of psychologists in the attempted curing of neurotic disorders. It need hardly be emphasized that the brief time at my disposal will make it inevitable that what I have to say will sound much more dogmatic than I would like it to be; I have to ask your indulgence in this respect, and request you to bear in mind all the obvious qualifying clauses which, if included in this paper, would swell it to three times its present size.

Few psychiatrists are likely to deny that all behaviour ultimately rests on an inherited basis, but even fewer would be prepared to assert that environmental influences played no part in the genesis and modification of behaviour. Once we are agreed that learning and conditioning are instrumental in determining the different kinds of reaction we may make to environmental stimulation, we will find it very difficult to deny that neurotic reactions, like all others, are *learned* reactions and must obey the laws of learning. Thus, I would like to make my first claim by saying that modern learning theory,[11] and the experimental studies of learning and conditioning carried out by psychologists in their laboratories are extremely relevant to the problems raised by neurotic disorders. If the laws which have been formulated are, not necessarily true, but at least partially correct, then it must follow that we can make deductions from them to cover the type of behaviour represented by neurotic patients, construct a model which will duplicate the important and relevant features of the patient and suggest new and possibly helpful methods of treatment along lines laid down by learning theory. Whether these methods are in fact an improvement over existing

methods is, of course, an empirical problem; a few facts are available in this connection and will be mentioned later. It is unfortunate that insistence on empirical proof has not always accompanied the production of theories in the psychiatric field—much needless work, and many heartbreaking failures, could have been avoided if the simple medical practice of clinical trials with proper controls had always been followed in the consideration of such claims.

How, then, does modern learning theory look upon neurosis? In the first place, it would claim that neurotic symptoms are *learned patterns of behaviour* which for some reason or other are *unadaptive*. The paradigm of neurotic symptom formation would be Watson's famous experiment with little Albert, an eleven months old boy who was fond of animals.[14] By a simple process of classical Pavlovian conditioning, Watson created a phobia for white rats in this boy by standing behind him and making a very loud noise by banging an iron bar with a hammer whenever Albert reached for the animal. The rat was the conditioned stimulus in the experiment, the loud fear-producing noise was the unconditioned stimulus. As predicted, the unconditioned response (fear) became conditioned to the C.S. (the rat), and Albert developed a phobia for white rats, and indeed for all furry animals. This latter feature of the conditioning process is of course familiar to all students as the generalization gradient[12]; an animal or a person conditioned to one stimulus also responds, although less and less strongly, to other stimuli further and further removed from the original one along some continuum.

The fear of the rat thus conditioned is unadaptive (because white rats are not in fact dangerous) and hence is considered to be a neurotic symptom; a similarly conditioned fear of snakes would be regarded as adaptive, and hence not as neurotic. Yet the mechanism of acquisition is identical in both cases. This suggests that chance and environmental hazards are likely to play an important part in the acquisition of neurotic responses. If a rat happens to be present when the child hears a loud noise, a phobia results; when it is a snake that is present, a useful habit is built up!

The second claim which modern learning theory would make is this. People

---

*This fact is also beginning to be more widely realized, and it is symptomatic that such well-known departments as that belonging to the New York Psychiatric Hospital, have followed the lead of the Institute of Psychiatry and discontinued the routine use of projective techniques like the Rorschach.

and animals differ in the speed and firmness with which conditioned responses are built up.[15] Those in whom they are built up particularly quickly and strongly are more likely to develop phobias and other anxiety and fear reactions than are people who are relatively difficult to condition.[2] Watson was lucky in his choice of subject; others have banged away with hammers on metal bars in an attempt to condition infants, but not always with the same success. Individual differences must be taken into account in considering the consequences of any course of attempted conditioning. Nor is the degree of conditionability the only kind of individual variability with which we are concerned. Learning theory tells us that the amount of reinforcement following any action determines in part the amount of conditioning that takes place.[16] Thus the louder the noise, the greater the fright of the infant, and the greater the fright, the stronger the phobia. But different children have different types of autonomic system, and the same amount of noise produces quite unequal amounts of autonomic upheaval in different children. Consequently, autonomic reactivity must also be considered; the more labile or reactive the child, the more likely he is to produce strongly conditioned fear reactions, anxieties and phobias. The individual differences in autonomic reactivity and in conditionability have been conceptualized as giving rise to two dimensions of personality, namely neuroticism and introversion respectively.[5] The more autonomically reactive, the more prone will the individual be to neurotic disorders. The more easily he forms conditioned responses, the more introverted will his behaviour be. Combine introversion and neuroticism, and you get the dysthymic individual, the person almost predestined to suffer from anxieties, conditioned fears and phobias, compulsions and obsessions, reactive depressions and so forth.

But this is only part of the story. Many conditioned responses are unadaptive, and consequently may embarrass the individual and even drive him into a mental hospital if sufficiently intense. Yet other conditioned responses are obviously necessary and desirable; indeed, many of them are indispensable for survival. It has been argued very strongly that the whole process of socialization is built up on the principle of conditioning[17]; the overt display of aggressive and sexual tendencies is severely punished in the child, thus producing conditioned fear and pain responses (anxiety) to situations in which the individual is likely to display such tendencies. He consequently refrains from acting in the forbidden manner, not because of some conscious calculus of hedonic pleasure which attempts to equate the immediate pleasure to be gained from indulgence with the remote probability of later punishment, but because only by not indulging, and by physically removing himself can he relieve the very painful conditioned anxiety responses to the whole situation. Anxiety thus acts as a mediating drive, a drive which may be exceedingly powerful by virtue of its combination of central, autonomic, skeletal, and hormonal reactions. This mediating role of anxiety, and its capacity to function as an acquired drive, have been subjected to many well conceived experimental studies, and the consensus of opinion appears to leave little doubt about the great value and predictive capacity of his conception.[18]

Let us now consider an individual who is deficient in his capacity to form quick and strong conditioned responses. He will be all the less likely to be subject to phobias and other anxieties, but he will also be less likely to form useful conditioned responses, or to become a thoroughly socialized individual. When this lack of socialization is combined with strong autonomic drive reactions (high neuroticism), such an individual is likely to show the neurotic symptomatology of the psychopath or the hysteric, and indeed, in our experimental work we have found that, as predicted, dysthymic patients, and normal introverts, are characterized by the quick and strong formation of conditioned responses, while psychopaths and normal extraverts are characterized by the weak and slow formation of conditioned responses.[19,20,2] Thus the deviation from the average in either direction may prove disastrous — too strong conditioning easily leads to dysthymic reactions, too weak conditioning easily leads to psychopathic and hysterical reactions. The logic of this whole approach leads me to postulate two great classes of neurotic symptoms which between them exhaust in principle all the possible abnormal reactions with which you are all familiar. On the one hand we have *surplus conditioned reactions,* i.e. reactions acquired along the lines I have adumbrated, and where the reaction is unadaptive, even though originally it may have been well suited to circumstances. On the other hand we have *deficient conditioned reactions,* i.e., reactions normally acquired by most individuals in society which are adaptive, but which because of defective conditioning powers have not been acquired by a particular person. It is necessary to emphasize that surplus conditioned reactions and deficient conditioned reactions are due to an interplay between such individual factors as conditionability and autonomic lability, on the one hand, and environmental conditions on the other. There will be no socialization for an individual who cannot form conditioned responses at all, but conversely, there will be no socialization for a person growing up on a desert island, however powerful his conditioning mechanism may happen to be. In this paper I have no time to deal with differences in the conditioning forces of the environment, and their relation to such factors as social class, but they should certainly not be forgotten.

Many other testable deductions, apart from the differential conditionability of dysthymics and hysterics, follow from such a formulation. Some of these deductions can be tested in the laboratory, and examples have been given in my book, *Dynamics of Anxiety and Hysteria.*[2] But others can be tested clinically, and for the sake of an example I shall give just one of these. I have shown how psychopathic reactions originate because of the inability of the psychopath, due to his low level of conditionability, to acquire the proper socialized responses. But this failure is not absolute; he conditions much less quickly and strongly than others, but he does condition. Thus, where the normal person may need 50 pairings of the conditioned and the unconditioned stimulus and where the dysthymic may need 10, the psychopath may require 100. But presumably in due course the 100 pairings will be forthcoming, although probably much later in life than the 10 of the dysthymic, or the 50 of the normal person, and then he will finally achieve a reasonable level of socialization. If this chain of reasoning is correct, it would lead us to expect that the diagnosis "psychopath" would by and large be confined to relatively young

people, say under thirty years of age; after thirty the course of life should have brought forth the required 100 pairings and thus produced the needed amount of socialization. As far as I can ascertain, clinical psychiatric opinion is in agreement with this prediction.

How does our theory compare with the psychoanalytic one? In the formation of neurotic symptoms, Freud emphasizes the traumatic nature of the events leading up to the neurosis, as well as their roots in early childhood. Learning theory can accommodate with equal ease traumatic single-trial learning, for which there is good experimental evidence,[21] but it can also deal with repeated sub-traumatic pain and fear responses which build up the conditioned reaction rather more gradually.[22] As regards the importance of childhood, the Freudian stress appears to be rather misplaced in allocating the origins of *all* neurosis to this period. It is possible that many neurotic symptoms find their origin in this period, but there is no reason at all to assume that neurotic symptoms cannot equally easily be generated at a later period provided conditions are arranged so as to favour their emergence.

The point, however, on which the theory here advocated breaks decisively with psychoanalytic thought of any description is in this. Freudian theory regards neurotic symptoms as adaptive mechanisms which are evidence of repression; they are "the visible upshot of unconscious causes."[23] Learning theory does not postulate any such "unconscious causes," but regards neurotic symptoms as simple learned habits; there is no neurosis underlying the symptom, but merely the symptom itself. *Get rid of the symptom and you have eliminated the neurosis.* This notion of purely symptomatic treatment is so alien to psychoanalysis that it may be considered the crucial part of the theory here proposed. I would like to explore its implications a little further later on.

From the point of view of learning theory, treatment is in essence a very simple process. In the case of surplus conditioned responses, treatment should consist in the extinction of these responses; in the case of deficient conditioned responses, treatment should consist in the building up of the missing stimulus-response connections. Yet this apparent simplicity should not mislead us into thinking that the treatment of neurotic disorders offers no further problems. It is often found in scientific research that the solution of the problems posed by applied science is as complex and difficult as is the solution of the problems posed by pure science; even after Faraday and Maxwell had successfully laid the foundations of modern theories of electricity it needed fifty years and the genius of Edison to make possible the actual application of these advances to the solution of practical problems. Similarly here: a solution in principle, even if correct, still needs much concentrated and high-powered research in the field of application before it can be used practically in the fields of cure, amelioration, and prophylaxis.

What are the methods of cure suggested by learning theory? I shall give two brief examples only, to illustrate certain principles; others have been given by G. Jones.[1] One method of extinguishing the neurotic response X to a given stimulus S is to condition another response R to S, provided that R and X are mutually incompatible. This method, called "reciprocal inhibition" by Wolpe,[24] harks back to Sherrington[25] of course, and may be illustrated by returning to our rat-phobic little boy. Essentially, what Watson had done was to condition a strong sympathetic reaction to the sight of the rat. If we could now succeed in establishing a strong parasympathetic reaction to the sight of the rat, this might succeed in overcoming and eliminating the sympathetic response. The practical difficulty arises that, to begin with at least, the already established conditioned response is of necessity stronger than the to-be-conditioned parasympathetic response. To overcome this difficulty, we make use of the concept of stimulus gradient already mentioned. The rat close by produces a strong conditioned fear reaction; the rat way out in the distance produces a much weaker reaction. If we now feed the infant chocolate while the rat is being introduced in the far distance the strong parasympathetic response produced by the chocolate-munching extinguishes the weak sympathetic response produced by the rat. As the conditioned parasympathetic response grows in strength, so we can bring the rat nearer and nearer, until finally even close proximity does not produce sympathetic reactions. The sympathetic reaction has been extinguished; the phobia has been

cured. This is in fact the method which was used experimentally to get rid of the experimentally induced fear,[26] and it has been used successfully by several workers in the field of child psychiatry. More recently Herzberg[27] in his system of active psychotherapy, and more particularly, Wolpe[24] in his psychotherapy by reciprocal inhibition, have shown that these principles can be applied with equal success to the severe neuroses of adult men and women—substituting other methods, of course, for the chocolate-munching, which is more effective with children than with adults.

As an example of the cure of deficient conditioned responses, let me merely mention *enuresis nocturna*, where clearly the usual conditioned response of waking to the conditioned stimulus of bladder extension has not been properly built up. A simple course of training, in which a bell rings loudly whenever the child begins to urinate, thus activating an electric circuit embedded in his bedclothes, soon establishes the previously missing connection, and the extremely impressive list of successes achieved with this method, as compared with the very modest success of psychotherapeutic methods, speaks strongly for the correctness of the theoretical point of view which gave rise to this conception.[28]

We thus have here, I would suggest, an alternative theory to the Freudian, a theory which claims to account for the facts at least as satisfactorily as does psychoanalysis, and which in addition puts forward quite specific suggestions about methods of treatment. I have called these methods "behaviour therapy" to contrast them with methods of psychotherapy.* This contrast of terms is meant to indicate two things. According

---

*The growth of the theoretical concepts and practical methods of treatment subsumed in the term "behaviour therapy" owes much to a large number of people. Apart from Pavlov and Hull, who originated the main tenets of modern learning theory, most credit is probably due to Watson, who was among the first to see the usefulness of the conditioned paradigm for the explanation of neurotic disorders; to Miller and Mowrer, who have done so much to bring together learning theory and abnormal human behaviour; to Spence, whose important contributions include the detailed analysis of the relation between anxiety and learning; and to Wolpe, who was the first to apply explicitly some of the laws of learning theory to the large-scale treatment of severe neurotics. If there is any novelty in my own

to psychoanalytic doctrine, there is a psychological complex, situated in the unconscious mind, underlying all the manifest symptoms of neurotic disorder. Hence the necessity of therapy for the psyche. According to learning theory, we are dealing with unadaptive behaviour conditioned to certain classes of stimuli; no reference is made to any underlying disorders or complexes in the psyche. Following on this analysis, it is not surprising that psychoanalysts show a preoccupation with psychological methods involving

---

treatment of these issues it lies primarily: (1) in the pulling together of numerous original contributions into a general theory and (2) in the introduction into this system of the concepts of neuroticism and extraversion-introversion as essential parameters in the description and prediction of behaviour. I would like to emphasize, however, that this contribution could not have been made had the ground work not been well and truly laid by the writers quoted above and by many more, only some of whom are quoted in the bibliography.

mainly *speech*, while behaviour therapy concentrates on actual *behaviour* as most likely to lead to the extinction of the unadaptive conditioned responses. The two terms express rather concisely the opposing viewpoints of the two schools. Below, in summary form, is a tabulation of the most important differences between psychotherapy and behaviour therapy.

What kind of answer would we expect from the Freudians? I think their main points would be these. They would claim, in the first place, that conditioning therapy has frequently been tried, but with very poor results; aversion therapies of alcoholism are often mentioned in this connection. They would go on to say that even where symptomatic treatments of this kind are apparently successful, as in enuresis, the symptom is likely to return, or be supplanted by some other symptom, or by an increase in anxiety. Finally, they would claim that even if in some cases the

TABLE 1

Psychotherapy	Behaviour Therapy
1. Based on inconsistent theory never properly formulated in postulate form.	Based on consistent, properly formulated theory leading to testable deductions.
2. Derived from clinical observations made without necessary control observations or experiments.	Derived from experimental studies specifically designed to test basic theory and deductions made therefrom.
3. Considers symptoms the visible upshot of unconscious causes ("complexes").	Considers symptoms as unadaptive conditioned responses.
4. Regards symptoms as evidence of *repression*.	Regards symptoms as evidence of faulty learning.
5. Believes that symptomatology is determined by defence mechanisms.	Believes that symptomatology is determined by individual differences in conditionability and autonomic lability, as well as accidental environmental circumstances.
6. All treatment of neurotic disorders must be *historically* based.	All treatment of neurotic disorders is concerned with habits existing at *present*; their historical development is largely irrelevant.
7. Cures are achieved by handling the underlying (unconscious) dynamics, not by treating the symptom itself.	Cures are achieved by treating the symptom itself, i.e. by extinguishing unadaptive C.Rs and establishing desirable C.Rs.
8. Interpretation of symptoms, dreams, acts, etc. is an important element of treatment.	Interpretation, even if not completely subjective and erroneous, is irrelevant.
9. Symptomatic treatment leads to the elaboration of new symptoms.	Symptomatic treatment leads to permanent recovery provided autonomic as well as skeletal surplus C.Rs are extinguished.
10. Transference relations are essential for cures of neurotic disorders.	Personal relations are not essential for cures of neurotic disorder, although they may be useful in certain circumstances.

therapies suggested might be successful, yet in the great majority of cases psychoanalysis would be the only method to produce lasting cures. Let me deal with these points one by one.

There is no doubt that conditioning treatment of alcoholism has often been tried, and that it has often failed. I have no wish to take refuge in a *tu quoque* argument by pointing out that alcoholism has been particularly difficult to treat by any method whatever, and that psychoanalytic methods also have been largely unsuccessful. I would rather point out that learning theory is an exact science, which has elaborated quite definite rules about the establishment of conditioned reflexes; it is only when these rules are properly applied by psychologists with knowledge and experience in this field that the question of success or failure arises. Thus it is quite elementary knowledge that the conditioned stimulus must precede the unconditioned stimulus if conditioning is to take place; backward conditioning, if it occurs at all, is at best very weak. Yet some workers in the field of alcoholism have used a method in which the unconditioned stimulus regularly preceded the conditioned stimulus; under these conditions learning theory would in fact predict the complete failure of the experiment actually reported! Again, the time relation between the application of the conditioned stimulus and the unconditioned stimulus is a very important one; it is controlled to very fine limits of hundredths of a sec. in psychological experimentation and it has been universally reported that conditioning in which any but the optimal time relation is chosen is relatively ineffective. Taking eye-blink conditioning as an example: it is found that a time interval of about ½ sec. is optimal and that with intervals of 2½ sec. no conditioning at all takes place.[29,30] No attention seems to have been paid to these points by most workers on alcoholism, who apply the conditioned and unconditioned stimuli in such a vague way that it is often impossible to find out what the actual time relations were. This lack of rigour makes it quite impossible to adduce these so-called experiments as evidence either in favour or against conditioning therapy.[31]

How about the return of symptoms? I have made a thorough search of the literature dealing with behaviour therapy with this particular point in view. Many psychoanalytically trained therapists using these methods have been specially on the outlook for the return of symptoms, or the emergence of alternative ones; yet neither they nor any of the other practitioners have found anything of this kind to happen except in the most rare and unusual cases.[17] Enuresis, once cured by conditioning therapy, remains cured as a general rule; relapses occur, as indeed one would expect in terms of learning theory under certain circumstances, but they quickly yield to repeat treatment. So certain of success are the commercial operators of this method that they work on a "money back if unsuccessful" policy; their financial solvency is an adequate answer to the psychoanalytic claim. Nor would it be true that alternative symptoms emerge; quite the contrary happens. The disappearance of the very annoying symptom promotes peace in the home, allays anxieties, and leads to an all-round improvement in character and behaviour. Similar results are reported in the case of major applications of behaviour therapy to adults suffering from severe neurotic disorders; abolition of the symptom does not leave behind some mysterious complex seeking outlet in alternative symptoms.[17] Once the symptom is removed, the patient is cured; when there are multiple symptoms, as there usually are, removal of one symptom facilitates removal of the others, and removal of all the symptoms completes the cure.[24]

There is one apparent exception to this rule which should be carefully noted because it may be responsible for some of the beliefs so widely held. Surplus conditioned reactions may themselves be divided into two kinds, autonomic and motor. Anxiety reactions are typical of the autonomic type of surplus conditioned reactions, whereas tics, compulsive movements, etc. are typical of motor conditioned reactions. What has been said about the complete disappearance of the symptom producing a complete disappearance of the neurosis is true only as far as the autonomic conditioned reactions are concerned. Motor reactions are frequently activated by their drive reducing properties *vis-à-vis* the historically earlier conditioned autonomic responses[17]; the extinction of the motor response without the simultaneous extinction of the conditioned autonomic response would only be a very partial cure and could not be recommended as being sufficient. As pointed out at the end of the previous paragraph, "removal of *all* the symptoms completes the cure," and clearly removal of the motor conditioned response by itself, without the removal of the autonomic conditioned response is only a very partial kind of treatment. Behaviour therapy requires the extinction of all non-adaptive conditioned responses complained of by the patient, or causally related to these symptoms.

But how frequently does this type of treatment result in cures? Again I have made a thorough search of the literature, with the following outcome. GP treatment, not making use of psychotherapy in any of its usual forms, results in a recovery of about two seriously ill neurotics out of three.[32] Eclectic psychotherapy results in a recovery of about two seriously ill neurotics out of three.[7] Psychotherapy by means of psychoanalysis fares slightly worse, but results are at a comparable level.[8] Results of behaviour therapy of seriously ill neurotics, as reported by Wolpe, are distinctly superior to this, over 90 per cent recovering.[24] This difference is highly significant statistically and it should be borne in mind that the number of sessions required by behaviour therapy is distinctly smaller than that required by psychotherapy, whether eclectic or psychoanalytic. (Wolpe reports an average of about 30 sittings for his cases.)

These results are encouraging, but of course, they must not be taken too seriously. Actuarial comparisons of this kind suffer severely from the difficulty of equating the seriousness of disorders treated by different practitioners, the equally obvious difficulty of arriving at an agreed scale for the measurement of "recovery," and the impossibility of excluding the myriad chance factors which may affect gross behaviour changes of the kind we are here considering. I would not like to be understood as saying that behaviour therapy has been *proved* superior to psychotherapy; nothing could be further from my intention. What I am claiming is simply that as far as they go—which is not very far—available *data* do not support in any sense the Freudian belief that behaviour therapy is doomed to failure, and that only psychoanalysis or some kindred type of treatment is adequate to relieve neurotic disorders.

This Freudian belief is precisely this—a belief; it has no empirical or rational foundation. I have no wish to set up a counter-belief, equally unsupported, to the effect that psychotherapy is doomed to failure and that only behaviour therapy is adequate to relieve neurotic disorders. What I would like to suggest is simply that a good case can be made out, both on the theoretical and the empirical level, for the proposition that behaviour therapy is an effective, relatively quick, and probably lasting method of cure of some neurotic disorders. This case is so strong that clinical trials would appear to be in order now to establish the relative value of this method as compared with other available methods, such as psychoanalysis, or electroshock treatment. Even more important, I think the evidence would justify psychiatrists in experimenting with the method, or rather set of methods, involved, in order to come to some preliminary estimate of their efficiency. I have noted with some surprise that many psychotherapists have refused to use such methods as conditioning therapy in enuresis, not on empirical grounds, but on *a priori* grounds, claiming that such mechanical methods simply could not work, and disregarding the large body of evidence available. Even in long established sciences *a priori* considerations carry little weight; in such a young discipline as psychology they are quite out of place. Only actual use can show the value of one method of treatment as opposed to another.

There is one point I would like to emphasize. Freud developed his psychological theories on the basis of his study of neurotic disorders and their treatment. Behaviour therapy, on the contrary, began with the thorough experimental study of the laws of learning and conditioning in normal people and in animals; these well-established principles were then applied to neurotic disorders. It seems to me that this latter method is in principle superior to the former; scientific advance has nearly always taken the form of making fundamental discoveries and then applying these in practice, and I can see no valid reason why this process should be inverted in connection with neurosis. It may be objected that learning theorists are not always in agreement with each other[11] and that it is difficult to apply principles about which there is still so much argument. This is only very partially true; those points about which argument rages are usually of academic interest rather than of practical importance. Thus, reinforcement theorists and contiguity theorists have strong differences of view about the necessity of reinforcement during learning and different reinforcement theorists have different theories about the nature of reinforcement. Yet there would be general agreement in any particular case about the optimum methods of achieving a quick rate of conditioning, or extinction; these are questions of fact and it is only with the interpretation of some of these facts that disagreements arise. Even when the disputes about the corpuscular or wavular nature of light were at their height, there was sufficient common ground between contestants regarding the facts of the case to make possible the practical application of available knowledge; the same is true of learning theory. The 10 per cent which is in dispute should not blind us to the 90 per cent which is not—disagreements and disputes naturally attract more attention, but agreements on facts and principles are actually much more common. Greater familiarity with the large and rapidly growing literature will quickly substantiate this statement.[12]

It is sometimes said that the model offered here differs from the psychoanalytic model only in the terminology used and that in fact the two models are very similar. Such a statement would be both true and untrue. There undoubtedly are certain similarities, as Mowrer[17] and Miller and Dollard[33] have been at pains to point out. The motivating role of anxiety in the Freudian system is obviously very similar in conception to the drive-producing conditioned autonomic responses of learning theory, and the relief from anxiety produced by hysterical and obsessional symptoms in Freudian terminology is very similar to the conditioned drive-reducing properties of motor movements. Similarly, a case could be made out in favour of regarding the undersocialized, non-conditionable psychopathic individual as being Id-dominated, and the dysthymic, over-conditionable individual as being Super-Ego dominated. Many other similarities will occur to the reader in going through these pages and indeed the writer would be the first to acknowledge the tremendous service that Freud has done in elucidating for the first time some of these dynamic relationships and in particular in stressing the motivating role of anxiety.

Nevertheless, there are two main reasons for not regarding the present formulation as simply an alternative differing from the psychoanalytic one only in the terminology used. In the first place, the formulation here given differs from the Freudian in several essential features, as can be seen most clearly by studying Table 1. Perhaps these differences are most apparent with respect to the deductions made from the two theories as to treatment. Psychoanalytic theory distrusts purely symptomatic treatment and insists on the removal of the underlying complexes. Behaviour theory on the other hand stresses the purely symptomatological side of treatment and is unconvinced of the very existence of "complexes." It might, of course, be suggested that there is some similarity between the Freudian "complex" and the "conditioned surplus autonomic reaction" posited by behaviour theory. That there is some similarity cannot be denied, but no one familiar with psychoanalytic writings would agree that the Freudian complex was not in essence a very different conception from the conditioned autonomic response, both from the point of view of its origins, as well as from the point of view of the appropriate method of extinction.

This brings me to the second great difference between the two models. What the Freudian model lacks above all, is an intelligible objectively testable *modus operandi* which can be experimentally studied in the laboratory, which can be precisely quantified and which can then be subjected to the formulation of strict scientific laws. The stress on such a mechanism, namely that of conditioning, is the most noteworthy feature of the model here advocated. It is entirely due to the great body of research which has been done in connection with the elaboration of laws of modern learning theory, that we are enabled to make fairly precise deductions resulting in different methods of treatment for patients suffering from neurotic disorders and it is with respect to this feature of the model that the relevant case histories and accounts of treatment should be read.[34,35,36]

It has sometimes been suggested that the criticisms which I have levelled against the psychotherapeutic schools because of their failure to provide adequate control groups to validate their claims regarding the curative properties of their methods, could justifiably be levelled against the accounts given by those who have used behaviour therapy and reported upon the effects achieved. Such a criticism would not be justified for two reasons. In the first place, the cases quoted are *illustrative of methods*, not *proofs of psychotherapeutic efficacy*; the only case in which claims regarding relative efficacy have been made contains a statistical comparison with the effects of psychoanalytic treatment of similar cases.[24] In the second place, the concept of "control" in scientific experiments is somewhat more than simply the provision of a control *group*; the control in an experiment may be *internal*. As an example, consider the experiment reported by Yates[36] on the extinction of 4 tics in a female patient by means of a rather novel and unusual method, namely that of repeated voluntary repetition of the tic by massed practice. Precise predictions were made as to the effects that should follow and these predictions were studied by using the fate of some of the tics as compared to the fate of other tics submitted to dissimilar treatment. Thus, practice for 2 tics might be discontinued for a fortnight, while practice on the other two would go on. By showing that the predictions made could thus be verified and the *rate of extinction* of the tics varied at will —in accordance with the experimental manipulation for such variables as massing of practice—a degree of control was achieved far superior to the simple assessment of significance produced in the comparison of two random groups submitted to different treatments. It is by its insistence on such experimental precision and the incorporation of experimental tests of the hypotheses employed, even during the treatment, that behaviour theory differs from psychotherapy.

There is one further method of pointing up the differences between the two theories and of deciding between them; I mention this matter with some hesitation because to many psychiatrists it seems almost sacrilegious to use animal experimentation in the consideration of human neurosis. However, Fenichel himself,[37] p. 19 has quoted "experimental neuroses" as support for the Freudian conception of neurotic disorders and it is with respect to these experiments that the contrast between the psychoanalytic and our own model may be worked out most explicitly. Fenichel maintains that the model of psychoneurosis "is represented by the artificial neuroses that have been inflicted upon animals by experimental psychologists. Some stimulus which had represented pleasant instinctual experiences or which has served as a signal that some action would now procure gratification is suddenly connected by the experimenter with frustrating or threatening experiences, or the experimenter decreases the difference between stimuli which the animal had been trained to associate with instinct gratification and threat respectively; the animal then gets into a state of irritation which is very similar to that of a traumatic neurosis. He feels contradictory impulses; the conflict makes it impossible for him to give in to the impulses in the accustomed way; the discharge is blocked, and this decrease in discharge works in the same way as an increase in influx: it brings the organism into a state of tension and calls for emergency discharges.

"In psychoneuroses some impulses have been blocked; the consequence is a state of tension and eventually some 'emergency discharges.' These consist partly in unspecific restlessness and its elaborations and partly in much more specific phenomena which represent the distorted involuntary discharges of those very instinctual drives for which a normal discharge has been interdicted. Thus we have in psychoneuroses, first a defense of the ego against an instinct, then a conflict between the instinct striving for discharge and the defensive forces of the ego, then a state of damming up and finally the neurotic symptoms which are distorted discharges as a consequence of the state of damming up—a compromise between the opposing forces. The symptom is the only step in this development that becomes manifest; the conflict, its history, and the significance of the symptoms are unconscious."

Hebb[38] has laid down certain requirements for attempting to demonstrate that experimental neurosis occurs in animals and Broadhurst[39,40] has examined the literature, and particularly that referred to by Fenichel, from this point of view. Here is his summary. "How does the large body of American work stand up to such an assessment? For the purposes of a recent review,[40] the available literature was examined in the light of Hebb's criteria. Noteworthy among this is the work of the group headed by Liddell,[41] one of the pioneers of conditioning methodology in the United States, who has used principally the sheep as his experimental subject; of Gantt,[42] whose long term study of the dog 'Nick' is well known; and of Masserman,[43] who has done extensive work using cats. This is not the place to enter into the details of this evaluation, which is reported elsewhere,[40] but the overall conclusion which was reached was that there are few instances in all this work of any cases of experimentally induced abnormalities of animal behaviour which meet all of Hebb's criteria. Let us take, for example, the work of Masserman, whose theoretical interpretation of abnormal behaviour need not concern us here except to note that it was the basis upon which he designed his experiments to produce 'conflict' between one drive and another. What he did was this. He trained hungry cats to respond to a sensory signal by opening a food box to obtain food. Then he subjected them to a noxious stimulus, a blast of air, or electric shock, just at the moment of feeding. The resulting changes in behaviour—the animals showed fear of the situation and of the experimenter, and refused to feed further—he identified as experimental neurosis. But the behaviour observed fails to fulfill more than one or two of Hebb's criteria and, moreover, certain deficiencies in the design of his experiments make it impossible to draw any satisfactory conclusions from them. Thus Wolpe[44] repeated part of Masserman's work using the essential control group which Masserman had omitted—that is, he gave the cats the noxious stimulus alone, without any 'conflict' between the fear motivation thus induced, and the hunger which, in Masserman's animals, operated as well—and found that the same behaviour occurred. It hardly needs to be said that a fear response to a threatening stimulus is not abnormal and cannot be regarded as an experimental neurosis.''

It is clear from the studies cited that Fenichel is quite wrong in claiming that ''experimental neurosis'' is in any way analogous to the Freudian model of human neurosis. It appears, therefore, that in so far as these studies are relevant at all they can be regarded as demonstrating nothing but simple conditioned fear responses of the kind called for by our theory. It is perhaps worthy of note that the failure of psychoanalysis to use control groups in the human field has extended to their work with animals, as in the case of Masserman quoted above. Fenichel's easy acceptance of data congruent with his hypothesis is paralleled by his failure to mention data contrary to the psychoanalytic viewpoint. By taking into account all the data it seems more likely that a correct conclusion will be reached.

I would now like to return to some of the points which I raised at the beginning of this paper. I argued then, that the special knowledge and competence of psychologists in mental hospitals was largely wasted because of concentration on and preoccupation with Freudian theories and projective types of test. I would now like to make a more positive suggestion and maintain that by virtue of their training and experience psychologists are (or should be) experts in the fields of conditioning and learning theory, laboratory procedures and research design. In suitable cases, surely their help would be invaluable in diagnostic problems, such as ascertaining a given patient's speed of conditioning, in the theoretical problem of constructing a model of his personality dynamics and in the practical problem of designing a suitable course of behaviour therapy which would take into account all the available information about the case.* I am not suggesting that psychologists should themselves necessarily carry out this course of treatment; it would appear relatively

---

*It will be clear that the function here sketched out for the psychologist demands that he be furnished with the necessary tools of his trade, such as soundproof rooms, conditioning apparatus and all the other techniques for delivering stimuli and measuring responses on a strictly quantified basis.[45] It is equally clear that such facilities do not exist in the majority of our mental hospitals. Until they do, the handicaps under which the clinical psychologists work at such institutions will be all but insurmountable, and no reasonable estimate of their potential usefulness can be formed. One might just as well employ an electroencephalographer and refuse to pay for the machine which he has been trained to use! It would be better to have a few, properly equipped departments than a large number of small, ill-equipped ones as at present. Even in the United States the position is bad; in this country it is worse. A relatively small capital investment would be likely to bear considerable fruit.

immaterial whether the therapy is carried out by one person or another, by psychologist or psychiatrist. Both types of procedure have been experimented with and both have shown equally promising results. Indeed, certain aspects of the therapy can obviously be carried out by less senior and experienced personnel, provided the course of treatment is reviewed periodically by the person in charge. Psychoanalysis lays much stress on what is sometimes called "transference," a devil conjured up only to be sent back to his usual habitat with much expenditure of time and energy.[37] Behaviour therapy has no need of this adjunct, nor does it admit that the evidence for its existence is remotely adequate at the present time. However that may be, relinquishing the personal relationship supposed to be indispensable for the "transference" relation allows us to use relatively unqualified help in many of the more time-consuming and routine parts of behaviour therapy. In certain cases, of course, personal relationships may be required in order to provide a necessary step on the generalization gradient; but this is not always true.*

From a limited experience with this kind of work, carried out by various members of my department, I can with confidence say two things. The direct application of psychological theories to the practical problem of effecting a cure in a particular person, here and now, acts as a very powerful challenge to the psychologist concerned, and makes him more aware than almost anything else of the strengths and weaknesses of the formulations of modern learning theory. And the successful discharge of this self-chosen duty serves more than almost anything else to convince his psychiatric colleagues that psychology can successfully emerge from its academic retreat and take a hand in the day-to-day struggle with the hundred-and-one problems facing the psychiatrist. It seems to me that the tragic fratricidal struggle between psychiatrists and psychologists, which has so exacerbated

relations between them in the United States, could easily be avoided here by recognizing the special competence of the psychologist in this particular corner of the field, while acknowledging the necessity of keeping the general medical care of the patient in the hands of the psychiatrist. I believe that most psychiatrists are too well aware of the precarious state of our knowledge in the field of neurotic disorders to do anything but welcome the help which the application of learning theory in the hands of a competent psychologist may be able to bring.

References

1. Jones, H. G. (1958). Neurosis and experimental psychology. *J. Ment. Sci., 104*, 55–62.
2. Eysenck, H. J. (1957). *Dynamics of Anxiety and Hysteria*. Routledge & Kegan Paul, London.
3. Eysenck, H. J. (1947). *Dimensions of Personality*. Routledge & Kegan Paul, London.
4. Eysenck, H. J. (1952). *The Scientific Study of Personality*. Routledge & Kegan Paul, London.
5. Eysenck, H. J. (1953). *The Structure of Human Personality*. Methuen, London.
6. Glover, E. (1955). *The Technique of Psychoanalysis*. Bailliere, London.
7. Eysenck, H. J. (1952). The effects of psychotherapy: an evaluation. *J. Cons. Psychol., 16*, 319–324.
8. Eysenck, H. J. (1960). The effects of psychotherapy. In *Handbook of Abnormal Psychology*. Ed. by H. J. Eysenck. Pitman, London.
9. Eysenck, H. J. (1953). *Uses and Abuses of Psychology*. Pelican, London.
10. Eysenck, H. J. (1958). Personality tests: 1950–1955. In *Recent Progress in Psychiatry*. Ed. by G. W. T. W. Fleming. J. & A. Churchill, London.
11. Hilgard, G. A. (1956). *Theories of Learning*. Appleton-Century, New York.
12. Osgood, C. E. (1953). *Method and Theory in Experimental Psychology*. Oxford Univ. Press, London.
13. Shoben, E. J. (1949). Psychotherapy as a problem in learning theory. *Psychol. Bull., 46*, 366–392.
14. Watson, J. B., and Rayner, R. (1920). Conditioned emotional reaction. *J. Exp. Psychol., 3*, 1–4.
15. Pavlov, I. P. (1927). *Conditioned Reflexes*. Oxford Univ. Press, London.
16. Spence, K. G., Haggard, P. F., and Ross, L. G. (1958). UCS intensity and the associated (habit) strength of the eyelid CR. *J. Exp. Psychol., 95*, 404–411.
17. Mowrer, O. H. (1950). *Learning Theory and Personality Dynamics*. Ronald Press, New York.
18. Miller, V. G. (1951). Learnable drives and rewards. *Handbook of Experimental Psychology*. Ed. by S. S. Spencer. Wiley, New York.
19. Eysenck, H. J. (1954). Zur Theorie der Person-

---

*As an example of this we may quote a case reported by Graham White. This concerns a child who became anorexic after the death of her father. The therapist adopted the father's role in a variety of circumstances, ranging in order from play with dolls' teasets to the actual eating situation, and reinforcing those reactions which were considered desirable. The theoretical rationale was that the father had become a conditioned stimulus on which eating depended.

lichkeitsmessung. *Z. Diag. Psychol. Personlichkeitsforsch.*, 2, 87–101, 171–187.

20. Eysenck, H. J. (1957). Los principios del condicionamiento y la teoria de la personalidad. *Riv. Psicol.*, 12, 655–667.

21. Hudson, B. B. (1950). One-trial learning in the domestic rat. *Genet. Psychol. Monogr.*, 41, 94–146.

22. Solomon, R. L., Kamin, L. J., and Wynne, L. C. (1953). Traumatic avoidance learning. *J. Abnorm. (Soc.) Psychol.*, 48, 291–302.

23. Munroe, R. L. (1955). *Schools of Psychoanalytic Thought*. Dryden Press, New York.

24. Wolpe, J. (1958). *Psychotherapy by Reciprocal Inhibition*. Stanford Univ. Press.

25. Sherrington, C. S. (1926). *The Integrative Action of the Central Nervous System*. Oxford Univ. Press, London.

26. Jersild, A. T., and Holmes, F. B. (1935). Methods of overcoming children's fears. *J. Psychol.*, 1, 25–83.

27. Herzberg, A. (1941). Short treatment of neuroses by graduated tasks. *Brit. J. Med. Psychol.*, 19, 36–51.

28. Mowrer, O. H., and Morer, W. A. (1938). Enuresis. A method for its study and treatment. *Amer. J. Orthopsychiat.*, 8, 436–447.

29. McAllister, W. R. (1953). Eyelid conditioning as a function of the CS-UCS interval. *J. Exp. Psychol.*, 45, 412–422.

30. McAllister, W. R. (1953). The effect on eyelid conditioning of shifting the CS-UCS interval. *J. Exp. Psychol.*, 45, 423–428.

31. Frank, C. M. (1958). Alcohol, alcoholics and conditioning: a review of the literature and some theoretical considerations. *J. Ment. Sci.*, 104, 14–33.

32. Denker, P. G. (1946). Results of treatment of psychoneuroses by the general practitioner. A follow-up study of 500 cases. *N.Y. State J. Med.*, 46, 2164–2166.

33. Dollard, J., and Miller, V. G. (1950). *Personality and Psychotherapy*. McGraw-Hill, New York.

34. Jones, H. G. (1956). The application of conditioning and learning techniques to the treatment of a psychiatric patient. *J. Abnorm. (Soc.) Psychol.*, 52, 414–420.

35. Meyer, V. (1957). The treatment of two phobic patients on the basis of learning principles. *J. Abnorm. (Soc.) Psychol.*, 55, 261–266.

36. Yates, A. (1958). The application of learning theory to the treatment of tics. *J. Abnorm. (Soc.) Psychol.*, 56, 175–182.

37. Fenichel, O. (1945). *The Psychoanalytic Theory of Neurosis*. Kegan Paul, London.

38. Hebb, D. O. (1947). Spontaneous neurosis in chimpanzees: theoretical relations with clinical and experimental phenomena. *Psychosom. Med.*, 9, 3–16.

39. Broadhurst, P. L. (1958). The contribution of animal psychology to the concept of psychological normality-abnormality. *Proc. XII Internat. Congr. Appl. Psychol.*

40. Broadhurst, P. L. (1960). Abnormal animal behaviour. In *Handbook of Abnormal Psychology*. Ed. by H. J. Eysenck. Pitman, London.

41. Anderson, O. P., and Parmenter, A. (1941). A long-term study of the experimental neurosis in the sheep and dog. *Psychosom. Med. Monogr.*, 2, Nos. 3 and 4, 1–150.

42. Gantt, W. H. (1944). Experimental basis for neurotic behaviour. *Psychosom. Med. Monogr.*, 3, 1–211.

43. Masserman, J. K. (1943). *Behavior and Neurosis*. Univ. Press, Chicago.

44. Wolpe, J. (1952). Experimental neurosis as learned behaviour. *Brit. J. Psychol.*, 43, 243–268.

45. Eysenck, H. J. (1955). *Psychology and the Foundation of Psychiatry*. H. K. Lewis, London.

46. Estes, W. K. *et al* (1954). *Modern Learning Theory*. Appleton-Century, New York.

47. Hilgard, E. A., and Marquis, D. G. (1940). *Conditioning and Learning*. Appleton-Century, New York.

38. Psychological Therapy

JULIAN B. ROTTER

Many psychotherapists have stated in the past that psychotherapy is a process of learning. Learning is concerned with changes in behavior; psychotherapy is concerned with changes in behavior; learning and psychotherapy involve there-fore the same basic process. Having once stated this pious belief, they then ignore all of the principles of learning that seem fairly well established and proceed to explain therapy or to justify special techniques on the basis of principles strange to accepted learning theory. Cleaning out the unconscious, a force of self-integration, constructive will, transference, and the like become the governing principles of psychotherapy. Apparently personality change does not follow the same rules as that of learning to avoid a hot stove, to solve problems

From *Social Learning and Clinical Psychology*, Englewood Cliffs, N. J.: Prentice-Hall, 1954, pp. 335–351. Reprinted by permission. A more recent statement of Rotter's approach to psychotherapy and psychopathology, along with experimental reports, is presented in Rotter, J. B., Chance, J., and Phares, E. J.: *Applications of a Social Learning Theory of Personality*. New York, Holt, Rinehart, and Winston, 1972.

in arithmetic class, to acquire a foreign language, or to learn how to eat with a fork instead of one's fingers. Instead personality changes require the presence of a psychotherapist, who in some mysterious way acts as the necessary catalyst to any positive or adjustive changes.

It should be made clear at the outset that we reject this approach to psychotherapy. The changes that take place in or outside the therapy room follow the same laws and principles. The therapist himself has no special characteristic. The effect of new experiences either inside or outside the therapy room may result in better or poorer adjustment in either case. The therapist, as compared with a relative of the patient, may have some advantages in deliberately attempting to change the patient's behavior, but he also has some disadvantages. A change of attitude toward a child on the part of a parent may have more effect in changing the child's behavior than many hours of face-to-face therapy, smearing fingerpaints, and tearing apart dolls in the presence of a therapist.

In the previous chapters an expectancy-reinforcement theory of human learning has been described. It is not a completed theory, nor does it provide answers for all questions. It has many implications, however, for psychological treatment, and in this chapter we would like to make these implications clear. This will be attempted first by a general discussion of how behavior may be changed with particular reference to the function of a psychotherapist, and second by a discussion of current techniques in general usage and how they may be understood or modified from a social learning point of view. Although these two discussions may overlap each other, they may also serve to clarify each other. In our general discussion, we shall deal first with changing expectancies and then with changing reinforcement values.

CHANGING EXPECTANCIES

Mowrer, and Dollard and Miller have described in some detail why a maladjusted person does not learn adjustive behavior automatically. Since he is characterized by avoidant behaviors, the very nature of these avoidant behaviors keeps him out of situations or experiences where he may learn more adjustive behavior. He therefore continues to repeat the avoidant behavior as a way of dealing with the particular type of problem and never has an opportunity to learn alternative ways of behaving. Mowrer goes on to point out that although the avoidant behavior itself may lead to punishment, it is usually delayed punishment, which has less effect on reducing or eliminating the maladjustive or avoidant behavior than it would if it followed immediately. In general we would agree strongly with this position.

The person who first experiences punishment, failure, or frustration in a situation and then avoids similar situations not only has no opportunity to learn new, adjustive behavior in such a situation but continues to have a high expectancy for punishment or failure should he do anything but avoid the situation since he has no new experience of gratification or success in it. The avoidant behavior continues to result generally in the relative gratification of eliminating the punishment, rejection, failure, or whatever negative reinforcement is involved. Later punishments resulting from the avoidant behavior or related to it may not be associated at all with the avoidant behavior by the person involved. If the punishment is associated with the avoidant behavior, delay does not have a great significance, particularly as the maladjusted person develops beyond early childhood, but even then the punishments, though delayed, may not be as great as the punishment that is being avoided and the avoidant behavior will therefore continue. In addition to this, the maladjustive behaviors may serve other functions as well as direct avoidance of punishment or pain. They may bring attention, sympathy, protection, or other desirable reactions. Frequently psychologists misinterpret behavior of children as avoidant, fearful, or anxious when the behavior in question may more properly be thought of as a direct attempt to obtain some reinforcement from parents or others such as protection, attention, or concern. Very few children who are afraid of the dark have ever been hurt by the dark or as a result of being in darkness. They have learned, however, that the expression of such concern will get parents to stay with them when they go to bed. Perhaps this results in taking the parents away from rivals, either siblings or the other parent, or engaging the parents in some pleasant occupation such as telling stories or fondling. Similarly, very few children who are afraid of dogs have ever been bitten by one, but they have learned that their parents will show concern when they express such fears and will be willing to watch or play with a child when they might otherwise ignore him and take care of some other business. Adler was one of the first to point out how frequently such fears develop following the birth of another sibling but relatively independently of any specific traumatic experience. That the behavior itself is maladjustive in the long run is quite clear. Not only does the child limit his own potential for constructive behavior but the very child who is seeking to hold on to parents who may already favor him frequently loses the affection of these same parents as they turn to the displacing child, who is so frequently characterized as "so good natured," "less demanding," and so on. As a result the maladjustive child attempts more and more extreme behaviors to hold the attention and concern of the parents.

Maladjustive behavior, then, not only may be avoidant behavior in the sense of avoiding some previously experienced specific punishment but also may be a learned, direct way to obtain satisfactions with a history of reinforcement or gratification. In any case, we may say that the maladjusted person has an expectancy that his maladjustive behavior as seen from the outsider's point of view will lead to greater gratification (or less punishment) than would the behavior that the outsider sees as desirable, constructive, or adjustive.

One major problem in therapy, then, may be said to be that of lowering the expectancy that a particular behavior or behaviors will lead to gratifications or increasing the expectancy that alternate or new behaviors would lead to greater gratification in the same situation or situations. In general learning terms we might say we have the choice of either weakening the inadequate response, strengthening the correct or adequate response, or doing both.

Before discussing methods of changing expectancies, it might be worth while to reflect on the relative efficiency of weakening inadequate responses versus strengthening adequate responses. Research in learning in general has shown that praise or reward for a correct response is a much more effective learning device than punishment of an inadequate response. Generally a combination of both is most effective, but almost all the research tends to support the greater effectiveness of reward for correct response over punishment for incorrect response. Surprisingly enough, most psychotherapy practices now in common usage operate on the opposite principle, that the elimination of the bad response is much more important than the substitution or building up of a good response. By reflection, catharsis, insight, discussion, projection, transference, the therapist attempts to get his patient to eliminate his maladjustive behavior, but relatively little emphasis is placed upon alternative or adjustive responses to the same problem situations. Although many therapists accept the importance of the problem of developing adequate responses, they seem to feel that this problem must be pushed aside until one can rub out, eliminate, or erase the maladaptive responses; and yet they experience great difficulty in carrying out such a plan, primarily because the patient involved has nothing better to substitute and so he holds on to what he has. Although the implications of social learning theory are for the usefulness of reducing of the potential for maladaptive behavior, compared with other views toward psychotherapy, we place much greater emphasis on building up the potential for more adequate ways of dealing with the same problem situations. In keeping with this, we shall first discuss the problem of increasing the expectancy for gratification for alternative or new behaviors (including implicit defense behaviors), suggesting five ways in which this may be accomplished.

The most direct or simple way of increasing behavior potentials is through direct reinforcement. Frequently so-called adjustive behaviors are used by a maladjusted person, but not as a dominant response and sometimes only in particular situations. If it is possible to reinforce these directly, potentiality of the behaviors' recurring increases. With children this can perhaps be done most efficiently through parents, teachers, or other people who play an important role in the day-to-day environment. With adults it is more difficult for the therapist to reach these other people and effect changes in them; however, it is still probably true that attempts to change the behavior of people who are important in the patient's life space is neglected in the treatment of both children and adults. There is too much emphasis on what goes on in the therapy room and too little emphasis on what goes on in the day-to-day life situations. Where it might be possible to deal with wives, husbands, and even bosses, many therapists are likely to ignore these possibilities, either because they are overconcerned with what goes on in the therapy room in terms of their relationship with the patient, because they are timid in making or arranging for such contacts, or because they fear without actually investigating that the patient will resent such contacts or be afraid that his confidences are being violated. Sometimes these latter two reasons are sufficient justification for the therapist's not attempting to deal with anyone other than the patient. More frequently, they are assumed to be valid reasons for not dealing with others, without investigation and without any attempt to explain or interpret to the patient the potential value of such contacts, both to him and to the others involved.

However, the therapist in his day-to-day contacts does have the opportunity to respond positively or with positive reinforcement to the behavior of the patient. In fact, he does so probably to a much greater extent than he is aware. By the use of group therapy, he may also place the patient in a situation where both he and others may directly reward adjustive behavior on the part of the patient. More specifically he frequently rewards by expression and statement the patient's attempts to deal frankly with his problems, to look for new solutions, to lessen his frustrations with humor; moreover, by his very acceptance of the patient and his reassurance regarding potential change, he directly rewards the patient's behavior in attempting to do something about his problem. Unfortunately, sometimes he directly rewards behaviors that are not so adjustive, such as the patient's projecting blame on others, his fixating on childhood experiences, or his continuous self-concern.

Where the patient himself does not display behavior that the therapist might directly reinforce, alternative methods of behaving might be discussed with him so that he will attempt new behaviors, or at least behaviors that he has not used in these situations before or may not have used for some time. He may also be made aware of how others use different behaviors. Luchins, in his studies of set, has clearly demonstrated that one can by verbal techniques direct attention to cues which, although previously present, were not attended to. Similarly, the therapist can direct the patient's attention to the relationship between the behavior of others and the gratifications or subsequent rewards that others obtain. Sometimes that has been accomplished merely by the patient's being placed in a situation where he can observe these relationships or have an opportunity to observe that he may not have had before. Frequently the placement of a child with poor social skills into group situations may in itself result in the learning of much adequate social behavior. Where the therapist is depending upon face-to-face verbal discussions with the patient, one potential for learning new behaviors may come from the patient's discussions of other people important in his day-to-day living or in his past life and from the patient's attempts to understand these other people. Too often such discussions are centered upon the patient himself.

When alternative behaviors do not occur frequently enough to be reinforced directly in the patient's own behavior repertoire or in the people around him, and when such behaviors are not discovered by the patient himself in his discussing possible solutions, then the therapist may suggest them directly. He does this by discussing with the patient, if necessary, both how the specific behavior may be carried out and the potential consequences of the behavior. By his discussion of possible positive consequences for behaviors, he creates some expectancy on the patient's part that if he behaves in a particular way it will lead to a gratification. Expectancies created in such verbal, symbolic form are probably not as high as those where the patient attempts the behavior in some life situation and is directly reinforced by some person of importance to him. But as the therapist himself gains in reinforcement value, the potentiality increases that the patient will try out alternative behaviors in a life situation and thereby obtain some direct gratification.

Sometimes the therapist may discuss with the patient the previous use of behaviors that the patient has eliminated because they have led to punishment or frustration. In order to increase the patient's expectancy that such behaviors may lead to gratification, the therapist must discuss with the patient why the previous experiences of punishment or failure occurred in the past and are not likely to occur in the future, or why reinforcements or reactions may now be expected from peers other than those which were previously expected from parents. What the therapist is doing in this case is using the verbal kind of learning described earlier, where it is possible by the use of language to make abstractions from the experience of the patient himself to be used now in the understanding of new relationships (Adler would call this utilizing the patient's common sense). Only too frequently the therapist may be concerned more with the patient's learning some new, esoteric understanding of his behavior than with using the patient's common sense or the experience he shares with others to reinterpret the behavior that results from distortion and brings him discomfort.

It is the purpose of therapy not to solve all of the patient's problems, but rather to increase the patient's ability to solve his own problems. The rational techniques employed in some therapies frequently lead the patient to become expert at interpreting his own behavior or the behavior of others but provide him with little potentiality for change. The ineffectiveness of such techniques may be due in part to their failure to stress alternative ways of behaving or dealing with problems. From a social learning point of view, one of the most important aspects of treatment, particularly of face-to-face treatment, is to reinforce in the patient the expectancy that problems are solvable by looking for alternative solutions. The study by Schroder and Rotter demonstrates quite clearly that it is possible for such a behavior to be reinforced in an experimental sequence. There seems to be little reason to doubt that this behavior may also be reinforced in therapy.

Morton, in a study using extremely brief psychotherapy, was able to demonstrate that a technique based primarily on the principle of reinforcing attempts to solve problems by looking for alternative solutions showed clearly measurable improvement in adjustment. In one of the rare studies where a matched control group was used, Morton randomly selected one of a matched pair of college students both seeking help at the Occupational Opportunities Service and both referred by vocational counselors for personal counseling. He treated one of the pair and told the other that the facilities were extremely crowded and made an appointment for three months later. The therapy consisted of the patient's giving TAT stories, then going over some of the stories with the therapist to analyze them in terms of the nature of the problem faced by the central characters, the nature of the solution that was used in the story, and what other possible alternative solutions could be made. Unless the patient himself brought it up, no direct reference was made to the implications of the TAT stories for the patient's own problems. The patients were then asked to take the rest of the TAT stories home and to analyze them, following an outline given them by the therapist. These were brought back and, story by story, discussed with the therapist over a period of approximately four hours. In each case the emphasis was on alternative solutions and the potential effects of them. Before treatment the subjects had a long interview, a Mooney Problem Checklist, and an Incomplete Sentences Blank. Subjects were matched on the basis of this pretesting into pairs, the scoring being done objectively by people other than the therapist. Three months after the treatment the patients and the control subjects were again tested with the same techniques. The interview was rated by judges who did not know which were controls and which were experimental subjects, and the Incomplete Sentences Blank was likewise scored by judges who did not know the identity of the subjects. Using difference scores, Morton found that treated patients improved significantly more than the controls on both the interview and Incomplete Sentences Blank. On the Mooney Problem Checklist, the improvement approached significance.

An interesting sidelight on this study was that Morton found that the controls themselves improved significantly from test to retest, an improvement that is probably due not merely to regression but actually partly to the therapeutic effects of time. That is, many clients coming for therapy or for help come at a time when their problems are most pressing, and at least some of these clients, if held off, find solutions of their own. The implication, however, is of great significance for research on psychotherapy. It indicates quite clearly that a before-and-after measure of improvement cannot be relied upon to indicate accurately the efficiency of a treatment procedure unless a matched control group is used.

In summary, then, we have suggested some five ways in which the therapist attempts to increase the potentiality of alternative or adjustive behaviors' occurring as a function of an increased expectancy for some gratification or positive reinforcement. These include: (1) the direct reinforcement of the behavior, either by the therapist or by others, in which the therapist uses the knowledge of what reinforcements are of high value for the patient; (2) placing the patient, or helping him to find and enter, into situations where he may observe in others alternative behaviors and their consequences, or where by discussion and interpretation he can try to understand the behavior of others retrospectively; (3) dealing with the patient's own past history of alternative behaviors and reducing his expectancy that they will now result in the same frustrations or negative reinforcements as they did in the past, and verbally increasing his expectancy that these alternative behaviors will result in gratifications; (4) discussing with the patient possible alternatives apparently for the first time, including discussions of how the behaviors are actually carried out, and creating for him an expectancy that they may lead to gratification in life situations; (5) creating and reinforcing for the patient an expectancy that he may solve his problems more effectively by looking for and trying out alternative solutions or behaviors.

Lowering Expectancies for Reinforcement

As in the case of raising expectancies, in reducing them the therapist may also choose between direct reinforcement and some verbal technique. A direct method consists of failing to reinforce or to reward a behavior in the way that such a behavior has been rewarded before. It may be useful where the maladaptive behavior has in the past or still frequently leads to some direct satisfaction other than avoidance of punishment. By failing to react with concern, sympathy, protection, or attention, the therapist himself may reduce the potentiality of behaviors directed toward these goals. He may also deal with other people in the client's environment so that they, likewise, fail to reinforce the particular behaviors as they have done in the past. This is to imply not that the therapist should, in responding to these same behaviors, assume an attitude of stern rejection or so-called "neutrality," but rather that he should react to these same behaviors in some different way that is not reinforcing or at least not as reinforcing as the way most people have reacted in the past. His behavior may be mildly negatively reinforcing when his relationship is such that this negative reinforcement will not so weaken the relationship that he loses his case. For example, instead of listening and nodding sympathetically with implicit agreement to a long discourse of blame projection, he might instead, in a voice tinged more with curiosity than with acceptance, ask, "You feel that these problems are all the result of others' behavior?" Or to the child who falls down and announces proudly that he hurt himself, instead of showing concern and asking for the locus of the injury, the therapist might comment without concern "So I see," and then change the subject. Undoubtedly, these failures to reinforce behavior as the patient has had them reinforced in the past and still seeks to have them reinforced in the present places a strain upon the therapeutic relationship and the reinforcement value of the therapist for the patient. They should be engaged in only insofar as they are balanced by more positive rewards by the therapist and as the therapist determines by gradual means how much the therapeutic relationship can stand. Similarly, if a parent, a teacher, or someone else is given recommendations to cease particular kinds of reinforcements, they must also be given recommendations for positive reinforcements for alternative behaviors with at least equal, if not greater, emphasis placed upon the latter.

Expectancies for reinforcement may also be reduced by verbal analysis methods. As in the case of increasing expectancies for new behaviors, this analysis may take the form of contrasting the patient's life situation in the past with his present life situation in order to point out the carryover of expectations on his part that are not appropriate in the present situation. In the case of avoidant behaviors, the patient may discover for himself, as he discusses his past life, that the punishments and failures he has been avoiding are not now as likely to occur or are not at all likely to occur. His reduced expectancy for the punishment to occur will result in a correspondingly reduced expectancy that he is achieving any goal by his avoidant behavior. Similarly, through verbal discussion, the patient may discover by himself or through interpretation that his maladjustive behavior is successful only in delaying and not in truly avoiding the punishment.

Sometimes when the behavior is actually leading to reinforcement in life situations—for example, where it leads to domination of a spouse or parent or to concern and protection—it is necessary to reduce the expectancy for future reinforcement by verbal analysis. This will be discussed in the following section.

CHANGING REINFORCEMENT VALUES

Changing the value of external reinforcements or goals is essentially a problem of changing what we have called E_2, or the expectancy, based on the subject's past experience, that immediate reinforcements will lead to specific subsequent reinforcements. The problem should be, therefore, essentially the same as that of changing expectancies for the occurrence of a reinforcement; and in many respects it is the same problem, but additional practical difficulties are frequently present.

It seems a great deal easier to change the behavior that a person uses to reach a goal than to change the importance of the goal for him. This difficulty is very well illustrated by clinical attempts to change a stutterer's pattern of stuttering. It has been demonstrated clinically many times that it is possible to change the pattern of stuttering so that it has physiologically very little in common with the previous pattern—a person, for example, whose stuttering is characterized by long, tonic blocks may be taught rather

readily to stutter instead with bouncy, clonic blocks. Stutterers' effort and starter mechanisms may be shifted rather readily. On the other hand, it is much more difficult to "cure" these same people of stuttering. They are not as willing to give up the satisfactions or the goals toward which their stuttering is aimed as they are to change the method of reaching these goals. Similarly, many a wife would be willing to change the pattern by which she attempts to dominate her husband, but it is much more difficult for her to give up the goal of dominating for something else. There are several reasons for this. The values attached to the goals are frequently learned over a long period of time and have a history of many, many reinforcements. The relationships between the goals and other goals are much less frequently verbalized or easily perceived. People see their goals more as Allport has described them, as autonomous—"as goals in their own right."

The therapist frequently attempts to change goals that are still reinforced by many people in the same culture. For example, the therapist may fail to see that it is not the goal itself that is socially unacceptable or maladaptive but either the way in which the patient has learned to reach it or possibly the situations in which he attempts to reach it. A wife finds that dominating a husband who himself has some doubts regarding his masculinity leads to trouble, but becoming president of the local Ladies Aid Society does not. The therapist, implicitly or explicitly attempting to change the value of a patient's goal by implying that the value is a mistaken one for the society in which the patient lives, frequently neglects the fact that within that society there are times when the goal has the value the patient places upon it.

Before we discuss how reinforcement values or goal values are changed, a brief discussion of when it is appropriate to change such goals would be in order. It is not always true that an inadequate behavior implies an inadequate goal. The delinquent from a deprived neighborhood learns to steal cars because this may lead to peer recognition, and peer recognition is for him the major source of satisfaction. When such a child has a father who disappeared before his birth and a mother who is gone working during the day, his major source of satisfaction frequently comes from the recognition and acceptance of his peers or what is sometimes known as "the gang." Such a goal is a normal and healthy one. What is perhaps wrong is the particular group from which he seeks his recognition; in terms of a broader analysis, the difficulty lies in the social conditions rather than the individual adjustment of the children involved. At any rate, the problem is not to have the child give up his seeking of peer acceptance and recognition, but to change, either for him or for the whole group, the behaviors that lead to such peer acceptance and recognition.

For another child who may steal as a gesture of hostility or aggression toward a middle-class father who is himself strict and rejecting, the goal of successfully hurting the father may well be changed, since it leads in the long run to greater frustration and rejection for the child. Similarly, not all attention-getting or recognition-seeking behaviors or goals are maladaptive. The child who seeks attention in the classroom by creating a disturbance or by vomiting has learned inadequate behaviors, but constructive accomplishment is considered a quite acceptable way to get attention in the same classroom and it also leads to additional reinforcements. Frequently the problem is not so much one of eliminating a particular goal as one of reducing its relative preference value, particularly for specific situations. Recognition-seeking is an important part of our culture, but recognition-seeking to the exclusion of everything else, on the playground as well as in the classroom or in heterosexual relationships, leads to many subsequent frustrations.

Since the changing of expectancies for subsequent reinforcements is further removed from behavior directed toward the initial reinforcement, it is more difficult to obtain changes in behavior by changes in subsequent reinforcement without some interpretation. Effective direct reinforcement without interpretation is not impossible, but attempts are frequently inefficient since a change in the subsequent reinforcement (R_{b-n}) may not be associated by the subject with the problem behavior. For example, affection shown to a child after he has brought home a poor grade from school may be intended as acceptance of the poor grade to reduce the child's minimal goal, but

may be seen by the child in terms of his previous experience as simply a result of a particular mood on the part of the parent, or perhaps as a different kind of approach to motivate him to do better, unless some verbal connection is established by the parent. On the other hand, if the accepting behavior occurs several times, he will probably establish the relationship himself. Without the use of language, changing reinforcement values by direct reinforcements alone is a longer learning process than when the reinforcement follows directly and is obviously associated with the behavior. In other words, interpretation at some level seems both necessary and desirable in attempts to change goal values or need values.

We have stated before that, particularly with children, such attempts at verbal explanation have frequently been slighted. This is apparently due to the belief either that the child cannot learn verbally or that it is not important to verbalize the relationships between his own behavior and the behavior of others. Our own clinical experience as well as the obvious evidence that a child does learn on his own and can verbalize countless such relationships would suggest that when properly stated such explanations or interpretations may be extremely useful in a treatment program. They should, however, refer to things that actually have occurred to the child, either in the immediate past or often enough so that he has very clear referents for what is being discussed.

Like initial expectancies, reinforcement or goal values may be changed by verbal analysis of past experience, by current day-to-day living, or by future experience. Often people have goal values based either upon a misinterpretation of earlier experience or upon experience appropriate for an earlier life occasion but not for the present. An example of the former may be the child who perceives his sister as favored by his father and finds his mother essentially a cold, rejecting woman but apparently important to his father. Such a child might misperceive the relationships between the father's love and his own masculine characteristics and develop a goal of effeminacy, although such behaviors in themselves lead more to his father's rejection than to his love. An example of placing value on a goal because of earlier experience, now inappropriate, is that of the adult who succeeds in controlling or outdoing everyone he has face-to-face relationships with and is somewhat hurt and confused that no one likes him. Such a person may have been urged by parents to win in every competition, to be better than everyone else, and was rewarded with love when he succeeded. At one time the behavior was appropriate enough for obtaining the goal of the parents' love, but as the child developed this goal was generalized to the goal of love from others. In the present the behavior leads more to the frustration of that goal than to the satisfaction of it.

Since experiences in the present are related to the expectancies built up on the basis of the past, we may wish to weaken or reduce such expectancies by verbal methods. As in our early discussion of rewarding alternative approaches to obtaining satisfaction, reduction in expectancies built out of past experience is likely to succeed in changing behavior only if there are alternatives more likely to lead to satisfaction for the subject. In dealing with the present, then, we are concerned not only with reducing some goal values and helping the subject to grasp more clearly the relationships between his behavior and immediate and delayed reinforcements, but also with increasing the potential for new behaviors by increasing the reinforcement value for new goals, or goals that have previously had relatively low value. For example, we are concerned less, perhaps, with reducing the need for dependence in some patients than with the patients' perceiving the benefits or potential satisfactions that come from independence. Similarly, we are interested not merely in reducing the value of controlling, dominating, or succeeding over others but also in increasing the value of helping, cooperating with, accepting, or appreciating others.

In reducing goal values through the analysis of current or present life experiences, the problem is frequently one of helping the patient discover the relationship between his current goals and his current frustrations and dissatisfactions. Similarly, relationships can be seen between potential future dissatisfactions and current goals. The unrealistic or noncontributive goals of the present may lead to much frustration in the future, even though they currently

lead to only minor frustration. For example, the girl who wishes to be indulged and taken care of by a man may not mind the absence of suitors at age 22 while an indulgent father is still satisfying her needs, but might readily perceive the problem she might face when she is 35. Or the goals of avoiding masculine domination (stated otherwise, the goals of dominating men in both the social and sexual aspects) may lead to some immediate gratifications but to severe future frustrations.

However, the patients themselves are likely to be most interested in their current, day-to-day frustrations—the difficulty of holding a job, the quarreling with a marital partner, the expectancy of punishment for sexual transgression or hostile wishes—and the relationship of these frustrations to their goals; and discussion of the relationships provide the best opportunity for changing goal or need values.

Minimal Goal Levels and Reducing Reinforcement Values

It has been previously indicated that minimal goal levels are frequently too high in maladjusted people. The psychoanalysts have stressed the high moral goals or standards in the realm of sex. Johnson has stressed the maladjusted person's absolute notions of success. Adler has stressed the unrealistic goals of superiority or security of maladjusted people. We believe the reduction of such standards or goals is essentially a problem of increasing the reinforcement values of goals or reinforcements below the minimal goal, or of attaching positive subsequent reinforcements to reinforcements that have previously been followed by punishment or frustration. Lesser accomplishments may be followed by praise instead of exhortations to do better, punishments, or criticisms. Following hostile behavior, sexual deviation, or lying by acceptance and understanding rather than by severe punishment should reduce minimal goals of "moral" adequacy. As with increasing the reinforcement value of any goal, the use of direct reinforcements by the therapist or by others is one technique and verbal analysis is another.

All of the previous discussion regarding change of reinforcement values applies to minimal goals or to raising the value of goals below the minimal goal. However, the direct reinforcement of the therapist may have more effect in changing minimal goals than in some other instances of changing goal values, particularly where the therapist is able by acceptance to increase the reinforcement value of some reinforcement for which the patient previously anticipated punishment. By the fact that the therapist himself does not react with horror, chagrin, or criticism when the patient discusses his transgressions, errors, and inadequacies, he is able directly to lower the minimal goal of the patient.

Along with the direct behavior or reinforcements of the therapist, there is the possibility of discussing with the patient how his standards or high minimal goals have been set by misinterpretation of past experience or by the behavior of his parents or other adults important in his early development. Frequently it helps the patient to see and understand the present inappropriateness of such learned values as he learns to contrast the behavior of parents with that of the rest of the culture. He is able to accept this better as he learns to see the parent's behavior resulting from lack of knowledge or from the problems, frustrations, and maladjustments of these adults themselves.

Behavioral Theories

CRITICAL EVALUATION

Behavioral theorists of psychopathology borrow their concepts from experimental learning research; consequently, one would expect their work to be subject to little scientific faulting. The failure to live up to this expectation, according to some critics, points up the difficulty of transferring concepts from one field to another. Borrowing the rigorously derived concepts of laboratory research may be no more than a specious ennoblement of one's meagre accomplishments, a cloak of falsely appropriated prestige which duly impresses the naïve.

David Rapaport's review of Dollard and Miller's work suggests that their scientific sounding terminology is no more than a set of flimsy analogies of psychoanalytic theory, offering no new explanatory powers or insights; old wine in new bottles is still old wine, wine best left in its old container. Breger and McGaugh's penetrating critique of the logical and empirical foundations of the behavioral approach raises the question of whether the laboratory based concepts borrowed from the prestigious field of learning are genuinely useful in psychopathology or whether they are merely bandied about in an allegorical and superficial manner. They note further that the "basic" laws of learning are not so basic after all; much dissent exists among learning theorists as to which concepts and laws are "basic." They ask whether laws of learning should be applied to highly complex clinical processes when the existence of these laws in simple situations remains a matter of dispute.

39. A Critique of Dollard and Miller's "Personality and Psychotherapy"

DAVID RAPAPORT

This is a difficult volume (Dollard and Miller's *Personality and Psychotherapy*, 1950) to review, because it is hard to pin down its arguments. This for several reasons. First, it professes to be a collection of hypotheses and to use clinical material only to illustrate, and not to prove anything. Second, it is disarming in its admission of our general ignorance and of the need for further knowledge before a definitive theoretical structure can be built. Third, it is ambiguous in its alternating enthusiasm for and rejection of psychoanalytic premises, concepts and theories. Its ground in this respect is shifting and therefore difficult to come to grips with. Last but not least, it has been reviewed before by both psychologists and psychiatrists who, unlimited by familiarity either with learning theory or with psychotherapy, hailed it with the starry-eyed enthusiasm of wishful thinking.

There is one fixed point around which this book pivots, and this is learning theory. There is also a somewhat less fixed point, namely, the use of learning theory in order to explain phenomena of

From *Amer. J. Orthopsychiat.* 23: 204–208, 1953, by David Rapaport. Copyright, the American Orthopsychiatric Association, Inc. Reproduced by permission.

neurosis and therapy. These two ~~p~~ will be taken here as points of departu~~re~~.

Dollard and Miller suggest that th~~e~~ concepts of drive, cue, response, and reward (reinforcement) are "exceedingly important" for the understanding of all levels of acquired behavior. These concepts readily indicate that this theory of acquired behavior is a learning theory and, more particularly, one of the conditioned-response vintage. The authors guardedly dwell on the question whether these concepts are "essential" or just "important" for the understanding of acquired behavior (pp. 25-26). Nevertheless, their actual argument seems to assume that all behavior can be understood in terms of motivating drives, which elicit responses when the proper cues are present, and that cues and responses are linked to the drive and to each other by the success of the response, which both establishes and reinforces these links.

This theory sounds much like the psychoanalytic theory. At the same time, it appeals much more to "common sense" than the psychoanalytic theory. It is therefore tempting to demonstrate the shortcomings of this theory as a learning theory, and to show up its inadequacy in coping with the phenomena for which psychoanalytic theory was developed. This is, however, neither our task here, nor possible in a brief review. Instead, it should suffice to say that Dollard and Miller may leave their readers with an erroneous impression. They propound this theory of learning as if to say that those aspects of it which they present are well established, though other aspects of it may be still open to question. This is, however, not the case. The battle of cognitive vs. stimulus-response theories of learning is still on. Not long ago Tolman (1949) summarized his studies in an article entitled "There Is More Than One Kind of Learning"; he found that there are eight different kinds. Only recently the neuropsychologist Hebb (1949) has put forth evidence to show that neither the Gestalt nor the conditioned-response theories of learning do justice to many fundamental observations concerning learning, and particularly to the observation that early learning in infancy is qualitatively different in character from late learning. None of the learning theories have as yet integrated Piaget's (1952) genetic observations concerning learning. Last but not least, the most recent review

th~~e~~ all ~~~~ to ap~~~~ to the ~~~~ chotherapy~~~~ they had ma~~~~ applying the _th~~~~_ had made plain t~~~~ worker, etc., not~~~~ theory, that the con~~~~ psychotherapy and neu~~~~ say the least—far from being ~~~~ly accepted. It would have been ~~de~~sirable if they too, like Kendler (1951)—one of the adherents of this type of learning theory—would have spoken out candidly: "In spite of its relative sophistication, S-R reinforcement theory is still basically a primitive formulation. It would be unwise for S-R psychologists to try to 'sell it' for anything more than that" (p. 372). One would also wish the authors had brought to the attention of all who are not versed in the theories of learning that the problems of learning are just as complicated and just as unsolved as the problems of neurosis and psychotherapy. It is certainly to Dollard and Miller's credit that they even attempted to bring the problem of neurosis and the problem of learning to bear on each other. They vitiate their merit, however, by giving the impression that "normal learning" is already understood and that therefore its "laws" can now be applied to "pathological learning." It should be said in their defense, however, that they also stress that much can be learned about learning from patients; patients may oblige us where normals do not have the motivation to let us learn from them.

Dollard and Miller are emphatic that their use of clinical material should not be construed as proof or evidence for their hypotheses but only as concrete illustration of principles (p. 16). Thus we are given a series of principles of learning and a series of illustrations for them from everyday life as well as from clinical experience. Some of the examples of clinical phenomena are labeled with customary psychiatric or psychoanalytic terms, others with new terms. Surely, this again is a justified endeavor. It is in accord with the commonly accepted scientific pro-

apply to
...ying them to
...rent realm of ob-
...question which always
...ch endeavors is whether this
...et of concepts is more parsimonious
...than the one used heretofore to describe,
to explain and to predict in this realm.
Dollard and Miller in general do not attempt to offer any proof that their concepts and theory are preferable to those
of psychoanalysis. All they do is express
their hope that they are bringing a better
conceptual system into the field of
neurosis and psychotherapy than the one
used heretofore, slip in a few pejorative
assertions concerning some common
Freudian concepts, and praise their own
concepts as superior to the Freudian.
They could have argued explicitly and not
merely by implication that their theory
which was tested in animal and human experiment should also be "scientific" in the
field of neurosis and psychotherapy than
the prevailing, experimentally untested
theories. Their implicit argument dis-
regards the fact that their theory was developed to account for a very limited
range of animal behavior and an even
more limited range of human behavior. It
is therefore necessary to stress explicitly
that no proof is offered by the authors that
the conceptual system of psychoanalysis
at large is any better or worse for prediction of phenomena of neurosis and
psychotherapy than the conceptual system they champion and attempt to illustrate in this volume. There is an old
proverb which says, "When the angels
came down to earth, they too did eat."
When Miller and Dollard came down from
the experimental laboratory to clinical
material, their treatment of phenomena
and their use of concepts is certainly no
more rigorous than the psychiatrists' and
psychoanalysts' treatment of phenomena
and use of concepts. Indeed one may ask
whether theirs has as much consistency
and rigor as the latter.

It would be unfair to Dollard and
Miller to apply to their study the yardstick
of Freudian theory, even if they do
occasionally claim acceptance of this
theory. Yet it seems important to point
out one relationship between psychoanalysis and their theory. From the
beginning one of the outstanding
characteristics of psychoanalytic theory
has been its distinction between, on the

one hand, the *primary processes* which
are motivated by basic drives and which
in their operation display the so-called
Freudian mechanisms (condensation, displacement, symbolization, etc.) and, on
the other hand, the *secondary processes*
which follow the rules of logic and reality-
testing. In the course of the development
of psychoanalytic theory this distinction
developed into the distinction between the
ego and the id. The fluid transition between these two types of processes, their
interaction in adjustment, creativity, and
neurosis, etc., was brought into the
framework of psychoanalytic theory. It is
one of the merits of Dollard and Miller's
theory, as it is of Mowrer's recent theory,
that by the distinction between innate and
learned drives they attempt to do some
justice to the distinction between early
and late learning, between primary processes and secondary processes. (Earlier
learning theories disregarded this distinction entirely.) This merit is, however,
vitiated by the fact that, according to their
theories, both innate and learned drives
operate by the same reward-reinforcement
mechanism. The complexity of clinical
phenomena which led to the development
of psychoanalytic ego-psychology and
which also led to Allport's recognition
of functional autonomy within the
framework of his ego psychology, the
phenomena which made it necessary for
all ego psychologies to assume that the
ego has constitutional foundations of its
own, are not even envisaged by these
learning theories. Dollard and Miller's
"acquired secondary drives" and their
single reliance on the reward mechanism
of learning cannot come to grips with
these complexities, not even if the concept
of reward is formulated so broadly as to
include social rewards. It is characteristic
for Dollard and Miller's presentation that
phenomena of concern to psychoanalytic
ego-psychology are as a rule dealt with
tangentially and without apparent
awareness of the existence of psychoanalytic ego-psychology. This holds
for defenses, which are treated only in
the sense of "resistance" (pp. 265ff).
synthetic functions, differentiation functions, as well as "higher mental processes." It appears that Dollard and
Miller's understanding of psychoanalysis
is in most—if not in all—respects as of
1922, that is, of a date preceding Freud's
The Ego and the Id and *The Problem of*

Anxiety, as well as Anna Freud's *The Ego and the Mechanisms of Defense.* In this sense these authors are proponents of a peculiar psychoanalytic orthodoxy, which should be as unsatisfactory to any Neo-Freudian psychoanalyst or psychiatrist as it is to the psychoanalyst aware of the development in psychoanalytic ego-psychology. The contributions of Horney to our understanding of defenses, of Sullivan to our understanding of the self, of Fromm to our understanding of social and cultural factors, have as little place in the framework of this theory as anything Freud had to say after 1923, and as any of Anna Freud's, Hartmann's, Kris's, E. H. Erikson's, Redl's, and Bettelheim's contributions.

While we are all eager to reach a state where our theories will be borne out not only by clinical experience but verified also by experiment, we have to acknowledge the fact that the reason that our theories are no better than they are is not simply because we are not clever enough to develop rigorous operational concepts, but because our subject matter is complex and we are yet at the beginning of its exploration. Under such handicaps, not even scientists equipped with the methodology of operationalism and with experimental know-how, as Dollard and Miller certainly are, can develop a neat and simple theory for us. Indeed the more they try to make it neat and pat, the more cavalier they become in their disregard of clinical fact.

Finally, I can't help remarking that in an attempt as ambitious as this we could expect somewhat more clinical sophistication than is evident. A single example of the unfortunate combination of lack of clinical understanding with a mechanical application of an inapt theory, so characteristic of this volume, follows.

"Example of the problem of masturbation. Masturbation presents a special problem to the therapist because it is a response that frequently occurs and produces a marked reduction in drive but is not the socially most desirable form of sexual adaptation. It is an inferior form of adaptation because it *removes one of the strong rewards from marriage** which seems to provide the best all-around basis for personal adjustment.

"If the patient has too much fear to

---

*Italics mine—D. R.

try any heterosexual responses, masturbation may be good as the first step toward the goal of normal sexual behavior. When the patient first tries masturbation, the orgasm produced in this way will reward the general attempt to try sexual behavior, help to define the goal, and *give the patient a good chance to discover and extinguish some of his fears of sex.** We will expect this extinction to generalize and tend to weaken the fear motivating the inhibition of heterosexual behavior. On the other hand if the therapist shows any signs of *disapproval** at this stage, he will strengthen the patient's fear, and this fear will tend to generalize to all forms of sexual behavior.

"If the therapist *allows** masturbation to become established as more than a transitional habit, it will become so strongly reinforced that it may be hard to abandon. Furthermore it will tend to keep the sex drive so low that the heterosexual responses never can become stronger than their inhibitions. Finally, the patient may be having undesirable phantasies during masturbation. *Associating the strong sexual reward of the orgasm with the cues involved in these phantasies may increase his appetite for childish, perverse, or extramarital sex outlets.**

"This theoretical analysis yields several practical suggestions. If possible, it is better for the patient to move directly toward a heterosexual marital adjustment. If the patient's inhibitions are too strong for this to be possible, it may be necessary for the therapist to be *permissive** toward masturbation at first. After masturbation is started, it may be desirable for the therapist to try to *exert some control over the accompanying phantasies and direct them toward the heterosexual marital goal.* Finally, after the patient's inhibitions have been weakened enough so that he will be able to try better responses, it may be necessary *to discourage masturbation by pointing out the ways in which it is an inferior response"** (pp. 386-387).

I have to leave it to the reader to judge in what sense this example is consistent with the authors' initial statement: "We have concentrated our analysis on the one type of therapeutic practice with which we are familiar—namely Freudian. Even here, we have attempted to analyze only those features of theory and practice that we understood best" (p. viii).

References

Hebb, D. O. *Organization of behavior: A neuropsychological theory.* New York: Wiley, 1949.

Hilgard, E. R. *Theories of learning.* New York: Appleton-Century-Crofts, 1948.

Kendler, H. H. Reflections and confessions of a reinforcement theorist. *Psychol. Rev.,* 1951, *58,* 368–374.

Piaget, J. *Play, dreams and imitation in childhood.* New York: Norton, 1952.

Tolman, E. There is more than one kind of learning. *Psychol. Rev.,* 1949, *56,* 144–156.

40. Critique and Reformulation of "Learning-Theory" Approaches to Psychotherapy and Neurosis

LOUIS BREGER and JAMES L. McGAUGH

A careful look at the heterogeneous problems that are brought to psychotherapy points up the urgent need for new and varied theories and techniques. While some new methods have been developed in recent years, the field is still characterized by "schools" —groups who adhere to a particular set of ideas and techniques to the exclusion of others. Thus, there are dogmatic psychoanalysts, Adlerians, Rogerians, and, most recently, dogmatic behaviorists.

It is unfortunate that the techniques used by the behavior-therapy group (Bandura, 1961; Eysenck, 1960; Grossberg, 1964; Wolpe 1958) have so quickly become encapsulated in a dogmatic "school," but this seems to be the case. Before examining the theory and practice of behavior therapy, let us first distinguish three different positions, all of which are associated with the behaviorism or "learning-theory" label. These are: *(a)* Dollard and Miller (1950) as represented in their book, *(b)* the Wolpe-Eysenck position as represented in Wolpe's work (1958; Wolpe, Salter, & Reyna, 1964) and in the volume edited by Eysenck (1960), and *(c)* the Skinnerian position as seen in Krasner (1961) and the work that appears in the *Journal of the Experimental Analysis of Behavior.*

Dollard and Miller present an attempt to translate psychoanalytic concepts into the terminology of Hullian learning theory. While many recent behavior therapists reject Dollard and

Miller because of their identification with psychoanalysis and their failure to provide techniques distinct from psychoanalytic therapy, the Dollard-Miller explanation of neurotic symptoms in terms of conditioning and secondary anxiety drive is utilized extensively by Wolpe and his followers. Wolpe's position seems to be a combination of early Hullian learning theory and various active therapy techniques. He relies heavily on the idea of reciprocal inhibition, which is best exemplified by the technique of counter-conditioning. In line with this Hullian background, Wolpe, Eysenck, and others in this group use explanations based on Pavlovian conditioning. They define neurosis as "persistent unadaptive habits that have been conditioned (that is, learned) (Wolpe et al., 1964, p. 96)," and their explanation of neurosis stresses the persistence of "maladaptive habits" which are anxiety reducing.

The Skinnerian group (see Bachrach in Wolpe et al., 1964) have no special theory of neurosis; in fact, following Skinner, they tend to disavow the necessity of theory. Their approach rests heavily on *techniques* of operant conditioning, on the use of "reinforcement" to control and shape behavior, and on the related notion that "symptoms," like all other "behaviors," are maintained by their effects.

Our discussion will be directed to the Wolpe-Eysenck group and the Skinnerians, keeping in mind that some of the points we will raise are not equally applicable to both. Insofar as the Skinnerians disavow a theory of neurosis, for example, they are not open to criticism in this area.

It is our opinion that the current

From *Psychol. Bull. 63*: 338–358, 1965, by permission of the American Psychological Association and the authors.

arguments supporting a learning-theory approach to psychotherapy and neurosis are deficient on a number of grounds. First, we question whether the broad claims they make rest on a foundation of accurate and complete description of the basic data of neurosis and psychotherapy. The process of selecting among the data for those examples fitting the theory and techniques while ignoring a large amount of relevant data seriously undermines the strength and generality of the position. Second, claims for the efficacy of methods should be based on adequately controlled and accurately described evidence. And, finally, when overall claims for the superiority of behavioral therapies are based on alleged similarity to laboratory experiments and alleged derivation from "well-established laws of learning," the relevance of the laboratory experimental findings for psychotherapy data should be justified and the laws of learning should be shown to be both relevant and valid.

In what follows we will consider these issues in detail, beginning with the frequently voiced claim that behavior therapy rests on a solid "scientific" base. Next, we will examine the nature and adequacy of the learning-theory principles which they advocate. We will point out how their learning theory is unable to account for the evidence from laboratory studies of learning. That is to say, the laws or principles of conditioning and reinforcement which form the basis of their learning theory are insufficient explanations for the findings from laboratory experiments, let alone the complex learning phenomena that are encountered in psychotherapy. Then we will discuss how the inadequate conception of learning phenomena in terms of conditioned responses is paralleled by an equally inadequate conception of neurosis in terms of discrete symptoms. Within learning theory, conceptions of habit and response have been shown to be inadequate and are giving away to conceptions emphasizing "strategies," "plans," "programs," "schemata," or other complex central mediators. A central point of this paper is that conceptions of habit and response are also inadequate to account for neuroses and the learning that goes on in psychotherapy and must here too be replaced with conceptions analogous to strategies. Next we will turn our attention to an evaluation of the claims of

success put forth by the proponents of behavior therapy. Regardless of the adequacy of their theory, the claims that the methods work are deserving of careful scrutiny. Here we shall raise a number of questions centering around the issue of adequate controls. Finally, we shall attempt a reformulation in terms of more recent developments within learning, emphasizing the role of central processes.

SCIENCE ISSUE

Claims of scientific respectability are made with great frequency by the behavior therapists. Terms such as laboratory based, experimental, behavioral, systematic, and control are continually used to support their position. The validity of a theory or method must rest on empirical evidence, however. Thus, their use of scientific sounding terminology does not make their approach scientific, but rather seems to obscure an examination of the evidence on which their claims are based.

Let us examine some of this evidence. Bandura (1961) provides the following account of a typical behavior-therapy method (Wolpe's counter-conditioning):

On the basis of historical information, interview data, and psychological test responses, the therapist constructs an anxiety hierarchy, a ranked list of stimuli to which the patient reacts with anxiety. In the case of desensitization based on relaxation, the patient is hypnotized, and is given relaxation suggestions. He is then asked to imagine a scene representing the weakest item on the anxiety hierarchy and, if the relaxation is unimpaired, this is followed by having the patient imagine the next item on the list, and so on. Thus, the anxiety cues are gradually increased from session to session until the last phobic stimulus can be presented without impairing the relaxed state. Through this procedure, relaxation responses eventually come to be attached to the anxiety evoking stimuli (p. 144).

Without going into great detail, it should be clear from this example that the use of the terms stimulus and response are only remotely allegorical to the traditional use of these terms in psychology. The "imagination of a scene" is hardly an objectively defined stimulus, nor is something as general as "relaxation" a specifiable or clearly observable response. What the example shows is that counterconditioning is no more objective, no more controlled, and no more scientific than classical psychoanalysis, hypnotherapy, or treatment with tranquilizers. The claim to scientific respectability rests on the misleading use of terms such as stimulus, response, and conditioning, which have become associated with some of the methods of science because of their place in experimental psychology. But this implied association rests on the use of the same *words* and on the use of the same *methods*.

We should stress that our quarrel is not with the techniques themselves but with the attempt to tie these techniques to principles and concepts from the field of learning. The techniques go back at least as far as Bagby (1928), indicating their independence from "modern learning theory." Although techniques such as these have received little attention in recent years (except from the behavior therapists) they are certainly worth further consideration as potentially useful techniques.*

The use of the term conditioning brings us to a second point, that the claims to scientific respectability rest heavily on the attempts of these writers to associate their work with the prestigious field of learning. They speak of something called modern learning theory, implying that psychologists in the area of learning have generally agreed upon a large number of basic principles and laws which can be taken as the foundation for a "scientific" approach to psychotherapy. For example, Eysenck (1960) states:

Behavior therapy . . . began with the thorough experimental study of the laws of learning and conditioning in normal people and in animals; these well-established principles were then applied to neurotic disorders. . . . It may be objected that learning theorists are not always in agreement with each other and that it is difficult to apply principles about which there is still so much argument. This is only very partially true; those points about

which argument rages are usually of academic interest rather than of practical importance. . . . The 10% which is in dispute should not blind us to the 90% which is not—disagreements and disputes naturally attract more attention, but agreements on facts and principles are actually much more common. Greater familiarity with the large and rapidly growing literature will quickly substantiate this statement (pp. 14–15).

As we shall show in the next section, this assertion is untenable. "Greater familiarity with the large and rapidly growing literature" shows that the very core of "modern learning theory," as Eysenck describes it, has been seriously questioned or abandoned in favor of alternative conceptualizations. For example, the notion that the discrete response provides an adequate unit of analysis or that reinforcement can be widely used as an explanation of both learning and performance, or that mediational processes can be ignored are being or have been rejected. Eysenck's picture of the field as one with 90% agreement about basic principles is quite simply untrue. The references that Eysenck himself gives for this statement (Hilgard, 1956; Osgood, 1953) do not support the claim. Hilgard presented many theories, not one "modern learning theory," some of which (Gestalt, Tolman, Lewin) might just as easily be said to be in 90% disagreement with behavioristic conditioning approaches. In the same vein, Osgood's text was one of the first to give heavy emphasis to the role of mediation, in an attempt to compensate for the inadequacies of a simple conditioning or one-stage S-R approach. Eysenck seems largely unaware of the very problems within the field of learning which necessitated the introduction of mediational concepts, even by S-R theorists such as Osgood.

These inadequacies center, in part, around the problem of generalization. The problem of generalizing from the level of conditioning to the level of complex human behavior has been recognized for a long time (Lewin, 1951; Tolman, 1933). It is a problem that is crucial in simple laboratory phenomena such as maze learning where it has resulted in the introduction of a variety of mediational concepts, and it is certainly a problem when complex human behavior is being dealt with. For example, Dollard and Miller (1950) began their book with an attempt

---

*Another early application of behavioral techniques has recently been brought to our attention: Stevenson Smith's use of the Guthrie approach to learning in his work at the children's clinic at the University of Washington. Guthrie's interpretation of reinforcement avoids the pitfalls we discuss shortly, and contemporary behaviorists might learn something from a review of his work (see Guthrie, 1935).

to explain neurosis with simple conditioning principles. A careful reading of the book reveals, however, that as the behavior to be explained became more and more complex, their explanations relied more and more on mediational concepts, including language. The necessity for these mediators arises from the inadequacy of a simple *peripheral* S-R model to account for the generality of learning, the equivalence of responses, and the adaptive application of behavior in novel situations. We shall return to these points shortly; here we just wish to emphasize that the field of learning is not "one big happy family" whose problems have been solved by the widespread acceptance of a simple conditioning model. The claim to scientific respectability by reference back to established laws of learning is, thus, illusory.

LEARNING AND LEARNING THEORIES

We have already noted the differences between the Wolpe-Eysenck and the Skinnerian approaches; let us now examine the similarities. Three things stand out: the focus on the overt response, the reliance on a conditioning model, and the notion of reinforcement. First, there is the belief that the response, consisting of some discrete aspect of overt behavior, is the most meaningful unit of human behavior. While this should ideally refer to a specific contraction of muscles or secretion of glands, with the possible exception of Guthrie (1935), traditional S-R theorists have tended to define response in terms of an effect on the environment rather than as a specific movement of the organism. The problems raised by the use of the response as a basic unit, both in traditional learning phenomena and in the areas of neuroses and psychotherapy will be discussed in the section entitled, What is Learned? A second common assumption is that the concepts taken from conditioning, either as described by Pavlov or the operant conditioning of Skinner, can be used as explanatory principles. The assumption in question here is that conditioning phenomena are the simplest kinds of learning and that all other behavior can be explained in terms of these "simple" principles. We shall deal with the problems that arise from this source in a second section. The third

assumption is that rewards play an essential role in all learning phenomena. We shall consider the problems that stem from this assumption in a third section.

WHAT IS LEARNED?

Since its inception in the early twentieth century, behaviorism has taken overt stimuli and responses as its core units of analysis. Learning, as the behaviorist views it, is defined as the tendency to make a *particular response* in the presence of a *particular stimulus;* what is learned is a discrete response. Almost from its inception, however, this view has been plagued by a number of problems.

First, findings from studies of perception, particularly the fact of perceptual constancy, provide embarrassment for a peripheral S-R theory. Perceptual constancy findings show, for example, that the stimulus is much more than peripheral receptor stimulation. For example, once we have learned a song in a particular key (i.e., particular stimulus elements), we can readily recognize it or sing it in other keys. We are amazingly accurate in recognizing objects and events as being "the same" or equivalent, even though the particular stimulation they provide varies considerably on different occasions (Gibson, 1950). Although the bases of perceptual constancies (size, shapes, brightness, etc.) are not yet well understood, the facts of perceptual constancy—invariance in percept with variation in perceptual stimulation—are not in question. The related phenomenon of transposition has received considerable attention in animal experimentation. Animals, infrahuman as well as human, respond to relations among stimuli (Köhler, 1929). For a number of years, transposition was not considered to pose a serious problem for a peripheral S-R theory since it was thought that it could be adequately handled by principles of conditioning and stimulus generalization (Spence, 1937). This view has not been supported by later experiments, however (Lawrence & DeRivera, 1954; Riley, 1958). It now appears more likely that stimulus generalization is but a special case of the more general complex phenomenon of stimulus equivalence. The absolute theory of transposition was important and instructive because it revealed in clear relief the nature and limitations of a peripheral S-R approach to behavior. The effective stimulus is clearly more "central" than receptor excitation. The chapters on learning in the recent Koch series make it clear that workers in this area have seen the need for coming to terms with the facts of perception (Guttman, 1963; Lawrence, 1963; Leeper, 1963; Postman, 1963).

Second, the facts of response equivalence or response transfer posed the same kind of problem for a peripheral S-R view. A learned response does not consist merely of a stereotyped pattern of muscular contraction or glandular secretion. Even within the S-R tradition (e.g., Hull, Skinner) there has been a tendency to define responses in terms of environmental achievements. Anyone who has trained animals has recognized that animals can achieve the same general response, that is, make the same environmental change, in a variety of different ways once the response is learned. "What is learned," then, is not a mechanical sequence of responses but rather, *what needs to be done in order to achieve some final event*. This notion is not new; Tolman stressed it as early as 1932 when he wrote of "purposive behavior," and it has been strongly supported by a variety of experimental findings (e.g., Beach, Hebb, Morgan, & Nissen, 1960; Ritchie, Aeschliman, & Peirce, 1950). As this work shows, animals somehow seem to be able to bypass the execution of specific responses in reaching an environmental achievement. They can learn to go to particular places in the environment in spite of the fact that to do so requires them to make different responses from trial to trial. The learning of relatively specific responses to specific stimuli appears to be a special case which might be called stereotyped learning (canalization) rather than a basic prototype on the basis of which all other learning may be explained.

It should be noted further that even the stereotyped learning that forms the basic model of S-R conditioning does not hold up under closer scrutiny. First, once a subject has learned a stereotyped movement or response, he is still capable of achieving a goal in other ways when the situation requires it. Thus, while we have all learned to write our names with a particular hand in a relatively stereotyped fashion, we can switch to the other hand, or even write our name with a pencil

gripped in our teeth if we have to, in spite of the fact that we may not have made this specific response in this way before. Second, even a response that is grossly defined as constant, stable, or stereotyped does not appear as such a stereotyped pattern of muscular contractions when it is closely observed.* These findings in the area of response transfer indicate that a response seems to be highly variable and equipotential. This notion is, of course, quite old in the history of psychology, and it has been stressed repeatedly by numerous investigators including Lashley (see Beach et al., 1960), Osgood (1953), Tolman (1932), and Woodworth (1958).

The facts of both response transfer and stimulus equivalence seem much more adequately handled if we assume that what is learned is a *strategy* (alternatively called cognitive maps, programs, plans, schemata, hypotheses, e.g., Krechevsky, 1932) for obtaining environmental achievements. When we take this view, habits, in the traditional behaviorist sense, become a later stage of response learning rather than a basic explanation (building block) for later, more complex learning.

Perhaps this whole problem can be clarified if we look at a specific example such as language learning. As Chomsky (1959) has demonstrated in his excellent critique of Skinner's *Verbal Behavior* (1957), the basic facts of language learning and usage simply cannot be handled within an S-R approach. It seems clear that an adequate view of language must account for the fact that humans, at a rather early age, internalize a complex set of rules (grammar) which enable them to both recognize and generate meaningful sentences involving patterns of words that they may never have used before. Thus, in language learning, what is learned are not only sets of responses (words and sentences) but, in addition, some form of internal strategies or plans (grammar). We learn a grammar which enables us to generate a variety of English sentences. We do not merely learn specific English sentence habits. How this grammar or set of strategies is acquired, retained, and used in language comprehension and generation is a matter for serious research effort; but, it is clear that attempts to understand language learning on the basis of analogies from bar-pressing experiments

_____

*G. Hoyle, personal communication, 1963.

are doomed before they start. To anticipate, we will argue shortly that if we are to make an attempt to understand the phenomena of neurosis, using analogies from the area of learning, it will be much more appropriate to take these analogies from the area of psycholinguistics and language learning rather than, as has typically been done, from studies of classical and operant conditioning. That is, the focus will have to be on response transfer, equipotentiality, and the learning of plans and strategies rather than on stereotyped response learning or habituation.

USE OF A CONDITIONING MODEL

As we indicated earlier, when writers in the behaviorist tradition say "learning theory," they probably mean a conditioning theory; most of the interpretations of clinical phenomena are reinterpretations in terms of the principles of conditioning. Thus, a phobic symptom is viewed as a conditioned response, maintained by the reinforcement of a secondary fear drive or by a Skinnerian as a single operant maintained by reinforcement. Two types of conditioning are involved in these explanations by reduction. The first is Pavlovian or classical conditioning, frequently used in conjunction with later Hullian concepts such as secondary drive; the second is operant conditioning of the kind proposed by Skinner. The use of both of these models to explain more complex phenomena such as transposition, response transfer, problem solving, language learning, or neurosis and psychotherapy poses a number of difficulties.

The basic assumption that underlies the use of either kind of conditioning as an explanation for more complex phenomena is that basic laws of behavior have been established in the highly controlled laboratory situation and may thus be applied to behavior of a more complex variety. When we look at the way conditioning principles are applied in the explanation of more complex phenomena, we see that only a rather flimsy analogy bridges the gap between such laboratory defined terms as stimulus, response, and reinforcement and their referents in the case of complex behavior. Thus, while a stimulus may be defined as an electric shock or a light of a certain intensity in a classical conditioning experiment, Bandura (1961) speaks of the "imagination of a scene"; or, while a response may consist of salivation or a barpress in a conditioning experiment, behavior therapists speak of anxiety as a response. As Chomsky (1959) puts it, with regard to this same problem in the area of language:

He (Skinner in *Verbal Behavior*) utilizes the experimental results as evidence for the scientific character of his system of behavior, and analogic guesses (formulated in terms of a metaphoric extension of the technical vocabulary of the laboratory) as evidence for its scope. This creates the illusion of a rigorous scientific theory with a very broad scope, although in fact the terms used in the description of real-life and of laboratory behavior may be mere homonyms, with at most a vague similarity of meaning (p. 30).

A second and related problem stems from the fact that the behavior-therapy workers accept the findings of conditioning experiments as basic principles or laws of learning. Unfortunately, there is now good reason to believe that classical conditioning is no more simple or basic than other forms of learning. Rather, it seems to be a form of learning that is in itself in need of explanation in terms of more general principles. For example, a popular but naive view of conditioning is that of stimulus substitution—the view that conditioning consists merely of the substitution of a conditioned stimulus for an unconditioned stimulus. Close examination of conditioning experiments reveals that this is not the case, however, for the conditioned response is typically *unlike* the unconditioned response (Zener, 1937). Apparently, in conditioning, a new response is learned. Most of the major learning theorists have taken this fact into account in abandoning the notion of conditioning as mere stimulus substitution.

More than this, the most important theoretical developments using essentially Pavlovian conditioning principles have not even stressed overt behavior (Osgood, 1953). Hull and the neo-Hullians, for example, have relied quite heavily on Tolman's (1932) distinction between learning and performance, performance being what is observed while learning (conditioning) is but one essential ingredient contributing to any instance of observed performance. The most important, and perhaps the most sophisticated, developments in Hullian and neo-Hullian theory concern the attempts to explain complicated goal-directed behavior in terms of the conditioning of fractional responses. Unobserved, fractional responses (already we see the drift away from the overt behavior criteria of response) are assumed to serve a mediating role in behavior. Once a fractional response is conditioned in a particular situation, it is assumed to occur to the stimuli in that situation when those stimuli recur. The stimulus consequences of the fractional response referred to as the r_g are assumed to serve as guides to behavior either by serving as a cue or by activating responses or by serving to reinforce other responses by secondary reinforcement. The latter-day proponents of a conditioning point of view (Bugelski, 1956; Osgood, 1953) have come to rely more and more heavily on concepts like the fractional response to bridge the gap between stimulus and overt behavior and to account for the facts of response transfer, environmental achievements, and equipotentiality. What this indicates is that a simple conditioning paradigm which rests solely on observable stimuli and responses has proved inadequate even to the task of encompassing simple conditioning and maze-learning phenomena, and the workers within this tradition have come to rely more and more heavily on mediational (central, cognitive, etc.) concepts, although they still attempt to clothe these concepts in traditional conditioning garb. To add to the problem, a number of recent papers (Deutsch, 1956; Gonzales & Diamond, 1960) have indicated that the r_g interpretations of complex behavior are neither simple nor adequate.

When we look again at the way conditioning principles have been applied to clinical phenomena, we see an amazing unawareness of these problems that have been so salient to experimental and animal psychologists working with conditioning.

While the above discussion has been oriented primarily to classical conditioning, the general argument would apply equally well to those attempts to make the principles of learning derived from operant conditioning the basis of an explanation of neurosis and psychotherapy (as in Krasner, 1961). The Skinnerians have been particularly oblivious to the wide variety of problems that are entailed when one attempts to apply concepts and findings from laboratory learning experiments to other, and particularly more complex, phenomena. While we will deal more directly with their point of view shortly, a few comments might be in order now concerning their use of the operant-conditioning paradigm as a basis for the handling of more complex data. When Skinnerians speak of laws of learning, they have reference to the curves representing rate of responding of rats pressing bars (Skinner, 1938), and pigeons pecking (Ferster & Skinner, 1957) which are, in fact, a function of certain highly controlled contingencies such as the schedule of reinforcement, the amount of deprivation, the experimental situation itself (there is very little else to do in a Skinner box), and the species of animals involved. These experiments are of some interest, both as exercises in animal training under highly restricted conditions, and for what light they may shed on the more general question of partial reinforcement. It is dubious that these findings constitute laws of learning that can be applied across species (see Breland & Breland, 1961) or even to situations that differ in any significant way from the Skinner box.

USE OF REINFORCEMENT

Advocates of the application of learning theory to clinical phenomena have relied heavily on the "law of effect" as perhaps their foremost established principle of learning. We shall attempt to point out that a good deal of evidence from experimental animal studies argues strongly that, at the most, the law of effect is a weak law of performance.

Essentially, the controversy can be reduced to the question of whether or not reward is necessary for learning. The initial source of evidence indicating that it was not came from the findings of latent learning studies (Blodgett, 1929; Tolman & Honzik, 1930) in which it was found, for example, that rats who were allowed to explore a maze without reward made fewer errors when learning the maze than controls who had no opportunity for exploration. Thus, these early latent learning studies, as well as a variety of more recent ones (Thistlethwaite, 1951) indicate that learning can take place without reward but may not be revealed until a reward situation makes it appropriate to do so (or to put it another way, the reward elicits the performance but plays little role during learning). Other sources which point to learning without reward come from studies of perceptual learning (Hebb, 1949), imitation (Herbert & Harsh, 1944), language learning (Chomsky, 1959), and imprinting (Moltz, 1960).

Defenders of the point of view that reinforcement is necessary for learning have attempted to handle results such as these in a variety of ways. One has been by appealing to the concept of secondary reinforcement (e.g., a maze has secondary reinforcing properties which account for the learning during exploration). When this sort of thing is done, even with respect to experiments where attempts were made to minimize secondary reinforcements (Thistlethwaite, 1951), it seems clear that this particular notion of reinforcement has become incapable of disproof. Another way of handling these potentially embarrassing results has been by the invention of a new set of drives (curiosity drive, exploratory drive, etc.) but this too has a post hoc flavor to it, and one wonders what kind of explanation is achieved by postulating an "exploratory drive" to account for the fact that animals and humans engage in exploration. In fact, the assumption that exploration reduces an exploratory drive makes it difficult to explain why a rat's tendency to enter an alley of a maze *decreases* after he has explored the alley (Watson, 1961). Finally, there are those (particularly the Skinnerians) who tend to define reinforcement so broadly that neither the findings from latent learning nor any other source can prove embarrassing, since whenever learning has taken place this "proves" that there has been reinforcement. To better understand this problem, however, we had best look for a moment at the general problem of defining reinforcement in a meaningful way.

Obviously, if the view that reinforcement is necessary for learning is to have any meaning, what constitutes a reinforcement must be defined independently from the learning situation itself. There has been a great deal of difficulty in getting around a circular definition of the law of effect, and it might be worthwhile to examine some of the attempts that have been made in the past.

One of the best known was the attempt to relate the reinforcing properties of stimuli to their drive-reducing

characteristics (Hull, 1951). The drive-reduction model has had to be abandoned, however, because of evidence from a variety of areas including latent learning, sensory preconditioning (Brogden, 1939), and novelty and curiosity (Berlyne, 1960). Other evidence such as that of Olds and Milner (1954) on the effect of direct brain stimulation have strengthened the conviction that the drive-reduction interpretation of reinforcement is inadequate; and, in fact, original adherents of this view have begun to abandon it (e.g., Miller, 1959).

The other most frequent solution to the circularity problem has been by way of the "empirical law of effect," an approach typified by Skinner's definition of reinforcement as any stimulus that can be demonstrated to produce a change in response strength. Skinner argues that this is not circular since some stimuli are found to produce changes and others are not, and they can subsequently be classified on that basis. This seems to be a reasonable position if it is adhered to; that is, if care is taken to define reinforcement in terms of class membership *independently* of the observations that show that learning has taken place. When we examine the actual use of the term reinforcement by Skinner (see especially *Verbal Behavior,* 1957) and by other Skinnerians (Lundin, 1961), we find that care is only taken in this regard within the context of animal experiments, but that when the jumps are made to other phenomena, such as language and psychotherapy, care is usually *not* taken to define reinforcement independently from learning as indicated by response strength. This leads to a state of affairs where any observed change in behavior is said to occur *because of* reinforcement, when, in fact, the change in behavior is itself the only indicator of what the reinforcement has been. Chomsky (1959) reviews the use of the concept of reinforcement by Skinner with regard to language and reaches the following conclusion:

From this sample, it can be seen that the notion of reinforcement has totally lost whatever objective meaning it may ever have had. Running through these examples, we see that a person can be reinforced though he emits no response at all, and the reinforcing "stimulus" need not impinge on the reinforced person or need not even exist (it is sufficient that it be imagined or hoped for). When we read that a person plays what music he likes (165), says what he likes (165), thinks what he likes (438-9), reads what books he likes (163), etc., *because* he finds it reinforcing to do so, or that we write books or inform others of facts *because* we are reinforced by what we hope will be the ultimate behavior of reader or listener, we can only conclude that the term "reinforcement" has a purely ritual function. The phrase "X is reinforced by Y (stimulus, state of affairs, event, etc.)" is being used as a cover term for "X wants Y," "X likes Y," "X wishes that Y were the case," etc. Invoking the term "reinforcement" has no explanatory force, and any idea that this paraphrase introduces any new clarity or objectivity into the description of wishing, liking, etc., is a serious delusion [pp. 37-38].

This problem is exemplified in the area of psychotherapy by the attempts to use the studies of verbal conditioning (Krasner, 1958) as analogues to psychotherapy. First we should note that if these studies are taken at face value (i.e., if subjects are conditioned to increase the emission of certain responses because of reinforcement, without their awareness of this fact) it appears that a simple conditioning model is inadequate since subjects are presumably responding in terms of a class of responses (e.g., plural nouns, etc.) rather than in terms of a specific response (e.g., bar press), such classes implying response transfer and mediation. Second, and more to the point, a number of recent investigators (Eriksen, 1962) have begun to question whether verbal conditioning does occur without the subject's awareness. If it does not, the whole phenomenon begins to look like nothing more than a rather inefficient way to get subjects to figure out what the experimenter wants them to do (telling them directly to emit plural nouns would probably be much more efficient) after which they can decide whether they want to do it or not. In any case, there seems to be enough question about what goes on in verbal conditioning itself to indicate that it cannot be utilized as a more basic explanation for complex phenomena such as psychotherapy. Psychotherapists of many persuasions would agree that rewards of some kind are important in work with patients. Thus, the view that the psychotherapist is a "reinforcement machine" is trivial. The difficult problems are in specifying just what therapist activities are rewarding, in what ways, to what sorts of patients, and with what effects.

The above discussion should make clear that the use of the concept of reinforcement is only of explanatory usefulness when it is specified in some delimited fashion. As an empirical law of performance almost everyone in and out of psychology would accept it, including Lewin, Freud, Tolman, and others outside the traditional S-R movement. But this amounts to saying nothing more than that some events, when presented, tend to increase the probability of responses that they have followed. The hard job, but the only one that will lead to any meaningful use of the concept of reinforcement, is specifying what the various events called reinforcers have in common. Some have argued that since this is such a difficult task, we should restrict ourselves to listing and cataloging so-called reinforcers. But this is nearly impossible, in a general way, because reinforcers differ from individual to individual, from species to species, from situation to situation, and from time to time (the saying "one man's meat is another man's poison" is trite but true). Meaningful analysis must stem from a comprehensive study of the particular learning phenomena in question, whether it is language learning, the development of perceptual and perceptual-motor skills (Fitts, 1964; Hebb, 1949), the acquisition of particular species behavior patterns during critical periods of development (Scott, 1962), the learning of a neurosis, or the learning that takes place during psychotherapy. Experience with all of these phenomena has revealed that different kinds of events seem to be involved and that these can only be understood in the context of the phenomena in question. Lumping all these events together under the single term reinforcement serves to muddle rather than to clarify understanding.

The staunch reinforcement adherent might respond that all these complicated arguments may be true but we can ignore them, since all we are really interested in is predicting what the organism will do, and we can do this when we know the organism's reinforcement history. The answer to this is that the experimental literature does not support such a claim; rather, it shows that, in many instances, performance *cannot* be predicted on the basis of a knowledge of the history of reinforcement.

Latent learning studies indicate this

quite clearly. Perhaps of more interest are the findings of discrimination-reversal learning studies (Goodwin & Lawrence, 1955; Mackintosh, 1963). Here, we find that subjects that have been trained on a series of discrimination reversals learn to select the correct stimulus with very few errors even though they may have been rewarded *much more frequently and more recently for responding to another stimulus.* Similarly, in the double drive discrimination studies (Thistlethwaite, 1951) animals chose alleys leading to food when they were hungry and water when they were thirsty, even though they have been rewarded equally frequently on the alleys on previous trials. In other words, "what is learned" was not equivalent with "reinforcement history." The law of effect is not disproved by these studies; it is merely shown to be irrelevant.

To summarize: The "law of effect," or reinforcement, conceived as a *"law of learning,"* occupies a very dubious status. Like the principles of conditioning, it appears to be an unlikely candidate as an explanatory principle of learning. As a strong law of learning it has already been rejected by many of the theorists who previously relied on it. As an empirical "law of *performance"* it is noncontroversial, but usually so generally stated as to be of little explanatory value.

CONCEPTION OF NEUROSIS

In this section we will explicate the conception of neurosis that forms the basis of the behavior-therapy approach (particularly of the Wolpe-Eysenck group) and attempt to demonstrate its inadequacies both in terms of learning theory and as a way of accounting for the observed facts of neurosis. Our argument in the first instance will be that the conception of neurosis in terms of symptoms and anxiety parallels the general conception of learning in terms of overt responses, conditioning, and secondary drives, and suffers from the same inadequacies that we have outlined in preceding section. With regard to the facts of neurosis, we will argue that the behavior-therapy position is inadequate at a descriptive level as well as being conceptually incorrect. It should be pointed out again that we are discussing the explanation or theory of neurosis here and

not the techniques used by the behavior therapists. The strict Skinnerian may excuse himself at this point if he adheres to a "no-theory" position and is only concerned with the effects of environmental manipulation. Furthermore, certain techniques themselves may be useful and have some of the effects attributed to them regardless of the theory.

In its essence, the conception of neurosis put forth by the behavior therapists is that neuroses are conditioned responses or habits (including conditioned anxiety) and *nothing else,* though it should be noted that they do not adhere to this argument when they describe the success of their methods. Wolpe, for example, while ostensibly treating overt symptoms, describes his patients as becoming more productive, having improved adjustment and pleasure in sex, improved interpersonal relationships, and so forth. The argument that removal of a troublesome symptom somehow "generalizes" to all of these other areas begs the question. Their conception is typically put forth as an alternative to a psychodynamic viewpoint, which they characterize as resting on a distinction between symptoms and underlying causes (unconscious conflicts, impulses, defenses, etc.). They stress the point that inferences about underlying factors of this sort are unnecessary and misleading and that a more parsimonious explanation treats symptoms (which are typically equated with behavior or that which can be objectively observed) as the neurosis per se. They argue that by equating neurosis with symptoms, and symptoms, in turn, with habits (conditioned responses), they are able to bring "modern learning theory" with its "well-established laws" to bear on the understanding and treatment of neurosis.

As we have labored to show in the preceding section, the well-established laws of learning to which they refer have considerable difficulty within the area of simple animal behavior. More specifically, it seems clear that a wide variety of behaviors (from maze learning to more complex forms) cannot be adequately dealt with when the overt response and conditioned habit are the units of analysis. Furthermore, their learning position leads the behavior therapists into postulating an isomorphic relationship between antecedent learning and present behavior in which observed differences are accounted for in terms of principles of generalization. This is a key issue, and we shall explore it a little further at this time.

Much of the behaviorist conception of neurosis rests on a rejection of the distinction between symptoms and underlying causes (Eysenck, 1960) as typified by Yates' (1958) argument against "symptom substitution." By focusing attention on overt symptoms and banishing all underlying causes, however, the behavior therapists are faced with the same problem that has long confronted behaviorism; namely, the difficulty of explaining how *generality* of behavior results from specific learning experiences. The problem of *generality* (i.e., as exemplified by the facts of transposition and response transfer) has, in fact, brought about the downfall of peripheral S-R learning, of the conditioned habit as a basic unit, and tangentially, is leading to the dethroning of the law of effect. With regard to neurosis, this view has led the behavior therapists into the position where they must posit a specific learning experience for each symptom of a neurosis. They have partly avoided this problem by focusing their attention on those neuroses that can be described in terms of specific symptoms (bedwetting, if this is a neurosis, tics, specific phobias, etc.) and have tended to ignore those conditions which do not fit their model, such as neurotic depressions, general unhappiness, obsessional disorders, and the kinds of persistent interpersonal entanglements that characterize so many neurotics. This leaves them free to explain the specific symptom in terms of a specific learning experience, as, for example, when a fear of going outdoors is explained in terms of some previous experience in which the stimulus (outdoors) has been associated with (conditioned to) something unpleasant or painful and has now, through generalization, spread to any response of going outdoors. As our previous analysis should make clear, however, even a simple conceptualization such as this, in terms of stimuli, responses, and conditioning is extremely cumbersome and begs the important questions. Within an S-R framework, in which generalization occurs along the dimension of physical stimulus similarity, it is difficult, if not impossible, to show how a previous experience such as being frightened in the

country as a child could generalize to the "stimulus" outdoors without a great deal of *mediation* in which the concept of "outdoors" carried most of the burden of generalization. As we have pointed out, most workers in the field of learning recognize this and rely heavily on mediational concepts in their explanations of complex behavior. Dollard and Miller (1950), for example, return again and again to mediational explanations once they move beyond the "combat neuroses" which lend themselves more readily to a simple isomorphic explanation.

A second important facet of the behaviorist conception of neurosis is the use of the concept of anxiety as a secondary drive. Here, Wolpe and Eysenck and some others seem to follow the explanatory model laid down by Dollard and Miller. Anxiety is viewed as the main motivating force for symptoms and, in general, occupies a central place in their thinking. Briefly, it is worth pointing out that the concept of drive reduction, the distinction between primary drives and secondary drives, as well as the early thinking about the uniquely persistent qualities of fear-motivated behavior have had serious difficulty within learning theory (Watson, 1961; Solomon, 1964). The use of these concepts to explain clinical phenomena thus rests on an exceedingly shaky foundation.

Let us turn our attention now to the phenomena of neuroses. We shall try to point out that underlying the dispute over symptoms versus underlying causes is a real difference in definition that arises at the descriptive level, which, in a sense, antedates disagreements at the level of theory and explanation.

To keep the presentation simple, we will adopt the terms psychodynamic to refer to all those theorists and therapists, following Freud, whose view of neurosis and its treatment deals with motives (conscious and unconscious), conflict, etc. This covers a wide variety of workers, in addition to the more or less traditional followers of Freud, including Sullivan and his adherents (Fromm-Reichman, 1950), other neo-Freudians, and that broad group of psychiatrists and clinical psychologists who have been strongly influenced by the Freudian and neo-Freudian viewpoints even though they may not claim allegiance to any of the formal schools.

The point we wish to make here is

that disagreement between the behaviorist and psychodynamic viewpoints seems to rest on a very real difference at the purely descriptive or observational level. The behaviorist looks at a neurotic and sees specific symptoms and anxiety. The psychodynamicist looks at the same individual and sees a complex intra- and interpersonal mode of functioning which may or may not contain certain observable fears* or certain behavioral symptoms such as compulsive motor acts. When the psychodynamicist describes a neurosis, his referent is a cohering component of the individual's functioning, including his characteristic ways of interacting with other people (e.g., sweet and self-effacing on the surface but hostile in covert ways), his characteristic modes of thinking and perceiving (e.g., the hysteric who never "remembers" anything unpleasant, the obsessive whose memories are over-elaborated and circumstantial, etc.), characteristic modes of fantasy and dreaming, a variety of secondary gain features, and the like. Specific or isolatable symptoms may sometimes be a part of such an integrated neurotic pattern, but, even viewed descriptively, they in no sense constitute the neurosis per se.

So far, we have considered the behavior therapists' position at face value. In actuality, a good case can be made that they *behave* in a way which is quite inconsistent with their own position. A specific example, taken from one of Wolpe's own case descriptions, will illustrate this point, and, at the same time, show what the psychodynamicist sees when he looks at a neurotic. Wolpe (1960) presents the following case:

Case 5—An attractive woman of 28 came for treatment because she was in acute distress as a result of her lovers' casual treatment of her. Every one of very numerous love affairs had followed a similar pattern—first she would attract the man, then she would offer herself on a platter. He would soon treat her with contempt and after a time leave her. In general she lacked assurance, was very dependent, and was practically never free from feelings of tension and anxiety.

What is described here is a complex pattern of interpersonal relationships, psychological strategies and misunderstandings (such as the way she became involved with men, the way she communicated her availability to them, her dependency, etc.), expectations that she had (presumably that men would not react with contempt to her generosity, that being dependent might lead to being taken care of, etc.), and thoughts and feelings about herself (lack of assurance, acute distress, etc.). Many of the statements about her (e.g., the description of the course of her love affairs) are abbreviations for very complex and involved processes involving two people interacting over a period of time. It is this, the psychodynamicist would argue, that *is* the neurosis. The tension and anxiety may be a part of it in this particular case (though there might be other cases in which there is no complaint of anxiety but, rather, its reverse—seeming inability to "feel" anything)—but it is secondary and can be understood only in relation to the other aspects of the patient's functioning. Wolpe's case histories are classic testaments to the fact that he cannot, and does not, apply the symptom approach when working with actual data. As a further example, consider the argument against a symptom-substitution point of view (Yates, 1958) in which it is implied that anything other than symptoms is some sort of metaphysical inference. While it may be true that theories such as psychoanalysis deal with a number of inferential and higher-order constructs in their attempts to integrate the complex mass of data that constitutes a neurosis, it is also true that much more than symptoms exist at the level of observation. Secondary-gain features of a neurosis, in which it is apparent that a variety of goals may be served by a set of interchangeable symptoms are the rule in most neurotic individuals. We are not defending the view (attributed to psychoanalysis by Yates) that if one symptom is removed another pops up to take its place; rather, we are arguing that the empirical phenomena of neurosis does not fit the symptom or response theory, but is much more compatible with a theory built around central mediators. Whether unconscious conflicts and defense mechanisms are adequate ways of conceptualizing the problem is an entirely separate question. What is clear is that a view stressing central mediators in which

---

*The term anxiety is frequently used as a theoretical inference, i.e., a patient deals with personal material in an overly intellectual fashion, and this is described as a defense mechanism—intellectualization—whose purpose is to ward off anxiety.

specific responses are seen as equipotential means of reaching certain goals is necessary to encompass the data of neurosis just as it has proven necessary to encompass the phenomena of animal learning.

To sum up, it would seem that the behaviorists have reached a position where an inadequate conceptual framework forces them to adopt an inadequate and superficial view of the very data that they are concerned with. They are then forced to slip many of the key facts in the back door, so to speak, for example, when all sorts of fantasy, imaginary, and thought processes are blithely called responses. This process is, of course, parallel to what has gone on within S-R learning theory where all sorts of central and mediational processes have been cumbersomely handled with S-R terminology (e.g., Deutsch, 1956). Thus, we have a situation where the behavior therapists argue strongly against a dynamic interpretation of neurosis at some points and at other points behave as if they had adopted such a point of view. This inconsistency should be kept in mind in reading the next section in which we evaluate the claims of success put forth by the behaviorist group. Insofar as there is disagreement as to what constitutes the descriptive facts of neurosis, it makes little sense to compare the effectiveness of different methods. However, since the behaviorist group adopts very broad (or psychodynamic, if you will) criteria for improvement, and since their *techniques* may have some effectiveness, in spite of theoretical and conceptual inadequacies, it is crucial that we look carefully at the empirical results that they lay claim to.

CLAIMS OF SUCCESS

While much of the writing of the behavior therapists consists of arguments and appeals to principles of science and learning, the claims that are made for the success of the methods seem open to empirical analysis. No doubt a great deal of the appeal of behavior therapy lies right here. Here seem to be methods whose application can be clearly described (unlike such messy psychodynamic methods as "handling countertransference" or "interpreting resistance"), whose course

is relatively short, and which seem to achieve a large number of practical results in the form of removal of symptoms. Wolpe (1960), for example, presents the following data: of 122 cases treated with behavioral techniques, 44% were "apparently cured," 46% were "much improved," 7% were "slightly or moderately improved," and 3% were "unimproved." Combining categories, he claims 90% "apparently cured or much improved," and 10% "improvement moderate, slight or nil." (Criteria of improvement consists of "symptomatic improvement, increased productiveness, improved adjustment and pleasure in sex, improved interpersonal relationships and ability to handle ordinary psychological conflicts and reasonable reality stresses.")

He compares this with data from the Berlin Psychoanalytic Institute (Knight, 1941) which shows 62—40.5% in the first category and 38—59.5% in the second. Wolpe concludes, as have others (Bandura, 1961; Eysenck, 1960; Lazarus, 1963), that this demonstrates the superiority of the behavior therapy methods. The fact that the psychoanalytic method showed as much as 62% improvement is explained as being due to whatever accidental "reciprocal inhibition" occurred during the therapy. (There is, however, no analysis or description of how this might have happened.) The behavioral methods achieve superior results presumably because of the more explicit application of these techniques.

It is fair to say that if these results can be substantiated they present a very strong argument in favor of behavioral *techniques*—even granting the theoretical and empirical inconsistencies we have discussed. However, we must ask if these claims are any better substantiated than those made by the practitioners of other methods of psychotherapy. Insofar as claims such as Wolpe's are based on uncontrolled case histories, they may reflect the enthusiasm of the practitioner as much as the effect of the method. History shows that new methods of therapy (ECS, tranquilizing drugs, as well as various schools of psychotherapy) have been oversold by their original proponents. Thus, a careful look at what lies behind the claims of the behavior-therapy group is in order.

The following does not purport to be

a comprehensive review of the behavior-therapy literature. Rather, it is based on a survey of all the studies reported in the two reviews that have appeared (Bandura, 1961; Grossberg, 1964). The most striking thing about this large body of studies is that they are almost all case studies. A careful reading of the original sources reveals that only one study (Lang & Lazovik, 1963) is a controlled experiment, and here the subjects were not neurotics but normal college students. Thus, most of the claims (including those of Wolpe which have been widely quoted) must be regarded as no better substantiated than those of any other enthusiastic school of psychotherapy whose practitioners claim that their patients get better. Behavior therapy has appeared to differ on this score because of its identification with experimental psychology and with "well-established laws of learning." We have already dealt with this issue, so let us now turn to some problems in evaluating psychotherapy as a technique.

The problems here are essentially those of control, and they may be broken down into three areas: (a) sampling biases, (b) observer bias, and (c) problems of experimental control. While research in psychotherapy presents particular difficulties in controlling "experimental input," more sophisticated workers (Frank, 1959) have attempted to deal with at least the sampling and observer problems. It thus comes as somewhat of a surprise that the behavior-therapy workers, despite their identification with experimental psychology, base their claims on evidence which is almost totally lacking in any form of control. Let us examine these issues in greater detail.

Sampling Biases. Obviously a claim such as Wolpe's of 90% success has meaning only when we know the population from which the sample of patients was drawn and the way in which they were selected. Ideally, a comparison of treatment techniques would involve the random assignment of patient from a common population pool to alternative treatments. Since, in practice, this is rarely feasible, it is essential for anyone making comparisons of different treatment methods to, at the very least, examine the comparability of the populations *and* of the methods used in selecting from these populations. Neither Wolpe's data nor

that of Lazarus (1963) contains this evidence. Wolpe reports, for example, that:

> Both series (70 patients reported on in 1952 and 52 patients reported on in 1954 on which the 90% figure is based) include only patients whose treatment has ceased after they have been afforded a reasonable opportunity for the application of the available methods; i.e., they have had as a minimum both a course of instruction on the changing of behavior in the life situation and a proper initiation of a course of relaxation-desensitization. This minimum takes up to about 15 interviews, including anamestic interviews and *no patient who has had 15 or more interviews has been omitted from the series* [emphasis added].

We may conclude from this that some patients (how many we do not know) having up to 14 interviews have been excluded from the sample—a procedure highly favorable to the success of the method but which violates the simplest canons of sampling. Wolpe's final sample of 122 consists of those patients most likely to show improvement, since both they and he were satisfied enough with the first 14 (or less) interviews to warrant proceeding further. Those patients least likely to improve are those most likely to drop out early (14 sessions or less) and not be included in the computation of success rate. The fact that a large number of poor-prognosis patients would very likely be eliminated during these early sessions is supported by a variety of research findings (Strickland & Crowne, 1963), which show that most dropping-out of untreatable or unsuccessful cases occurs during the first 10 sessions. This serious sampling bias would be expected to spuriously inflate the percent showing improvement.

When we add this to whatever unknown factors operate to delimit the original population (presumably there is some self-selection of patients who seek out this form of treatment), it becomes apparent that little confidence can be given to the reports of success.

Observer Bias. Psychologists have long been aware that human beings are fallible observers, particularly when they have predispositions or vested interests to protect. In controlled studies, we try to protect judges from their own biases by not acquainting them with the hypotheses, or with the nature of the groups they are judging, or by using blind and double-blind designs. This problem is particularly acute with regard to psychotherapy because both therapist and patient have investments of time, involvement, competence, and reputation to protect. For these reasons, workers in the area have become extremely skeptical of claims put forth for any method which rests on the uncontrolled observation of the person administering the treatment. At a minimum we expect some sort of external evidence. Beyond this minimum we hope for an independent judge who can compare differentially treated groups without knowing which is which.

In addition, there is the problem of the patient's freedom to report effects which may be seriously curtailed when all his reports go directly to the person who has treated him. It seems reasonable to assume that some patients are prevented from expressing dissatisfaction with treatment when they must report directly to the therapist, either because they do not want to hurt his feelings, or are afraid, or are just saying what they think is being demanded of them, or are being polite, or for some other reason. Again, it would be highly appropriate to provide the patients with the opportunity of reporting results in a situation as free from such pressure as possible.

Examination of the 26 studies reviewed by Bandura reveals a surprising lack of concern with these problems. Of the 26 studies sampled, only 12 report evaluation of results by persons other than the treating therapist; four of these use ratings of the hospital staff (who may be acquainted with the treatment), four use mothers or parents reporting on their children to the treating therapist, one is a wife reporting on her husband to the therapist, and three use a second observer. Obviously, whatever factors enter in to cause observer and reporter biases are allowed full reign in most of these cases. While we cannot conclude from this that the reported results are *due to* observer and reporter biases (as is clearly indicated with the sampling biases), it is impossible to rule them out. Furthermore, a great deal of evidence from many areas of psychology leads us to be very skeptical of claims in which biases of this sort go uncontrolled.

Experimental Control. While control of sampling and observer effects are basic to a wide variety of research activities, including field and clinical research, more exacting control over experimental conditions has long been the sine qua non of the laboratory methods of experimental psychology. The power of the experimental method stems, in part, from keeping careful control over all but a few conditions, which are experimentally varied, with the subsequent effects of these variations being observed. Since psychotherapy is not a controlled experiment, it is probably unfair to expect this type of control. However, there are more and less accurate descriptions of what goes on during any form of therapy, and we can demand as accurate a description as possible in lieu of experimental control. Thus, while we are led to believe that methods, such as counterconditioning, extinction of maladaptive responses, methods of reward, and the like, are applied in a manner analogous to their laboratory counterparts—examination of what is *actually done* reveals that the application of the learning techniques is embedded in a wide variety of activities (including many of the traditional therapy and interview techniques) which make any attribution of effect to the specific learning techniques impossible. Let us consider a few examples. From Wolpe (1960):

Case 4—The patient had 65 therapeutic interviews, unevenly distributed over 27 months. The greater part of the time was devoted to discussions of how to gain control of her interpersonal relationships and stand up for herself. She had considerable difficulty with this at first, even though it had early become emotionally important to her to please the therapist. But she gradually mastered the assertive behavior required of her, overcame her anxieties and became exceedingly self-reliant in all interpersonal dealings, including those with her mother-in-law.

From Lazarus and Rachman (1957) on systematic desensitization:

Case 1—The patient was instructed in the use of assertive responses and deep (nonhypnotic) relaxation. The first anxiety hierarchy dealt with was that of dull weather. Starting from "a bright sunny day" it was possible for the subject to visualize "damp overcast weather" without anxiety after 21 desensitization sessions, and 10 days after the completion of this hierarchy, she was able to report that, "the weather is much better, it doesn't even bother me to look at the weather when I wake up in the morning" (previously depressing). . . . During the course of therapy, part of the reason for the development of the anxiety state in this patient was unearthed. When she was 17 years old she had become involved in a love affair with a married man 12 years her senior. This affair had been conducted in an extremely discreet manner for 4 years, during which time she had suffered from recurrent guilt feelings and shame—so much so, that on one occasion she had attempted suicide by throwing herself into a river. It was her custom to meet her lover after work *in the late afternoon.* The dull weather can be accounted for, as this affair took place in London.

From Rachman (1959):

Interview No. 12. The patient having received a jolt in her love relationship, this session was restricted to a sort of nondirective, cathartic discussion. No desensitizing was undertaken because of A.G.'s depressed mood and obvious desire to "just talk."

These excerpts have been presented because they seem representative of the practices of the behavioral therapists. As can be seen, the number and variety of activities that go on during these treatment sessions is great, including, in these few examples, discussions, explanations of techniques and principles, explanations of the unadaptiveness of anxiety and symptoms, hypnosis of various sorts, relaxation practice and training with and without hypnosis, "nondirective cathartic discussions," "obtaining an understanding of the patient's personality and background," and the "unearthing" of a 17-year-old memory of an illicit affair. The case reports are brief and presented anecdotally so that it is really impossible to know what else went on in addition to those things described. What should be abundantly clear from these examples is that there is no attempt to restrict what goes on to learning techniques. Since it seems clear that a great variety of things do go on, any attribution of behavior change to specific learning techniques is entirely unwarranted.

In summary, there are several important issues that must be differentiated. First, a review of both learning theory and of the empirical results of behavior therapy demonstrates that they can claim no special scientific status for their work on either ground. Second, there are important differences of opinion concerning the type of patient likely to be affected by behavior therapy. Grossberg (1964), for example, states that: "Behavior

therapies have been most successful when applied to neurotic disorders with specific behavioral manifestations (p. 81)." He goes on to point out that the results with alcoholism and sexual disorders have been disappointing and that the best results are achieved with phobias and enuresis. He later states that "desensitization only alleviates those phobias that are being treated, but other coexisting phobias remain at high strength, indicating a specific treatment effect (p. 83)." Wolpe et al. (1964), on the other hand, argue that: "The conditioning therapist differs from his colleagues in that he *seeks out* the precise stimuli to anxiety, and finds himself able to break down almost every neurosis into what are essentially *phobic systems* (p. 11)." The best controlled study (Lang & Lazovik, 1963) indicates that "desensitization is very effective in reducing the intense fear of snakes held by normal subjects, though it can be questioned whether this is a phobia in the clinical sense."

Thus, there seems to be some evidence that these *techniques* (as techniques and not as learning theory) are effective with certain conditions.* We feel that this bears stressing because psychotherapy has come to be narrowly defined in terms of dynamic, evocative, and nondirective methods, placing unnecessary limitations on the kind of patient suitable for psychotherapy. First, we must note that behavior techniques are not new (as Murray, 1964, points out in a recent article). Freud and Breuer used similar techniques prior to the development of psychoanalysis, Bagby described a number of these methods in 1928, and therapy based on techniques designed to eliminate undesirable responses was used for many years by Stevenson Smith at the University of Washington Clinic. While most of these techniques have been superseded by the various forms of dynamic psychotherapy, recent work (Frank, 1961) suggests that the time may be ripe for taking a fresh look at a variety of methods such as hypnosis, suggestion,

---

*Just how many neurotics fit the phobia and/or specific symptom model is a complicated question, the answer to which depends in part on what one's own point of view leads one to look for. For example, an informal census of the first 81 admissions to the University of Oregon Psychology Clinic in 1964 revealed only 2 patients who could be so classified.

relaxation, and other approaches of a more *structured nature* in which the therapist takes a *more active role*. Needless to say, this fresh look would best proceed unencumbered by an inadequate learning theory and with some minimal concern for control. As an example of a nondynamic approach to patient management, we refer to the work of Fairweather (1964) and his colleagues.

REFORMULATION

Up to this point our analysis has been primarily critical. We have tried to show that many of the so-called principles of learning employed by workers with a behaviorist orientation are inadequate and are not likely to provide useful explanations for clinical phenomena. In this section we will examine the potential value of ideas from different learning conceptions. Before proceeding, however, we would like to discuss briefly the issue of the application of "laws," principles, and findings from one area (such as animal experimentation) to another (such as neurosis and psychotherapy). The behaviorists have traditionally assumed that principles established under highly controlled conditions, usually with animal subjects, form a scientific foundation for a psychology of learning. Yet when they come to apply these principles to human learning situations, the transition is typically bridged by rather flimsy analogies which ignore crucial differences between the situations, the species, etc. Recently, Underwood (1964) has made the following comments concerning this problem:

> Learning theories as developed in the animal-learning laboratory, have never seemed . . . to have relevance to the behavior of a subject in learning a list of paired associates. The emphasis upon the role of a pellet of food or a sip of water in the white rat's acquiring a response somehow never seemed to make contact with the human *S* learning to say VXK when the stimulus DOF was presented [p. 74].

We would add that the relevance is at least equally obscure in applications of traditional S-R reinforcement theory to clinical phenomena.

We do *not* wish, however, to damn any and all attempts to conceptualize clinical phenomena in terms of principles of learning developed outside the clinic. On the contrary, recent work in learning may suggest certain theoretical models which may prove useful in conceptualizing the learning processes involved in psychotherapy and the development of neuroses. Whether these notions can form the basis for a useful learning conceptualization of clinical phenomena will depend upon the ingenuity with which they are subsequently developed and upon their adequacy in encompassing the facts of neurosis and psychotherapy. Further, we would like to stress that their association with experimental work in the field of learning does not give them any a priori scientific status. Their status as explanatory principles in the clinical area must be empirically established within that area. In what follows, then, we will outline some ideas about learning and make some suggestions concerning their relevance to clinical problems.

Our view of learning centers around the concepts of information storage and retrieval. Learning is viewed as the process by which information about the environment is acquired, stored, and categorized. This cognitive view is, of course, quite contrary to the view that learning consists of the acquisition of specific responses; responses, according to our view, are mediated by the nature of the stored information, which may consist of facts or of strategies or programs analogous to the grammar that is acquired in the learning of a language. Thus, "what is learned" may be a system for generating responses as a consequence of the specific information that is stored. This general point of view has been emphasized by Lashley (see Beach et al., 1960), by Miller, Galenter, and Pribram (1960), in the form of the TOTE hypothesis, and by a number of workers in the cognitive learning tradition (Tolman, 1951; Woodworth, 1958). Recently it has even been suggested as a necessary formulation for dealing with that eminently S-R area, motor skills (Adams, 1964; Fitts, 1964).

This conception of learning may be useful in the clinical area in two ways; one, in formulating a theoretical explanation for the acquisition or development of neurosis, symptoms, behavior pathology, and the like, and, two, in conceptualizing psychotherapy as a learning process, and suggesting new methods stemming from this learning model.

A conceptualization of the problem of neurosis in terms of information storage and retrieval is based on the fundamental idea that what is learned in a neurosis is a set of central strategies (or a program) which guide the individual's adaptation to his evironment. Neuroses are not symptoms (responses) but are strategies of a particular kind which lead to certain observable (tics, compulsive acts, etc.) and certain other less observable, phenomena (fears, feelings of depression, etc.). The whole problem of symptom substitution is thus seen as an instance of response substitution or response equipotentiality, concepts which are supported by abundant laboratory evidence.

Similarly, the problem of a learning conceptualization of unconscious phenomena may be reopened. Traditional S-R approaches have equated the unconscious with some kind of avoidance of a verbalization response. From our point of view, there is no reason to assume that people can give accurate descriptions of the central strategies mediating much of their behavior any more than a child can give a description of the grammatical rules which govern the understanding and production of his language. As a matter of fact, consciousness may very well be a special or extraordinary case—the rule being "unawareness" of the mediating strategies—which is in need of special explanation, rather than the reverse. This view avoids the cumbersome necessity of having to postulate specific fear experiences or the persistence of anxiety-motivated behavior, as has typically been done by S-R theorists with regard to unconscious phenomena. It also avoids equating the unconscious with the neurotic, which is a virtue since there is so much that goes on within "normal" individuals that they are unaware of. It further avoids the trap of attributing especially persistent and maladaptive consequences to painful experiences. As Solomon (1964) points out, the existing evidence does not support the view that punishment and pain lead unequivocally to anxiety and maladaptive consequences.

The view of learning we have outlined does not supply a set of ready-made answers to clinical problems that can be applied from the laboratory, but it indicates what sort of questions will have to be answered to achieve a meaningful learning conceptualization of neurosis and symptoms. Questions such as "What are the conditions under which strategies are acquired or developed?" stress the fact that these conditions may be quite different from the final observed behavior. That is to say, a particular symptom is not necessarily acquired because of some learning experience in which its stimulus components were associated with pain or fear-producing stimuli. Rather, a symptom may function as an equipotential response, mediated by a central strategy acquired under different circumstances. As an example, consider Harlow's (1958, 1962) monkeys who developed a number of symptoms, the most striking being sexual impotence (a much better animal analogue of human neurosis than those typically cited as experimental neuroses [Liddell, 1944]). Their longitudinal record, or "learning history," indicates that the development of this abnormal "affectional system," as Harlow terms it, is dependent on a variety of nonisomorphic experiences, including the lack of a mother-infant relationship and the lack of a variety of peer-play experiences.

These brief examples are only meant to give a flavor of where a learning conception of neurosis which stresses the acquisition of strategies will lead. A chief advantage of this view is that it has *generality* built in at the core, rather than imported secondarily, as is the case with S-R concepts of stimulus and response generalization.

Let us now turn our attention to the very difficult problem of applying learning concepts to psychotherapy. Basically, we would argue that the development of methods and techniques is largely a function of the empirical skill and ingenuity of the individual-craftsman-therapist. Even a carefully worked-out and well-established set of learning principles (which we do not have at this time) would not necessarily tell us how to modify acquired strategies in the individual case—just as the generally agreed-upon idea that rewards affect performance does not tell us what will be an effective reward in any specific instance.

Bearing these cautions in mind, we might still address ourselves to the question of what applications are suggested by the learning approach we have presented. As a first suggestion, we might consider the analogy of learning a new language. Here we see a process that parallels psychotherapy insofar as it involves modifying or developing a new set of strategies of a pervasive nature. A careful study of the most effective techniques for the learning of a new language might yield some interesting suggestions for psychotherapy. Learning a new language involves the development of a new set of strategies for responding—new syntax as well as new vocabulary. Language learning *may or may not* be facilitated by an intensive attempt to make the individual *aware* of the strategies used, as is done in traditional language instruction which teaches old-fashioned grammer, and as is done, analogously, in those psychotherapies which stress insight. Alternatively, language learning sometimes seems most rapid when the individual is immersed in surroundings (such as foreign country) where he hears nothing but the new language and where his old strategies and responses are totally ineffective.

Using this as a model for psychotherapy, we might suggest something like the following process: First, a careful study should be done to delineate the "neurotic language," both its vocabulary and its grammar, of the individual. Then a situation might be constructed (e.g., a group therapy situation) in which the individual's existing neurotic language is not understood and in which the individual must develop a new "language," a new set of central strategies, in order to be understood. The detailed working out of such a procedure might very well utilize a number of the techniques that have been found effective in existing therapies, both group and individual, and in addition draw on some new techniques from the fields of psycholinguistics and language learning.

These are, of course, but initial fragmentary guesses, and they may be wrong ones. But we believe that the conceptions on which these guesses are based are sufficiently supported by recent learning research to warrant serious attention. Although this reconceptualization may not lead immediately to the development of effective psychotherapeutic techniques, it may at least provide a first step in that direction.

References

Adams, J. A. Motor skills. In P. R. Farnsworth (Ed.), *Annual Review of Psychology*, 1964, *15*, 181–202.

Bagby, E. *The psychology of personality*. New York: Holt, 1928.

Bandura, A. Psychotherapy as a learning process. *Psychological Bulletin*, 1961, *58*, 143–159.

Beach, F. A., Hebb, D. O., Morgan, C. T., and Nissen, H. *The neuropsychology of Lashley*. New York: McGraw-Hill, 1960.

Berlyne, D. E. *Conflict, arousal, and curiosity*. New York: McGraw-Hill, 1960.

Blodgett, H. C. The effect of introduction of reward upon the maze performance of rats. *University of California Publications in Psychology*, 1929, *4*, 113–134.

Breland, K., and Breland, M. The misbehavior of organisms. *American Psychologist*, 1961, *16*, 681–684.

Brogden, W. J. Sensory preconditioning. *Journal of Experimental Psychology*, 1939, *25*, 323–332.

Bugelski, B. R. *The psychology of learning*. New York: Holt, 1956.

Chomsky, N. Review of B. F. Skinner, *Verbal behavior*. *Language*, 1959, *35*, 26–58.

Deutsch, J. A. The inadequacy of Hullian derivations of reasoning and latent learning. *Psychological Review*, 1956, *63*, 389–399.

Dollard, J., and Miller, N. E. *Personality and psychotherapy*. New York: McGraw-Hill, 1950.

Eriksen, C. W. (Ed.) *Behavior and awareness*. Durham, N. C.: Duke Univer. Press, 1962.

Eysenck, H. J. (Ed.) *Behaviour therapy and the neuroses*. New York: Pergamon Press, 1960.

Fairweather, G. W. *Social psychology in treating mental illness: An experimental approach*. New York: Wiley, 1964.

Ferster, C. B., and Skinner, B. F. *Schedules of reinforcement*. New York: Appleton-Century-Crofts, 1957.

Fitts, P. M. Perceptual-motor skill learning. In A. W. Melton (Ed.), *Categories of human learning*. New York: Academic Press, 1964, pp. 244–285.

Frank, J. D. Problems of controls in psychotherapy as exemplified by the psychotherapy research project of the Phipps Psychiatric Clinic. In E. A. Rubenstein and M. B. Parloff (Eds.), *Research in psychotherapy*. Washington, D. C.: American Psychological Association, 1959.

Frank, J. D. *Persuasion and healing: A comparative study of psychotherapy*. Baltimore: Johns Hopkins Press, 1961.

Fromm-Reichmann, Frieda. *Principles of intensive psychotherapy*. Chicago: Univer. Chicago Press, 1950.

Gibson, J. J. *The perception of the visual world*. Boston: Houghton Mifflin, 1950.

Gonzales, R. C., and Diamond, L. A test of Spence's theory of incentive motivation. *American Journal of Psychology*, 1960, *73*, 396–403.

Goodwin, W. R., and Lawrence, D. H. The functional independence of two discrimination habits associated with a constant stimulus situation. *Journal of Comparative and Physiological Psychology*, 1955, *48*, 437–443.

Grossberg, J. M. Behavior therapy: A review. *Psychological Bulletin*, 1964, *62*, 73–88.

Guthrie, E. R. *The psychology of learning*. New York: Harper, 1935.

Guttman, N. Laws of behavior and facts of perception. In S. Koch (Ed.), *Psychology: A study of a science*. Vol. 5. New York: McGraw-Hill, 1963. pp. 114–179.

Harlow, H. F. The nature of love. *American Psychologist*, 1958, *13*, 673–685.

Harlow, H. F. The heterosexual affectional system

in monkeys. *American Psychologist,* 1962, *17,* 1–9.

Hebb, D. O. *The organization of behavior: A neurophysiological theory.* New York: Wiley, 1949.

Herbert, M. J., and Harsh, C. M. Observational learning by cats. *Journal of Comparative Psychology,* 1944, *37,* 81–95.

Hilgard, E. R. *Theories of learning.* New York: Appleton-Century-Crofts, 1956.

Hull, C. L. *Essentials of behavior.* New Haven: Yale Univer. Press, 1951.

Knight, R. P. Evaluation of the results of psychoanalytic therapy. *American Journal of Psychiatry,* 1941, *98,* 434.

Kohler, W. *Gestalt psychology.* New York: Liveright, 1929.

Krasner, L. Studies of the conditioning of verbal behavior. *Psychological Bulletin,* 1958, *55,* 148–170.

Krasner, L. The therapist as a social reinforcement machine. In H. H. Strupp (Ed.), *Second research conference on psychotherapy.* Chapel Hill, N. C.: American Psychological Association, 1961.

Krechevsky, I. The genesis of "hypotheses" in rats. *University of California Publications in Psychology,* 1932, *6,* 45–64.

Lang, P. J., and Lazovik, A. D. Experimental desensitization of a phobia. *Journal of Abnormal and Social Psychology,* 1963, *66,* 519–525.

Lawrence, D. H. The nature of a stimulus: Some relationships between learning and perception. In S. Koch (Ed.), *Psychology: A study of a science.* Vol. 5. New York: McGraw-Hill, 1963. pp. 179–212.

Lawrence, D. H., and DeRivera, J. Evidence for relational transposition. *Journal of Comparative and Physiological Psychology,* 1954, *47,* 465–471.

Lazarus, A. A. The results of behaviour therapy in 126 cases of severe neurosis. *Behaviour Research and Therapy,* 1963, *1,* 69–80.

Lazarus, A. A., and Rachman, S. The use of systematic desensitization in psychotherapy. *South African Medical Journal,* 1957, *32,* 934–937.

Leeper, R. L. Learning and the fields of perception, motivation, and personality. In S. Koch (Ed.), *Psychology: A study of a science.* Vol. 5. New York: McGraw-Hill, 1963. pp. 365–487.

Lewin, K. *Field theory in social science.* New York: Harper, 1951. Ch. 4, pp. 60–86.

Liddell, H. S. Conditioned reflex method and experimental neurosis. In J. McV. Hunt (Ed.), *Personality and the behavior disorders.* New York: Ronald Press, 1944. Ch. 12.

Lundin, R. W. *Personality: An experimental approach.* New York: MacMillan, 1961.

Mackintosh, N. J. Extinction of a discrimination habit as a function of overtraining. *Journal of Comparative and Physiological Psychology,* 1963, *56,* 842–847.

Miller, G. A., Galanter, E. H., and Pribram, K. H. *Plans and the structure of behavior.* New York: Holt, Rinehart, & Winston, 1960.

Miller, N. E. Liberalization of basic S-R concepts: Extension to conflict behavior, motivation, and social learning. In S. Koch (Ed.), *Psychology: A study of a science.* Vol. 2. New York: McGraw-Hill, 1959. pp. 196–292.

Moltz, H. Imprinting, empirical basis, and theoretical significance. *Psychological Bulletin,* 1960, *57,* 291–314.

Murray, E. J. Sociotropic learning approach to psychotherapy. In P. Worchel and D. Byrne (Eds.), *Personality change.* New York: Wiley, 1964. pp. 249–288.

Olds, J., and Milner, P. Positive reinforcement produced by electrical stimulation of septal area and other regions of rat brain. *Journal of Comparative and Physiological Psychology,* 1954, *47,* 419–427.

Osgood, C. E. *Method and theory in experimental psychology.* New York: Oxford Univer. Press, 1953.

Postman, L. Perception and learning. In S. Koch (Ed.), *Psychology: A study of a science.* Vol. 5. New York: McGraw-Hill, 1963. pp. 30–113.

Rachman, S. The treatment of anxiety and phobic reactions by systematic desensitization psychotherapy. *Journal of Abnormal and Social Psychology,* 1959, *58,* 259–263.

Riley, D. A. The nature of the effective stimulus in animal discrimination learning: Transposition reconsidered. *Psychological Review,* 1958, *65,* 1–7.

Ritchie, B. F., Aeschliman, B., and Peirce, P. Studies in spatial learning. VIII. Place performance and the acquisition of place dispositions. *Journal of Comparative and Physiological Psychology,* 1950, *43,* 73–85.

Rotter, J. B. *Social learning and clinical psychology.* New York: Prentice-Hall, 1954.

Scott, J. P. Critical periods in behavioral development. *Science,* 1962, *138,* 949–958.

Skinner, B. F. *The behavior of organisms: An experimental analysis.* New York: Appleton-Century-Crofts, 1938.

Skinner, B. F. *Verbal behavior.* New York: Appleton-Century-Crofts, 1957.

Solomon, R. L. Punishment. *American Psychologist,* 1964, *19,* 239–253.

Spence, K. W. The differential response in animals to stimuli varying within a single dimension. *Psychological Review,* 1937, *44,* 430–440.

Strickland, Bonnie R., and Crowne, D. P. The need for approval and the premature termination of psychotherapy. *Journal of Consulting Psychology,* 1963, *27,* 95–101.

Thistlethwaite, D. A critical review of latent learning and related experiments. *Psychological Bulletin,* 1951, *48,* 97–129.

Tolman, E. C. *Purposive behavior in animals and men.* New York: Appleton-Century, 1932.

Tolman, E. C. Sign gestalt or conditioned reflex? *Psychological Review,* 1933, *40,* 391–411.

Tolman, E. C. *Collected papers in psychology.* Berkeley: Univer. California Press, 1951.

Tolman, E. C., and Honzik, C. H. Introduction and removal of reward and maze performance in rats. *University of California Publications in Psychology,* 1930, *4,* 257–275.

Underwood, B. J. The representativeness of rote verbal learning. In A. W. Melton (Ed.), *Categories of human learning.* New York: Academic Press, 1964. pp. 47–78.

Watson, A. J. The place of reinforcement in the explanation of behavior. In W. H. Thorpe and O. L. Zangwill, *Current problems in animal behavior.* Cambridge: Cambridge Univer. Press, 1961.

Wolpe, J. *Psychotherapy by reciprocal inhibition.* Palo Alto: Stanford Univer. Press, 1958.

Wolpe, J. Reciprocal inhibition as the main basis of psychotherapeutic effects. In H. J. Eysenck (Ed.), *Behaviour therapy and the neuroses.* New York: Pergamon Press, 1960. pp. 88–113.

Wolpe, J., Salter, A., and Reyna, L. J. (Eds.) *The*

conditioning therapies. New York: Holt, Rinehart, & Winston, 1964.

Woodworth, R. S. *Dynamics of behavior.* New York: Holt, 1958.

Yates, A. J. Symptoms and symptom substitution. *Psychological Review,* 1958, *65,* 371–374.

Zener, K. The significance of behavior accompanying conditioned salivary secretion for theories of the conditioned response. *American Journal of Psychology,* 1937, *50,* 384–403.

Part V

Sociocultural Theories

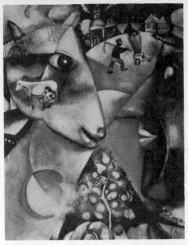

Marc Chagall—*I and the Village* (1911). (Courtesy, The Museum of Modern Art, New York.)

INTRODUCTION

Whether or not the label, "the third mental health revolution," applies appropriately to the theories presented in this section, there can be little doubt that they represent a marked departure in orientation from views described earlier in the text. No longer are the individual patient's behaviors, self-concepts, or defense mechanisms the point of focus; rather, it is the community and the cultural setting that have taken center stage; that is, the wider social forces which shape and color the patient's life and which, in turn, he shapes and colors. The "clinical model" is no longer salient, having been supplanted by the "public health model"; and with it has come a shift toward preventive programs, therapeutic hospital communities, crisis intervention therapies, social-action research, and the like.

Beginning with Dorothea Dix's demands for public responsibility in mental health in the mid-nineteenth century, and coalescing with the "mental hygiene" movement and the writings of sociocultural theorists such as Emile Durkheim and Franz Boaz early this century, the foundations of the "third revolution" were well set prior to its resurgence in the 1960's. Spurred by increased support from Federal sources and the growing disenchantment with traditional treatment approaches, the views of social and community theorists have attracted a large group of vigorous, action-oriented adherents.

ORIENTATION

Not infrequently, one hears colleagues state unequivocally that social theories have little or no relevance to psychopathology, that, at best, they furnish an intriguing, if distorting, backdrop against which the more salient processes of psychological dynamics may be viewed. Melvin Sabshin touches on this issue in his illuminating paper, but then provides the reader with both an historical review of the field and an analysis of the essential elements that comprise our current body of community and social psychiatric theories. Moving from this broad sweep to a sharp focus, Alexander Leighton outlines a series of specific theoretical propositions in his article, and then articulates them with various sources of data that can be examined empirically as a check on their utility as heuristic tools.

41.   Theoretical Models in Community and Social Psychiatry

MELVIN SABSHIN

Juxtaposing the words "theory" and "community psychiatry" may appear hopelessly paradoxical, for community psychiatry undoubtedly conveys to many an image of long overdue action, of meeting social responsibility, and of departing the ivory or aluminum tower for the real world. To some the image may be just as pragmatic but tainted by professional grandiosity and political chicanery. These images, whether pro or con, have a distinctly American flavor, not surprising since community psychiatry in this mid-decade is strikingly typical of our national attempts at massive and occasionally restless solutions of social problems. The action-oriented viewpoint is so pervasive that a discussion of theory may seem to be merely a delaying tactic. Having had some experience with pragmatic community psychiatrists and their equally action-oriented detractors, I wish to avoid sounding like a history professor addressing a national political convention, just be-

fore the first balloting, on the relationships of de Tocqueville and Jefferson as they pertain to candidate selection. Community psychiatry is like a swirling modern convention blaring with noise and spirit that is being beamed to large numbers of friends and neutrals and the opposition party. Bellak hails it as "the third psychiatric revolution" in his new book (1). Dunham (5), clearly alarmed, calls it "the newest therapeutic bandwagon," and a hundred other slogans are in the process of being manufactured as the anti-community psychiatry groups begin to notice each other. It is painful for psychiatrists to accept how much of our activity reflects segmentalized ideological positions or can be characterized as a "movement" in the sense that Freud uses the term in "The History of the Psychoanalytic Movement" (10). In a recent paper (6) and in a forthcoming book (22), several colleagues and I have summarized our own studies of psychiatric ideologies and institutions. The overwhelming majority of the four hundred psychiatrists studied considered themselves to be reasonably and broadly eclectic, even though their questionnaire scores and, more important, their behavior often indicated strongly partisan positions. The readiness

From Melvin Sabshin, "Theoretical Models in Community and Social Psychiatry," in Roberts, L., Halleck, S., and Loeb, M.B., editors, *Community Psychiatry* (Madison: The University of Wisconsin Press; © 1966 by the Regents of the University of Wisconsin), pp. 15-30.

to accept or dismiss community psychiatry seems as closely related to these partisan stands as to any other factor, although to my knowledge this relationship has not yet been investigated. The progress of community psychiatry is hampered by interprofessional jurisdictional issues as well as intraprofessional concerns. Sociologists, social workers, social psychologists, and public health experts have raised serious questions regarding the psychiatrist's fitness for leading community psychiatry or community mental health programs. The level of alarm rises precipitously when the language employed by the psychiatrist suggests treatment of a collectivity in a massive experiment in social engineering. Implications have been seen in these suggestions of everything from the threat of a society regimented in an Orwellian fashion to a communist or an extreme rightist plot. That community psychiatry has been able to develop despite these divergent opinions, conflicting perspectives, and sinister implications is, in my opinion, largely a result of the enormity of unmet mental health needs and the determined, though awkward, effort of a group of professions to realign themselves so as to meet these needs. The social reorganization of many of our psychiatric hospitals in the 1950's, the report of the Joint Commission on Mental Illness and Health (14), and the late President's now historic message on mental health have paved the way, and the time is now propitious for such a realignment.

This is not the first time in the twentieth century that the United States has seemed ready for a community approach. The period antedating the flowering of the child guidance movement in the 1920's also saw the enthusiastic entry of the mental health professions into the wider area of social process. The pioneering efforts of Healy, Bronner, Levy, and others marked the birth of child psychiatry, and the city of Chicago played a prominent part in the early nurturence of this field in the halcyon days at the Institute for Juvenile Research. Healy's deep interest in problems of delinquency led him and his colleagues out of the consulting rooms and into the arena of public action. From this arena ultimately evolved the child guidance clinics and the search for a preventive approach. It is not surprising that some of the older genera-

tion of child psychiatrists view the current trends in community psychiatry as a repetition of days gone by. During the course of a half-century, however, the child guidance movement gradually lost the momentum of its preventive approach and, at least until quite recently, also lost its major commitment to a community perspective. This loss of momentum was primarily a result of too much emphasis on pragmatics and too little emphasis on research. The lessons for community psychiatry today are patent.

This conference, as its title indicates, is devoted to defining community psychiatry. But other terms and labels will be used which may be hard to distinguish from community psychiatry: social psychiatry, comprehensive psychiatry, community mental health, preventive psychiatry, administrative psychiatry, public health psychiatry, community organization, community planning. The possibility of placing adjectives before the word "psychiatry" seems to be infinite. Stephen E. Goldston of the Training and Manpower Resources Branch of the National Institute of Mental Health has recently compiled a list of selected definitions (11) of terms related to community psychiatry which is useful in appreciating the complexity of the perspectives on this field. I will limit my own definitions to the areas of social psychiatry and community psychiatry. The framework within which these definitions will be formulated is certainly not unique, but I believe that it differs from others at least in its emphasis on and possible usefulness for theory and research. Since my conceptual model of community psychiatry involves its being subsumed under social psychiatry, I shall first discuss social psychiatry, then define community psychiatry, and, finally, attempt to weave them together.

In a previous paper (18) outlining the historical evolution of social psychiatry, I have traced its roots in broad, ameliorative movements. In Germany after World War I, for example, there was a sudden burst of interest in social psychiatry. As Dreikurs (4) has indicated, textbooks of social psychiatry appeared, and psychiatrists worked in courts, schools, and government much as did Healy and his collaborators in this country. Ten years later German social psychiatry came to a sudden halt with the rise of

Naziism. Leighton (16) has pointed out that social psychiatry has somewhat different meanings in America and abroad, particularly in England. He states, "In the United States the term usually brings to mind preventive community programs, industrial and forensic psychiatry, group therapy, and participation of psychiatry in administrative medicine, the utilization of the social milieu in treatment, and the study of social factors in the etiology and dynamics of mental illness. In England, social psychiatry is more likely to connote an emphasis on social amelioration as reflected in the development of various treatment services; it has been less closely related to general developments in the social sciences." In the United States, however, social psychiatry is coming increasingly to connote a demarcated theoretical and research area. Redlich and Pepper (17), for example, have stated, "Our own brief definition, influenced by Rennie, defines social psychiatry as the study of psychiatric disorders and psychiatric therapy, hopefully including prevention, within a social setting. This implies that social psychiatry is defined as an exploration of social systems and culture and their impact on psychiatric phenomena rather than as a type of psychiatric practice." Redlich and Pepper's emphasis is on study and exploration; Wilmer, on the other hand, emphasizes a pattern of psychiatric practice in the first part of his description of social psychiatry (23): "an area where physicians qualified as trained psychiatrists . . . utilize selective contributions of social psychology, medicine, and psychiatry in the prevention and treatment of emotional and mental illness; in the rehabilitation, socialization, and acculturation of the sick from any cause whatsoever." Wilmer (23) goes on to include theoretical aspects when he states that social psychiatry is also involved "in the scientific study of etiologies, hypotheses, theories, and treatment concepts under field or operating conditions. . . ." Similarly, Harris (11) has defined social psychiatry as "that part of psychiatry concerned with various aspects of society as it relates to emotional disturbance. Insofar as it is similar to social psychology, its emphasis is probably more theoretical than practical." My own definition essentially concurs with that of Harris but goes beyond it at least in one specific sense. I have defined social psychiatry (18) as an emergent theoretical and research field in which sophisticated employment of both social science and psychiatric variables is necessary for understanding a problem and, ultimately, for finding medically useful solutions to it. By "sophisticated" I mean that the independent and dependent variables, whether they stem from social science or from psychiatry, will be based on mature, professional understanding of both areas; and by "emergent," that the social psychiatry of the future should become increasingly sophisticated in developing interactional and transactional models and hypotheses. Most current studies employ a simple interactional design in which attempts are made to correlate social and psychiatric phenomena. Hollingshead and Redlich's study (12) of the interaction of social stratification and diagnostic categorization of psychiatric patients is prototypic of current social psychiatric research. Not only does it represent an interactional, rather than a transactional, model, but the independent social variables and the dependent psychiatric variables, though adequate, are vulnerable to criticism since they lack specificity or precision. Studies in the area of social class and mental illness should, in the future, become more sophisticated and increasingly focused, and should move towards predictive statements. Epidemiological studies will also require increasing precision to fit within my definition of social psychiatry. A repetition of Faris and Dunham's (7) pioneering effort in correlating gross residential locale in an urban context with the prevalence rates of specific psychoses would not, without refining the variables, constitute sophisticated social psychiatric research in the 1960's. The utilization of relatively unsophisticated experimental design in studying the dependent variables should also be increasingly questioned. Sociologists have frequently tended to be somewhat naive in their use of psychiatric dependent variables, just as psychiatrists have occasionally been slipshod in their use of cultural and social variables. One excellent illustration of the latter has been the search for anthropological evidence to support a particular psychiatric hypothesis. The mourning process as formulated by psychiatrists is often assumed to possess essentially universalistic characteristics. Transcultural evidence has been utilized to support this postulation, but there has been little interest in broadening or altering the basic hypothesis to take into account dependent cultural variables that do not conform to the original hypothesis. Hospital psychiatry affords us a number of excellent examples of good social psychiatric research. That studies on the interaction of social milieu and process or outcome of therapy are becoming increasingly sophisticated is evidenced by recent efforts to develop more complex transactional designs (15). My definition of social psychiatry is obviously quite close to some of the earlier definitions of social psychology. Social psychiatry is encountering some of the same problems that social psychology experienced in its early years, but I would predict that social psychiatry, like social psychology, will become increasingly specific. Although I have emphasized the theoretical and research aspects of social psychiatry, I believe that it differs from social psychology in all of the issues determining the differences between psychiatry and psychology. Thus, social psychiatry is slightly more pragmatic than social psychology and necessarily maintains ties with many applied areas.

One of the most unfortunate consequences of the division of psychiatrists into various ideological subgroupings involves the fact that the advent of social psychiatry posed new dilemmas for psychiatrists oriented toward somatotherapy and psychotherapy. The social psychiatrists who speak as if the human beings were born with a *tabula rasa,* and who view therapy exclusively within a framework of altering social structure, readily lend themselves to criticism, most notably and visibly today from the psychoanalysts. The relationship between social psychiatry and psychoanalysis affords an excellent example of the dangers of conflicting sectarian approaches. Extremists in social psychiatry and psychoanalysis view each other with marked suspicion. Some social and community psychiatrists hold psychoanalysis largely responsible for moving American psychiatry out of the mainstream of its responsibilities for the care of those with major mental illnesses. A few psychoanalysts, on the other hand, have become concerned and even suspicious about the tendency of social psychiatrists to dilute or, if you will, inundate the intrapsychic with the cultural and the social. Several psychoanalysts involved in training psychiatric residents have repeatedly pointed out that trainees can utilize social process as a defense against involvement with patients and hence as a device to avoid commitment to therapeutic endeavors. Many psychoanalysts are guarded about the present role of social science in psychiatry because they tend to equate undue interest on the social level with so-called "revisionism" in psychoanalysis. It is my conviction, however, that a sophisticated social psychiatry that avoids the cul-de-sac of a *tabula rasa* model and attempts to provide meaningful links between social process and psychological events has no essential disagreement with the science of psychoanalysis. It also has no basic quarrel with the biological aspects of mental health and illness. I have attempted in one study (19) to correlate aspects of the social setting with response to psychopharmacological agents; in another (20) I have tried to demonstrate how a number of parameters in the social setting affected psychophysiological variables in the psychosomatic laboratory. Illustrations could be cited to demonstrate the application of the social psychiatric perspective to an array of psychiatric problems, issues, and settings. Clearly, social psychiatry as I have defined it is also pertinent to the study of group process; it provides an organizational framework for approaches to family diagnosis and therapy; it is relevant for the recently revived field of transcultural psychiatry; and it provides, as well, a broader theoretical perspective from which to view both hospital and community psychiatry. It is somewhat paradoxical that friction exists between advocates of hospital psychiatry and those in community mental health programs since both, it seems to me, rely heavily on social psychiatric theory. It is impossible to practice good hospital psychiatry today without paying attention to both the broad and the specific impacts of the milieu on the diagnostic and treatment processes, just as it is impossible to be a community psychiatrist without taking a serious interest in both the particularities of the community and their impact on those who live in it. Obviously, most of the friction comes from polar groups who either view with alarm the rapid dissolution of the large state hospitals or are impatient with progress in increasing the permeability between hospital and community. The interaction of the hospital and community approaches is analogous to the relationship of social psychiatry and psychoanalysis, which have much more in common than they have in opposition and are clearly related not only in their links with social psychiatry but in their functional interaction. This is most evident in situations where community psychiatry is centered about a multipurpose institute that provides not only inpatient and transitional services (such as day hospital and halfway houses) but home visits and clinic care. Furthermore, many research linkages exist between community and hospital psychiatry. Comparative analyses of the impact of various aspects of therapeutic services, for example, have already proven useful. It is to be hoped that this kind of research will increase in both scope and breadth.

In describing the relationship of social psychiatry and community psychiatry, I have indicated a model in which a general research field (social psychiatry) is related to one of its subparts (community psychiatry) which, though it has specific functions, is not merely an applied area. Before this model is elaborated, an alternative viewpoint should be considered. In discussing community psychiatry, one of its most experienced practitioners, Viola Bernard (2), has stated, "Community psychiatry and social psychiatry are often used interchangeably and we believe with considerable justification. We recognize many areas of overlap between the two. However, in distinguishing between them, we think that community psychiatry tends to signify a greater emphasis on applied practice at the community level, as well as the investigations and program evaluations which underlie and keep shaping its service operations, while social psychiatry has come to connote a more exclusive emphasis on theory and research rather than practice. Therefore, community psychiatry in encompassing both is viewed as the more comprehensive designation." While I agree with Bernard that social psychiatry places greater emphasis on theory and research and that community psychiatry must involve

service operations, I cannot agree that community psychiatry, in encompassing both theory and practice, is the more comprehensive designation. Such a view, I believe, is not only contrary to our usual distinctions between the more basic areas and the applied areas but tends to weaken the argument for social psychiatry's central position in relation to a number of other areas, such as hospital psychiatry. My conceptual model views social psychiatry as a sun with a number of planets in orbit around it. Each of the planets interacts with the others as well as with the sun. While Bernard is careful not to imply, as others have done, that community psychiatry is only an applied area and that social psychiatry is its theoretical source, she places greater emphasis on an applied definition of community psychiatry than I find optimal. The pragmatic model of community psychiatry has a number of weaknesses. In discussing the child guidance movement I described the ultimate weakening of an area oversaturated with faith, hope, and enthusiasm. If community psychiatry becomes an applied field exclusively, it may well not live up to its promise. One danger is that the applied model may tend to attract less capable individuals than a model that offers theoretical generativity as well as exciting service opportunities. In a paper presented recently to a conference on training in community psychiatry, I stated that (21): "What we need most is to attract first-class individuals to community psychiatry, including those who will become the models for future trainees." I went on to emphasize that our very best trainees will be excited and intrigued by a new idea, but that they can make no long-term commitment to a field that, though full of action, lacks substance. Community psychiatry could not, under such circumstances, compete with other aspects of psychiatry, and it must compete in the professional market place for the available talent. My emphasis has been misinterpreted if I appear to be saying that community psychiatry should not have a service base. On the contrary, community psychiatry cannot exist without such a base, but the pendulum has moved much too far in that direction.

Community psychiatry, as I would define it, involves the utilization of the techniques, methods, and theories of social psychiatry and other behavioral sciences to investigate and to meet the mental health needs of a functionally or geographically defined population over a significant period of time, and the feeding back of information to modify the central body of social psychiatric and other behavioral science knowledge. Part of this statement is borrowed from Caplan (3), who has essentially defined community psychiatry as the process of meeting the mental health needs of a functionally or geographically defined population. While Caplan is deeply committed to the evolution of theoretical models in community psychiatry and has contributed as much to such models as any psychiatrist, his definition places insufficient stress on a feedback system in which social psychiatric concepts and methods can be brought into play and, consequently, significantly affected by community psychiatry. Duhl's definition also lacks emphasis on the rich research possibilities of community psychiatry. Duhl (11) defines community psychiatry as "concern with optimizing the adaptive potential and psychosocial life skills as well as lessening the amount of pathology in population groups (communities, functional groups, etc.) by population-wide programs of prevention, case-finding, care, treatment, and rehabilitation. The individual becomes important not only as an individual problem but also as a flag of a more general psychiatric need of a population group." Like Caplan, Duhl has been influenced by the public health model of community psychiatry. While both Caplan and Duhl are exceedingly broad in vision and scope, their public health model seems to imply that the major task of community psychiatry involves the ready-made application of models of primary, secondary, and tertiary prevention. I agree wholeheartedly that this is an important part of community psychiatry, but I take issue with those who equate community psychiatry exclusively with a public health preventive approach. Hume, for example, states (13), "Community psychiatry does not take positive mental health as its focus. Rather the focus of community psychiatry is upon prevention." I object to the rigidity inherent in this limitation of community psychiatry, and to the resulting difficulty of generating alternative models. I also object to a model that does not recognize community psychiatry's

emergence as an area devoted to the formulation of new hypotheses.

A community center jointly developed by the Chicago Board of Health, the Illinois Department of Mental Health, and the University of Illinois department of psychiatry is an example of a program in community psychiatry committed equally to service and to research. Although the center has been in operation for less than a year, it has already been responsible for a number of interesting developments. The area within which the center functions is a classic example of the geographically defined community model. It is a section on the south side of Chicago called Woodlawn, whose 82,000 inhabitants, of whom almost 100 per cent are Negro, live within a clear-cut geographic boundary. Woodlawn's population is not homogenous but falls into two general categories: a stable, home-owning, middle-class population that resides in the western area; and a complex concatenation of groups that reside, in some instances in slum areas, in the east. Leadership at the center is provided by three psychiatrists, all of whom have moved to Chicago within the past year and hold appointments in the university department of psychiatry where they are now providing significant leadership in training. The center itself is located in an office building in a densely populated part of Woodlawn. It consists of a suite of comfortable offices, conference rooms, waiting rooms, and secretarial space. It was apparent from its very inception, however, that the center would not and could not be a traditional psychiatric clinic. Instead, it has undertaken to provide consultative services to a broad network of agencies within the area. It has now passed through the first stage of entry into the community. Progress has occasionally been stormy, but a viable dialogue has developed with broad segments of the community's leadership and a strong advisory committee has been drawn from the Woodlawn area to provide local sanction. Contact has been established with legal agencies, religious groups, school officials, social agencies, physicians, neighborhood clubs and organizations, recreational groups, and the major political groups within the geographic boundaries. Meetings with these groups have resulted in frank discussions about the community's fears and expectations of the psychiatrists' role, and a number of stereotypes have been at least partially erased. The dialogue has not been a one-way process; we have received even more of an education than we have provided.

While it has been clearly recognized that the development of service operations is of paramount importance, center leadership has undertaken the difficult and ambitious project of working out sanctions to give strong emphasis to research operations. While this task has still to be completed, close ties with a department of psychiatry afford a medium for its successful accomplishment. The directors of the center* are also engaged in delineating research proposals that promise to aid the service functions. They are now developing, for example, a plan to study the way teachers tag first grade students as emotionally disturbed. Following the social psychiatric perspective, they are interested in the teachers who do the tagging and the setting in which they make their decisions. Not only the ecological characteristics of tagged and untagged children, but the very process of tagging, requires study. Obviously, the psychological status of the children must also be carefully investigated, and psychiatrically sophisticated instruments have been developed for this purpose. The second step in this research will involve following up the tagged students and comparing them with an adequate control group. Intervention of various types, including attempts at changing the setting, the teachers, the family, and the children, will then be utilized to ascertain which, if any, of these interventions may alter the deleterious consequences of being or becoming a child labeled as emotionally disturbed. The group at the center has also studied broad epidemiological and ecological characteristics of individuals requiring psychiatric hospitalization, and of Woodlawn adolescents classified as delinquents. These epidemiological surveys are rich in implications for social psychiatric theory and are useful, as well, in developing guidelines for services such as providing aid for citizens who require full or partial hospitalization. The group at the Woodlawn center has also been deeply interested in the process by which the community defines deviance or mental illness. A number of social agencies in the Woodlawn area have their own definitions of deviant behavior. The welfare department, for example, has developed a special list of people receiving aid because of what the department feels are clear-cut psychological problems. The police have also classified various types of psychological deviation, and center personnel were surprised at the amount of relevant behavioral data the police had obtained.

The issue of the community's definition of deviance, illness, and health touches on one of psychiatry's central theoretical and research problems: the development of an adequate theoretical model for defining mental health. Psychiatry lags behind several other medical disciplines in possession of adequate samples of nomothetic and of normative data. Although concepts of mental health and illness have clearly been correlated with current forms of psychiatric practice, we have lacked the practical means as well as adequate models for establishing what is healthy. At the turn of the century, when psychiatry was essentially a hospital specialty, it was fairly simple to be concerned only with cases of gross psychopathology and to assume that the remaining 99 per cent of the population were mentally healthy, since health was defined as the antonym of gross psychopathology. Psychoanalysis changed this concept considerably. Freud thought of normality or health as an "ideal fiction" (9). Not all analysts agree with Freud's concept, but it is apparent that psychoanalysis has not been able to develop a convincing theory of mental health. With a few significant exceptions, psychoanalysts have not been deeply interested in empirical normative studies, especially studies of adult populations. One of the reasons that the collection of normative data on adult populations has not developed into a major research concern has been the implicit assumptions that the population seen by the psychoanalyst is a representative sample, and that the range of behavior seen in psychoanalytic practice is a good cross-section of the type of clinical problems existing in the various strata of American life. In my opinion, the bulk of the evidence goes in the other direction. Psychoanalysis has studied a limited segment of the American population, and

---

*Drs. Sheldon Schiff, Sheppard Kellam, and Edward Futterman.

what is needed now is the collection of empirical data, by psychoanalysts as well as others, on populations who do not come to our offices. Community psychiatry is in a unique position to provide such data. I do not mean data that merely echo our current theoretical models. Epidemiological studies that report a very high percentage of psychiatric disease in any particular population probably reflect the lack of clarity in our conceptualization of health and illness. We need new tools, new concepts, and new observations of individuals in new settings. Functionally as well as geographically organized community psychiatric centers will help fulfill this need. Psychiatrists are moving in increasing numbers to functionally defined communities, which may vary from a group of small industries to a group of labor unions interested in their community's mental health needs. Studies might involve the mental health needs of members of the Peace Corps, American Indians moved from the reservation, or students attending a university. Psychiatrists working in collegiate health programs have a unique opportunity to study the interaction of the collegiate milieu and the problems it creates or fails to create or ameliorate in the adolescents who pass through its doors. Social psychiatric studies such as these (8) have contributed and may contribute further to our knowledge of both psychopathology and normal coping mechanisms.

The mental health center sponsored by the University of Illinois represents only one possibility for the development of a community psychiatric program. It is to be hoped that there will be considerable heterogeneity in the evolution of these programs, so that comparative analysis will become both possible and feasible. If the Montefiore Hospital in New York City is able to achieve its goal of serving the census tract surrounding it, it can make a unique contribution to community psychiatry. A family court may be an ideal setting for the development of a community psychiatric program. In Massachusetts a number of such court centers have been developed where the leadership is not only sophisticated about psychiatric phenomena but also knowledgeable about family law and the complexities of the court setting. Each of these types of community mental health centers has unique problems as well as unique opportunities to broaden our knowledge about etiology and treatment.

It is relatively simple to advocate the evolution of theoretical models; it is quite another thing to develop new models in actuality. What I have attempted here is to indicate the directions that development of a new model of community psychiatry should take. Psychiatry has entered a new phase of realignment within the social fabric of our culture, and the tasks this entails cannot be accomplished without meaningful collaboration with other disciplines. Community psychiatry and social psychiatry are far too broad in scope to be limited to the confines of a single discipline. In moving toward these new directions we must, of course, be prepared to take risks, but there are limits to risk taking, and reasonable boundaries must be established. In the long run I am convinced that the clarifications and definitions we now lack will be provided by a new generation of investigators and clinicians who will have been stimulated to enter community psychiatry if our generation helps to make it an exciting field.

References

1. Bellak, Leopold, ed. *Handbook of Community Psychiatry and Community Mental Health.* New York, Grune & Stratton, 1964.
2. Bernard, Viola W. "Education for Community Psychiatry in a University Medical Center." In *Handbook of Community Psychiatry and Community Mental Health,* edited by Leopold Bellak. New York, Grune & Stratton, 1964, pp. 82–123.
3. Caplan, Gerald. "Community Psychiatry—Introduction and Overview." In *Concepts of Community Psychiatry,* edited by Stephen E. Goldston. Washington, D.C., U.S. Dept. of Health, Education, and Welfare, 1965, pp. 3–18.
4. Dreikurs, Rudolf. Early experiments in social psychiatry. *Int. J. Soc. Psychiat.* 7:141–47. 1961.
5. Dunham, H. W. Community psychiatry: The newest therapeutic bandwagon. *A.M.A. Arch. Gen. Psychiat.* 12:303–13, 1965.
6. Ehrlich, D., and Sabshin, M. A study of sociotherapeutically oriented psychiatrists. *Amer. J. Orthopsychiat.* 34:469–80, 1964.
7. Faris, Robert E. L., and Dunham, H. W. *Mental Disorders in Urban Areas.* Chicago, Univ. of Chicago Press, 1939.
8. Farnsworth, Dana L. *Mental Health in College and University.* Cambridge, Harvard Univ. Press, 1957.
9. Freud, Sigmund. "Analysis Terminable and Interminable" (first published in 1937). *Collected Papers,* Vol. V, edited by Ernest

Jones. London, The Hogarth Press, 1950, pp. 316–57.

10. Freud, Sigmund. "On the History of the Psychoanalytic Movement" (first published in 1914). *Collected Papers,* Vol. I, edited by Ernest Jones. London, The Hogarth Press, 1949, pp. 287–359.

11. Goldston, Stephen E. "Selected Definitions." In *Concepts of Community Psychiatry,* edited by Stephen E. Goldston. Washington, D.C., U.S. Dept. of Health, Education, and Welfare, 1965, pp. 195–204.

12. Hollingshead, A. B., and Redlich, F. C. *Social Class and Mental Illness.* New York, Wiley, 1958.

13. Hume, Portia B. "Principles and Practice of Community Psychiatry: The Role and Training of the Specialist in Community Psychiatry." In *Handbook of Community Psychiatry and Community Mental Health,* edited by Leopold Bellak. New York, Grune & Stratton, 1964, pp. 65–82.

14. Joint Commission of Mental Illness and Health. *Action for Mental Health.* New York, Basic Books, 1961.

15. Kellam, Sheppard T., Durell, Jack, and Shader, Richard. Measurement of staff attitudes and the clinical course of patients on a psychiatric ward. Paper presented at a meeting of The Association for the Advancement of Psychotherapy, Los Angeles, California, May 3, 1964.

16. Leighton, Alexander H. *My Name is Legion.* New York, Basic Books, 1959.

17. Redlich, F. C., and Pepper, Max P. Social psychiatry. *Amer. J. Psychiat. 116:*611–16, 1960.

18. Sabshin, Melvin. Current perspectives in social psychiatry. Paper presented before the Illinois Psychiatric Society, Chicago, Illinois, April 18, 1962.

19. Sabshin, Melvin, and Eisen, Sydney B. The effects of ward tension on the quality and quantity of tranquilizer utilization. *Ann. N.Y. Acad. Sci. 67:*746–56, 1957.

20. Sabshin, Melvin, *et al.* Significance of pre-experimental studies in the psychosomatic laboratory. *A.M.A. Arch. Neurol. Psychiat. 78:*207–19, 1957.

21. Sabshin, Melvin. "Theory and Practice of Community Psychiatry Training in the Medical School Setting." In *Concepts of Community Psychiatry,* edited by Stephen E. Goldston. Washington, D.C., U.S. Dept. of Health, Education, and Welfare, 1965, pp. 49–56.

22. Strauss, A., Schatzman, L., Bucher, R., Ehrlich, D., and Sabshin, M. *Psychiatric Ideologies and Institutions.* New York, The Free Press of Glencoe, 1964.

23. Wilmer, Harry A. *Social Psychiatry in Action.* Springfield, Illinois, Thomas, 1958.

42. Relationship of Sociocultural Integration and Disintegration to Mental Health

ALEXANDER H. LEIGHTON

The propositions outlined in what follows are current best guesses. They are impressions derived from the research of my colleagues and myself and they are supported by some evidence. Their main purpose, however, is to direct attention toward areas of further inquiry.

THE PROPOSITIONS

1. Events during the entire course of life have potential for precipitating psychiatric disorder.

2. Psychiatric symptoms, once they have emerged, generally become a part of the individual's personality structure, and it is not often that they disappear entirely.

3. The social and psychological dis-

ability resulting from symptoms, on the other hand, does fluctuate markedly, from none or minimal to severe.

4. Contemporary sociocultural processes and situations can produce a high level of disability or, conversely, can markedly reduce the level of disability due to psychiatric symptoms.

5. The sociocultural conditions that tend most to foster symptoms and disability are those that place the individual at a disadvantage in terms of love, guides to decision-making, having a place in the social system, maintaining a degree of self-determination, and feeling respect for what he is and does.

6. Because of the above, a certain minimal degree of integration in a sociocultural system is a necessary condition for the mental health of the constituent members.

7. Sociocultural disintegration is largely responsible for the high prevalence

From J. Zubin and F. Freyhan, *Social Psychiatry,* New York: Grune & Stratton, 1968, pp. 1–7. Reprinted by permission of Grune & Stratton and the author.

of psychiatric disorder in lower socioeconomic groups, in situations of cross-cultural conflict, and in rapidly changing societies, such as those in underdeveloped countries.

THE NATURE OF THE TERMS

Although the words in which these propositions are stated have been carefully chosen, and reworked over a period of years, it does not follow that reader and author will see the same meanings in them. Everybody agrees that there are social phenomena and psychiatric phenomena, and most people think it probable that causal links exist between them, but no appropriate standard system of categorizing the phenomena and referring to concepts has been generally adopted. Witness the various meaning of words like "culture" and "depression." There has been controversy, for example, over the frequency, or even existence, of depression among Africans. The evidence is apparently quite different depending on whether or not you insist that guilt is part of the definition. Without guilt, depression is common, with guilt it is rare. But then, what is the meaning of the word "guilt"?

If I say "anxiety" and am heard by a student of Freud, a student of Sullivan and a student of Skinner—what various circuits start in these three separate brains in response to the same word? What does "insight" mean to a clinical psychiatrist, and what to an experimental psychologist interested in cognitive process?

Social psychiatry is so rumpled by these matters of words that at times one is led into despair. Perhaps, after all, the subject is just not studiable in any scientific sense. Certainly, there are those who say it is a matter of viewpoint, that everything is relative.

An alternative to despair and taking refuge in the relativity of all perceptions is to adopt working terms bound together in a systematic set of definitions. Within such a framework it is possible for one to approach more and more closely to knowing what he means by the words he is using. If the framework is shared by a group, the members reduce the noise in their communications. Linnaeus once said, "Names are the first letters of all knowledge . . . because without them nothing can be learned."

It is worth noting in passing that he and his successors did pretty well in preparing the way for demonstrating a great theory—organic evolution. Without their success in deriving a system of defining species, it is unlikely that Darwin would have been able to write the *Origin of Species*.

All this is preamble to saying that my colleagues and I have tried to develop a consistent system of words and definitions and that the propositions have their origin and meaning in this system.

A way of categorizing psychiatric disorders has been worked out, together with criteria of recognition and rules for decision making in classification. The same has been done with regard to social factors, although thus far somewhat less thoroughly. It is only within these categories and rules that the propositions have their meaning. Another typology with different rules could well use the same words to convey radically different meaning. Much, for example, hangs on what one intends and understands by the word "symptom": is it a phenomenon commonly but not inevitably associated with psychological disturbance? Or, is it a manifestation of an underlying disease, such that if there is no disease then there can be no symptom?

NOTATIONS ON A SYSTEM FOR CATEGORIZING PSYCHIATRIC DISORDERS

Inasmuch as descriptions of the rules and definitions are already in print,[1,2] comment here may be limited to two points: our system gives particular attention to symptoms which may be designated as those behavior patterns commonly but not exclusively seen in psychiatric disorders; and, secondly, it gives attention to the degree to which an individual is impaired or disabled by these patterns. This is the basis of the words "psychiatric disorders," "symptoms" and "disability" in the propositions.

In research that underlies the propositions, the system has been utilized in the study of probability samples of adults drawn from the general population, without regard to whether or not treatment for psychiatric disorder has ever occurred. Relevant data about the individuals have been gathered by questionnaire, by observation and from collateral sources. This we call the "survey." The gathering is generally by trained interviewers rather than psychiatrists, while the evaluation of the data on each individual is done by psychiatrists trained in the technique.

Various tests of logic and reliability have been run, and also tests of validity against clinical standards. The major test of logic has been the translation of the system to a computer program.[3] Reliability tests have included comparing the independent evaluations by different psychiatrists of the same data and also the performance of the same psychiatrist with the same data carried out at two different points in time. While agreement is encouraging and respectable all around, the results do cry for improvement of the system and the technique.

Validity—in the sense of agreement of survey technique with independent clinical appraisal—is at about the same level as the reliability tests.[4]

Against this background we may now observe that the first proposition is saying that if you define the phenomena with which psychiatrists commonly deal in terms of manifest symptoms and degrees of disability, then it appears that disorder can be evoked by life experience at virtually any age.

This does not deny that the difficulty may have been engendered at a very early age, but it focuses attention on when apparent difficulty emerges and postulates that this can be, and often is, a response to life experiences.

The second, third and fourth propositions accept the view that personality is an emergent, and state that many kinds of symptom patterns become an integral and enduring part of the whole. Such, however, does not necessarily constitute disorder. Thus, one person may have a chronic tendency to anxiety, another to hypochondriacal preoccupations, still another to wary suspiciousness, and so on, without any of this amounting to disorder. At times, however (and this can be in response to experiences), the symptom patterns flower forth in disabilities that interfere with work and the fulfillment of every-day social roles.

The fifth proposition outlines the kinds of experiences proposed as most likely to produce manifest disorder. While they may remind one a bit of someone's

ideal for the "good life," they are in fact the product of systematic observation and the comparing of different kinds of human situations. They are furthermore the survivors from a larger range of possibilities. It is interesting, incidentally, to examine the list for what it does not include.

SOCIOCULTURAL DISINTEGRATION

With the six and seventh propositions we come to the consideration of social process; we move from looking at the bee and his experiences to looking at the hive.

There are many ways of looking at the human hive—culture, socioeconomic class, etc.—but the dimension of integration-disintegration is selected here because it has turned out to have strong association with psychiatric disorder frequency and because it has some theoretical interest and explanatory power. We are again, however, confronted with the problem of terms. "Integration" and "disintegration" are words with many and diverse meanings. They become useful for our purposes only when narrowed down to a limited set of working definitions that have the possibility of systematic relationship to the manner of designating psychiatric disorders.

The model on which these working definitions are based is the small community regarded as a functioning system. Such communities have fairly clear-cut margins, and most of the people who make up their populations spend most of their lives in them, passing through the arc from birth to death. Such a model emphasizes these semi-autonomous, quasi-organismic properties of the hive, and visualizes functional prerequisites of the whole such as:

Family formation and perpetuation;
Systems for obtaining subsistence;
Protection against weather, disease and attack; and
The ability to make collective decisions in the face of new, confronting situations.

It is to these functional prerequisites that the words "integration" and "disintegration" refer. More specifically they refer to the results obtained when certain operational indicators are applied. A description of these indicators and the methods of using them would be a lengthy matter comparable to presenting the entire system for designating psychiatric disorders, but since here too there has been publication,[5] a few of the items can serve as illustrations:

Proportion of intact families in the community;
Proportion of effective associations;
Proportion of leaders;
Effectiveness of the communications network.

This then is the context and meaning of disintegration. The association with psychiatric disorder that our studies have found in North America and Africa[2] is limited to these types of communities and to these systems of designating psychiatric disorder and social process.

These are rather severe limits, obviously. Much of the world does not live in the model-type village, and our conceptual system is parochial. Why should we even be interested?

For one thing, a lot of the world does live in such villages.

For another, the association was not found accidentally, but predicted on the basis of a body of theory. The prediction was that if the hive fails markedly in its functions as a hive, there will be an increase in the prevalence of psychiatric disorder among the bees. The body of theory that leads to this expectation is one that has been lifted and synthesized from the public domain. It constitutes a logical network whereby explanations can be traced that link areas as far apart as unconscious processes in the individual and the massive processes of social systems.[6]

The network's more immediate and relevant use is to provide a logical ladder between social and cultural factors, and psychiatric disorders. The finding of the association between disintegration and disorder frequency strengthens the frame of reference and provides a gateway for further investigation.

A third reason for interest is that it may be possible to extrapolate from the village model to the vaster urban societal systems in which so many people live. This means some reformulation of the basic notion, but it still seems plausible to suppose that towns and cities must fulfill functional prerequisites of a society if they are to survive. The question arises as to whether the crucial unit, from the point of view of mental health, is the whole city, or a sub-system such as a ghetto, a socioeconomic class, an occupational group, or a kin and friendship network. In a city, more than in the model village, any given individual has the opportunity of participating in several different societal systems. Depending on circumstances, this can be a stress or a resource; the systems in which he participates may have a disjunctive impact on him because of conflicting demands, even though each system is itself integrated; or he may be able to escape the stress of one disintegrated system (e.g., residential area) by withdrawal and participation in others (e.g., work or kin network).

It appears likely that there are various patterns of sociocultural disintegration in a variety of contexts, and my colleagues and I are attracted by the possibility that there is a common process underlying these that is of maximal significance for mental health and psychiatric disorder. Consider, for example, poverty, and the well-known association of poverty with a high frequency of people who have psychiatric disorder. Failure of social prerequisites—disintegration—is a common but not inevitable accompaniment of poverty. We have in view now a group in Tunis that is far more poverty-stricken than any we have studied on this continent, but it is not disintegrated. We would predict that this will be reflected in its mental health. The relationships may be expressed thus:

Poverty is a condition of risk with respect to the development of social disintegration; social disintegration in turn is a condition of risk with respect to the emergence of psychiatric disorders.

The picture is similar in the matter of cultural change: cultural change does not of itself produce an increase of psychiatric disorder in populations, but it may and often does produce social disintegration which then operates so as to increase psychiatric disorder. The situation can be supposed similar where rapid social change occurs as a result of technological innovation. Migration is another example.

These are the ideas contained in proposition seven.

As a conclusion, let me say that the matter of relating social process and psychological process is of considerable theoretical interest. It has also, however, practical implications. These may be rather distant in realization, but they are nonetheless important, and they have to do with developing strategies of preventive psychiatry through deliberate alterations in social and cultural processes.

References

1. Leighton, D. C. et al.: The Character of Danger. New York, Basic Books, 1963.

2. Leighton, A. H. et al.: Psychiatric Disorders Among the Yoruba. Ithaca, N. Y., Cornell University Press, 1963.

3. Smith, W. G., Taintor, Z. C., and Kaplan, Ellen Brauer: Computer evaluations in psychiatric epidemiology. Social Psychiatry 1:174–181, 1967.

4. Leighton, A. H., Leighton, D. C., and Danley, R. A.: Validity in mental health surveys. Canad. Psychiat. Ass. J. 11:167–178, 1966.

5. Leighton, A. H.: My Name is Legion. New York, Basic Books, 1959.

6. Leighton, A. H.: Psychiatric disorder and social environment: an outline for a frame of reference. In Bergen, B. J. and Thomas, C. S. (Eds.): Issues and Problems in Social Psychiatry: A Book of Readings. Springfield, Ill., Charles C Thomas, 1966, pp. 155–197.

ETIOLOGY AND DEVELOPMENT

Why do mental disorders occur? Is it a defective neurochemical, an unresolved oedipus, an inability to act in accord with one's personal values, a lack of exposure to the proper regimen of positive reinforcements? Each group of theorists presented earlier in the text provides a rationale for their pet notions. Perhaps it is none of these. Instead, can it be the social environment that proves primary? Perhaps many of the components we observe in our patients merely reflect the operation of social influences, cultural mores and styles, as well as simple economics.

Ernest Gruenberg contends that much of what we see clinically is a product of social forces which impede or facilitate mental health. Howard Becker furnishes a concrete and dramatic portrayal of the operation of these forces, tracing the complex of cultural and economic influences that shape the course of becoming "deviant."

43. From Practice to Theory—Community Mental-Health Services and the Nature of Psychoses[*]

ERNEST M. GRUENBERG

Summary

Experiments with comprehensive (community) psychiatric services have resulted in a striking reduction in chronic cases of what may be termed "social-breakdown syndrome" (S.B.S.). This practical experience can be referred back to theory, to throw new light on the textbook description of psychoses and on standard psychiatric training programmes. The pathogenesis of S.B.S. can be thought of in seven stages—from the time when an individual's ability comes to be at odds with what society expects of him, via a vague diagnostic label resulting in exclusion from society into mental hospital, and ending in expedient compliance with hospital conditions. Preventive measures along this pathway can best be achieved by a team, responsible for the continuing care of the patient.

*Abbreviated version of address delivered at the annual meeting of the Royal Medico-Psychological Association in Plymouth, on July 10, 1968. Reprinted from The Lancet, April 5, 1969, pp. 721–724 with permission of author and publishers.

INTRODUCTION

An old adage has it that "It ain't ignorance so much that causes all this world's troubles —it's folks *knowing* things which just ain't so."

Certain notions about psychoses which persist in our textbooks and classrooms cannot be reconciled with the lessons learned from practical experience: they persist because we "know" things about the psychoses which just "ain't so".

Most descriptions of the nature of psychoses continue to identify chronic disorganised behaviour, combativeness, suicidal tendencies, deterioration, and vegetable existence as direct manifestations of certain psychotic disorders. Yet when patients with these psychotic disorders are treated in comprehensive, community-based psychiatric services which provide continuity of care, these behavioural distortions develop much more rarely, and when they do these patterns almost always last only a short time.

Early British comprehensive psychiatric services,[1,7] developed in the 1940s by T. P. Rees,[5] Duncan Macmillan,[3,4] and G. M. Bell[2] from their "open hospitals", showed a remarkable decrease both in hospital census and in "social-breakdown syndrome" (S.B.S.). S.B.S. is the deterioration in social functioning associated with mental disorders which can be prevented both by less harmful responses to those disorders and by changed community attitudes toward the mentally ill and their treatment.[8,9] We now have more definitive evidence from studies of a similar type of programme in Dutchess County, New York, which owed its inspiration to these British pioneering efforts.[10,13] The Dutchess County data indicate a striking benefit in preventing long-term S.B.S. among the 100,000 people aged 16–65 who reside in the service area. Under the old system this population produced annually about 20 S.B.S. episodes which continued 4 years or more. Under the new patterns of caring for cases of severe mental disorders this population has produced annually only about half as many such S.B.S. episodes, indicating a saving of at least 40 man-years of severe disability for each year the new system is in operation.

New patterns of patient-care do make a difference in the symptoms that psychotic patients manifest. But even many who know of these advances do not see their full implications.

Even people working in new types

of programmes are not aware that they are applying new and better ways of organising treatment; they think they are implementing shifts brought about since 1955 by the "tranquillising" drugs. Certainly these new drugs make it easier to care for psychotic patients—both because they directly affect the patient's behaviour and because they have a placebo effect on the physicians administering them. I am impressed both by the pre-drug experiences in community care and by the post-drug experiences at Graylingwell, Plymouth, Fort Logan and Dutchess County, but many colleagues have ignored, or been sceptical of (or even indifferent to), the fact that very similar results had been obtained by Macmillan and Rees before these tranquillising drugs were available.

It is a pity that this body of experience has not become incorporated into our writings on the psychoses and into our training programme. Our standard descriptions of the psychoses and their manifestations should incorporate information on how sensitive these manifestations are to the way in which people with psychotic disorders are cared for. Before these fruits of practical experience are incorporated into our texts and instructional material we may require a theory as to why these manifestations are so sensitive to the organisation of psychiatric care. To help meet this need, I would like to suggest some mechanisms by which these dramatic changes in the course of psychotic disorders could have been achieved. Specifying these mechanisms may help make acceptable and respectable the truths that have been learned from practice.

[1]In the Mental Hospital. *Lancet,* London, 1957.
[2]Bell, G. M. *Int. J. Soc. Psychiat.* 1955, *1*, 42.
[3]Macmillan, D. *in* Proceedings of the Thirty-fourth Annual Conference of the Milbank Memorial Fund, 1957, part 1, p. 29. Milbank Memorial Fund, New York, 1958.
[4]MacMillan, D. *Lancet,* 1963, i, 567.
[5]See *ibid.* p. 13.
[6]Conolly, J. The Indications of Insanity. 1830. London, 1964 (reprinted).
[7]Maclay, W. S. *Can. Med. Ass. J.* 1958, *78*, 909.
[8]Control of Mental Disorders. American Public Health Association, 1962.
[9]Gruenberg, E. M. *Am. J. Psychiat.* 1967, *123*, 12,
[10]Hunt, R. C. *in* An Approach to the Prevention of Disability from Chronic Psychoses; part 1, p. 9. Milbank Memorial Fund, New York, 1958.
[11]New York State Hospital Directors *in* Proceedings of the Thirty-sixth Annual Conference of the Milbank Memorial Fund, 1959, p. 11. Milbank Memorial Fund, New York, 1960.
[12]Gruenberg, E. M. (editor) Evaluating the Effectiveness of Community Mental Health Services. Mental Health Materials Center, New York, 1966.
[13]Gruenberg, E. M., Bennet, C. I., Snow, H. B. *in* Social Psychiatry, ARMND (edited by F. C. Redlich); vol. XLVII. Baltimore, 1969.

SOCIAL-BREAKDOWN SYNDROME

People with different psychotic disorders exhibit similar disturbances of social functioning. New patient-care arrangements almost eliminated the worst patterns of disordered social functioning and halved the frequency with which new chronic cases start. Thus we can infer two types of symptoms: the direct consequences of mental disorder and the secondary complications whose appearance and continuation depend on circumstances and are apparently preventable. Those secondary manifestations which are mainly prevented by using the best-known systems of care are called the social-breakdown syndrome.

Manifestations. The S.B.S. covers a wide range of overt disturbed behaviour —withdrawal, self-neglect, dangerous behaviour, shouting, self-harm, failure to work, and failure to enjoy recreation being the main manifestations. Either troublesome behaviour or functional performance deficit may predominate. Troublesome manifestations occur with or without functional loss. Severity ranges widely. (Hallucinations, confusion, phobias and other subjective experiences are not included in our studies because, first, many patients in improved programmes continue to describe these symptoms and, second, because our field-study techniques cannot yet systematically investigate subjective experiences. This exclusion does not prejudge the possibility that these too may often be secondary manifestations in the same sense, readily modified by the social environment.)

Course. Most S.B.S. episodes last but a few weeks, some a few months, and (today) only rarely do episodes last for years. The onset is sometimes insidious, the course indolent, the end the vegetative state described in textbooks. More commonly onset occurs in a single, explosive leap, beginning with violent behaviour or the sudden termination of all ordinary social roles, often accompanied by a confused or clouded state. Spontaneous remission often occurs in days or weeks. Other cases progress for a while and then arrest for a long period at a particular stage, which is sometimes followed by recovery. Some other cases pursue a remitting course. First episodes and relapses show similar patterns.

Occurrence. S.B.S. cases are found in psychiatric inpatients and in people in need of hospital admission. In fact, the syndrome evidently begins outside the hospitals, the components of S.B.S. being the common justifications for admission (leading, as they do, to the conclusion that the candidate is "incapable of caring for himself" or is "dangerous to self or others"). Thus S.B.S. describes the severe burdens the community experiences in dealing with these individuals, and these burdens account for the decision to extrude them from the community. S.B.S. also describes common reasons for keeping a patient in hospital,

an indication that hospital admission does not always terminate S.B.S.

Pathogenesis. The pathogenesis of S.B.S. might be described in seven steps, leading to the chronically deteriorated picture formerly seen in the back wards of mental hospitals. The S.B.S. describes the way in which the relationship between a person and his social environment breaks down. The syndrome seems to emerge as a result of a spiralling crescendo of interactions between the patient and the people in his immediate social environment.

THE PUSH. This first step is common in ordinary life; it consists of a discrepancy between what a person can do and what he is expected to do. These discrepancies are generally transient: they are eliminated by a change in performance, by escaping from the demanding environment, by a change in environmental demands, or by an "explanation" which relieves the individual of the responsibility for the discrepancy.

HEIGHTENED SUGGESTIBILITY. When the discrepancy persists, the individual on whom the demand is being placed is held responsible for the failure to perform as demanded. On this point the individual and those making the demand must be in agreement. Finding no other "explanation" he wonders what is "wrong" with him. A diffuse uncertainty regarding his own nature and value system develops in relationship to environmental pressures which produces hesitancy or impulsiveness (or both). He has become more dependent on current cues from the environment regarding right and wrong. His increased sense of uncertainty about himself, his values, and his customary ways of dealing with life produce a readiness to consider new ways of doing things, new ways of looking at things, new ways of looking at himself. This is the precondition for constructive changes in attitude and behaviour which, when the environment is suitable, leads to corrective modifications of functioning. Every psychotherapist, every army sergeant, and every job supervisor has seen this process; such behavioural modifications are part of normal life. But a special danger is created when the individual accepts that the environment's expectations are appropriate but cannot modify his behaviour in the expected way. A common way to deny that the expectations are appropriate is to conclude that those making the demands on the individual have misunderstood his true nature—they are asking something appropriate, but they are asking it of the wrong kind of person. He decides that for this task he is too young, too old, too short, too tall, too blind, too crippled, or too ignorant to be expected to do what was asked. The failing individual's sense of responsibility for his failure to comply with the demands is relieved, and since he no longer holds himself responsible for the discrepancy I refer to these explanations as exculpating. (As will emerge below, the discovery of suitable exculpating explanations can play a large role in the process of preventing S.B.S.) When the discrepancy between environmental demand and individual performance is not thus terminated, the individual takes an unsatisfactory step to rectify the situation which serves only to arouse fears of resentment, further putting him out of gear with the people around him. This produces an increased need to modify his behaviour to satisfy increasingly urgent demands. But his response to this still more tense situation has the opposite effect, resulting in still more misunderstanding and hostility. This process of action-reaction, reaction to the reaction, and reaction to that, goes on either towards an explosion and social extrusion of the individual or to his progressive withdrawal from interaction, and hence from his usual roles and functions.

LABELLING. He is then labelled as "not quite right", leading to a vague or rejecting "diagnosis" such as "schizophrenic" or "psychotic" or just plain "mentally ill" and to the recommendation that he be admitted to hospital.

EXTRUSION. Admission to hospital can itself contribute to the further development of S.B.S. Most damaging is formal commitment, with the petitioning mechanism through which those closest to the failing individual join with the community establishment to engage in the labelling process.

INSTITUTIONALISATION. An overly sheltering hospital environment can further encourage the process of S.B.S. pathogenesis. In his community he may have been expected to do things he could not do, but in the traditional hospital he is expected to do nothing except what he is told to do (or, of course, to try to run away). Whatever the patient's behaviour, no-one expresses surprise. He is called "sick" and is told that he must be cared for. Thus he is morally relieved of responsibility for his failures at the price of being identified as having a condition which makes his own impulses, thoughts, and speech largely irrelevant to any practical activities of daily life.

COMPLIANCE AND ISOLATION. The S.B.S. progresses another step when the patient, while still viewing himself as "different" from the other patients, complies with the hospital's rules of accepted behaviour to stay out of trouble. He becomes isolated from his former ties. The family is told that everything necessary will be done by the staff; visiting is restricted to a few hours; staff members familiar with the patient's case will probably be unavailable to the family.

IDENTIFICATION. Next the patient comes to identify with fellow patients, anticipate staff demands, "fit in" and become a "good patient". Sometimes he fits into one of the available rebellious roles for which the hospital is equally prepared. In time, whatever his former capacities were, his ability to carry out ordinary social exchanges and work tasks decreases and becomes awkward from disuse. The end of this process is most readily seen in the mental hospital's chronic wards.

Prevention. Outlining the pathway to S.B.S. helps plan intervention at each step to arrest progress and reverse the pathogenic processes. Expert assistance should be given to reduce distressing discrepancies, either by improving the patient's performance, or by modifying his environment's expectations, or both. Expectations can be modified by reorienting lay people in the sick person's environment to a more realistic view of the patient's capacities. This may require a clear description of a patient's handicap or defect. This will automatically alter expectations—a man called "blind" is not expected to teach painting. These handicaps should be described clearly and simply so as to avoid abstract symbols such as "psychosis" which can arouse vague fears as to what he might do and thus justify extrusion from the community. The patient must also be given this interpretation of his handicap.

Admission to hospital, when indicated, is least damaging if the patient retains responsibility for himself as far as possible, and if he enters voluntarily. In the hospital he can be helped to maintain a self-respecting, self-governing role. All tendencies toward uniform procedures must be opposed (locked doors, fixed bathing-hours, and so on). The clinician not only arranges for the patient's clinical programme but also acts to interrupt and reverse the pathogenesis of the S.B.S.

Such preventive measures are most easily executed when a single professional team takes comprehensive responsibility for the whole course of treatment (continuity of care). This team needs close ties with the whole complex of community services and access to a full psychiatric service (inpatient, outpatient, and transitional forms of treatment).

Differential Diagnosis. Some S.B.S. components also arise by other mechanisms as direct consequences of physical illness (mutism, incontinence, orientation loss) or social disorganisation or panic (combativeness, loss of initiative). Some subcultures apparently require combativeness and irresponsibility.

We can readily ascertain the presence or absence of the syndrome's components through well-developed definitions of these components and data-gathering techniques, but we cannot always determine which cases to attribute to the pathogenic pathway described above and which to attribute to a physical handicap. When recovery follows a social reablement programme it is tempting, but fallible, to attribute the patient's disturbance to the sociogenic mechanism; when social reablement fails, attribution to physical handicaps is equally fallible.

Unlike the "institutional neurosis" concept,[14] the S.B.S. concept recognises that advanced cases can present without the aid of institutions or psychiatrists; many such episodes terminate after a brief spell of hospital treatment. When medical research reveals an unintended hazard associated with hospital treatment (as with cross-infection), it seeks means of avoiding these hazards while preserving the hospital's assets.

DISCUSSION

Treatment conditions for people with psychotic disorders which favour the S.B.S. development continue despite the past two decades' drastic improvements in many British and American mental hospitals. Comprehensive community mental-health programmes offering continuity of care have advanced most in certain provincial services, while destructive patterns from the past persist too frequently in affluent private services, many university services and other prestigious places. (Perhaps "high standards" and high staff ratios produce excessively rigid divisions of staff and agency functions.[15])

Many hope that the new mental-health centres in the U.S.A. will assign comprehensive responsibility to one treatment team for each patient. This concept of the S.B.S., and its pathogenesis, supports this movement by specifying what these teams might prevent.

Time will tell whether the mental health centres reduce chronic mental disability. The outcome is by no means certain since most plans emphasise the availability of comprehensive services (no matter how nominal their coordination might be); they do not concentrate on ensuring continuity of attention through the provision of a single team which cares for each patient throughout his illness.

[14]Barton, R. Institutional Neurosis. Bristol, 1959.

[15]*Milbank Meml. Fund Q*. 1064, *42*, no. 3, part 2.

44.　Becoming a Marihuana User

HOWARD S. BECKER

The use of marihuana is and has been the focus of a good deal of attention on the part of both scientists and laymen. One of the major problems students of the practice have addressed themselves to has been the identification of those individual psychological traits which differentiate marihuana users from nonusers and which are assumed to account for the use of the drug. That approach, common in the study of behavior categorized as deviant, is based on the premise that the presence of a given kind of behavior in an individual can best be explained as the result of some trait which predisposes or motivates him to engage in the behavior.[1]

This study is likewise concerned with accounting for the presence or absence of marihuana use in an individual's behavior. It starts, however, from a different premise: that the presence of a given kind of behavior is the result of a sequence of social experiences during which the person acquires a conception of the meaning of the behavior, and perceptions and judgments of objects and situations, all of which make the activity possible and desirable. Thus, the motivation or disposition to engage in the activity is built up in the course of learning to engage in it and does not antedate this learning process. For such a view it is not necessary to identify those "traits" which "cause" the behavior. Instead, the problem becomes one of describing the set of changes in the person's conception of the activity and of the experience it provides for him.[2]

This paper seeks to describe the sequence of changes in attitude and experience which leads to *the use of marihuana*

for pleasure. Marihuana does not produce addiction, as do alcohol and the opiate drugs; there is no withdrawal sickness and no ineradicable craving for the drug.[3] The most frequent pattern of use might be termed "recreational." The drug is used occasionally for the pleasure the user finds in it, a relatively casual kind of behavior in comparison with that connected with the use of addicting drugs. The term "use for pleasure" is meant to emphasize the noncompulsive and casual character of the behavior. It is also meant to eliminate from consideration here those few cases in which marihuana is used for its prestige value only, as a symbol that one is a certain kind of person, with no pleasure at all being derived from its use.

The analysis presented here is conceived of as demonstrating the greater explanatory usefulness of the kind of theory outlined above as opposed to the predispositional theories now current. This may be seen in two ways: (1) predispositional theories cannot account for that group of users (whose existence is admitted)[4] who do not exhibit the trait or traits considered to cause the behavior and (2) such theories cannot account for the great variability over time of a given individual's behavior with reference to the drug. The same person will at one stage be unable to use the drug for pleasure, at a later stage be able and willing to do so, and, still later, again be unable to use it in this way. These changes, difficult to explain from a predispositional or motivational theory, are readily understandable in terms of changes in the individual's conception of the drug as is the existence of "normal" users.

The study attempted to arrive at a general statement of the sequence of changes in individual attitude and experience which have always occurred when the individual has become willing and able to use marihuana for pleasure and which have not occurred or not been

From *The American Journal of Sociology,* LIX (November, 1953), 235–242. Reprinted by permission of the University of Chicago Press and the author. ©1953 by The University of Chicago. All rights reserved.

[1]See, as examples of this approach, the following: Eli Marcovitz and Henry J. Meyers, "The Marihuana Addict in the Army," *War Medicine,* VI (December, 1944), 382–91; Herbert S. Gaskill, "Marihuana, an Intoxicant," *American Journal of Psychiatry,* CII (September, 1945), 202–4; Sol Charen and Luis Perelman, "Personality Studies of Marihuana Addicts," *American Journal of Psychiatry,* CII (March, 1946), 674–82.

[2]This approach stems from George Herbert Mead's discussion of objects in *Mind, Self, and Society* (Chicago: University of Chicago Press, 1934), pp. 277–80.

[3]Cf. Roger Adams, "Marihuana," *Bulletin of the New York Academy of Medicine,* XVIII (November, 1942), 705–30.

[4]Cf. Lawrence Kolb, "Marihuana," *Federal Probation,* II (July, 1938), 22–25; and Walter Bromberg, "Marihuana: A Psychiatric Study," *Journal of the American Medical Association,* CXIII (July 1, 1939), II.

permanently maintained when this is not the case. This generalization is stated in universal terms in order that negative cases may be discovered and used to revise the explanatory hypothesis.[5]

Fifty interviews with marihuana users from a variety of social backgrounds and present positions in society constitute the data from which the generalization was constructed and against which it was tested.[6] The interviews focused on the history of the person's experience with the drug, seeking major changes in his attitude toward it and in his actual use of it and the reasons for these changes. The final generalization is a statement of that sequence of changes in attitude which occurred in every case known to me in which the person came to use marihuana for pleasure. Until a negative case is found, it may be considered as an explanation of all cases of marihuana use for pleasure. In addition, changes from use to nonuse are shown to be related to similar changes in conception, and in each case it is possible to explain variations in the individual's behavior in these terms.

This paper covers only a portion of the natural history of an individual's use of marihuana,[7] starting with the person having arrived at the point of willingness to try marihuana. He knows that others use it to "get high," but he does not know what this means in concrete terms. He is curious about the experience, ignorant of what it may turn out to be, and afraid that it may be more than he has bargained for. The steps outlined below, if he undergoes them all and maintains the attitudes developed in them, leave him willing and able to use the drug for pleasure when the opportunity presents itself.

I

The novice does not ordinarily get high the first time he smokes marihuana, and several attempts are usually necessary to induce this state. One explanation of this may be that the drug is not smoked "properly," that is, in a way that insures sufficient dosage to produce real symptoms of intoxication. Most users agree that it cannot be smoked like tobacco if one is to get high:

Take in a lot of air, you know, and . . . I don't know how to describe it, you don't smoke it like a cigarette, you draw in a lot of air and get it deep down in your system and then keep it there. Keep it there as long as you can.

Without the use of some such technique[8] the drug will produce no effects, and the user will be unable to get high:

The trouble with people like that [who are not able to get high] is that they're just not smoking it right, that's all there is to it. Either they're not holding it down long enough, or they're getting too much air and not enough smoke, or the other way around or something like that. A lot of people just don't smoke it right, so naturally nothing's gonna happen.

If nothing happens, it is manifestly impossible for the user to develop a conception of the drug as an object which can be used for pleasure, and use will therefore not continue. The first step in the sequence of events that must occur if the person is to become a user is that he must learn to use the proper smoking technique in order that his use of the drug will produce some effects in terms of which his conception of it can change.

Such a change is, as might be expected, a result of the individual's participation in groups in which marihuana is used. In them the individual learns the proper way to smoke the drug. This may occur through direct teaching:

I was smoking like I did an ordinary cigarette. He said, "No, don't do it like that." He said, "Suck it, you know, draw in and hold it in your lungs till you . . . for a period of time."

I said, "Is there any limit of time to hold it?"

He said, "No, just till you feel that you want to let it out, let it out." So I did that three or four times.

---

[5]The method used is that described by Alfred R. Lindesmith in his *Opiate Addiction* (Bloomington: Principia Press, 1947), chap. i. I would like also to acknowledge the important role Lindesmith's work played in shaping my thinking about the genesis of marihuana use.

[6]Most of the interviews were done by the author. I am grateful to Solomon Kobrin and Harold Finestone for allowing me to make use of interviews done by them.

[7]I hope to discuss elsewhere other stages in this natural history.

[8]A pharmacologist notes that this ritual is in fact an extremely efficient way of getting the drug into the blood stream (R. P. Walton, *Marihuana: America's New Drug Problem* [Philadelphia: J. B. Lippincott, 1938], p. 48).

Many new users are ashamed to admit ignorance and, pretending to know already, must learn through the more indirect means of observation and imitation:

I came on like I had turned on [smoked marihuana] many times before, you know. I didn't want to seem like a punk to this cat. See, like I didn't know the first thing about it—how to smoke it, or what was going to happen, or what. I just watched him like a hawk—I didn't take my eyes off him for a second, because I wanted to do everything just as he did it. I watched how he held it, how he smoked it, and everything. Then when he gave it to me I just

came on cool, as though I knew exactly what the score was. I held it like he did and took a poke just the way he did.

No person continued marihuana use for pleasure without learning a technique that supplied sufficient dosage for the effects of the drug to appear. Only when this was learned was it possible for a conception of the drug as an object which could be used for pleasure to emerge. Without such a conception marihuana use was considered meaningless and did not continue.

II

Even after he learns the proper smoking technique, the new user may not get high and thus not form a conception of the drug as something which can be used for pleasure. A remark made by a user suggested the reason for this difficulty in getting high and pointed to the next necessary step on the road to being a user:

I was told during an interview, "As a matter of fact, I've seen a guy who was high out of his mind and didn't know it."

I expressed disbelief: "How can that be, man?"

The interviewee said, "Well, it's pretty strange, I'll grant you that, but I've seen it. This guy got on with me, claiming that he'd never got high, one of those guys, and he got completely stoned. And he kept insisting that he wasn't high. So I had to prove to him that he was."

What does this mean? It suggests that being high consists of two elements: the presence of symptoms caused by marihuana use and the recognition of these symptoms and their connection by the user with his use of the drug. It is not enough, that is, that the effects be present; they alone do not automatically provide the experience of being high. The user must be able to point them out to himself and consciously connect them with his having smoked marihuana before he can have this experience. Otherwise, regardless of the actual effects produced, he considers that the drug has had no effect on him: "I figured it either had no effect on me or other people were exaggerating its effects on them, you know. I thought it was probably psychological, see." Such persons believe that the whole thing is an illusion and that the

wish to be high leads the user to deceive himself into believing that something is happening when, in fact, nothing is. They do not continue marihuana use, feeling that "it does nothing" for them.

Typically, however, the novice has faith (developed from his observation of users who do get high) that the drug actually will produce some new experience and continues to experiment with it until it does. His failure to get high worries him, and he is likely to ask more experienced users or provoke comments from them about it. In such conversations he is made aware of specific details of his experience which he may not have noticed or may have noticed but failed to identify as symptoms of being high:

I didn't get high the first time. . . . I don't think I held it in long enough. I probably let it out, you know, you're a little afraid. The second time I wasn't sure, and he [smoking companion] told me, like I asked him for some of the symptoms or something, how would I know, you know. . . . So he told me to sit on a stool. I sat on—I think I sat on a bar stool—and he said, "Let your feet hang," and then when I got down my feet were real cold, you know.

And I started feeling it, you know. That was the first time. And then about a week after that, sometime pretty close to it. I really got on. That was the first time I got a big laughing kick, you know. Then I really knew I was on.

One symptom of being high is an intense hunger. In the next case the novice becomes aware of this and gets high for the first time:

They were just laughing the hell out of me because like I was eating so much. I just scoffed [ate] so much food, and they were just laughing at me, you know. Sometimes I'd be looking at them, you know, wondering why they're laughing, you know, not knowing what I was doing. [Well, did they tell you why they were laughing eventually?] Yeah, yeah, I come back, "Hey, man, what's happening?" Like, you know, like I'd ask, "What's happening?" and all of a sudden I feel weird, you know. "Man, you're on, you know. You're on pot [high on marihuana]." I said, "No, am I?" Like I don't know what's happening.

The learning may occur in more indirect ways:

I heard little remarks that were made by other people. Somebody said, "My legs are rubbery," and I can't remember all the remarks that were made because I was very attentively listening for all these cues for what I was supposed to feel like.

The novice, then, eager to have this feeling, picks up from other users some concrete referents of the term "high" and applies these notions to his own experience. The new concepts make it possible for him to locate these symptoms among his own sensations and to point out to himself a "something different" in his experience that he connects with drug use. It is only when he can do this that he is high. In the next case, the contrast between two successive experiences of a user makes clear the crucial importance of the awareness of the symptoms in being high and re-emphasizes the important role of interaction with other users in acquiring the concepts that make this awareness possible:

[Did you get high the first time you turned on?] Yeah, sure. Although, come to think of it, I guess I really didn't. I mean, like that first time it was more or less of a mild drunk. I was happy, I guess, you know what I mean. But I didn't really know I was high, you know what I mean. It was only after the second time I got high that I realized I was high the first time. Then I knew that something different was happening.

[How did you know that?] How did I know? If what happened to me that night would of happened to you, you would've known, believe me. We played the first tune for almost two hours—one tune! Imagine, man! We got on the stand and played this one tune, we started at nine o'clock. When we got finished I looked at my watch, it's a quarter to eleven. Almost two hours on one tune. And it didn't seem like anything.

I mean, you know, it does that to you. It's like you have much more time or something. Anyway, when I saw that, man, it was too much. I knew I must really be high or something if anything like that could happen. See,

and then they explained to me that that's what it did to you, you had a different sense of time and everything. So I realized that that's what it was. I knew then. Like the first time, I probably felt that way, you know, but I didn't know what's happening.

It is only when the novice becomes able to get high in this sense that he will continue to use marihuana for pleasure. In every case in which use continued, the user had acquired the necessary concepts with which to express to himself the fact that he was experiencing new sensations caused by the drug. That is, for use to continue, it is necessary not only to use the drug so as to produce effects but also to learn to perceive these effects when they occur. In this way marihuana acquires meaning for the user as an object which can be used for pleasure.

With increasing experience the user develops a greater appreciation of the drug's effects; he continues to learn to get high. He examines succeeding experiences closely, looking for new effects, making sure the old ones are still there. Out of this there grows a stable set of categories for experiencing the drug's effects whose presence enables the user to get high with ease.

The ability to perceive the drug's effects must be maintained if use is to continue; if it is lost, marihuana use ceases. Two kinds of evidence support this statement. First, people who become heavy users of alcohol, barbiturates, or opiates do not continue to smoke marihuana, largely because they lose the ability to distinguish between its effects and those of the other drugs.[9] They no longer know whether the marihuana gets them high. Second, in those few cases in which an individual uses marihuana in such quantities that he is always high, he is apt to get this same feeling that the drug has no effect on him, since the essential element of a noticeable difference between feeling high and feeling normal is missing. In such a situation, use is likely to be given up completely, but temporarily, in order that the user may once again be able to perceive the difference.

---

[9]"Smokers have repeatedly stated that the consumption of whiskey while smoking negates the potency of the drug. They find it very difficult to get 'high' while drinking whiskey and because of that smokers will not drink while using the 'weed' " (cf. New York City Mayor's Committee on Marihuana, *The Marihuana Problem in the City of New York* [Lancaster, Pa.: Jacques Cattell Press, 1944], p. 13).

III

One more step is necessary if the user who has now learned to get high is to continue use. He must learn to enjoy the effects he has just learned to experience. Marihuana-produced sensations are not automatically or necessarily pleasurable. The taste for such experience is a socially acquired one, not different in kind from acquired tastes for oysters or dry martinis. The user feels dizzy, thirsty; his scalp tingles; he misjudges time and distances; and so on. Are these things pleasurable? He isn't sure. If he is to continue marihuana use, he must decide that they are. Otherwise, getting high, while a real enough experience, will be an unpleasant one he would rather avoid.

The effects of the drug, when first perceived, may be physically unpleasant or at least ambiguous:

It started taking effect, and I didn't know what was happening, you know, what it was, and I was very sick. I walked around the room, walking around the room trying to get off, you know; it just scared me at first, you know. I wasn't used to that kind of feeling.

In addition, the novice's naive interpretation of what is happening to him may further confuse and frighten him, particularly if he decides, as many do, that he is going insane:

I felt I was insane, you know. Everything people done to me just wigged me. I couldn't hold a conversation, and my mind would be wandering, and I was always thinking, oh, I don't know, weird things, like hearing music different. . . . I get the feeling that I can't talk to anyone. I'll goof completely.

Given these typically frightening and unpleasant first experiences, the beginner will not continue use unless he learns to re-define the sensations as pleasurable:

It was offered to me, and I tried it. I'll tell you one thing. I never did enjoy it at all. I mean it was just nothing that I could enjoy. [Well, did you get high when you turned on?] Oh, yeah, I got definite feelings from it. But I didn't enjoy them. I mean I got plenty of reactions, but they were mostly reactions of fear. [You were frightened?] Yes. I didn't enjoy it. I couldn't seem to relax with it, you know. If you can't relax with a thing, you can't enjoy it, I don't think.

In other cases the first experiences were also definitely unpleasant, but the person did become a marihuana user. This oc-

curred, however, only after a later experience enabled him to redefine the sensations as pleasurable:

[This man's first experience was extremely unpleasant, involving distortion of spatial relationships and sounds, violent thirst, and panic produced by these symptoms.] After the first time I didn't turn on for about, I'd say, ten months to a year. . . . It wasn't a moral thing; it was because I'd gotten so frightened, bein' so high. An' I didn't want to go through that again, I mean, my reaction was, "Well, if this is what they call bein' high, I don't dig [like] it." . . . So I didn't turn on for a year almost, accounta that. . . .

Well, my friends started, an' consequently I started again. But I didn't have any more, I didn't have that same initial reaction, after I started turning on again.

[In interaction with his friends he became able to find pleasure in the effects of the drug and eventually became a regular user.]

In no case will use continue without such a redefinition of the effects as enjoyable.

This redefinition occurs, typically, in interaction with more experienced users who, in a number of ways, teach the novice to find pleasure in this experience which is at first so frightening.[10] They may reassure him as to the temporary character of the unpleasant sensations and minimize their seriousness, at the same time calling attention to the more enjoyable aspects. An experienced user describes how he handles newcomers to marihuana use:

Well, they get pretty high sometimes. The average person isn't ready for that, and it is a little frightening to them sometimes. I mean, they've been high on lush [alcohol], and they get higher that way than they've ever been before, and they don't know what's happening to them. Because they think they're going to keep going up, up, up till they lose their minds or begin doing weird things or something. You have to like reassure them, explain to them that they're not really flipping or anything, that they're gonna be all right. You have to just talk them out of being afraid. Keep talking to them, reassuring, telling them it's all right. And come on with your own story, you know: "The same thing happened to me. You'll get to like that after awhile." Keep coming on like that; pretty soon you talk them out of being scared. And besides they see you doing it and nothing horrible is happening to you, so that gives them more confidence.

---

[10]Charen and Perelman, *op. cit.*, p. 679.

The more experienced user may also teach the novice to regulate the amount he smokes more carefully, so as to avoid any severely uncomfortable symptoms while retaining the pleasant ones. Finally, he teaches the new user that he can "get to like it after awhile." He teaches him to regard those ambiguous experiences formerly defined as unpleasant as enjoyable. The older user in the following incident is a person whose tastes have shifted in this way, and his remarks have the effect of helping others to make a similar redefinition:

A new user had her first experience of the effects of marihuana and became frightened and hysterical. She "felt like she was half in and half out of the room" and experienced a number of alarming physical symptoms. One of the more experienced users present said, "She's dragged because she's high like that. I'd give anything to get that high myself. I haven't been that high in years."

In short, what was once frightening and distasteful becomes, after a taste for it is built up, pleasant, desired, and sought after. Enjoyment is introduced by the favorable definition of the experience that one acquires from others. Without this, use will not continue, for marihuana will not be for the user an object he can use for pleasure.

In addition to being a necessary step in becoming a user, this represents an important condition for continued use. It is quite common for experienced users suddenly to have an unpleasant or frightening experience, which they cannot define as pleasurable, either because they have used a larger amount of marihuana than usual or because it turns out to be a higher-quality marihuana than they expected. The user has sensations which go beyond any conception he has of what being high is and is in much the same situation as the novice, uncomfortable and frightened. He may blame it on an overdose and simply be more careful in the future. But he may make this the occasion for a rethinking of his attitude toward the drug and decide that it no longer can give him pleasure. When this occurs and is not followed by a redefinition of the drug as capable of producing pleasure, use will cease.

The likelihood of such a redefinition occurring depends on the degree of the individual's participation with other users. Where this participation is intensive, the individual is quickly talked out of his feeling against marihuana use. In the next case, on the other hand, the experience was very disturbing, and the aftermath of the incident cut the person's participation with other users to almost zero. Use stopped for three years and began again only when a combination of circumstances, important among which was a resumption of ties with users, made possible a redefinition of the nature of the drug:

It was too much, like I only made about four pokes, and I couldn't even get it out of my mouth, I was so high, and I got real flipped. In the basement, you know, I just couldn't stay in there anymore. My heart was pounding real hard, you know, and I was going out of my mind; I thought I was losing my mind completely. So I cut out of this basement, and this other guy, he's out of his mind, told me, "Don't, don't leave me, man. Stay here." And I couldn't.

I walked outside, and it was five below zero, and I thought I was dying, and I had my coat open; I was sweating, I was perspiring. My whole insides were all . . . , and I walked about two blocks away, and I fainted behind a bush. I don't know how long I laid there. I woke up, and I was feeling the worst, I can't describe it at all, so I made it to a bowling alley, man, and I was trying to act normal, I was trying to shoot pool, you know, trying to act real normal, and I couldn't lay and I couldn't stand up and I couldn't sit down, and I went up and laid down where some guys that spot pins lay down, and that didn't help me, and I went down to a doctor's office. I was going to go in there and tell the doctor to put me out of my misery . . . because my heart was pounding so hard, you know. . . . So then all week end I started flipping, seeing things there and going through hell, you know, all kinds of abnormal things. . . . I just quit for a long time then.

[He went to a doctor who defined the symptoms for him as those of a nervous breakdown caused by "nerves" and "worries." Although he was no longer using marihuana, he had some recurrences of the symptoms which led him to suspect that "it was all his nerves."] So I just stopped worrying, you know; so it was about thirty-six months later I started making it again. I'd just take a few pokes, you know. [He first resumed use in the company of the same user-friend with whom he had been involved in the original incident.]

A person, then, cannot begin to use marihuana for pleasure, or continue its use for pleasure, unless he learns to define its effects as enjoyable, unless it becomes and remains an object which he conceives of as capable of producing pleasure.

IV

In summary, an individual will be able to use marihuana for pleasure only when he goes through a process of learning to conceive of it as an object which can be used in this way. No one becomes a user without (1) learning to smoke the drug in a way which will produce real effects; (2) learning to recognize the effects and connect them with drug use (learning, in other words, to get high); and (3) learning to enjoy the sensations he perceives. In the course of this process he develops a disposition or motivation to use marihuana which was not and could not have been present when he began use, for it involves and depends on conceptions of the drug which could only grow out of the kind of actual experience detailed above. On completion of this process he is willing and able to use marihuana for pleasure.

He has learned, in short, to answer "Yes" to the question: "Is it fun?" The direction his further use of the drug takes depends on his being able to continue to answer "Yes" to this question and, in addition, on his being able to answer "Yes" to other questions which arise as he becomes aware of the implications of the fact that the society as a whole disapproves of the practice: "Is it expedient?" "Is it moral?" [11] Once he has acquired the ability to get enjoyment out of the drug, use will continue to be possible for him. Considerations of morality and expediency, occasioned by the reactions of society, may interfere and inhibit use, but use continues to be a possibility in terms of his conception of the drug. The act becomes impossible only when the ability to enjoy the experience of being high is lost, through a change in the user's conception of the drug occasioned by certain kinds of experience with it.

In comparing this theory with those which ascribe marihuana use to motives or predispositions rooted deep in individual behavior, the evidence makes it clear that marihuana use for pleasure can occur only when the process described above is undergone and cannot occur without it. This is apparently so without reference to the nature of the individual's personal makeup or psychic problems. Such theories assume that people have stable modes of response which predetermine the way they will act in relation to any particular situation or object and that, when they come in contact with the given object or situation, they act in the way in which their makeup predisposes them.

This analysis of the genesis of marihuana use shows that the individuals who come in contact with a given object may respond to it at first in a great variety of ways. If a stable form of new behavior toward the object is to emerge, a transformation of meanings must occur, in which the person develops a new conception of the nature of the object. [12] This happens in a series of communicative acts in which others point out new aspects of his experience to him, present him with new interpretations of events, and help him achieve a new conceptual organization of his world, without which the new behavior is not possible. Persons who do not achieve the proper kind of conceptualization are unable to engage in the given behavior and turn off in the direction of some other relationship to the object or activity.

This suggests that behavior of any kind might fruitfully be studied developmentally, in terms of changes in meanings and concepts, their organization and reorganization, and the way they channel behavior, making some acts possible while excluding others.

---

[11] Another paper will discuss the series of developments in attitude that occurs as the individual begins to take account of these matters and adjust his use to them.

[12] Cf. Anselm Strauss, "The Development and Transformation of Monetary Meanings in the Child," *American Sociological Review*, XVII (June, 1952), 275–86.

Sociocultural Theories

PATHOLOGICAL PATTERNS

Thomas Scheff's penetrating analysis of the more traditional notions of mental disorder sets the stage for a series of propositions concerning the role of cultural influences in maintaining diverse forms of "deviance." In this paper, Scheff argues for the view that sociological concepts such as residual deviance, conformity, and social control can account, in great measure, for the pathological behavior of patients and, particularly, their tendency to retain these behaviors in conventional institutional settings. Focusing on a more specific phase of hospital life, notably the inpatient experience, Erving Goffman portrays, in an insightful reportorial style, the web of direct, as well as subtle, influences that determine the patient's role and conception of himself.

45. The Role of the Mentally Ill and the Dynamics of Mental Disorder

THOMAS J. SCHEFF

Although the last two decades have seen a vast increase in the number of studies of functional mental disorder, there is as yet no substantial, verified body of knowledge in this area. A quotation from a recent symposium on schizophrenia summarizes the present situation:

During the past decade, the problems of chronic schizophrenia have claimed the energy of workers in many fields. Despite significant contributions which reflect continuing progress, *we have yet to learn to ask ourselves the right questions.*[1]

Many investigators apparently agree; systematic studies have not only failed to provide answers to the problem of causation, but there is considerable feeling that the problem itself has not been formulated correctly.

One frequently noted deficiency in psychiatric formulations of the problem is the failure to incorporate social processes into the dynamics of mental disorder. Although the importance of these processes is increasingly recognized by psychiatrists, the conceptual models used in formulating research questions are basically concerned with individual rather than social systems. Genetic, biochemical, and psychological investigations seek different causal agents, but utilize similar models: dynamic systems which are located within the individual. In these investigations, social processes tend to be relegated to a subsidiary role, because the model focuses attention on individual differences, rather than on the social system in which the individuals are involved.

Recently a number of writers have sought to develop an approach which would give more emphasis to social processes. Lemert, Erikson, Goffman, and Szasz have notably contributed to this approach.[2] Lemert, particularly, by rejecting the more conventional concern

From *Sociometry*, 1963, 26, 436–453. Reprinted by permission.

[1]Nathanial S. Apter, "Our Growing Restlessness with Problems of Chronic Schizophrenia," in Lawrence Appleby, *et al.*, *Chronic Schizophrenia*, Glencoe, Ill.: Free Press, 1958.

[2]Edwin M. Lemert, *Social Pathology*, New York: McGraw-Hill, 1951; Kai T. Erikson, "Patient Role and Social Uncertainty—A Dilemma of the Mentally Ill," *Psychiatry*, 20 (August, 1957), pp. 263–274; Erving Goffman, *Asylums*, New York: Doubleday-Anchor, 1961; Thomas S. Szasz, *The Myth of Mental Illness*, New York: Hoeber-Harper, 1961.

with the origins of mental deviance, and stressing instead the potential importance of the societal reaction in stabilizing deviance, focuses primarily on mechanisms of social control. The work of all of these authors suggests research avenues which are analytically separable from questions of individual systems and point, therefore, to a theory which would incorporate social processes.

The purpose of the present paper is to contribute to the formulation of such a theory by stating a set of nine propositions which make up basic assumptions for a social system model of mental disorder. This set is largely derived from the work of the authors listed above, all but two of the propositions (#4 and #5) bring suggested, with varying degrees of explicitness, in the cited references. By stating these propositions explicitly, this paper attempts to facilitate testing of basic assumptions, all of which are empirically unverified, or only partly verified. By stating these assumptions in terms of standard sociological concepts, this paper attempts to show the relevance to studies of mental disorder of findings from diverse areas of social science, such as race relations and prestige suggestion. This paper also delineates three problems which are crucial for a sociological theory of mental disorder: what are the conditions in a culture under which diverse kinds of deviance become stable and uniform; to what extent, in different phases of careers of mental patients, are symptoms of mental illness the result of conforming behavior; is there a general set of contingencies which lead to the definition of deviant behavior as a manifestation of mental illness? Finally, this paper attempts to formulate special conceptual tools to deal with these problems, which are directly linked to sociological theory. The social institution of insanity, residual deviance, the social role of the mentally ill, and the bifurcation of the societal reaction into the alternative reactions of denial and labeling, are examples of such conceptual tools.

These conceptual tools are utilized to construct a theory of mental disorder in which psychiatric symptoms are considered to be violations of social norms, and stable "mental illness" to be a social role. The validity of this theory depends upon verification of the nine propositions listed below in future studies, and should, therefore, be applied with caution, and with appreciation for its limitations. One such limitation is that the theory attempts to account for a much narrower class of phenomena than is usually found under the rubric of mental disorder; the discussion that follows will be focused exclusively on stable or recurring mental disorder, and does not explain the causes of single deviant episodes. A second major limitation is that the theory probably distorts the phenomena under discussion. Just as the individual system models under-stress social processes, the model presented here probably exaggerates their importance. The social system model "holds constant" individual differences, in order to articulate the relationship between society and mental disorder. Ultimately, a framework which encompassed both individual and social systems would be desirable. Given the present state of knowledge, however, this framework may prove useful by providing an explicit contrast to the more conventional medical and psychological approaches, and thus assisting in the formulation of sociological studies of mental disorder.

THE SYMPTOMS OF "MENTAL ILLNESS" AS RESIDUALLY DEVIANT BEHAVIOR

One source of immediate embarrassment to any social theory of "mental illness" is that the terms used in referring to these phenomena in our society prejudge the issue. The medical metaphor "mental illness" suggests a determinate process which occurs within the individual: the unfolding and development of disease. It is convenient, therefore, to drop terms derived from the disease metaphor in favor of a standard sociological concept, deviant behavior, which signifies behavior that violates a social norm in a given society.

If the symptoms of mental illness are to be construed as violations of social norms, it is necessary to specify the type of norms involved. Most norm violations do not cause the violator to be labeled as mentally ill, but as ill-mannered, ignorant, sinful, criminal, or perhaps just harried, depending on the type of norm involved. There are innumerable norms, however, over which consensus is so complete that the members of a group appear to take them for granted. A host of such norms surround even the simplest conversation: a person engaged in conversation is expected to face toward his partner, rather than directly away from him; if his gaze is toward the partner, he is expected to look toward his eyes, rather than, say, toward his forehead; to stand at a proper conversational distance, neither one inch away nor across the room, and so on. A person who regularly violated these expectations probably would not be thought to be merely ill-bred, but as strange, bizarre, and frightening, because his behavior violates the assumptive world of the group, the world that is construed to be the only one that is natural, decent, and possible.

The culture of the group provides a vocabulary of terms for categorizing many norm violations: crime, perversion, drunkenness, and bad manners are familiar examples. Each of these terms is derived from the type of norm broken, and ultimately, from the type of behavior involved. After exhausting these categories, however, there is always a residue of the most diverse kinds of violations, for which the culture provides no explicit label. For example, although there is great cultural variation in what is defined as decent or real, each culture tends to reify its definition of decency and reality, and so provide no way of handling violations of its expectations in these areas. The typical norm governing decency or reality, therefore, literally "goes without saying" and its violation is unthinkable for most of its members. For the convenience of the society in construing those instances of unnamable deviance which are called to its attention, these violations may be lumped together into a residual category: witchcraft, spirit possession, or, in our own society, mental illness. In this paper, the diverse kinds of deviation for which our society provides no explicit label, and which, therefore, sometimes lead to the labeling of the violator as mentally ill, will be considered to be technically *residual deviance*.

THE ORIGINS, PREVALENCE AND COURSE OF RESIDUAL DEVIANCE

The first proposition concerns the origins of residual deviance. *1. Residual deviance arises from fundamentally diverse sources*. It has been demonstrated that some types of mental disorder are the result of organic causes. It appears likely, therefore, that there are genetic, biochemical or physiological origins for residual deviance. It also appears that residual deviance can arise from individual psychological peculiarities and from differences in upbringing and training. Residual deviance can also probably be produced by various kinds of external stress: the sustained fear and hardship of combat, and deprivation of food, sleep, and even sensory experience.[3] Residual deviance, finally, can be a volitional act of innovation or defiance. The kinds of behavior deemed typical of mental illness, such as hallucinations, delusions, depression, and mania, can all arise from these diverse sources.

The second proposition concerns the prevalence of residual deviance which is analogous to the "total" or "true" prevalence of mental disorder (in contrast to the "treated" prevalence). *2. Relative to the rate of treated mental illness, the rate of unrecorded residual deviance is extremely high*. There is evidence that grossly deviant behavior is often not noticed or, if it is noticed, it is rationalized as eccentricity. Apparently, many persons who are extremely withdrawn, or who "fly off the handle" for extended periods of time, who imagine fantastic events, or who hear voices or see visions, are not labeled as insane either by themselves or others.[4] Their deviance, rather, is unrecognized, ignored, or rationalized. This pattern of inattention and rationalization will be called "denial."[5]

In addition to the kind of evidence cited above there are a number of epidemiological studies of total prevalence. There are numerous problems in interpreting the results of these studies; the major difficulty is that the definition

---

[3]Philip Solomon, *et al.* (eds.), *Sensory Deprivation*, Cambridge: Harvard, 1961; E. L. Bliss, *et al.*, "Studies of Sleep Deprivation—Relationship to Schizophrenia," *A.M.A. Archives of Neurology and Psychiatry, 81* (March, 1959), 348–359.

[4]See, for example, John A. Clausen and Marian R. Yarrow, "Paths to the Mental Hospital," *Journal of Social Issues, 11* (December, 1955), pp. 25–32; August B. Hollingshead and Frederick C. Redlich, *Social Class and Mental Illness*, New York: Wiley, 1958, pp. 172–176; and Elaine Cumming and John Cumming, *Closed Ranks*, Cambridge: Harvard, 1957, pp. 92–103.

[5]The term "denial" is used in the same sense as in Cumming and Cumming, *ibid.*, Chap. VII.

of mental disorder is different in each study, as are the methods used to screen cases. These studies represent, however, the best available information and can be used to estimate total prevalence.

A convenient summary of findings is presented in Plunkett and Gordon.[6] This source compares the methods and populations used in eleven field studies, and lists rates of total prevalence (in percentages) as 1.7, 3.6, 4.5, 4.7, 5.3, 6.1, 10.9, 13.8, 23.2, 23.3, and 33.3.

How do these total rates compare with the rates of treated mental disorder? One of the studies cited by Plunkett and Gordon, the Baltimore study reported by Pasamanick, is useful in this regard since it includes both treated and untreated rates.[7] As compared with the untreated rate of 10.9 per cent, the rate of treatment in state, VA, and private hospitals of Baltimore residents was .5 per cent.[8] That is for every mental patient there were approximately 20 untreated cases located by the survey. It is possible that the treated rate is too low, however, since patients treated by private physicians were not included. Judging from another study, the New Haven study of treated prevalence, the number of patients treated in private practice is small compared to those hospitalized: over 70 per cent of the patient located in that study were hospitalized even though extensive case-finding techniques were employed. The over-all treated prevalence in the New Haven study was reported as .8 per cent, which is in good agreement with my estimate of .7 per cent for the Baltimore study.[9] If we accept .8 per cent as an estimate of the upper limit of treated prevalence for the Pasamanick study, the ratio of treated to untreated cases is 1/14. That is, for every treated patient we should expect to find 14 untreated cases in the community.

One interpretation of this finding is that the untreated patients in the community represent those cases with less severe disorders, while those patients with severe impairments all fall into the treated group. Some of the findings in the Pasamanick study point in this direction. Of the untreated patients, about half are classified as psychoneurotic. Of the psychoneurotics, in turn, about half again are classified as suffering from minimal impairment. At least a fourth of the untreated group, then, involved very mild disorders.[10]

The evidence from the group diagnosed as psychotic does not support this interpretation, however. Almost all of the cases diagnosed as psychotic were judged to involve severe impairment, yet half of the diagnoses of psychosis occurred in the untreated group. In other words, according to this study there were as many untreated as treated cases of psychoses.[11]

On the basis of the high total prevalence rates cited above and other evidence, it seems plausible that residual deviant behavior is usually transitory, which is the substance of the third proposition. *3. Most residual deviance is "denied" and is transitory.* The high rates of total prevalence suggest that most residual deviancy is unrecognized or rationalized away. For this type of deviance, which is amorphous and uncrystallized, Lemert uses the term "primary deviation."[12] Balint describes similar behavior as "the unorganized phase of illness."[13] Although Balint assumes that patients in this phase ultimately "settle down" to an "organized illness," other outcomes are possible. A person in this stage may "organize" his deviance in other than illness terms, e.g., as eccentricity or genius, or the deviant acts may terminate when situational stress is removed.

The experience of battlefield psychiatrists can be interpreted to support the hypothesis that residual deviance is usually transitory. Glass reports that combat neurosis is often self-terminating if the soldier is kept with his unit and given only the most superficial medical attention.[14]

[6]Richard J. Plunkett and John E. Gordon, *Epidemiology and Mental Illness*, New York: Basic Books, 1960.
[7]Benjamin Pasamanick, "A Survey of Mental Disease in an Urban Population, IV, An Approach to Total Prevalence Rates," *Archives of General Psychiatry*, 5 (August, 1961), pp. 151–155.
[8]*Ibid.,* p. 153.
[9]Hollingshead and Redlich, *op. cit.,* p. 199.

[10]Pasamanick, *op. cit.,* pp. 153–154.
[11]*Ibid.*
[12]Lemert, *op. cit.,* Chap. 4.
[13]Michael Balint, *The Doctor, His Patient, and the Illness*, New York: International Universities Press, 1957, p. 18.
[14]Albert J. Glass, "Psychotherapy in the Combat Zone," in *Symposium on Stress*, Washington, D.C.: Army Medical Service Graduate School, 1953. Cf. Abraham Kardiner and H. Spiegel, *War Stress and Neurotic Illness*, New York: Hoeber, 1947, Chaps. III–IV.

Descriptions of child behavior can be interpreted in the same way. According to these reports, most children go through periods in which at least several of the following kinds of deviance may occur; temper tantrums, head banging, scratching, pinching, biting, fantasy playmates or pets, illusory physical complaints, and fears of sounds, shapes, colors, persons, animals, darkness, weather, ghosts, and so on.[15] In the vast majority of instances, however, these behavior patterns do not become stable.

If residual deviance is highly prevalent among ostensibly "normal" persons and is usually transitory, as suggested by the last two propositions, what accounts for the small percentage of residual deviants who go on to deviant careers? To put the question another way, under what conditions is residual deviance stabilized? The conventional hypothesis is that the answer lies in the deviant himself. The hypothesis suggested here is that the most important single factor (but not the only factor) in the stabilization of residual deviance is the societal reaction. Residual deviance may be stabilized if it is defined to be evidence of mental illness, and/or the deviant is placed in a deviant status, and begins to play the role of the mentally ill. In order to avoid the implication that mental disorder is merely role-playing and pretence, it is first necessary to discuss the social institution of insanity.

SOCIAL CONTROL: INDIVIDUAL AND SOCIAL SYSTEMS OF BEHAVIOR

In *The Myth of Mental Illness,* Szasz proposes that mental disorder be viewed within the framework of "the game-playing model of human behavior." He than describes hysteria, schizophrenia, and other mental disorders as the "impersonation" of sick persons by those whose "real" problem concerns "problems of living." Although Szasz states that role-playing by mental patients may not be completely or even mostly voluntary, the implication is that mental disorder be viewed as a strategy chosen by the individual as a way of obtaining help from others. Thus, the term "impersonation" suggests calculated and deliberate shamming by the patient. In his comparisons of hysteria, malingering, and cheating, although he notes differences between these behavior patterns, he suggests that these differences may be mostly a matter of whose point of view is taken in describing the behavior.

The present paper also uses the role-playing model to analyze mental disorder, but places more emphasis on the involuntary aspects of role-playing than Szasz, who tends to treat role-playing as an individual system of behavior. In many social psychological discussions, however, role-playing is considered as a part of a social system. The individual plays his role by articulating his behavior with the cues and actions of other persons involved in the transaction. The proper performance of a role is dependent on having a cooperative audience. This proposition may also be reversed: having an audience which acts toward the individual in a uniform way may lead the actor to play the expected role even if he is not particularly interested in doing so. The "baby of the family" may come to find this role obnoxious, but the uniform pattern of cues and actions which confronts him in the family may lock in with his own vocabulary of responses so that it is inconvenient and difficult for him not to play the part expected of him. To the degree that alternative roles are closed off, the proffered role may come to be the only way the individual can cope with the situation.

One of Szasz's very apt formulations touches upon the social systemic aspects of role-playing. He draws an analogy between the role of the mentally ill and the "type-casting" of actors.[16] Some actors get a reputation for playing one type of role, and find it difficult to obtain other roles. Although they may be displeased, they may also come to incorporate aspects of the type-cast role into their self-conceptions, and ultimately into their behavior. Findings in several social psychological studies suggest that an individual's role behavior may be shaped

---

[15]Frances L. Ilg and Louise B. Ames, *Child Behavior,* New York: Dell, 1960, pp. 138–188.

[16]Szasz, *op. cit.,* p. 252. For discussion of type-casting see Orrin E. Klapp, *Heroes, Villains and Fools,* Englewood Cliffs, New Jersey: Prentice-Hall, 1962, pp. 5–8 and *passim.*

by the kinds of "deference" that he regularly receives from others.[17]

One aspect of the voluntariness of role-playing is the extent to which the actor believes in the part he is playing. Although a role may be played cynically, with no belief, or completely sincerely, with whole-hearted belief, many roles are played on the basis of an intricate mixture of belief and disbelief. During the course of a study of a large public mental hospital, several patients told the author in confidence about their cynical use of their symptoms—to frighten new personnel, to escape from unpleasant work details, and so on. Yet these *same* patients, at other times, appear to have been sincere in their symptomatic behavior. Apparently it was sometimes difficult for them to tell whether they were playing the role or the role was playing them. Certain types of symptomatology are quite interesting in this connection. In simulation of previous psychotic states, and in the behavior pattern known to psychiatrists as the Ganser syndrome, it is apparently almost impossible for the observer to separate feigning of symptoms from involuntary acts with any degree of certainty.[18] In accordance with what has been said so far, the difficulty is probably that the patient is just as confused by his own behavior as is the observer.

This discussion suggests that a stable role performance may arise when the actor's role imagery locks in with the type of "deference" which he regularly receives. An extreme example of this process may be taken from anthropological and medical reports concerning the "dead role," as in deaths attributed to "bone-pointing." Death from bone-pointing appears to arise from the conjunction of two fundamental processes which characterize all social behavior. First, all individuals continually orient themselves by means of responses which are perceived in social interaction: the individual's identity and continuity of experience are dependent on these cues.[19] Secondly, the individual has his own vocabulary of expectations, which may in a particular situation either agree with or be in conflict with the sanctions to which he is exposed. Entry into a role may be complete when this role is part of the individual's expectations, and when these expectations are reaffirmed in social interaction. In the following pages this principle will be applied to the problem of the causation of mental disorder.

What are the beliefs and practices that constitute the social institution of insanity?[20] And how do they figure in the development of mental disorder? Two propositions concerning beliefs about mental disorder in the general public will now be considered.

4. Stereotyped imagery of mental disorder is learned in early childhood. Although there are no substantiating

---

[17]Cf. Zena S. Blau, "Changes in Status and Age Identification," *American Sociological Review, 21* (April, 1956), pp. 198–203; James Benjamins, "Changes in Performance in Relation to Influences upon Self-Conceptualization," *Journal of Abnormal and Social Psychology, 45* (July, 1950), pp. 473–480; Albert Ellis, "The Sexual Psychology of Human Hermaphrodites," *Psychosomatic Medicine, 7* (March, 1945), pp. 108–125; S. Liberman, "The Effect of Changes in Roles on the Attitudes of Role Occupants," *Human Relations, 9* (1956), pp. 385–402. For a review of experimental evidence, see John H. Mann, "Experimental Evaluations of Role Playing," *Psychological Bulletin, 53* (May, 1956), pp. 227–234. For an interesting demonstration of the inter-relations between the symptoms of patients on the same ward, see Sheppard G. Kellam and J. B. Chassan, "Social Context and Symptom Fluctuation," *Psychiatry, 25* (November, 1962), pp. 370–381.

[18]Leo Sadow and Alvin Suslick, "Simulation of a Previous Psychotic State," *A.M.A. Archives of General Psychiatry, 4* (May, 1961), pp. 452–458.

[19]Generalizing from experimental findings, Blake and Mouton make this statement about the process of conformity, resistance to influence, and conversion to a new role:

. . . an individual requires a stable framework, including salient and firm reference points, in order to orient himself and to regulate his interactions with others. This framework consists of external and internal anchorages available to the individual whether he is aware of them or not. With an acceptable framework he can resist giving or accepting information that is inconsistent with that framework or that requires him to relinquish it. In the absence of a stable framework he actively seeks to establish one through his own strivings by making use of significant and relevant information provided within the context of interaction. *By controlling the amount and kind of information available for orientation, he can be led to embrace conforming attitudes which are entirely foreign to his earlier ways of thinking.*

Robert R. Blake and Jane S. Mouton, "Conformity, Resistance and Conversion," in *Conformity and Deviation,* Irwin A. Berg and Bernard M. Bass (eds.), New York: Harper, 1961, pp. 1–2. For a recent and striking demonstration of the effect on social communication in defining internal stimuli, see Stanley Schachter and Jerome E. Singer, "Cognitive, Social, and Physiological Determinants of Emotional State," *Psychological Review, 69* (September, 1962), pp. 379–399.

[20]The Cummings describe the social institution of insanity (the "patterned response" to deviance) in terms of denial, isolation, and insulation. Cumming and Cumming, *loc. cit.*

studies in this area, scattered observations lead the author to conclude that children learn a considerable amount of imagery concerning deviance very early, and that much of the imagery comes from their peers rather than from adults. The literal meaning of "crazy," a term now used in a wide variety of contexts, is probably grasped by children during the first years of elementary school. Since adults are often vague and evasive in their responses to questions in this area, an aura of mystery surrounds it. In this socialization the grossest stereotypes which are heir to childhood fears, e.g., of the "boogie man," survive. These conclusions are quite speculative, of course, and need to be investigated systematically, possibly with techniques similar to those used in studies of the early learning of racial stereotypes.

Assuming, however, that this hypothesis is sound, what effect does early learning have on the shared conceptions of insanity held in the community? There is much fallacious material learned in early childhood which is later discarded when more adequate information replaces it. This question leads to hypothesis No. 5. 5. *The stereotypes of insanity are continually reaffirmed, inadvertently, in ordinary social interaction.*

Although many adults become acquainted with medical concepts of mental illness, the traditional stereotypes are not discarded, but continue to exist alongside the medical conceptions, because the stereotypes receive almost continual support from the mass media and in ordinary social discourse. In newspapers, it is a common practice to mention that a rapist or a murderer was once a mental patient. This negative information, however, is seldom offset by positive reports. An item like the following is almost inconceivable:

Mrs. Ralph Jones, an ex-mental patient, was elected president of the Fairview Home and Garden Society in their meeting last Thursday.

Because of highly biased reporting, the reader is free to make the unwarranted inference that murder and rape occur more frequently among ex-mental patients than among the population at large. Actually, it has been demonstrated that the incidence of crimes of violence, or of any crime, is much lower among ex-mental patients than among the general population.[21] Yet, this is not the picture presented to the public.

Reaffirmation of the stereotype of insanity occurs not only in the mass media, but also in ordinary conversation, in jokes, anecdotes, and even in conventional phrases. Such phrases as "Are you crazy?", or "It would be a madhouse," "It's driving me out of my mind," or "It's driving me distracted," and hundreds of others occur frequently in informal conversations. In this usage insanity itself is seldom the topic of conversation; the phrases are so much a part of ordinary language that only the person who considers each word carefully can eliminate them from his speech. Through verbal usages the stereotypes of insanity are a relatively permanent part of the social structure.

In a recent study Nunnally demonstrated that reaffirmation of stereotypes occurs in the mass media. In a systematic and extensive content analysis of television, radio, newspapers and magazines, including "confession" magazines, they found an image of mental disorder presented which was overwhelmingly stereotyped.

. . . media presentations emphasized the bizarre symptoms of the mentally ill. For example, information relating to Factor I (the conception that mentally ill persons look and act different from "normal" people) was recorded 89 times. Of these, 88 affirmed the factor, that is, indicated or suggested that people with mental-health problems "look and act different": only one item denied Factor I. In television dramas, for example, the afflicted person often enters the scene staring glassy-eyed, with his mouth widely ajar, mumbling incoherent phrases or laughing uncontrollably. Even in what would be considered the milder disorders, neurotic phobias and obsessions, the afflicted person is presented as having bizarre facial expressions and actions.[22]

DENIAL AND LABELING

According to the analysis presented here, the traditional stereotypes of mental

[21]Henry Brill and Benjamin Malzberg, "Statistical Report Based on the Arrest Record of 5354 Male Ex-patients Released from New York State Mental Hospitals During the Period 1946-48," mimeographed document available from the authors; L. H. Cohen and H. Freeman, "How Dangerous to the Community are State Hospital Patients?", *Connecticut State Medical Journal*, 9 (September, 1945), pp. 697–701.
[22]Jum C. Nunnally, Jr., *Popular Conceptions of Mental Health*, New York: Holt, Rinehart and Winston, 1961, p. 74.

disorder are solidly entrenched in the population because they are learned early in childhood and are continuously reaffirmed in the mass media and in everyday conversation. How do these beliefs function in the processes leading to mental disorder? This question will be considered by first referring to the earlier discussion of the societal reaction to residual deviance.

It was stated that the usual reaction to residual deviance is denial, and that in these cases most residual deviance is transitory. The societal reaction to deviance is not always denial, however. In a small proportion of cases the reaction goes the other way, exaggerating and at times distorting the extent and degree of deviation. This pattern of exaggeration, which we will call "labeling," has been noted by Garfinkel in his discussion of the "degradation" of officially recognized criminals.[23] Goffman makes a similar point in his description of the "discrediting" of mental patients.[24] Apparently under some conditions the societal reaction to deviance is to seek out signs of abnormality in the deviant's history to show that he was always essentially a deviant.

The contrasting social reactions of denial and labeling provide a means of answering two fundamental questions. If deviance arises from diverse sources —physical, psychological, and situational—how does the uniformity of behavior that is associated with insanity develop? Secondly, if deviance is usually transitory, how does it become stabilized in those patients who became chronically deviant? To summarize, what are the sources of uniformity and stability of deviant behavior?

In the approach taken here the answer to this question is based on hypotheses Nos. 4 and 5, that the role imagery of insanity is learned early in childhood, and is reaffirmed in social interaction. In a crisis, when the deviance of an individual becomes a public issue, the traditional stereotype of insanity becomes the guiding imagery for action, both for those reacting to the deviant and, at times, for the deviant himself. When societal agents and persons around the deviant

react to him uniformly in terms of the traditional stereotypes of insanity, his amorphous and unstructured deviant behavior tends to crystallize in conformity to these expectations, thus becoming similar to the behavior of other deviants classified as mentally ill, and stable over time. The process of becoming uniform and stable is completed when the traditional imagery becomes a part of the deviant's orientation for guiding his own behavior.

The idea that cultural stereotypes may stabilize primary deviance, and tend to produce uniformity in symptoms, is supported by cross-cultural studies of mental disorder. Although some observers insist there are underlying similarities, most agree that there are enormous differences in the manifest symptoms of stable mental disorder *between* societies, and great similarity *within* societies.[25]

These considerations suggest that the labeling process is a crucial contingency in most careers of residual deviance. Thus Glass, who observed that neuropsychiatric casualties may not become mentally ill if they are kept with their unit, goes on to say that military experience with psychotherapy has been disappointing. Soldiers who are removed from their unit to a hospital, he states, often go on to become chronically impaired.[26] That is, their deviance is stabilized by the labeling process, which is implicit in their removal and hospitalization. A similar interpretation can be made by comparing the observations of childhood disorders among Mexican-Americans with those of "Anglo" children. Childhood disorders such as *susto* (an illness believed to result from fright) sometimes have damaging outcomes in Mexican-American children.[27] Yet the deviant behavior involved is very similar to that which seems to have high incidence among Anglo children, with permanent impairment virtually never occurring. Apparently through cues from his elders the Mexican-American child, behaving initially much like his Anglo counterpart, learns to enter the

[23]Harold Garfinkel, "Conditions of Successful Degradation Ceremonies," *American Journal of Sociology, 61* (March, 1956), pp. 420–424.

[24]Goffman, "The Moral Career of the Mental Patient," in *Asylums, op. cit.,* pp. 125–171.

[25]P. M. Yap, "Mental Diseases Peculiar to Certain Cultures: A Survey of Comparative Psychiatry," *Journal of Mental Science, 97* (April, 1951), pp. 313–327; Paul E. Benedict and Irving Jacks, "Mental Illness in Primitive Societies," *Psychiatry, 17* (November, 1954), pp. 377–389.

[26]Glass, *op. cit.*

[27]Lyle Saunders, *Cultural Differences and Medical Care,* New York: Russell Sage, 1954, p. 142.

sick role, at times with serious consequences.[28]

ACCEPTANCE OF THE DEVIANT ROLE

From this point of view, then, most mental disorder can be considered to be a social role. This social role complements and reflects the status of the insane in the social structure. It is through the social processes which maintain the status of the insane that the varied deviances from which mental disorder arises are made uniform and stable. The stabilization and uniformization of residual deviance are completed when the deviant accepts the role of the insane as the framework within which he organizes his own behavior. Three hypotheses are stated below which suggest some of the processes which cause the deviant to accept such a stigmatized role.

6. *Labeled deviants may be rewarded for playing the stereotyped deviant role.* Ordinarily patients who display "insight" are rewarded by psychiatrists and other personnel. That is, patients who manage to find evidence of "their illness" in their past and present behavior, confirming the medical and societal diagnosis, receive benefits. This pattern of behavior is a special case of a more general pattern that has been called the "apostolic function" by Balint, in which the physician and others inadvertently cause the patient to display symptoms of the illness the physician thinks the patient has.[29] Not only physicians but other hospital personnel and even other patients, reward the deviant for conforming to the stereotypes.[30]

7. *Labeled deviants are punished when they attempt the return to conventional roles.* The second process operative is the systematic blockage of entry to nondeviant roles once the label has been publicly applied. Thus the ex-mental patient, although he is urged to rehabilitate himself in the community, usually finds himself discriminated against in seeking to return to his old status, and on trying to find a new one in the occupational, marital, social, and other spheres.[31] Thus, to a degree, the labeled deviant is rewarded for deviating, and punished for attempting to conform.

8. *In the crisis occurring when a primary deviant is publicly labeled, the deviant is highly suggestible, and may accept the proffered role of the insane as the only alternative.* When gross deviancy is publicly recognized and made an issue, the primary deviant may be profoundly confused, anxious, and ashamed. In this crisis it seems reasonable to assume that the deviant will be suggestible to the cues that he gets from the reactions of others toward him.[32] But those around him are also in a crisis; the incomprehensible nature of the deviance, and the seeming need for immediate action lead them to take collective action against the deviant on the basis of the attitude which all share—the traditional stereotypes of insanity. The deviant is sensitive to the cues provided by these others and begins to think of himself in terms of the stereotyped role of insanity, which is part of his own role vocabulary also, since he, like those reacting to him, learned it early in childhood. In this situation his behavior may begin to follow the pattern suggested by his own stereotypes and the reactions of others. That is, when a primary deviant organizes his behavior within the framework of mental disorder, and when his organization is validated by others, particularly prestigeful others such as physicians, he is "hooked" and will proceed on a career of chronic deviance.

The role of suggestion is noted by Warner in his description of bone-pointing magic:

The effect of (the suggestion of the entire community on the victim) is obviously drastic. An analogous situation in our society is hard to imagine. If all a man's near kin, his father,

[28]For discussion, with many illustrative cases, of the process in which persons play the "dead role" and subsequently die, see Charles C. Herbert, "Life-influencing Interactions," in *The Physiology of Emotions,* Alexander Simon, *et al.,* eds., New York: Charles C Thomas, 1961.

[29]Balint, *op. cit.,* pp. 215–239. Cf. Thomas J. Scheff, "Decision Rules, Types of Error and Their Consequences in Medical Diagnosis," *Behavioral Science, 8* (April, 1963), pp. 97–107.

[30]William Caudill, F. C. Redlich, H. R. Gilmore, and E. B. Brody, "Social Structure and the Interaction Processes on a Psychiatric Ward," *American Journal of Orthopsychiatry, 22* (April, 1952), pp. 314–334.

[31]Lemert, *op. cit.,* provides an extensive discussion of this process under the heading of "Limitation of Participation," pp. 434–440.

[32]This proposition receives support from Erikson's observations: Kai T. Erikson, *loc. cit.*

mother, brothers and sisters, wife, children, business associates, friends and all the other members of the society, should suddenly withdraw themselves because of some dramatic circumstance, refusing to take any attitude but one of taboo . . . and then perform over him a sacred ceremony . . . the enormous suggestive power of this movement . . . of the community after it has had its attitudes (toward the victim) crystallized can be somewhat understood by ourselves.[33]

If we substitute for black magic the taboo that usually accompanies mental disorder, and consider a commitment proceeding or even mental hospital admission as a sacred ceremony, the similarity between Warner's description and the typical events in the development of mental disorder is considerable.

The last three propositions suggest that once a person has been placed in a deviant status there are rewards for conforming to the deviant role, and punishments for not conforming to the deviant role. This is not to imply, however, that the symptomatic behavior of persons occupying a deviant status is always a manifestation of conforming behavior. To explain this point, some discussion of the process of self-control in "normals" is necessary.

In a recent discussion of the process of self-control, Shibutani notes that self-control is not automatic, but is an intricate and delicately balanced process, sustainable only under propitious circumstances.[34] He points out that fatigue, the reaction to narcotics, excessive excitement or tension (such as is generated in mobs), or a number of other conditions interfere with self-control; conversely, conditions which produce normal bodily states, and deliberative processes such as symbolization and imaginative rehearsal before action, facilitate it.

One might argue that a crucially important aspect of imaginative rehearsal is the image of himself that the actor projects into his future action. Certainly in American society, the cultural image of the "normal" adult is that of a person endowed with self-control ("will-power," "backbone," "strength of character," etc.). For the person who sees himself as

endowed with the trait of self-control, self-control is facilitated, since he can imagine himself enduring stress during his imaginative rehearsal, and also while under actual stress.

For a person who has acquired an image of himself as lacking the ability to control his own actions, the process of self-control is likely to break down under stress. Such a person may feel that he has reached his "breaking-point" under circumstances which would be endured by a person with a "normal" self-conception. This is to say, a greater lack of self-control than can be explained by stress tends to appear in those roles for which the culture transmits imagery which emphasizes lack of self-control. In American society such imagery is transmitted for the roles of the very young and very old, drunkards and drug addicts, gamblers, and the mentally ill.

Thus, the social role of the mentally ill has a different significance at different phases of residual deviance. When labeling first occurs, it merely gives a name to primary deviation which has other roots. When (and if) the primary deviance becomes an issue, and is not ignored or rationalized away, labeling may create a social type, a pattern of "symptomatic" behavior in conformity with the stereotyped expectations of others. Finally, to the extent that the deviant role becomes a part of the deviant's self-conception, his ability to control his own behavior may be impaired under stress, resulting in episodes of compulsive behavior.

The preceding eight hypotheses form the basis for the final causal hypothesis. *9. Among residual deviants, labeling is the single most important cause of careers of residual deviance.* This hypothesis assumes that most residual deviance, if it does not become the basis for entry into the sick role, will not lead to a deviant career. Most deviant careers, according to this point of view, arise out of career contingencies, and are therefore not directly connected with the origins of the initial deviance.[35] Although there are a wide var-

[33]W. Lloyd Warner, *A Black Civilization,* rev. ed., New York: Harper, 1958, p. 242.

[34]T. Shibutani, *Society and Personality,* Englewood Cliffs, N.J.: Prentice-Hall, 1961, Chapter 6, "Consciousness and Voluntary Conduct."

[35]It should be noted, however, that these contingencies are causal only because they become part of a dynamic system: the reciprocal and cumulative inter-relation between the deviant's behavior and the societal reaction. For example, the more the deviant enters the role of the mentally ill, the more he is defined by others as mentally ill; but the more he is

iety of contingencies which lead to labeling rather than denial, these contingencies can be usefully classified in terms of the nature of the deviant behavior, the person who commits the deviant acts, and the community in which the deviance occurs. Other things being equal, the severity of the societal reaction to deviance is a function of, first, the degree, amount, and visibility of the deviant behavior, second, the power of the deviant, and the social distance between the deviant and the agents of social control; and finally, the tolerance level of the community, and the availability in the culture of the community of alternative nondeviant roles.[36] Particularly crucial for future research is the importance of the first two contingencies (the amount and degree of deviance), which are characteristics of the deviant, relative to the remaining five contingencies, which are characteristics of the social system.[37] To the extent that these five factors are found empirically to be independent determinants of labeling and denial, the status of the mental patient can be considered a partly ascribed rather than a completely achieved status. The dynamics of treated mental illness could then be profitably studied quite apart from the individual dynamics of mental disorder.

CONCLUSION

This paper has presented a sociological theory of the causation of stable mental disorder. Since the evidence advanced in support of the theory was scattered and fragmentary, it can only be suggested as a stimulus to further discussion and research. Among the areas pointed out for further investigation are field studies of the prevalence and duration of residual deviance; investigations of stereotypes of mental disorder in children, the mass media, and adult conversations; studies of the rewarding of steretyped deviation, blockage of return to conventional roles, and of the suggestibility of primary deviants in crises. The final causal hypothesis suggests studies of the conditions under which denial and labeling of residual deviation occur. The variables which might effect the social reaction concern the nature of the deviance, the deviant himself, and the community in which the deviation occurs. Although many of the hypotheses suggested are largely unverified, they suggest avenues for investigating mental disorder different than those that are usually followed, and the rudiments of a general theory of deviant behavior.

---

defined as mentally ill, the more fully he enters the role, and so on. By representing this theory in the form of a flow chart, Walter Buckley pointed out that there are numerous such feedback loops implied here. For an explicit treatment of feedback, see Edwin M. Lemert, "Paranoia and the Dynamics of Exclusion," *Sociometry, 25* (March, 1962), pp. 2–20.

[36]*Cf.* Lemert, *op. cit.,* pp. 51–53, 55–68; Goffman, "The Moral Career of the Mental Patient," in *Asylums, op. cit.,* pp. 134–135; David Mechanic, "Some Factors in Identifying and Defining Mental Illness," *Mental Hygiene, 46* (January, 1962), pp. 66–74; for a list of similar factors in the reaction to physical illness, see Earl L. Koos, *The Health of Regionville,* New York: Columbia University Press, 1954, pp. 30–38.

[37]*Cf.* Thomas J. Scheff, "Psychiatric and Social Contingencies in the Release of Mental Patients in a Midwestern State," forthcoming; Simon Dinitz, Mark Lefton, Shirley Angrist, and Benjamin Pasamanick, "Psychiatric and Social Attributes as Predictors of Case Outcome in Mental Hospitalization," *Social Problems, 8* (Spring, 1961), pp. 322–328.

46.　The Inmate World

ERVING GOFFMAN

It is characteristic of inmates that they come to the institution as members, already full-fledged, of a *home world,* that is, a way of life and a round of activities taken for granted up to the point of admission to the institution.[1] It is useful to look at this culture that the recruit brings with him to the institution's door—his *presenting culture*, to modify a psychiatric phrase—in terms especially designed to highlight what it is the total institution will do to him. Whatever the stability of his personal organization, we can assume it was part of a wider supporting framework lodged in his current social environment, a round of experience that somewhat confirms a conception of self that is somewhat acceptable to him and a set of defensive maneuvers exercisable at his own discretion as a means of coping with conflicts, discreditings and failures.

Now it appears that total institutions do not substitute their own unique culture for something already formed. We do not deal with acculturation or assimilation but with something more restricted than these. In a sense, total institutions do not look for cultural victory. They effectively create and sustain a particular kind of tension between the home world and the institutional world and use this persistent tension as strategic leverage in the management of men. The full meaning for the inmate of being "in" or "on the inside" does not exist apart from the special meaning to him of "getting out" or "getting on the outside."

The recruit comes into the institution with a self and with attachments to supports which had allowed this self to survive. Upon entrance, he is immediately stripped of his wonted supports, and his self is systematically, if often unintentionally, mortified. In the accurate language of some of our oldest total institutions, he is led into a series of abasements, degradations, humiliations, and profanations of self. He begins, in other words, some radical shifts in his *moral career,* a career laying out the progressive changes that occur in the beliefs that he has concerning himself and significant others.

In total institutions there will also be a system of what might be called *secondary adjustments,* namely, technics which do not directly challenge staff management but which allow inmates to obtain disallowed satisfactions or allowed ones by disallowed means. These practices are variously referred to as: the angles, knowing the ropes, conniving, gimmicks, deals, ins, etc. Such adaptations apparently reach their finest flower in prisons, but of course other total institutions are overrun with them too.[2] It seems apparent that an important aspect of secondary adjustments is that they provide the inmate with some evidence that he is still, as it were, his own man and still has some protective distance, under his own control, between himself and the institution. In some cases, then, a secondary adjustment becomes almost a kind of lodgment for the self, a churinga in which the soul is felt to reside.[3]

The occurrence of secondary adjustments correctly allows us to assume that the inmate group will have some kind of a *code* and some means of informal social control evolved to prevent one inmate from informing staff about the secondary adjustments of another. On the same grounds we can expect that one dimension of social typing among inmates will turn upon this question of security, leading to persons defined as "squealers," "finks," or "stoolies" on one hand, and persons

---

Excerpted from "Characteristics of Total Institutions: Introduction," *Symposium on Preventive and Social Psychiatry,* U.S. Government Printing Office, 1958, pp. 43–49.

[1] There is reason then to exclude orphanages and foundling homes from the list of total institutions, except insofar as the orphan comes to be socialized into the outside world by some process of cultural osmosis, even while this world is being systematically denied him.

[2] See, for example, Norman S. Hayner and Ellis Ash, "The Prisoner Community as a Social Group," *American Sociological Review,* Vol. 4, 1939, p. 364 ff. under "Conniving Processes;" also, Morris G. Caldwell, "Group Dynamics in the Prison Community," *Journal of Criminal Law,* Criminology and Police Science, Vol. 46, pp. 650–651.

[3] See, for example, Melville's extended description of the fight his fellow seamen put up to prevent the clipping of their beards in full accordance with Navy regulations. Herman Melville, *White Jacket,* New York, Grove Press, n.d., pp. 333–347.

defined as "right guys" on the other.[4] It should be added that where new inmates can play a role in the system of secondary adjustments, as in providing new faction members or new sexual objects, then their "welcome" may indeed be a sequence of initial indulgences and enticements, instead of exaggerated deprivations.[5] Because of secondary adjustments we also find *kitchen strata*, namely, a kind of rudimentary, largely informal, stratification of inmates on the basis of each one's differential access to disposable illicit commodities; so also we find social typing to designate the powerful persons in the informal market system.[6]

While the privilege system provides the chief framework within which reassembly of the self takes place, other factors characteristically lead by different routes in the same general direction. Relief from economic and social responsibilities—much touted as part of the therapy in mental hospitals—is one, although in many cases it would seem that the disorganizing effect of this moratorium is more significant than its organizing effect. More important as a reorganizing influence is the *fraternalization process*, namely, the process through which socially distant persons find themselves developing mutual support and common *counter-mores* in opposition to a system that has forced them into intimacy and into a single, equalitarian community of fate.[7] It seems that the new recruit frequently starts out with something like the staff's popular misconceptions of the character of the inmates and then comes to find that most of his fellows have all the properties of ordinary decent human beings and that the stereotypes associated with their condition or offense are not a reasonable ground for judgment of inmates.[8]

If the inmates are persons who are accused by staff and society of having committed some kind of a crime against society, then the new inmate, even though sometimes in fact quite guiltless, may come to share the guilty feelings of his fellows and, thereafter, their well-elaborated defenses against these feelings. A sense of common injustice and a sense of bitterness against the outside world tends to develop, marking an important movement in the inmate's moral career. This response to felt guilt and massive deprivation is most clearly illustrated perhaps in prison life:[9]

By their reasoning, after an offender has been subjected to unfair or excessive punishment and treatment more degrading than that prescribed by law, he comes to justify his act which he could not have justified when he committed it. He decides to "get even" for his unjust treatment in prison and takes reprisals through further crime at the first opportunity. *With that decision he becomes a criminal.*

A more general statement[10] may be taken from two other students of the same kind of total institution: "In many ways, the inmate social system may be viewed as providing a way of life which enables the inmates to avoid the devastating psychological effects of internalizing and converting social rejection into self rejection. In effect, it permits the inmate to reject his rejectors rather than himself."

The mortifying processes that have been discussed and the privilege system represent the conditions that the inmate must adapt to in some way, but however pressing, these conditions allow for differ-

[4]See, for example, Donald Clemmer, "Leadership Phenomenon in a Prison Community," *Journal of Criminal Law, Criminology and Police Science,* Vol. 28, 1938, p. 868.

[5]See, for example, Ida Ann Harper, "The Role of the 'Fringer' in a State Prison for Women," *Social Forces,* Vol. 31, 1952, pp. 53–60.

[6]For concentration camps, see the discussion of "Prominents" throughout Elie A. Cohen, *Human Behavior in the Concentration Camp,* London, Jonathan Cape, 1954; for mental hospitals, see Ivan Belknap, *Human Problems of a State Mental Hospital,* New York, McGraw-Hill, 1956, p. 189. For prisons, see the discussion of "Politicos" in Donald Clemmer, *The Prison Community,* Christopher Publishing House, Boston, 1940, pp. 277–279, 298–309; also Hayner, *op. cit.,* p. 367; and Caldwell, *op. cit.,* pp. 651–653.

[7]For the version of this inmate solidarity to be found in military academies, see, Sanford M. Dornbush, "The Military Academy as an Assimilating Institution," *Social Forces,* Vol. 33, 1955, p. 318.

[8]An interesting example of this re-evaluation may be found in a conscientious objector's experience with nonpolitical prisoners, see Alfred Hassler, *Diary of a Self-Made Convict,* Henry Regnery, Chicago, 1954, p. 74, 117. In mental hospitals, of course, the patient's antagonism to staff obtains one of its supports from the discovery that, like himself, many other patients are more like ordinary persons than like anything else.

[9]Richard McCleery, *The Strange Journey,* University of North Carolina Extension Bulletin, Vol. 32, 1953, p. 24. Italics are McCleery's.

[10]Lloyd W. McCorkle and Richard Korn, "Resocialization Within Walls," *The Annals,* May 1954, p. 88. See also p. 95.

ent ways of meeting them. We find, in fact, that the same inmate will employ different lines of adaptation or tacks at different phases in his moral career and may even fluctuate between different tacks at the same time.

First, there is the process of *situational withdrawal.* The inmate withdraws apparent attention from everything except events immediately around his body and sees these in a perspective not employed by others present. This drastic curtailment of involvement in interactional events is best known, of course, in mental hospitals, under the title of "regression." Aspects of "prison psychosis" or "stir simpleness" represent the same adjustment, as do some forms of "acute depersonalization" described in concentration camps. I do not think it is known whether this line of adaptation forms a single continuum of varying degrees of withdrawal or whether there are standard discontinuous plateaus of disinvolvement. It does seem to be the case, however, that, given the pressures apparently required to dislodge an inmate from this status, as well as the currently limited facilities for doing so, we frequently find here, effectively speaking, an irreversible line of adaptation.

Second, there is the *rebellious line.* The inmate intentionally challenges the institution by flagrantly refusing to cooperate with staff in almost any way.[11] The result is a constantly communicated intransigency and sometimes high rebel-morale. Most large mental hospitals, for example, seem to have wards where this spirit strongly prevails. Interestingly enough, there are many circumstances in which sustained rejection of a total institution requires sustained orientation to its formal organization and hence, paradoxically, a deep kind of commitment to the establishment. Similarly, when total institutions take the line (as they sometimes do in the case of mental hospitals prescribing lobotomy[12] or army barracks prescribing the stockade) that the recalcitrant inmate must be broken, then, in their way, they must show as much special devotion to the rebel as he has shown to them. It should be added, finally, that

while prisoners of war have been known staunchly to take a rebellious stance throughout their incarceration, this stance is typically a temporary and initial phase of reaction, emerging from this to situational withdrawal or some other line of adaptation.

Third, another standard alignment in the institutional world takes the form of a kind of *colonization.* The sampling of the outside world provided by the establishment is taken by the inmate as the whole, and a stable, relatively contented existence is built up out of the maximum satisfactions procurable within the institution.[13] Experience of the outside world is used as a point of reference to demonstrate the desirability of life on the inside; and the usual tension between the two worlds collapses, thwarting the social arrangements based upon this felt discrepancy. Characteristically, the individual who too obviously takes this line may be accused by his fellow inmates of "having found a home" or of "never having had it so good." Staff itself may become vaguely embarrassed by this use that is being made of the institution, sensing that the benign possibilities in the situation are somehow being misused. Colonizers themselves may feel obliged to deny their satisfaction with the institution, if only in the interest of sustaining the countermores supporting inmate solidarity. They may find it necessary to mess up just prior to their slated discharge, thereby allowing themselves to present involuntary reasons for continued incarceration. It should be incidentally noted that any humanistic effort to make life in total institutions more bearable must face the possibility that doing so may increase the attractiveness and likelihood of colonization.

Fourth, one mode of adaptation to the setting of a total institution is that of *conversion.* The inmate appears to take over completely the official or staff view of himself and tries to act out the role of the perfect inmate. While the colonized inmate builds as much of a free community as possible for himself by using the limited facilities available, the convert takes a more disciplined, moralistic, monochromatic line, presenting himself as someone whose institutional enthusiasm is

[11]See, for example, the discussion of "The Resisters," in Edgar H. Schein, "The Chinese Indoctrination Program for Prisoners of War," *Psychiatry,* Vol. 19, 1956, pp. 166–167.

[12]See, for example, Belknap, *op. cit.,* p. 192.

[13]In the case of mental hospitals, those who take this line are sometimes called "institutional cures" or are said to suffer from "hospitalitis."

always at the disposal of the staff. In Chinese POW camps, we find Americans who became "pros" and fully espoused the Communist view of the world.[14] In army barracks there are enlisted men who give the impression that they are always "sucking around" and always "bucking for promotion." In prisons there are "square johns." In German concentration camps, longtime prisoners sometimes came to adapt the vocabulary, recreation, posture, expressions of aggression, and clothing style of the Gestapo, executing their role of straw-boss with military strictness.[15] Some mental hospitals have the distinction of providing two quite different conversion possibilities—one for the new admission who can see the light after an appropriate struggle and adapt the psychiatric view of himself, and another for the chronic ward patient who adopts the manner and dress of attendants while helping them to manage the other ward patients with a stringency excelling that of the attendants themselves.

Here, it should be noted, is a significant way in which total institutions differ. Many, like progressive mental hospitals, merchant ships, TB sanitariums and brainwashing camps, offer the inmate an opportunity to live up to a model of conduct that is at once ideal and staff-sponsored— a model felt by its advocates to be in the supreme interests of the very persons to whom it is applied. Other total institutions, like some concentration camps and some prisons, do not officially sponsor an ideal that the inmate is expected to incorporate as a means of judging himself.

While the alignments that have been mentioned represent coherent courses to pursue, few inmates, it seems, carry these pursuits very far. In most total institutions, what we seem to find is that most inmates take the tack of what they call *playing it cool*. This involves a somewhat opportunistic combination of secondary adjustments, conversion, colonization and loyalty to the inmate group, so that in the particular circumstances the inmate will have a maximum chance of eventually getting out physically and psychically undamaged.[16] Typically, the inmate will support the counter-mores when with fellow inmates and be silent to them on how tractably he acts when alone in the presence of staff.[17] Inmates taking this line tend to subordinate contacts with their fellows to the higher claim of "keeping out of trouble." They tend to volunteer for nothing, and they may even learn to cut their ties to the outside world sufficiently to give cultural reality to the world inside but not enough to lead to colonization.

I have suggested some of the lines of adaptation that inmates can take to the pressures that play in total institutions. Each represents a way of managing the tension between the home world and the institutional world. However, there are circumstances in which the home world of the inmate was such, in fact, as to *immunize* him against the bleak world on the inside, and for such persons no particular scheme of adaptation need be carried very far. Thus, some lower-class mental hospital patients who have lived all their previous life in orphanages, reformatories and jails, tend to see the hospital as just another total institution to which it is possible to apply the adaptive technics learned and perfected in other total institutions. "Playing it cool" represents for such persons, not a shift in their moral career, but an alignment that is already second nature.

The professional criminal element in the early periods of German concentration camps displayed something of the same immunity to their surroundings or even found new satisfactions through fraternization with middle-class political prisoners.[18] Similarly, Shetland youths recruited

[14]Schein, *op. cit.,* pp. 167–169.

[15]See, Bruno Bettelheim, "Individual and Mass Behavior in Extreme Situations," *Journal of Abnormal and Social Psychology,* Vol. 38, 1943, pp. 447–451. It should be added that in concentration camps, colonization and conversion often seemed to go together. See, Cohen, *op. cit.,* pp. 200–203, where the role of the "Kapo" is discussed.

[16]See the discussion in Schein, *op. cit.,* pp. 165–166 of the "Get-Alongers," and Robert J. Lifton, "Home by Ship: Reaction Patterns of American Prisoners of War Repatriated From North Korea," *American Journal of Psychiatry,* Vol. 110, 1954, p. 734.

[17]This two-facedness, of course, is very commonly found in total institutions. In the state-type mental hospital studied by the writer, even the few elite patients selected for individual psychotherapy, and hence in the best position for espousal of the psychiatric approach to self, tended to present their favorable view of psychotherapy only to the members of their intimate cliques. For a report on the way in which Army prisoners concealed from fellow offenders their interest in "restoration" to the Army, see the comments by Richard Cloward in Session 4 of *New Perspectives for Research on Juvenile Delinquency,* ed. by Helen L. Witmer and Ruth Kotinsky, U.S. Department of Health, Education and Welfare, Children's Bureau Bulletin, 1955, especially p. 90.

[18]Bettelheim, *op. cit.,* p. 425.

into the British merchant marine are not apparently threatened much by the cramped arduous life on board because island life is even more stunted; they make uncomplaining sailors because from their point of view they have nothing much to complain about. Strong religious and political convictions may also serve perhaps to immunize the true believer against the assaults of a total institution, and even a failure to speak the language of the staff may cause the staff to give up its efforts at reformation, allowing the nonspeaker immunity to certain pressures.[19]

---

[19]Thus, Schein, *op. cit.*, p. 165 fn., suggests that Puerto Ricans and other non-English-speaking prisoners of war in China were given up on and allowed to work out a viable routine of menial chores.
Source: Harvey L. Smith and Jean Thrasher, "Roles, Cliques and Sanctions: Dimensions of Patient Society," *International Journal of Social Psychiatry,* 9:184–191, 1963.

Sociocultural Theories

THERAPY

No paper can more appropriately follow the preceding article by Goffman than that of Maxwell Jones, the leading exponent of "milieu therapy." In the presentation published here, Jones outlines the structure of hospital therapy he has evolved over the past two decades, an approach characterized by the assumption of an active role on the part of patients in programs designed for their own rehabilitation as members of society. Broadening the scope of community-oriented mental health, Klein and Lindemann (the latter one of the earliest exponents of the community approach) detail the rationale and procedures involved in providing what has since been termed social-preventive and crisis-intervention services.

47. The Therapeutic Community: Milieu Therapy

MAXWELL JONES

The decentralization of large state hospitals into small, semi-autonomous units serving discrete geographical areas may prove to have many benefits for patient management and treatment. The improvement of communications both intra and extramurally, manifested by the establishment of closer ties between patients, staff and relatives, and with outside agencies, can be seen as advantageous. The smaller treatment units also allow for easier examination and modification of roles, role-relationships and the over-all culture on the unit.

This process can be developed further and a very different picture emerges when the above trends are developed and the sociocultural process becomes an integral part of treatment. The resultant picture is often called a therapeutic community or the process described as milieu therapy. I have elsewhere (21) described a therapeutic community as distinctive among other comparable treatment centers in the way the institution's total resources, both staff and patients, are self-consciously pooled in furthering

treatment. This implies, above all, a change in the usual status of patients. In collaboration with the staff, they now become active participants in the therapy of themselves and other patients and in other aspects of the over-all hospital work—in contrast to their relatively more passive, recipient role in conventional treatment regimes.

SOCIAL STRUCTURE

The social structure of a therapeutic community is characteristically different from the more traditional hospital ward or decentralized unit. The term implies that the whole community of staff and patients is involved at least partly in treatment and administration. The extent to which this is practicable or desirable will depend on many variables including the attitude of the leader and the other staff, the type of patients being treated, and the sanctions afforded by higher authority. The emphasis on free communication in and between both staff and patient groups and on permissive attitudes which encourage free expression of feeling imply a democratic equalitarian rather than a traditional hierarchical social organization (68).

From Maxwell Jones, *Social psychiatry: In the community, in hospitals, and in prisons.* Springfield, Ill.: Charles C Thomas, 1962. Pp. 53–71. Reprinted by permission.

Staff and patient roles and role-relationships are the subject of frequent examination and discussion. This is devised to increase the effectiveness of roles and sharpen the community's perception of them. Thus, it may be felt that a nurse's role is clarified and rendered more effective if she ceases to wear a uniform. It may take months of study and discussion to decide that, say, a nurse requires on an average four months on a ward before she feels secure enough to discard her uniform. To share this discussion with the patients is to increase their awareness of the difficulties of a nursing role and may modify their relationship to the nurses. The aim is to achieve sufficient role flexibility so that the role at any one time reflects the expectations of behavior of both staff and patients collectively.

The examination and clarification of roles inevitably sharpens the role prescription but may at the same time lead to some role blurring. This is not contradictory. Thus, it may seem appropriate that nurses as well as social workers should visit patients' homes. The former might accompany patients on home visits to help in the rehabilitation process to the outside world and to encourage the family member to attend ward group meetings. The social worker might visit the home with the patient's approval but not in his presence. Her visit might be mainly to try and engage the family members in treatment which would be complementary to the patient's treatment in hospital.

The over-all culture in a ward or psychiatric unit represents the accumulation through time of the attitudes, beliefs and behavior patterns, common to a large part of the unit. This is arrived at as a result of considerable inquiry into the nature of these attitudes and an attempt is made to modify them to meet the treatment needs of the patients. In this context the term "therapeutic culture" is sometimes perhaps hopefully used. The tendency is for these cultural patterns to be most clearly established in the more stable and permanent members of the community, i.e., the staff.

Examples of such attitudes contributing to a therapeutic culture or treatment ideology would be an emphasis on active rehabilitation, as against "custodialism" and segregation; "democratization" in contrast to the old hierarchies and formalities of status differentiation; "permis-siveness" in contrast to the stereotyped patterns of communication and behavior; and "communalism" as opposed to highly specialized therapeutic roles often limited to the doctor (69).

A basic aspect of the social organization of a therapeutic community is the establishment of daily community meetings. By a community meeting, we mean a meeting of the entire patient staff population who are working together in a single geographical area. My colleagues and I have found it practicable to hold meetings of this kind with as many as eighty patients and twenty to thirty staff. It is our opinion that the upper limit for the establishment of a therapeutic community in the sense that the term is used here is around 100 patients. The term group therapy as opposed to community therapy is used in the more conventional sense. A relatively small group of patients who are treated by their own doctor or therapist in a group setting will often represent a subgroup of the total community who have been selected on clinical grounds, age, intelligence, motivation, et cetera. In my experience, it is desirable for community meetings to be followed by group meetings. In the community meetings, the tensions in the ward or unit at a particular time will be ventilated and will activate a great deal of material within the individual patient. Many of the tensions cannot easily be worked through in a community meeting but if this is followed by a group meeting, it would seem to act as a useful stimulus to communication in the smaller meeting.

THE COMMUNITY MEETING

A ward or treatment unit of, say, eighty or ninety patients have to live together and, although of course they split off into small sub-groups or even withdraw to a relatively isolated position, the patients must inevitably interact with each other in varying degrees. In a community meeting the staff is exposed to some of the social forces which normally operate on the ward. Harry Wilmer (70) has described in great detail ward meetings of this kind involving very disturbed schizophrenic patients.

The first problem to consider is the attitude of the staff. In general, they will view this type of meeting with very mixed feelings. The charge nurse, or charge aide, may see this as depriving her of her cherished exclusive daily interview with the doctor which, in the past, may have done much to relieve her of her own anxieties. In the past she often became "the therapist" of the ward, describing activities of a disturbing kind to the doctor and recommending "treatment" which not infrequently he was only too glad to accept, failing to realize that the "treatment" he was sanctioning was sometimes to relieve the anxiety of the nurse rather than the patient. Thus, the use of shock treatment or sedatives or transfer of patients to another ward has frequently been centralized in the nursing role. The attitudes of other staff members, although obviously important, may never have been examined and the more junior aides especially may have come to feel that they were excluded from much of the interest in the work and that their own status was devalued. However, the establishment of a daily community meeting does very little to improve the situation if the staff, other than the doctor, feel that it is a waste of time and liable to create more, rather than less, disturbance among the patients. The charge nurse or aide may find that she hesitates to say to the whole community what she feels about patient behavior, fearing consciously or unconsciously that some of her prejudices or tendency to have favorites may become apparent to all. Moreover, her authority may be questioned by some of her aides, who may point out the irrationality or inconsistency of some of her decisions. On the other hand, the aides may well feel incapable of communicating in public, fearing ridicule or possibly even later reprisals from their own senior staff.

Perhaps most important, this kind of situation calls for a more responsible role on the part of the nursing staff than they have been used to playing. In this context, the aide may talk frequently about her desire for further education and speak resentfully about the poor quality of the inservice training, if any, but the other side of the coin is that frequently she is afraid of change. In fact, she may prefer the passive-dependent role which gives her the relative absence of responsibility and also, of course, an opportunity to grumble quite legitimately about her devalued position. The important point is that no community meeting is likely to be very effective until such time as the unit personnel really believe that it has value, not only for the patients but for themselves.

Clearly the nature of the patient population is extremely important. In a busy admission unit with a rapid turnover of patients, it is difficult to get any continuity of culture. Some patients may begin to appreciate daily meetings just at the time when they have to leave. Many more will probably never see anything in this for them before they leave the ward to return home or are transferred to one of the long-stay wards. Our own experience would indicate that one really needs at least a nucleus of moderately long-stay patients to help the newer patients to perceive the community meeting as a place where they can, from the start, expect to get an answer to some of their difficulties and/or insight into their own behavior. Daily community meetings will tend to produce in both patients and staff an increasing awareness of the nature and predisposing factors behind disturbed behavior. This in turn tends to produce changes in the social structure of the ward so that further disturbances can be in part prevented and better handled where they occur. It may become clear that patients leave the handling of "incidents" entirely to the nursing staff. At the same time, the nursing staff may be criticized for their actions in these disturbances, some patients feeling that they have been too perfunctory or too rough or used restraints when they were not necessary and so on.

In such a discussion, the likelihood is that many of the patients will bring forward factors about the incident which change its significance for all concerned. They often see where the patient's behavior had been misunderstood by the staff and the tendency is for the patients slowly to become more responsible in relation to the handling and even restraint of their peers. Thus, the passive-dependent attitude which is so often associated with the role of the patient comes to be modified in the direction of more active participation in relation to acting out behavior or other incidents, and becomes much more closely identified with the staff role. Another example of this is the way in which the patients and staff respond to a patient leaving the community meeting. In many instances, the incident passes apparently unnoticed, but if the doctor or other staff member begins to draw attention to the fact that so-and-so leaves at some significant point and suggests that the departure has something to do with the patient's anxiety, then the unit personnel tends to become more sensitive to the meaning of behavior. In time, the patients will probably come to talk about doing something to bring the anxious member back into the community meeting where his anxiety can be examined.

A sharing of responsibility for patient behavior is particularly important in relation to the night staff. Unfortunately, they are frequently the ones who are not present at community meetings or the discussions which should, in our opinion, always follow a community meeting. Communication to them must be through the morning or evening shifts, with overlap. The latter themselves tend to be isolated from the morning teaching programs. The interest of the evening and night shifts can be aroused most effectively by the duty doctor explaining much of the significance of community meetings and telling them how much any written or verbal feedback that they care to offer is appreciated. However, their anxieties about the day staff and their lack of familiarity with the treatment culture may make this difficult. Also, being left alone on the ward with patients about whom they may know very little and who may cause them considerable anxiety often makes them feel that their point of view might be distorted or misunderstood if it is handled by people other than themselves. In rare instances, the night staff or evening shift may be so interested that they choose to stay on or arrive early to participate in the ward community meeting in which case their difficulties can be expressed directly to the patients and staff.

Patient Councils are popular and found in many hospital organizations. The function of these ward councils varies very considerably but in the main, in our experience, they are limited to the handling of practical ward details, such as privileges, arrangements for ward cleaning, rosters, and so on. Nevertheless, they tend through time to assume increasing responsibilities. In our opinion, they should not assume too much responsibility unaided and should be supervised by staff and the content of the discussions in their Council meetings fed back to the community meetings. It seems to us that much good can come from the development of patient responsibility skillfully supervised. Nevertheless, it would be foolish to assume that this kind of development occurs without considerable conflict.

If the Patient Council is allowed to develop responsibilities without having staff to turn to in times of need, and without an adequate "feedback" of their Council meetings, it is more than likely that they will find themselves isolated and resented by their peers. They may come to assume all the characteristics of authority figures and much of the hostility which was previously directed toward the staff is now directed towards them. It is for reasons like this that we feel that the staff should be present at Council meetings and when necessary point out what is happening. A staff member might feel a need to point out that certain decisions ought to be fed through the patient community as a whole before being finalized by the Council. If the Council does not feed back its deliberations and difficulties to the community meeting, there is a danger that their role may become misunderstood; thus, their peers may come to feel that the Council is no longer made up of members of the patient group but rather by people who are "ganging up" with the staff and are in some kind of alien authoritative relationship with themselves.

In our experience, the Council, and particularly the chairman, may find this difficulty so real that deterioration in his clinical condition may occur. In general, one could say that through time the staff responsibilities can be transferred in part to the patient population and particularly to the Patient Council with real benefit in creating a more varied and responsible role for the patients. At the same time, the general principle could be formulated that the degree of responsibility that the patients can usefully assume is inversely related to the degree of disorganization within a ward. Thus, at times of relatively satisfactory organization, with appropriate leaders within the patient population and free communications, the amount of responsibility which can be safely transferred to the patients is maximal whereas in times of disorganization, when the group ego, if one likes to use the term, is weak, then the staff must assume increasing responsibility for decision-making and the general direction of patient management (71).

THE STAFF MEETING OR "POST MORTEM"

With the increasing interest in the social environment of the patient, the role of the ward psychiatrist becomes more complex. It is not enough to be a competent diagnostician and individual therapist; he must now learn how to recognize and modify the social organization and culture of his ward, as well as the complexities of group treatment. Ideally, this would entail exposure to the teaching of experienced psychiatrists and social scientists. It is rare for a resident to get social science teaching outside a university hospital or clinic. However, the growing interest in the social dimension in mental hospital psychiatry is manifested by books on the social organization of mental hospitals, and the psychiatrist in training is increasingly referring to such studies (64, 63, 62). Nevertheless, it seems to me that whatever training skills are available, the most effective way of teaching this aspect of psychiatry is in the living situation on the ward.

This can best be accomplished by a daily community meeting as already described and lasting about an hour immediately followed by a "post mortem" involving all staff members. This affords an opportunity to examine the response of the various personnel with different skills, expectations, and prejudices, who have been exposed to the same interactional scene in the community meeting. We find that for training purposes a staff meeting or a "post mortem" of this kind should last for about an hour. In this setting, it is possible to discuss the perceptions and feelings of the staff retrospectively in relation to the community meeting and also to examine their interaction during the staff meeting.

Let us assume that all staff who come in contact with the patient in a therapeutic role will be present at both meetings. In the "post mortem," they will, in varying degrees, be able to express both their analysis of certain aspects of the community meeting and their subjective feelings. If we take a frequently recurring problem, such as authority, the aides may perceive this in terms of their own desire to con-

form to a strict authority system where implementation of the requirements of higher authority are of prime importance. The cleanliness of the ward, the observation of smoking rules, and the avoidance of incidents, are necessary if they are to avoid undue anxiety. In this context, they will tend to express, directly or indirectly, views which support the maintenance of patient discipline. At the other extreme, the doctors, if they have had considerable training and experience in examining the social interaction on a ward, may perceive untidiness or dirt on the ward as symptoms of disorganization among the patients and want to examine this as a form of communication. To do this at all skillfully, the anxieties of the aides will have to be given due consideration, and the realities of their position faced frankly.

In discussion, it may emerge that the aides are uncomfortable at community meetings, feel that they take up far too much of their time, and are responsible in part for the untidiness of the ward. They may point out that continued disapproval from higher authorities may result in possible loss of employment. The reality of this fear may be reinforced by the fact that their supervisors are themselves not trained in social psychiatry and may apply a value system to their area of responsibility which is at variance with the developing culture on the unit. It may be that a long-term plan involving training seminars with the supervisors will be a necessary adjunct to the effective functioning of the unit if the situation is to be rendered therapeutic. At the same time, it may appear that the anxiety of the aides stems in part from their personality difficulties attributable to their relatively inadequate education and lack of sophistication which hampers them in their role relationship with more highly trained personnel. They may deal with this by denial and rationalization, blaming the frequency of community meetings and lack of discipline for the unsatisfactory state of affairs. A situation of this kind is not infrequent and the mere gain in insight on the part of an aide may not in itself be enough. It may take a long period of education and support, if not of therapy, to tide them over the transition from their previous image of a structured, simplified role to that of a therapeutic one.

What has been said about the role of the aide in a ward problem bearing on authority would apply in different ways to all the roles and role-relationships on the unit.

The charge nurse may have particular difficulties in that, by contrast with the aide, she has a relatively higher status and a professional image which implies knowledge which frequently she does not possess. In the United States, she may have had no formal training in psychiatry other than a short affiliation as a student nurse. Most R.N.'s have been trained in a fairly strict, authoritarian culture and have little experience in the examination of roles and role-relationships, the sharing of responsibility, and the concept of group decisions or group treatment. She may resent both the loss of her relatively exclusive relationship with the doctor and the staff's examination of her handling of patients' problems. In the "post mortem," it may become clear that when she feels threatened by patients, she resorts to devices such as recommending shock treatment, transferring the patient to another ward, or "regressing" to an authoritarian disciplinary role. Like the aide, she, too, has the problem of a nursing authority structure. She is expected to satisfy the needs of personnel who have no direct contact with the ward and who view things from their own particular nursing perspective. Unless nursing supervisors and the higher echelons of nursing can themselves become identified with community programs, then confusion of roles is almost inevitable. The ward views the problems as material for treatment whereas the nursing hierarchy tend to view them as administrative problems, calling for immediate action. One device frequently used by the nursing profession is to transfer a nurse to another ward if there are repeated ward problems. By doing this, of course, nothing is learned from the disturbance on the ward, but, from the point of view of administration, the problem is got rid of by transfer.

I have found it possible, even in a large state hospital, to use situations of this kind as learning experiences for all personnel concerned. The Director of Nursing and her senior colleagues have been extremely willing to participate in seminars involving the ward problems so that even if a nurse has been transferred it is still possible to re-create the situation in retrospect and see what alternative answers could have been found to the problem. Whether this should be done by inviting senior nursing personnel to the unit "post mortem" meeting or whether it calls for a separate administrative learning situation is still, I think, an open question and much would depend upon the circumstances. The essential point is that the unit doctor should be involved so that he is in a position to gain experience in dealing with problems involving extraward personnel and differing role perceptions. Nurses from the Department of Education may, with advantage, also be involved in this kind of learning experience. If they have student nurses on a ward, they tend to teach them in a situation which is removed from the actual ward interaction. If, however, the Nursing Education personnel themselves become involved in community meetings and find a functional role on the ward, they are then in a position to discuss the interactional scene with their students in the staff meeting and in their own teaching seminars. In this way, their own perceptions of what went on and what they would normally teach their students can be examined by other trained personnel and Nursing Education puts itself in the position of having a continuous educational experience, instead of tending to become stereotyped.

Moreover, the staff meeting is an ideal setting in which to work through some of the problems inherent in the role relationships between medical, nursing service, and nursing education personnel. All three have a significant relationship with the student nurse and unless a serious attempt is made to work through this relationship, the student may find herself confused, and, at times, victimized. What she wants above all is someone to turn to when she is in emotional difficulties with her patients. My feeling is that in the kind of program we are discussing, she will be able to turn to the charge nurse, to the Nursing Education supervisor, or to the ward personnel, including the doctor, social worker, psychologist, and so on, all of whom should be in a position to understand certain aspects of the problems of nurse-patient relationships on the ward. This implies a degree of role blurring which is perhaps unusual. At the same time, it implies a degree of sophistication through time of all ward personnel which tends to evolve through daily staff meetings when the problems of treatment, ward management, interpersonal relationships, including staff relationships, are under constant scrutiny and discussion.

What I have said about the roles of the personnel in direct contact with the patient applies equally to the more peripheral roles, including the social worker and psychologist. It seems to me that it is equally important that their relationships with patients, whether as social case-workers or as therapists or group workers, should be discussed freely with the total unit staff personnel. This implies that roles are constantly being modified and that a psychologist or social worker on Unit A need not necessarily have a similar role on Unit B. In fact, it seems a pity if professional personnel become identified with their own professional subgroup rather than with the Unit on which they are working. All this implies a considerable degree of skill and sophistication on the part of the unit leader who, at the present time, is usually, or perhaps invariably, the psychiatrist. There seems to me no adequate reason why this responsibility should continue to rest with the psychiatrist unless he has the kind of training and skill which we are discussing. This leadership role could reasonably be given to one of the other staff personnel provided, of course, that the purely medical matters were left, as they must be, to the doctor.

In order to become competent in handling the various role-relationships and management problems which we have been discussing, the psychiatrist is forced to attempt to examine the problems of the various personnel and see them from not only his own but from the other points of view. Whether group consensus can be seen as a satisfactory way of resolving problems, if indeed it is ever achieved, is an open question, but the attempt to examine problems in various dimensions is a rich learning experience. Obviously, it is much better if this whole procedure is supervised by a social scientist with experience in psychiatry or a psychiatrist who has considerable experience in group work and the social science field. Such training will help him to make optimal use of his staff and the social environment generally and, where psychiatrists are concerned, will be invaluable preparation for a possible future role as a mental hospital administrator.

COMMUNITY TREATMENT

If one assumes that the patient population has certain treatment potentials which can be developed under constant medical and professional supervision, then one has to set up a structure whereby the patient contribution can be maximized. The immediate objection can be raised that the patients are ill and it is unfair or unrealistic to expect them to help in treatment and make decisions involving a good deal of responsibility; in any case, this is the job that the staff is paid to do. On the other hand, it can be argued that perhaps the most outstanding characteristic of newly admitted patients is their feeling of depression and despair and, if possible, they must be helped to deal with this. A former colleague, Gil Elles, a psychoanalyst working at the therapeutic community at Henderson Hospital, London (formerly the Social Rehabilitation Unit at Belmont Hospital), described the handling of this problem as follows (72).

The community has developed techniques for dealing with this problem at a conscious level and at the same time has become aware of the unconscious mechanisms which are all the time operating to prevent individual, group, or community from becoming overwhelmed by this despair. In the first instance emphasis is placed on trying to lessen the force of unconscious guilt which drives the psychopath compulsively into trouble again and again, and seriously inhibits his capacity to learn by experience. With the new patient this takes the form of making known to the community his problem so that at the earliest possible moment in treatment he is accepted for what he *is* rather than what he would *like* to be, or what he fears himself to be. In this way, it is hoped that the deep-seated guilt is somewhat diminished and the patient's ego strengths are increased and made more available to him.

In the second place every patient has a dual role both of trying to accept and give treatment. Therefore through the second part of his role his self regard is fortified enabling him to feel less of a failure because he is expected to help and understand others. Thus, in the long run he is able to feel less threatened in admitting some part of his own desperation about himself.

In the third instance and following on from these initial community attitudes despair is limited by improving communication within the individual and between individuals in their various groups. The community has a culture whereby feelings are shared very openly and the reasons for such feelings examined in great detail. To do this the day has to be geared so that every community activity is associated with a long period for discussion about it. Furthermore, the various activity groups are so interrelated that the maximum contact in as many social roles as possible is provided for each patient in the community. In effect this experience tends to build up in each individual a more integrated picture of himself, firstly as seen by others, and finally when accepted by him as part of his own self-evaluation.

What has happened in such situations following admission is that a reduction of the violence and fragmentation of the individual splitting processes has taken place. This means that the despairing patient's urgent need to project wholesale the unacceptable parts of himself —good as well as bad—has been diminished in the first place by the community's attitude of understanding and acceptance. This enables the patient to be aware of new strength so long as he remains a member of the community. By establishing firm bonds through patient-staff and patient-patient interaction which all the while is looked at and discussed a framework is then secondarily built up that is strong enough to carry the weight of a personal depression of a more mature order. Thus some patients for the first time experience both an outer security and an inner despair which allows them to feel and to understand the emotions of remorse and pity, followed by a longing for and a belief in their own ability to repair and restore the fabric of damaged relationships. For such a patient this means that authority figures are gradually perceived as less threatening and other relationships as more lasting. Thus the patient in internalizing a conscience now less punitive can accept both more responsibility and more success.

This question of elaborating the role of a patient to one of therapist is, I think, one of the fundamental tenets of community treatment procedure. This concept is often mistakenly seen as handing over ultimate responsibility to the patients. This, in my opinion, is not practicable and that what one wishes to do is to give the patients the optimal responsibility compatible with their over-all capacity at any one time and that in no sense does the staff or the doctor in charge relinquish his ultimate authority which merely remains latent to be invoked when necessary. It is the application of this principle which calls for considerable experience and skill. As an example, a community may be functioning at a fairly high level of effectiveness and the patients may be able to take over a considerable amount of responsibility and then, on a particular day, four or

five of the most responsible and successfully treated members leave to be replaced by four or five new patients who may be in the state of considerable disorganization.

The loss of patient leadership within the ward and the effect of the new intake may be such that ward functioning is materially altered and the staff have to play a much more active and controlling role than they were previously doing (71). This is not fundamentally different from what happens in an individual or a group treatment session when the lack of ego strength or anxiety level is such that the therapist feels it necessary to be largely supportive for a time. I am talking about patient responsibility of a higher order than one usually understands by the term "patient government." Patient government is usually restricted to decisions on relatively minor matters of ward organization and activities. What I have in mind is decisions shared with the staff and involving such matters as the discharge of patients or transfer to other wards or what disciplinary action should be taken in the case of deviant behavior. This sharing of serious responsibility with the staff is, I think, one of the most important ways in overcoming the lack of confidence, low self-estimate, and overdependency which all too frequently are characteristic of the psychiatric patient in the hospital ward. This responsibility can also be carried over to the patients' work roles (22).

It is ideal if one can do production work for the community and have patient foremen, timekeepers, et cetera. If one is fortunate enough to have the freedom to build up a therapeutic community from the point of view of the patients' social and treatment needs, then I think one must inevitably end up with a structure which deviates markedly from the more usual pattern in which the organization is essentially staff-centered and often is determined by traditions from the past which have little relevance to current treatment methods and practices. As an example, one finds that in a ward where the patients have a great deal of identification with responsible roles and with treatment, they will come to the aid of the night nurse in the event of disturbed patient behavior, instead of leaving it entirely for the staff to deal with. In this context also, the patients come to feel much more able to bear with highly disturbed behavior among their peers because the community meetings help them to understand the meaning of the disturbed behavior and give them a better idea of how to relate in a helpful and understanding way to the sick member.

The daily examination of behavior and current problems means that the patients become aware of the factors which lie behind behavior and learn a great deal about each other's problems. In any type of hospital, they are forced to relate to other patients and staff at ward level whether they like it or not, and it seems reasonable to try to help them to have a positive role to play and a much better insight into what is going on in themselves and in those around them. In my experience, it is possible to get patients and staff at all levels to appreciate some of the phenomena that occur on the unit and in the daily community meetings. The progression that occurs in these meetings through time has many points in common with ordinary group treatment. In the first instance, the patients in the community meeting tend to look to the staff for leadership and are glad when some general topic is raised which has no personal significance. As time progresses, they begin to talk about some of their deeper feelings and to test out the staff reactions in this direction. Assuming adequate skills on the part of the staff, they become used as transference figures with advantage to the treatment process. The same applies to the transference onto various members of the patient population.

The concepts of manifest and latent content, the unconscious, and ego defenses come to be understood in much the way that occurs in a small group. It may be necessary to have additional seminars for the aides who are less well-trained than the other staff members and to whom the change of role implicit in this discussion is greater than that required of any other staff member. For the staff meeting, concepts like feedback from informal staff-patient groups and difficulties occurring during the night between patients and night staff can be usefully communicated to the group. Ideally, of course, one would hope that nursing personnel rotate so that the night staff have opportunity to participate in the learning experience afforded to the day staff, more particularly the morning shift.

The meetings I am describing are clearly less specifically therapeutic and more concerned with everyday behavior and ward management than is the typical therapeutic group of six or eight patients of a selected kind. Nevertheless, I think that the community meetings of up to eighty patients and staff have a particular place in institutional therapy, particularly in bringing about the establishment of what one might call a therapeutic culture. By this, I mean that the day-after-day examination of the problems existing on a ward and the consideration of the roles of all staff members and of the patients leads through time to considerable modification of the ward structure. Not only that, but the traditional attitudes and beliefs can come in for scrutiny and we are in a position to ask ourselves why we do what we do when we do. A learning experience of the kind I am describing is far from easy and clearly causes the staff considerable anxiety (20).

Often, the doctors themselves are the people who have had less training than either social workers or psychologists and in any case their training in a general hospital has tended to give them a feeling of considerable authority and even omnipotence. To have their performance in these daily meetings questioned by their juniors and other professional colleagues can be extremely painful but is undoubtedly a valuable learning experience if the personality of the individual allows this to happen. Nevertheless, there are many people who are not suited for this kind of community practice and I think that one has to make this clear from the start. My feeling is that every resident should be afforded the opportunity of learning therapy of this kind but that many of them will not feel comfortable in this type of community situation and will prefer to operate in the more traditional, authoritarian role. I see nothing wrong with this as I think that in any case a ward will tend to develop along the lines prescribed by the most senior member—that is, at present, the doctor. I would like to think that doctors trained in this way who are able to assimilate this kind of orientation will be well-prepared for future roles as hospital superintendents and to some extent, I think it can be seen as a very valuable training for community psychiatry. My own experience is that the doctor who can relate to his ward personnel and to the patients in an easy and relaxed way and who can listen to their communications is very frequently the doctor, who in outpatient departments or in community psychiatry automatically feels at home meeting the patient in his social setting along with his own family group.

From what has already been said it is clear that training and treatment overlap. In the case of the staff meetings, whether for the total staff or seminars for the less experienced members, many intra-staff difficulties inevitably arise. In general, it is probably wiser to limit examination of these difficulties to situations bearing on the treatment of patients. This makes the discussion relatively objective and the motivation to help the patient at all costs weighs heavily. Thus, in a rivalry situation between two nurses about a patient it would be desirable to uncover or clarify the situation or the patient would almost certainly suffer (73). However, the indications of a covert homosexual problem in a staff member would best be ignored unless it produced obvious difficulties in relationships with the patients. In that case, therapy might well be indicated but should be done by an outside psychiatrist.

The over-all culture of the ward can modify the treatment ideology enormously. Take the question of sedation. Many patients arrive at hospital loaded with sedatives or tranquilizing drugs prescribed by their local doctor. If the culture of the ward is against sedation except under clearly specified conditions, then this may modify the new patient's expectation in a surprisingly short time. The same argument applies to the establishment of many potentially therapeutic attitudes (e.g., the desirability of invoking the patient's active participation in treatment rather than encouraging a passive-dependent attitude to the hospital).

As has already been pointed out, the development of a therapeutic culture will necessitate frequent, preferably daily, meetings of the entire patient and staff population. In this way the community is faced day in, day out, with the living problems of the patients. These reflect the problems which affected the patients outside and resulted in their hospitalization. By discussing these collectively the staff become involved in some measure with the patients' ward life and are, at the very least, in a better position to modify ward routine, or administrative procedure and so indirectly enhance treatment.

References

20. Greenblatt, M., Levinson, D. L., & Williams, R. H. (Eds.) *The patient and the mental hospital*. Glencoe, Ill.: Free Press, 1957. Chapter 14: The absorption of new doctors into a therapeutic community.

21. Jones, M. Towards a clarification of the therapeutic community concept. *British Journal of Medicine and Psychology*, 1959, *32*, 200–205.

22. Jones, M. Social rehabilitation with emphasis on work therapy as a form of group therapy. *British Journal of Medicine and Psychology*, 1960, *33*, 67–71.

62. Greenblatt, M., York, R. H., & Brown, E. L. *From custodial to therapeutic patient care in mental hospitals*. New York: Russell Sage Foundation, 1955.

63. Belknap, I. *Human problems of a state mental hospital*. New York: McGraw-Hill, 1956.

64. Caudill, W. *The psychiatric hospital as a small society*. Cambridge, Mass.: Harvard University Press, 1958.

68. Rapaport, R., & Rapaport, R. Permissiveness and treatment in a therapeutic community, *Psychiatry*, 1959, *22*, 57–64.

69. Rapaport, R. *Community as doctor*. Springfield, Ill.: Charles C Thomas, 1960.

70. Wilmer, H. *Social psychiatry in action*. Springfield, Ill.: Charles C Thomas, 1958.

71. Parker, S. Disorganization on a psychiatric ward. *Psychiatry*, 1959, *22*, 65–80.

72. Elles, G. Research into the aftercare needs of discharged patients. Unpublished paper, 1961.

73. Stanton, A. H., & Schwartz, M. S. *The mental hospital*. New York: Basic Books, 1954.

48.   Preventive Intervention in Individual and Family Crisis Situations

DONALD C. KLEIN and ERICH LINDEMANN

Impetus for this work came from Lindemann's (5) study of bereavement. He postulated that there are both adaptive and maladaptive ways of meeting a range of emotional hazards during the life cycle, each one of which may have significant consequences for later psychologic soundness and ability to cope. A multidisciplinary team was assembled to examine this basic premise from the standpoint of the clinical-psychiatric professions, social science, and public health. A series of interrelated studies and service operations was carried out over a five-year period in the community of Wellesley, Massachusetts, a suburban town fifteen miles west of Boston (6, 8).

In 1953 the community assumed responsibility for the program. By that time there had been developed a relatively well coordinated pattern of services in the areas of both primary and secondary prevention. Services now include planning and consultation with lay and professional groups, mental health education, and a short-term clinical service. The latter will be described in more detail later. Research activities continue to focus attention upon diverse aspects of the community as an emotionally relevant human environment, especially upon those aspects that appear to be emotionally hazardous to certain segments of the population.

An *emotionally hazardous situation* (or emotional hazard) refers to any sudden alteration in the field of social forces within which the individual exists, such that the individual's expectations of himself and his relationships with others undergo change. Major categories of hazards include: (1) a loss or threatened loss of a significant relationship; (2) the introduction of one or more new individuals into the social orbit; (3) transitions in social status and role relationships as a consequence of such factors as (*a*) maturation (e.g., entry into adolescence), (*b*)

achievement of a new social role (e.g., marriage), or (*c*) horizontal or vertical social mobility (e.g., job promotion). In all instances, it is believed, the hazardous circumstance is patterned by institutional and other sociocultural arrangements.

The term *crisis* is reserved for the acute and often prolonged disturbance that may occur in an individual or social orbit as the result of an emotional hazard. The crisis of the individual is often a manifestation of a group crisis; conversely, the development of an intrapersonal crisis may lead to a crisis situation for the group of which the individual is a significant member. Nevertheless, the two states are not universally coexistent and it is essential to distinguish between them in this work. As will be noted later, we have been particularly interested in discovering and understanding those circumstances wherein marked emotional distress or intrapersonal crisis has reflected or been precipitated by an alteration of the individual's relevant human environment.

Emotional predicament is used in the most generic sense to encompass the distressed individuals, the crisis situation, and the emotional hazard, all of which must be assessed in any comprehensive appraisal of a predicament situation.

Studies of mental health issues in a community setting have led to the two growing convictions with which this chapter is concerned. Still being tested by experience is the first belief that general clinical services that emphasize prevention and health promotion can in time be made available to the general population. The quest for such a clinical service, aimed at general maintenance of mental health, has been going on not only in Wellesley since 1948 but also at the mental health service of the Massachusetts General Hospital since 1953. These centers are concerning themselves with: (1) the enlargement and altered application of clinical skills at times of psychologic crisis; (2) the establishment of the most appropriate settings for such services; (3) the education of prospective recipients so that their expectations become increasingly congruent with available services. The strategy of this type of service

From Chapter 13, "Preventive Intervention in Individual and Family Crisis Situations," by Donald C. Klein and Erich Lindemann, in *Prevention of Mental Disorders in Children* by Gerald Kaplan, ©1961 by Barie Books, Inc. Publishers, New York.

is clear: namely, to encourage in the community the utilization of clinically trained mental health personnel for health checkups, anticipation of health hazards, and help with the many common emotional predicaments that usually are not brought to the attention of psychiatry until after some form of major or minor illness has developed. The tactics whereby such a strategy may be realized are still being developed and refined. This paper represents an early formulation of experiences and resulting theoretical ideas.

The second emphasis suggests that mental health services can be deployed most effectively when it is possible for them to concentrate upon specific subgroups at the times of heightened tensions that are occasioned by specific life challenges. Two such specific programs have been pursued to date in Wellesley. Each has been based upon research carried out after initial tentative identification of the hazard in question. These investigations, in each instance, attempted to describe the nature of the emotionally hazardous situation itself, the institutional or community context in which it was experienced, and the impact it was apt to have upon those experiencing it.

A CLINICAL SERVICE FOR PREDICAMENTS*

Preventively oriented clinical work (for which the term *direct preventive intervention* has been used) seems most often indicated in predicaments where there is a crisis of recent onset that is experienced with a sense of immediacy and urgency by those involved because it is having a major effect on one or more individuals in the immediate social orbit. It is rarely successful when a crisis has resulted finally in a chronically disturbed state of the individual and the group.

Brief work with predicament† has been likened to the situation of exerting a gentle push against someone standing upon one leg. The "disequilibrium" can be maintained only temporarily. The other leg eventually will come down, whether

or not one pushes. The opportunities for direct intervention during the predicament period, as implied in the analogy, are twofold: first, to ensure that the psychological "other leg" comes down on firm ground; second, to exert pressure in such a fashion that the individual is encouraged to move in a desirable direction as the foot descends and equilibrium is re-established.

The analogy also suggests that in working with a crisis a maximum of change may be possible with a minimum of effort, as compared with intervention in a noncrisis situation when, so to speak, both feet are planted firmly on the ground. At the very least, it may be possible to carry out primary prevention by helping to restore the equilibrium existing prior to the crisis before the situation leads to some form of emotional pathology. Beyond this goal, however, is the opportunity in some cases to foster a more desirable equilibrium between an individual and his immediate human environment than had existed before. It is the second, in many ways more ambitious goal that leads to a form of preventive intervention that can be differentiated from the several brief psychotherapies or ego therapies that have been developed over the past few decades. Preventive intervention shares with such remedial efforts the need to make a careful assessment of the intrapsychic structure and dynamics of personality. However, it extends the assessment to an equally important appraisal of the individual's social role and of the significant role relationships in which he is involved. Hence the weight of emphasis shifts from the individual alone to the individual enmeshed in a social network. The unit of inquiry, planning, and intervention is, therefore, not the individual patient alone but rather the individual and one or more of the social orbits of which he is a member. The essential difference is one of emphasis and focus.

By judicious use of staff time and avoidance of long-term treatment responsibilities with those already sick, it has been possible to maintain a service that is available promptly to all those requesting help, without resort to selective intake or waiting lists. The assessment of each predicament is initiated within a few days of the request for service. In Wellesley it is now possible to carry out some work in the area of primary prevention with

---

*Direct preventive intervention in individual and family predicaments usually includes aspects of both primary and secondary prevention. For the purposes of this presentation, however, only the former aspects will be discussed.

†G. Caplan, Personal communication.

about 40 to 50 per cent of the cases. Those in need of and desiring long-term treatment are helped to find it elsewhere. A few situations in which chronic pathology is involved are carried on a follow-up basis, often in collaboration with one or more such professional caretaking resources as a physician, clergyman, or family case worker in the community.*

The ability of the clinical service to work preventively at times of crisis is greatly enhanced by the development of close, effective working relationships with a variety of professional caretakers in the community. An intensive program of education and interpretation with both professional and lay groups has led to ever-increasing community understanding and acceptance of the goals of primary prevention. Thus it has become possible to "cast the net" somewhat broadly over the population and to be available to an increasingly high proportion of those coping with emotional hazards before a psychiatric casualty has ensued.

In the following sections, for purposes of convenience in the presentation, the work is summarized in four categories: (1) appraisal of the predicament; (2) planning the intervention; (3) altering the balance of forces; (4) resolving the crisis and anticipatory planning.

APPRAISAL OF THE PREDICAMENT

As in most clinical work, the analysis of the problem and the development of a relationship proceed more or less simultaneously. The clinical alliance formed with the client as the appraisal of the predicament proceeds is basically no different from that developed in other contexts. One attempts to mobilize the ego resources of the client by overtly and explicitly enlisting him in the assessment of the predicament. He is invited to look at his own feelings and those of others in the situation, and in a successful alliance becomes a collaborator in the process of

---

*It seemed important to make this comparison with psychotherapy in the interests of those readers whose specialty is clinical diagnosis and treatment. However, the reader is asked to bear in mind that the target of preventive intervention is always a social grouping. Thus, the focus of intervention is on the interrelatedness of some or all members of an interpersonal network, often especially on those most able to effect change in the social orbit.

problem appraisal. The client's attention is also directed to the healthy aspects of the situation. By mobilizing the strengths of the individual through the clinical alliance, the attempt is made to help him to a more realistic appraisal of the predicament and of the potential inner and outer resources at his disposal.

The clinical appraisal of a predicament situation is usually somewhat more extensive than the diagnosis of individual pathology. In the analysis it is necessary to keep in mind such areas as:

1. A historical review of the interpersonal relationships in question;
2. A consideration of the personalities of those involved in the relationships, when possible by direct clinical study;
3. Some attention to the dynamics of the social orbit, both in terms of its internal patterns and its interactions with the outer world;
4. An identification of possible emotional hazards to which the individuals concerned have been exposed over the several years preceding the crisis.

PLANNING THE NATURE OF THE INTERVENTION

The process of arriving at a plan for intervention rests upon several considerations. First of all, the clinician must determine the extent to which a crisis exists, since, as was mentioned earlier, direct preventive intervention over a short period of time has not been found to be appropriate for chronic disturbances without crisis. Having so determined, the worker attempts to evaluate the actual or potential impact of the emotionally hazardous circumstances upon his client and upon other individuals in the social orbit. This step is important if one is to differentiate between symptoms that are the direct result of the impact of the hazard on the "patient" (i.e., the one in distress) and those that result from the manner in which all or part of the social orbit is attempting to cope with the hazard. If the latter, the focus of intervention in some instances must be extended to include other members of the group. Finally, the focus of intervention will depend upon the assessment of the strengths and resources available to those involved. Thus, in some instances the working through of the predicament is carried out not with the symptomatic member of the group but with one or more other persons who seem potentially in the best position to help the group cope in a healthier way with the predicament.

The work of planning the nature of the intervention is usually carried out by an extended staff team drawn from several professions. At present each predicament is discussed in conference with such other members of the staff as participants in an ecological study of neighborhoods in the community, mental health consultants familiar with each of the public schools and their clientele, team members responsible for contacts with other caretaking agencies, such as physicians, family case workers, and clergymen. In this fashion, knowledge of neighborhood patterns, community resources, and current community concerns that may have relevance to the specific predicament is added to the planning of the clinical team.

ALTERING THE BALANCE OF FORCES

As indicated earlier, the decision regarding those who will be seen during the intervention must be made primarily upon clinical grounds and rests largely upon the motivations of those involved. Those wishing direct help are offered it whenever possible. Others are sometimes seen because of the strengths they represent. Still others are occasionally seen because it is judged that their well-being may be impaired as the intervention alters the interpersonal patterns of the group. Such persons may require considerable help and support through the problem-solving phase. Otherwise, they may develop increased distress, which may be so great as to cause them to oppose needed changes or, by posing a new hazard, throw the groups again into crisis.

It should thus be clear that preventive intervention is not designed to bring about major changes in personality structure or profound alterations in psychic dynamics. It rather concerns itself, insofar as possible, with the restoration of a reasonably healthy equilibrium in a social orbit. Certain behavioral changes can and do occur within individuals as the result of alterations in their immediate human environment or perceptions of it (15). It is also possible within the limited framework of preventive intervention to help individuals

bring into play previously learned behavior patterns not being employed in the present. Though certain important intraindividual changes may occur through resolution of the crisis, it seems most appropriate and useful to think of possible changes in terms of the balance of forces within social orbits. At the present time, such alterations are tentatively classified into four groupings: (1) repeopling social space: (2) redistribution of role relationships within the group; (3) developing alternative means for interpersonal need satisfaction; (4) redefinition of the predicament.

Repeopling the Social Space

Many predicament situations arise as the result of disruptions in relationships of the kind typified by bereavement. When one or more persons have been abruptly removed from the social orbit, a crisis may erupt because interindividual demands upon group members undergo marked shifts and needs, previously satisfied through relationships no longer available, are brought to others in the group. The latter, with its newly shifting, often unpredictable patterns, may not be able to satisfy the emotional needs, often greatly heightened in intensity, presented by one or more of those bereaved. By "repeopling the social space" one means the effort to help the individual remove psychologic obstacles to the establishment of satisfactory relationships outside the group in order (1) to reduce pressures on others in the social system and (2) to facilitate the development of satisfactory object relationships with a wider range of people so as to render the person somewhat less vulnerable to separations in the future.

An example of such an effort involved contact with a mother during the period of time she was seeking a divorce from her husband, who had left the home. Presenting problem was mother's inability to handle her thirteen-year-old daughter, who had become suddenly defiant while, at the same time, showing a heightened dependence upon mother. The disturbed relationship appeared to have been precipitated by the father's departure. Mother's emotional distress was too great to permit her to help her daughter. In the course of a few months it was possible to discuss with mother the profound emotional impact upon her of the separation and divorce. She was encouraged to examine her altered interpersonal relationships and to accept the possibility of forming new ones. She took an evening school course and found a new, more congenial job, while reaching out for new social contacts through her church. Meanwhile, as her intense involvement with daughter was reduced, the latter's overdependent demands disappeared and her hostility was reduced somewhat, though mother continued to complain of the girl's occasional disobedience.

Redistribution of Role Relationships Within the Group

Predicaments often arise when, as the result of new demands upon one or more members of a group, previous patterns are no longer satisfactory. Every family, for instance, undergoes repeated alterations in parent-to-parent and parent-child relations as children develop and assume new roles and status. Occasionally, however, one or more members find it impossible to change, and serious individual and group tensions arise as old patterns persist and become increasingly maladaptive. Focus of intervention at such times may be upon the encouragement of the development of more appropriate patterns. Sifneos (14) describes a predicament in which a twenty-three-year-old student was helped in two interviews to develop an improved relationship with his overprotective mother following the student's prolonged hospitalization with tuberculosis.

Developing Alternative Means For Need Satisfaction

The goal of this approach is to help the individual secure outlets for strivings that cannot be satisfied within his present social orbit. In some cases, indeed, the very strivings of the individual or reactions resulting from their frustration, though not necessarily pathologic for the individual in question, have proved to be a pathogenic force for the group (2). Where such needs are neither entirely inappropriate nor overly intense, it often is possible for other outlets to be found in the community.

A typical situation is that of the college graduate mother who found that her strong professional career needs could no longer be set aside when her youngest child entered kindergarten. She became depressed and irritable, and consulted the service when the teacher reported the daughter in kindergarten cried frequently and seemed generally unhappy in school. The underlying predicament of the young mother struggling with the conflict between career needs and the guilt engendered by feelings of responsibility to the family is not uncommon in a suburban middle-class community. In this instance, the predicament was handled by supporting the mother as she came to recognize the conflict in which she found herself. She worked through her feelings sufficiently to seek a part-time job as a laboratory technician. Given much support and affection by the teacher, the daughter gradually became more outgoing and was happily adjusted to school by the end of the year.

Redefinition of the Predicament

Successful preventive intervention usually includes the attempt to help the individual alter his perception of the predicament. It is, however, almost essential to do so when the client is immobilized by the secondary tensions that often arise when the individual feels he has been made the passive victim of inner or outer forces not under his control. For some, such redefinition is all that is needed. With increased understanding and reduced feelings of helplessness, the individual is then able to bring his own strengths and social skills to bear upon the problem.

RESOLVING THE CRISIS AND ANTICIPATORY PLANNING

The clinical service is so conceived that, while predicament situations may be resolved, a "case" is never closed. The mental health center, concerned as it is with the population of the community, is always open for contact by any individual in that population. As a specific series of encounters draws to a close, it is made clear that the service will be available in the future should a similar or other difficulty arise. The attempt is made to interrupt the contact at a point where the proposed limited goals have been optimally attained and where a feeling of continued confidence exists towards clinician and agency. It is hoped that the image of the worker as a sympathetic but objective person may help the client assume a similar attitude when future challenges are met.

The ending phase usually is marked by a review with the client of what has been accomplished by him in the analysis and working through of the predicament.

Implications are drawn, when possible, to preferred modes of coping with future emotional hazards. In some instances arrangements are made for one or more follow-up visits or telephone contacts.

Modest success in the effort to maintain an open door policy is indicated by the fact that many individuals and families have used the service on two or more occasions for help with different predicaments. It has been observed that some families, when using the service on a later occasion, have shown both increased capacity for insight and readiness to use the kind of help offered.

RELATIONSHIP TO EGO THERAPIES AND GROUP DYNAMICS

Some distinction was made earlier between preventive intervention and various kinds of brief or ego therapies. It must also be clear from the foregoing that certain similarities exist. It is perhaps most accurate to state that preventive intervention represents an attempt to integrate elements of ego therapy and aspects of group analysis, most especially those focused upon role relationship patterns and communication processes. It is, indeed, hypothesized that the ability of the individual to cope with the problem may, by adding to his sense of personal worth and competence, increase his ability to deal with future stress—a capacity of the ego that we have termed "stability" (3).

Similarly, it would appear that success of the group in crisis resolution may add significantly to its integrative ability and morale in the face of new challenges. Rather than simply restoring a previous group equilibrium, it often seems possible to help those involved to develop an even more suitable distribution of roles and functions than had previously been possible. Therefore, direct preventive intervention, as it has developed over the past several years, has tended to combine elements of ego therapy with those aspects of group work that stress the integrative, morale-building processes in group life.

EVALUATION AND DISCUSSION

A full-scale evaluation of preventive intervention is for obvious reasons very difficult and, in any case, must await a fuller development of the method itself. However, the clinical assessment of work with individual cases has reflected what seems to be a reasonable degree of success in most instances. Sifneos summarizes his impressions of 108 cases seen for preventive intervention in Wellesley as follows:

> Most . . . faced hazardous situations. Most . . . were aware of painful emotions, and unable to deal with them successfully, had developed emotional crises. In some cases their reactions to these crises turned out to be fairly successful and with psychiatric help they quickly returned to a state of emotional equilibrium. In other cases a series of maladaptive reactions progressively lead to the development of psychiatric symptoms. They required long psychotherapy and at times hospitalization (14).

A surprisingly high proportion of predicaments involves the occurrence of *multiple hazards*. A rapid succession of several crises, such as multiple bereavements over a short period of time, often lead to requests for preventive intervention. These situations are reminiscent of the popular expression, "It never rains but what it pours!" which suggests that difficulties, however minor or resolvable individually, are apt to be inundating if confronted in series. By contrast, it is noteworthy that successful mastery of emotional hazards oftentimes appears to enhance emotional stability, by which we mean the ability to cope with later challenges. We have wondered whether a matter of timing is involved. It is possible that family and other groups require periods of equilibrium during which patterned modes of interpersonal behavior can become more or less habituated, freeing each individual to devote his energies to personal growth, meeting the needs of others in the social orbit, work, reaching out for new experiences and relationships, and the like. Otherwise, psychologic "vigilance" and a resulting tension state must be maintained over unduly long time periods. A series of emotional hazards may interfere with the development of habituated modes of interpersonal behavior in the group, with the end result of heightened irritability, decreased efficiency, inability to meet the psychologic needs of others, physiologic damage and, in some instances, ultimate psychologic collapse.

It is hoped that in the years to come an increasingly high proportion of requests will be made by clients for *anticipatory guidance* and health planning. Community-wide education and interpretation of the preventive nature of the mental health service have led in past years to contacts with a few families wishing help with imminent hazards. These families understood and accepted the concept of primary prevention in mental health. They came because they wished to forestall, if possible, emotional difficulties that they believed might result from some impending stress.

A compelling instance involved a mother, suffering from terminal cancer, who was concerned about the impact of the illness and death upon her nine-year-old daughter. The girl had been suffering from nightmares in which the girl, her house, and her family were threatened with destruction by gigantic, indescribable animals. The nightmares in an otherwise apparently happy and well-adjusted child worried the mother. The latter wished to be sure that her husband and daughter would be helped through their bereavement, if such help were needed. A few contacts with the father and child were made during the final weeks of the illness. The mother herself was seen regularly as long as her condition permitted, both at home and in hospital. Following mother's death, the father was seen three times over a two-month period. The nightmares disappeared and follow-up contacts indicated that the family unit was successfully reintegrated without impairment of the daughter's mental health.

The efforts described above may to some appear to reflect the current trend toward abandonment of the never totally accurate distinction between the intrapsychic focus of psychoanalysis and the environmental focus of social work. There is more involved, however, than the simple summation of intrapsychic and environmental preoccupations. Rather, there is emerging an interactional orientation viewing the individual organism both from a developmental perspective and from the standpoint of the reciprocal nature of relationships between individuals. Modern dynamic role theory has provided some needed theoretic underpinnings. It has also been increasingly imperative to extend the search to *patterns* of interplay between individuals, groups, organizations, institutions, and, in the final analysis, values in the population.

Some may have felt that the focus on individual-environment equilibrium has been unduly tinted by the blackness of bereavement (from whose study came much of the early impetus). Is life to be viewed mainly as a series of emotionally hazardous circumstances? Is the individual to be seen as hurtling from one dire psychologic threat to another? The authors have attempted to indicate that they look upon emotional hazards in broad, population-oriented terms. To paraphrase an old adage: "Many men's meat may be a few men's poison." The term *hazard* is used to indicate that, under certain circumstances, some events may induce emotional crises in some (ultimately predictable) proportion of those exposed. The fact is that certain experiences are at least temporarily disorganizing for most. On this observation is founded the essentially optimistic bias of the work. The disorganization offers the opportunity to re-examine and, if necessary, abandon old ways of coping. It provides motivation for change, for the assumption of new, emotionally more satisfying roles and relationships.

One can conceive possible danger in the widespread adoption of a word as negatively tinged as hazard. It is that there might be induced a tendency to avoid change and eschew new experience in the hope of escaping psychic injury. In view of parental anxieties ascribed to emphasis upon the traumatic experiences of early childhood, such a concern seems plausible. Experience indicates, however, that the orientation tends to be supportive rather than anxiety-producing. It organizes life experience meaningfully, just as concepts of nutrition and disease transmission have helped lay people take scientifically valid as versus magical precautions against disease. Furthermore, it enables professional caretakers as well as mental health personnel to participate more meaningfully in the supportive structure of communities.

Such a supportive structure would, on the one hand, provide certain safeguards against dangers and, on the other hand, make available the tools (psychologic, social, and physical) necessary for meeting the challenges and opportunities afforded by the hazardous circumstance. This twofold concept of environmental supports underlies the work herein described. We are indebted to Dr. Barbara Biber for a useful analogy. The supports at time of emotional hazard can be likened to parental responsibilities at a beach picnic: on the one hand, to keep the child from such dangers as drowning or becoming lost; on the other hand, to provide those tools best suited to the child's opportunity to use the environment to the optimum, as for example planning ahead to bring along the long-handled shovel that allows the child to dig holes far deeper than he could possibly accomplish in park or sandbox. Thus, it is clear that hazards provide opportunities for promotion of emotional growth as well as the occasions for preventive measures.

References

1. Gruber, S. The concept of task-orientation in the analysis of play behavior of children entering kindergarten. *Am. J. Orthopsychiat., 24:* 326, 1954.
2. Gruenberg, E. "Socially Shared Psychopathology." In Leighton, A., Clausen, J., and Wilson, R. (eds.), *Explorations in Social Psychiatry.* New York: Basic Books, 1957.
3. Klein, D. Some concepts concerning the mental health of the individual. *J. Consult. Psychol., 24:* 4, 1960.
4. Klein, D., and Ross, A. "Kindergarten Entry: A Study of Role Transition and its Effects on Children and Their Families." In Krugman, M. (ed.), *Orthopsychiatry and the School.* New York: Amer. Orthopsychiatric Association, 1958.
5. Lindemann, E. Symptomatology and management of acute grief. *Am. J. Psychiat., 101:* 141, 1944.
6. Lindemann, E. "The Wellesley Project for the Study of Certain Problems in Community Mental Health." In *Interrelations between the Social Environment and Psychiatric Disorders.* New York: Milbank Memorial Fund, 1953.
7. McGinnis, M. The Wellesley project of pre-school emotional assessment. *J. Psychiat. Soc. Work, 23:* 135, 1954.
8. Naegele, K. "A Mental Health Project in a Boston Suburb." In Paul, B. (ed.), *Health, Culture, and Community: a Book of Cases.* New York: Russell Sage Foundation, 1956.
9. Rosenberg, P., and Fuller, M. Dynamic analysis of the student nurse. *Group Psychother., 10:* 22, 1957.
10. Rosenberg, P., and Fuller, M. Human relations seminar: A group work experiment in nursing education. *Ment. Hyg., 39:* 406, 1955.
11. Rosenberg, P., and Fuller, M. Human relations seminar for nursing students. *Nursing Outlook, 5:* 724, 1957.
12. Rosenberg, P., and Fuller, M. Seminar is student nurses' safety valve. *Modern Hospital, 85:* 53, 1955.
13. Ross, A., and Lindemann, E. "A Follow-up Study of a Predictive Test of Social Adaptation in Preschool Children." In Caplan, G. (ed.), *Emotional Problems of Early Childhood.* New York: Basic Books, 1955.
14. Sifneos, P. A concept of "emotional crisis." *Ment. Hyg., 44* (2): 169, 1960.
15. Stanton, A., and Schwartz, M. *The Mental Hospital.* New York: Basic Books, 1954.
16. Vaughan, W., and Faber, E. Field methods and techniques—the systematic observation of kindergarten children. *Human Organization, 11:* 33, 1952.

Sociocultural Theories

CRITICAL EVALUATION

Critical papers by an eminent sociologist, Warren Dunham, and a highly esteemed psychoanalyst, Lawrence Kubie, close our presentation of sociocultural theories. Both men have had distinguished careers and bring their broad experience to bear on questions of whether social and community approaches are feasible or efficacious. More specifically, they ask: Will there be acceptance of the ideologies and proposals of these new professional leaders in the community? What solid evidence is there that abstract psychological principles will generate changes in the social system that are "better" than those currently in existence? Is a program geared to shorter hospitalization, closer to the patient's home, demonstrably superior to traditional approaches? What sound and proven theories do the community psychiatrist and psychologist possess to justify faith in their plans?

49. Community Psychiatry: The Newest Therapeutic Bandwagon

H. WARREN DUNHAM

The proposal to add community psychiatry to the ever-widening list of psychiatric specialties deserves a critical examination. Thus, my purpose in this paper is fourfold. First, I intend to examine the nature of community psychiatry as it is taking shape. Second, I want to consider our continuing uncertainty about mental illness which is manifested in a widening of its definition. Third, I discuss some of the historical landmarks and cultural forces that have brought about the proposal for this new subspecialty of psychiatry. Finally, I examine some of its hidden aspects with respect to the future role of psychiatry.

COMMUNITY PSYCHIATRY—THE NEWEST SUBSPECIALTY

Let us begin by examining the nature of community psychiatry that is appar-ently emerging as judged by a mounting chorus of voices from those who jump on any bandwagon as long as it is moving. In doing this I will focus first on community psychiatry in relation to community mental health and the various programs, plans, and social actions that are currently getting under way, with emphases that are as varied as the cultural-regional contrasts of American society.

A pattern concerned with maximizing treatment potential for the mentally ill is gradually taking shape. This newest emphasis points to a declining role of the traditional state hospital and the rise of the community mental health center with all of the attendant auxiliary services essential for the treatment of the mentally ill. In its ideal form the community mental health center would provide psychiatric services, both diagnostic and treatment, for all age groups and for both inpatients and outpatients in a particular community. In addition, the center would have attached closely to it day and night hospitals, convalescent homes, rehabilitative programs or, for that matter, any service

From *Archives of General Psychiatry*, 1965, *12*, 303–313. Copyright 1965, American Medical Association. Reprinted by permission.

that helps toward the maximizing of treatment potential with respect to the characteristics of the population that it is designed to serve. Also attached to this center would be several kinds of research activities aimed at evaluating and experimenting with old and new therapeutic procedures. In the background would still be the state hospital which would, in all likelihood, become the recipient for those patients who seemingly defy all efforts with available therapeutic techniques to fit them back into family and community with an assurance of safety to themselves and others. This reorganization of psychiatric facilities as a community mental health program also implies an increased and workable coordination of the diverse social agencies in the community toward the end of detecting and referring those persons who need psychiatric help.

This ideal structure does appear to be oriented toward the urban community. Therefore, the need arises to clarify the size and type of the population that would be served. Further, a breakdown of the population into the several age and sex categories along with several projected estimates of the number of mentally ill persons that will occur in these population categories would be required. Estimates should be made for the psychoneuroses, the psychoses, the psychopathies, the mentally retarded, and the geriatrics cases that will be found in a community.

Indeed, we should attempt to mobilize and to organize our psychiatric resources in such a manner that they will maximize our existing therapeutic potential for any community. At all events, such a structure seems to suggest to certain professionals at the National Institute of Mental Health that if there comes into existence a realistic community mental health program, there must be a community psychiatry that knows how to use it. While the logic here escapes me, it seems to be quite clear to Viola Bernard who states that, "Recognition of the need to augment the conventional training for mental health personnel to equip them for the newer function of community mental health practice parallels wide-scale trends toward more effective treatment methods at the collective level to augment one-to-one clinical approaches" (3). Dr. Bernard goes on to say that community psychiatry can be regarded as a subspe-

cialty of psychiatry and that it embraces three major subdivisions—social psychiatry, administrative psychiatry, and public health psychiatry.

While Dr. Bernard may see clearly the nature of a community psychiatry that transcends the traditional one-to-one clinical approach, this is not the case with departments of psychiatry in some medical schools as the recent National Institute of Mental Health survey attests (10). In reviewing the limited literature it is all too clear that different conceptions abound as to what community psychiatry is and while these conceptions are not always inconsistent they nevertheless attest to the fact that the dimensions of the proposed new subspecialty are by no means clear-cut. These conceptions range all the way from the idea that community psychiatry means bringing psychiatric techniques and treatments to the indigent persons in the community to the notion that community psychiatry should involve the education of policemen, teachers, public health nurses, politicians, and junior executives in mental hygiene principles. A mere listing of some of the conceptions of what has been placed under the community psychiatry umbrella will give a further notion of this uncertainty. Community psychiatry has been regarded as encompassing (1) the community base mental hospital, (2) short-term mental hospitalization, (3) attempts to move the chronically hospitalized patient and return him to the community, (4) the integration of various community health services, (5) psychiatric counseling and services to nonpsychiatric institutions such as schools, police departments, industries, and the like, (6) the development of devices for maintaining mental patients in the community, (7) reorganization and administration of community mental health programs, and finally (8) the establishment of auxiliary services to community mental hospitals, such as outpatient clinics, day hospitals, night hospitals, home psychiatric visits, and the utilization of auxiliary psychiatric personnel in treatment programs (10).

Perhaps we can come close to what someone visualizes as the content of community psychiatry by quoting an announcement of an opening for a fellowship in community psychiatry in Minnesota. In the announcement the program is described as follows: "One year of diversified training and experience, including all aspects of community organization, consultation, and training techniques, administration, research and mass communication media.'' Such a psychiatric residency program certainly represents a great difference from the more traditional training program and points to a type of training that might be more fitting for a person who wants to specialize in community organization.

There is no clearer support for this conception than Leonard Duhl's paper (6) where he discusses the training problems for community psychiatry. In this paper he speaks of three contracts that the psychiatrist has, the traditional one with the patient, the more infrequent one with the family, and still more infrequent one with the community. In connection with his community contract, the psychiatrist states, according to Duhl, ''I will try to lower the rate of illness and maximize the health of this population.'' Duhl continues, and I quote, because the direction is most significant.

In preparing psychiatrists for these broadened contracts, a new set of skills must be communicated. For example, he must learn how to be consultant to a community, an institution, or a group without being patient-oriented. Rather, he must have the community's needs in central focus. He must be prepared for situations where he is expected to contribute to planning for services and programs, both in his field and in others, that are related: what information is needed; how it is gathered; what resources are available and so forth. Epidemiology, survey research and planning skills must be passed on to him. He must be prepared to find that people in other fields, such as the legislature often affect a program more than his profession does. He must find himself at home in the world of economics, political science, politics, planning, and all forms of social action (6, p. 6).

While these remarks of Bernard and Duhl may not represent any final statement as to what community psychiatry will become, they point to a probable direction that this newest addition to psychiatric subspecialties may take. However, in this conception of the community psychiatrist as a person skilled in the techniques of social action there lie so many uncertainties, unresolved issues, and hidden assumptions that it is difficult to determine where it will be most effective to start the analysis, with the role of the psychiatrist or with the nature of the community.

Perhaps sociologists can garner some small satisfaction in the fact that the psychiatrist finally has discovered the community—something that the sociologist has been studying and reporting on for over half a century in the United States. However, once the psychiatrist makes this discovery he must ask himself what he can do with it in the light of his professional task, how the discovery will affect his traditional professional role, and how working on or in the community structure can improve the mental health level of its people. Now, it seems that those leaders of psychiatry who are proposing this new subspecialty imply several things at the same time and are vague about all of them. They seem to be saying, in one form or another, the following:

1. We, psychiatrists, must know the community and learn how to work with the various groups and social strata composing it so that we can help to secure and organize the necessary psychiatric facilities that will serve to maximize the treatment potential for the mentally ill.

2. We must know the community because the community is composed of families which, through the interaction of their members, evolve those events and processes that in a given context have a pathic effect upon some of the persons who compose them.

3. We must know the community in order to develop more effective methods of treatment at the ''collective level,'' to eliminate mentally disorganizing social relationships, and to achieve a type of community organization that is most conducive to the preservation of mental health.

4. We must know the community if we are ever to make any headway in the prevention of mental illness. For we hold that in the multiple groups, families, and social institutions which compose the community, there are numerous unhealthy interpersonal relationships, pathological attitudes and beliefs, cultural conflicts and tensions, and unhealthy child training practices that make for the development of mental and emotional disturbances in the person.

An analysis of our first implication shows that no new burden is placed upon the psychiatrist but it merely emphasizes his role as a citizen—a role that, like any person in the society, he always has had. It merely emphasizes that the psychiatrist will take a more active part in working with other professionals in the community such as lawyers, teachers, social workers, ministers, labor leaders, and business men in achieving an organization of psychiatric facilities that will maximize the therapeutic potential in a given community. To be sure it means that in working with such persons and groups, he will contribute his own professional knowledge and insights in the attempt to obtain and to organize the psychiatric facilities in such a manner as to achieve a maximum therapeutic potential. Thus, this is hardly a new role for the psychiatrist. It only becomes sharper at this moment in history when a social change in the care and treatment of the mentally ill is impending, namely, a shift from a situation that emphasized the removal of the mental patient from the community to one that attempts to deal with him in the community and family setting and to keep active and intact his ties with these social structures.

The second implication is routine in the light of the orientation of much of contemporary psychiatry. Here, attention is merely called to the theory that stresses the atypical qualities of the family drama for providing an etiological push for the development of the several psychoneuroses, character disorders, adult behavior disturbances and in certain instances, psychotic reactions. Thus, it follows that to change or correct the condition found in the person, some attention must be paid to the family as a collectivity, in order to grasp and then modify those attitudes, behavior patterns, identifications, and emotional attachments that supposedly have a pathogenic effect on the family members. From the focus on the family the concern then extends to the larger community in an attempt to discover the degree to which the family is integrated in or alienated from it.

However, it is in the third implication that many probing questions arise. For here the conception is implicit that the community is the patient and consequently, the necessity arises to develop techniques that can be used in treating the community toward the end of supplementing the traditional one-to-one psychiatric relationship. This position also implies a certain etiological view, namely, that within the texture of those institutional arrangements that make up the community there exist dysfunctional processes, subcultures with unhealthy value complexes, specific institutional tensions, various ideological conflicts along age, sex, ethnic, racial and political axes, occasional cultural crises, and an increasing tempo of social change that in their functional interrelationships provide a pathogenic social environment. Thus, when these elements are incorporated into the experience of the persons, especially during their early and adolescent years, they emerge as abnormal forms of traits, attitudes, thought processes, and behavior patterns. In a theoretical vein, this is the Merton (17) paradigm wherein he attempts to show the diverse modes of adaptation that arise as a result of the various patterns of discrepancy between institutional means and cultural goals.

The influence of the social milieu in shaping, organizing, and integrating the personality structure, of course, has been recognized for a long time. What is not so clear, however, is the manner in which such knowledge can be utilized in working at the community level to treat the mental and emotional maladjustments that are continually appearing. In addition, the nature and function of those factors in the social milieu contributing to the production of the bona fide psychotics are by no means established.

These issues point to some very pressing queries. What are the possible techniques that can be developed to treat the "collectivity"? Why do psychiatrists think that it is possible to treat the "collectivity" when there still exists a marked uncertainty with respect to the treatment and cure of the individual case? What causes the psychiatrist to think that if he advances certain techniques for treating the "collectivity," they will have community acceptance? If he begins to "treat" a group through discussions in order to develop personal insights, what assurances does he have that the results will be psychologically beneficial to the persons? Does the psychiatrist know how to organize a community along mentally hygienic lines and if he does, what evidence does he have that such an organization will be an improvement over the existing organization? In what institutional setting or in what cultural milieu would the psychiatrist expect to begin in order to move toward more healthy social relationships in the community? These are serious questions and I raise them with reference to the notion that the community is the patient.

If a psychiatrist thinks that he can organize the community to move it toward a more healthy state I suggest that he run for some public office. This would certainly add to his experience and give him some conception as to whether or not the community is ready to be moved in the direction that he regards as mentally hygienic. If he should decide on such a step he will be successful to the extent that he jokingly refers to himself as a "head shrinker" and that he becomes acceptable as "one of the boys." But if he does, he functions as an independent citizen, in harmony with our democratic ethos, bringing his professional knowledge to bear on the goal he has set for himself and his constituents. However, successful or not, he will certainly achieve a new insight concerning the complexity involved in treating the community as the patient.

While I have poked at this proposition from the standpoint of politics, let me consider it with respect to education. If this becomes the medium by which the pathology of the community is to be arrested, one can assume that it means adding to and raising the quality of the educational system in the community. The dissemination of psychiatric information with respect to signs and symptoms, the desirability of early treatment, the natural character of mental illness, the therapeutic benefits of the new drugs, and the correct mental hygiene principles of child training have been going on not only through the usual community lectures and formal educational channels but also by means of the mass media—radio, television, the newspapers, and the slick magazines. I hasten to add, however, that this may not be to the advantage of the community, for it may do nothing else but raise the level of anxiety among certain middle-class persons, who, when they read an article on the correct procedure for bringing up children realize that they have done all the wrong things. Also, the media are frequently sources of misinformation and sometimes imply a promise that psychiatry cannot fulfill.

Further, I observe that in this proposal for a community psychiatry, the psychiatrist seems to be enmeshed in the same cultural vortex as is the professor.

For it is becoming fashionable for a professor to measure his success in having hardly any contact with students—he is too busy on larger undertakings, research, consultations, conferences, and the like. Likewise, some psychiatrists think that they have arrived if they have no contact with patients. For example, I have heard of one psychiatrist who has not seen a patient for several years—he spends his time educating teachers, nurses, policemen, business men, and the laity in psychiatric principles.

The third and fourth implications of the new focus provided by community psychiatry are closely related because each position partially views the structures and processes of the community as containing certain etiological elements that make for the development of certain types of mental and emotional illness. However, the third implication, as we have shown, points to the development of treatment techniques on the collective level, while the fourth emphasizes that knowledge of the community is essential if mental illness is ever to be prevented.

There is no doubt that the word prevention falling on the ears of well-intentioned Americans, is just what the doctor ordered. It is so hopeful that no one, I am sure, will deny that if we can prevent our pathologies this is far better than sitting back and waiting for them to develop. But, of course, there is a catch. How are we going to take the first preventive actions if we are still uncertain about the causes of mental disorders? How do we know where to even cut into a community's round of life? And if we did cut in, what assurance do we have that the results might not be completely the opposite to those anticipated? Of course, there is always secondary prevention —that is, directing our efforts to preventing a recurrence of illness in persons who have once been sick. This is a laudable goal but in connection with mental and emotional disturbances we are still uncertain as to the success of our original treatment efforts.

PREVENTION OF BEHAVIORAL PATHOLOGY—SOME PREVIOUS EFFORTS

There is no doubt that the possibility of prevention is something that will continue to intrigue us for years to come. Therefore, it is not without point to take a look at several other programs that, while they have not all been exclusively oriented toward the treatment of the community, have been launched with the hope of preventing the occurrence of certain unacceptable behavior on the part of the members of a community. I cite two experiments which are widely known with respect to the prevention of delinquency.

The first is Kobrin's statement concerning the 25 year assessment of the Chicago Area Project (15). Kobrin has presented us with a straightforward, modest, and sophisticated account of the accumulated experience provided by this project in the efforts to bring about a greater control of delinquency in certain areas of Chicago. This project has been significant on several counts, but in my judgment its greatest significance was that it helped to initiate various types of community organizational programs that logically proceeded from an empirically developed theory of delinquency. This theory, in general, viewed delinquency as primarily a "breakdown of the machinery of spontaneous social control." The theory stressed that delinquency was adaptive behavior on the part of adolescents in their peer groups in their efforts to achieve meaningful and respected adult roles, "unaided by the older generation and under the influence of criminal models for whom the intercity areas furnish a haven." This theory, in turn, rests upon certain postulates of sociological theory which emphasize that the development and control of conduct are determined by the network of primary relationships in which one's daily existence is embedded.

The significance of this experiment was that this theory of delinquency provided a rationalization for cutting into the community at certain points and seeking persons there who were ready to organize themselves to secure a higher level of welfare for themselves and their children. The results of this experiment are relevant to those advocators of the preventive function of a community psychiatry because there was not only the difficulty of determining what actually had been accomplished in the way of the prevention of delinquency but also a difficulty in assessing the experience in relation to community welfare.

Kobrin, in his opening sentence has stated this problem most cogently.

The Chicago Area Project shares with other delinquency prevention programs the difficulty of measuring its success in a simple and direct manner. At bottom this difficulty rests on the fact that such programs, as efforts to intervene in the life of a person, a group, or a community, cannot by their very nature, constitute more than a subsidiary element in changing the fundamental and sweeping forces which create the problems of groups and of persons or which shape human personality. Decline in rates of delinquents—the only conclusive way to evaluate delinquency prevention —may reflect influences unconnected with those of organized programs and are difficult to define and measure (15).

The point here is that in a carefully worked out plan based upon an empirically constructed theory it is difficult to determine what has been achieved. One can hazard the observation that if this is true with respect to delinquent behavior where mounting evidence has always supported the idea that its roots are deeply enmeshed in the network of social relationships, how much more difficult it will be in the field of psychiatry to make an assessment in preventive efforts when we are much more uncertain concerning the etiological foundations of those cases which appear in psychiatric offices, clinics, and hospitals.

The well-known Cambridge-Somerville Youth Study (19) provides the second example of a delinquency prevention program. While this study did not focus upon the community as such but rather on certain persons therein, it did proceed from a conception of a relationship between a person's needs and a treatment framework for administering to those needs. In this study an attempt was made to provide a warm, human, and continuing relationship between an assigned counsellor and a sample of delinquents and to withhold this relationship from another comparable matched sample. These relationships with most of the boys in the treatment group lasted for approximately eight years. At the conclusion of the experiment there was an attempt to assess the results. These were mainly negative. The number of boys in the treatment group appearing before the crime prevention bureau of the police department were slightly in excess of the number of boys making such appearances in the control group. The only positive note was that the boys in the control group were somewhat more active as recidivists than were the boys in the treatment group.

Although the results of this study were inconclusive and told us nothing particularly about the communities to which these boys were reacting, they did document the failure of one type of relationship therapy to reduce delinquency. While these results provide no final word they do point up the necessity for the various techniques in psychiatry to first acquire a far greater effectiveness than they now possess before starting to operate on a community level where there will be a great deal of fumbling in the dark before knowing exactly what to do.

It seems most appropriate in the light of the task envisioned for community psychiatry to call attention to the professional excitement that was engendered when the Commonwealth Fund inaugurated a child-guidance program in 1922. The Child Guidance Clinic was hailed as a step that eventually should have far-reaching consequences. For who saw fit to deny at that time in the light of certain prevailing theories and the optimism provided by the cultural ethos of the United States that if emotional, mental, and behavioral disturbances were ever to be arrested and prevented at the adult level it would be necessary to arrest these tendencies at their incipient stage, namely, in childhood. This all appears most logical and reasonable. However, 40 years after the opening of the first child guidance clinic we have such clinics in almost every state and they are very much utilized as evidenced by the long waiting lists. Nevertheless, not only does juvenile delinquency remain a continuing community problem but also the adult incidence rates of at least the major psychoses appear to remain approximately constant during this period, especially if the study by Goldhamer and Marshall (9) is accepted as valid.

I cite these three different kinds of experience primarily for the purpose of emphasizing the necessity to review our past efforts in attacking certain behavioral problems at a community level and also to point to some of the difficulties that are inherent in any proposal that emphasizes the development of psychiatric treatment techniques for the "collective level."

THE WIDENING DEFINITION OF MENTAL ILLNESS

Efforts in the direction of carving out a subspecialty of psychiatry known as community psychiatry take place in a cultural atmosphere which has seen a definite attempt to widen the definition of what constitutes mental illness. This is shown by the tendency in our society to place any recognized deviant behavior into the sick role. By doing this we not only supposedly understand them, but we can also point to therapies which will be appropriate for their treatment. Thus, the past two decades have witnessed attempts to place in the sick role delinquents, sex offenders, alcoholics, drug addicts, beatniks, communists, the racially prejudiced, and in fact, practically all persons who do not fit into the prevailing togetherness that we like to think characterizes middle-class American life. The danger here is that we only add to our state of confusion because the line between who is sick and who is well becomes increasingly a waving, uncertain one. Thus, we appear to be constantly moving the cutting point toward the end of the continuum that would include those persons who in some subcultural milieus are accepted as normal.

There is much current statistical evidence that supports this notion of a widening definition for mental illness. For example, if one examines the community epidemiological surveys of mental illness in the 1930's and compares them with the community epidemiological surveys in the 1950's one is struck with the fact that four to five times more cases are reported in the latter years (18, p. 90). In my own epidemiological study of schizophrenia, where I have examined many epidemiological studies from all over the world I have noted the great differences that are reported with respect to total mental disorders in the surveys, a marked decrease in the differences between the surveys when only psychoses are reported and a still further decrease in the rate variations when the reports are based upon only one mental disorder, namely, schizophrenia. In this latter case, the variations are slight and all of the rates are quite close together. One might point to the Mid-town Manhattan Survey (20) where two psychiatrists reviewing symptom schedules on a sample population as collected by field workers found that approximately 80 per cent of the sample were suffering from some type of psychiatric symptom. This extreme figure can be contrasted with the 20 per cent reported as incapacitated. The providing of adequate psychiatric services for even the latter figure would place an impossible burden on any community.

Several factors help to explain this widening definition of mental illness which has been so apparent during the past two decades. One factor, of course, has been the adaptation of psychiatry to office practice following World War II (1). Another factor is that the mounting frustration resulting from the failures to achieve therapeutic results with the bona fide psychotics has led to a widening of the psychiatric net in order to include those persons with minor emotional disturbances who are more responsive to existing treatment techniques. These people are suffering from what has been termed "problems of living," and they do not represent the bona fide mentally ill cases (22). In this connection it is interesting to note that George W. Albee, at an American Medical Association meeting in Chicago, stated:

What we clearly do not need more of in the mental health profession are people who go into private practice of psychotherapy with middle-aged neurotics in high income suburbs. While there are humanitarian and ethical reasons for offering all the help we possibly can to individuals afflicted with mental disorders, it seems unlikely that we will ever have the manpower to offer individual care on any kind of manageable ratio of therapists to sufferers.

In the light of Albee's observation it is instructive to note Paul Hoch's evaluation of the therapeutic accomplishments of mental health clinics in New York State (11). With respect to psychotherapeutic techniques he states:

I do not mean to deny that psychotherapy brings relief to those suffering from emotional disorders or that it may not be the treatment of choice in certain cases. What I am questioning is the preoccupation with intensive psychotherapy in clinics which are part of the community health program. After more than fifty years of its utilization we still have no foolproof measure of its effectiveness, of its superiority over other forms of treatment or even that a long term is better than brief psychotherapy (11).

He goes on to point out that while in the previous year 30,000 patients were released from the state hospital, nevertheless, only 8 per cent of the cases that were terminated by psychiatric clinics came from inpatient facilities. He notes also that the volume of patients being treated in the state hospitals is greater than ever before, in spite of an almost unanimous need to develop alternatives to state hospital care. His evidence supports this contention of a widening definition of mental illness, implying that the outpatient clinics are not treating cases that are likely to need hospital care but are treating numerous cases that are experiencing emotional problems. These are, for the most part, tied up with the daily round of human existence and can never be completely eliminated except in a societal utopia. One conclusion appears inescapable—the more clinics, the more patients. In addition, this widening definition of mental illness has served as a type of fuel for the development of the idea of a community psychiatry.

SOME HIDDEN ASPECTS FOR THE FUTURE ROLE OF PSYCHIATRY

In this account I have pointed to the several conceptions which seem to be implied in the development of a community psychiatry. I have emphasized that the tying of community psychiatry with the several evolving plans throughout the country to reorganize the mental health facilities toward the end of maximizing treatment potential is a significant move. While there is the question as to whether community psychiatry extends beyond current psychiatric practices there may be a gain in identifying the psychiatrist more closely with the different community services and breaking down the isolation in which both the psychoanalytic practitioner and the hospital practicing psychiatrist have been enmeshed. This would move the psychiatrist not only closer to the patient but what is more important, closer to the entire network of interpersonal relationships of the family and the community in which the patient is involved.

However, it is in the other visions that have been held up for community psychiatry wherein I think, as I have indicated, great difficulties are in the offing. Here I am most skeptical concerning the adequacy of our knowledge to develop significant techniques for treating social collectivities or for developing techniques on the community level that will really result in a reduction of mental disturbances in the community. It seems that such expectations are likely to remove the psychiatrist still further from the more bona fide cases of mental illnesses that develop within the community context. Much of his effort will be spent on dealing with the noncritical cases. This trend has already been going on for some time as I have indicated in discussing the widening definition of mental illness. Until we have a more sound knowledge which will indicate that the minor emotional disturbances are likely to develop into the more serious types of mental disturbances we will be dissipating much of our collective psychiatric efforts.

Then, too, there is another hidden aspect of these projected conceptions of community psychiatry which deserves careful exploration. I refer to the implication that the psychiatrist will be able to move into the ongoing power structure of a community. The profession must confront the issue as to whether its effectiveness will be less or greater if some of its members should succeed in obtaining roles within the power structure of any community. Here, I would suggest that such a psychiatrist would find himself in a system where his professional effectiveness would be considerably reduced because he would be involved in a series of mutual obligations and expectations in relation to the other persons composing the power structure. He would thus lose the role that in general characterizes the professional in other areas, that of being an adviser and a consultant with respect to any psychiatric problems or issues that the groups, institutions, and associations of the community confront. What I am trying to indicate is that in becoming a part of the power structure he is likely to lose more than he gains. That is, his gains would be in respect to power, personal prestige, and recognition but his losses would be in the growing rustiness of his diagnostic and therapeutic skills with patients.

Another implication of these aspects of community psychiatry is the fact that psychiatrists are being pushed in a direction not entirely of their own making. The national efforts and monies that are being directed to the states and communities for the reorganization of the mental health facilities have engendered a high degree of excitement among professional social workers, mental health educators, psychiatric nurses, and numerous well-intentioned persons who see new professional opportunities for service and careers. Thus, the psychiatrist is led to think, because of these pressures, that he should prepare himself with new skills in order to provide the required leadership to these various professionals who are planning to work toward this new vision to maximize the treatment potential in the community for the mentally ill.

Finally, there is the implication that psychiatry is being utilized to move us closer in the direction of the welfare state. This may not be undesirable in itself but it seems most essential that psychiatrists should be aware of the role that they are asked to play. We can anticipate that while the doctor-patient relationship will still be paramount in most medical practice the psychiatrist is likely to move into roles unforeseen but which will be required by the new structural organization of psychiatric facilities with the proposal for a community psychiatry. In such new roles the psychiatrists may become agents for social control, thus sacrificing the main task for which their education has fitted them.

In this paper I have attempted to show the link between community psychiatry and the new evolving community mental health programs. While one can see in this linkage a most significant development I am somewhat skeptical toward those emphases in community psychiatry which aim at the development of treatment techniques on the community level. In discussing the widening definition of mental illness I have tried to show that this is one of the crucial factors that has accounted for this movement toward a new type of psychiatric specialty. I have seen, in this widening definition, an opportunity to overcome a frustration that engulfs psychiatrists with respect to their inability to make much therapeutic headway with the traditional mental cases. Finally, I have attempted to consider some of the hidden implications for psychiatry in the proposal for this new psychiatric specialty.

References

1. Barton, W. E. Presidential address—Psychiatry in transition. *Amer. J. Psychiat.*, 1962, *119:* 1–15.
2. Belknap, I. *Human problems of state mental hospital.* New York: McGraw-Hill, 1956.
3. Bernard, V. Some interrelationships of training for community psychiatry, community mental health programs and research in social psychiatry. In *Proceedings of Third World Congress of psychiatry.* Montreal, Canada: McGill University and University of Toronto Press, 1961. Vol. 3, pp. 67–71.

4. Caudill, W. *Psychiatric hospital as a small society.* Cambridge: Harvard University Press, 1958.

5. Cumming, J., and Cumming, E. *Closed ranks: Experiment in mental health education.* Cambridge: Harvard University Press, Commonwealth Fund, 1957.

6. Duhl, L. J. Problems in training psychiatric residents in community psychiatry. Paper read before the Institute on Training in Community Psychiatry at University of California, Texas, Columbia, and Chicago, mimeographed, Fall-Winter, 1963–1964.

7. Dunham, H. W. *Sociological theory and mental disorder.* Detroit: Wayne State University Press, 1959, Chap. 6.

8. Dunham, H. W., and Weinberg, S. K. *Culture of state mental hospital.* Detroit: Wayne State University Press, 1960.

9. Goldhamer, H., and Marshall, A. *Psychoses and civilization.* Glencoe, Ill.: Free Press, 1953.

10. Goldston, S. E. Training in community psychiatry: Survey report of medical school departments of psychiatry. *Amer. J. Psychiat.*, 1964, *120:*789–92.

11. Hoch, P. H. In therapeutic accomplishments of mental health clinics. *Ment. Hyg. News.* June, 1963, pp. 1–3.

12. Joint Commission on Mental Illness and Health. *Action for Mental Health.* New York: Basic Books, 1961.

13. Jones, M. *Therapeutic community: New treatment method in psychiatry.* New York: Basic Books, 1953.

14. Kennedy, J. F. Message from President of United States relative to mental illness and mental retardation: February 5, 1963. *Amer. J. Psychiat.*, 1964, *120:*729–37.

15. Kobrin, S. Chicago area project—25-year assessment. *Ann. Amer. Acad. Political Soc. Sci.*, 1959, *322:*20–29.

16. Menninger, W. *Psychiatry in troubled world.* New York: Macmillan, 1948.

17. Merton, R. K. Social structures and anomie. In *Social theory and social structure.* Glencoe, Ill.: Free Press, 1949. pp. 125–50.

18. Plunkett, R. J., and Gordon, J. E. *Epidemiology and mental illness.* New York: Basic Books, 1960.

19. Powers, E., and Witmer, H. *Experiment in prevention of delinquency.* New York: Columbia University Press, 1951.

20. Srole, L., et al. *Mental health in metropolis: Midtown Manhattan study,* vol. 1. New York: McGraw-Hill, 1962.

21. Stanton, A., and Schwartz, M. S. *Mental hospital: Study of institutional participation in psychiatric illness and treatment.* New York: Basic Books, 1954.

22. Szasz, T. S. *Myth of mental illness: Foundations of theory of personal conduct.* New York: Harper, 1961.

23. Thompson, C. B. Psychiatry and social crisis. *J. Clin. Psychopath.*, 1946, 7:697–711.

50. Pitfalls of Community Psychiatry

LAWRENCE S. KUBIE

Much that will be presented here was anticipated by some of our distinguished predecessors. In 1932, after the late Dr. Frankwood Williams had been the Medical Director of the National Committee for Mental Hygiene for 17 years, he resigned and published an article entitled "Is There a Mental Hygiene?"[1] His objections to the mental hygiene movement of those days anticipates and parallels many of my concerns over today's fanfare for community psychiatry.

A comparable earlier episode is described in the *History of Medical Psychology* by Zilboorg and Henry.[2] They wrote of Ferrus, one of the more progressive French psychiatrists of the first half of the 19th century. In his struggles to ameliorate the conditions of the care of patients, Ferrus visited Gheel and other centers, including the hospital of an English contemporary, John Connolly, who had introduced the concept of "non-restraint" into psychiatric thinking.

Ferrus was an outspoken person. He told the Belgian king in plain language that the Gheel colony for the mentally sick of which Belgium was so proud offered little of which to be proud. Upon his return to France, he described the cruelty which prevailed in the colony and remarked that the treatment there was nil and that the only thing the insane had was detrimental.[2(p387)]

He also reported that he saw at Connolly's own hospital "in a well-padded cell a furious epileptic submitting to 'non-restraint'; ie, four powerful guards holding the arms and limbs of the unfortunate patient."[2(pp387-388)] Evidently Ferrus was not only liberal but also objective and critical. We should attempt to be equally objective and equally critical today in our

From *Archives of General Psychiatry, 18,* 257–266, 1968. Copyright 1968, American Medical Association. Reprinted by permission.

evaluation of what we are calling "community psychiatry."

Then if we leap from the early 19th and early 20th centuries to recent decades we find that before the words *Community Psychiatry* had become a popular banner there was much informed concern with the topic. In the summer of 1948 under the auspices of Harvard University a conference on mental hygiene was held in Cambridge. The panel included Drs. Karl A. Menninger, Harry C. Solomon, Carl Rogers, and others. The deliberations of this panel have never been published as a whole, but one contribution subsequently appeared in *Mental Hygiene*.[3] This is worth mentioning because it spelled out in detail the problems of community psychiatry without using the term; eg, the problems of staffing and of duration, the techniques of community education in mental hygiene, the techniques for evaluating results, the problems of sampling, the cost of a 15-year program to test the value of combining mental health education with early psychodiagnosis and early psychotherapy in a carefully chosen stable community. The current literature on community psychiatry hardly refers to these basic problems.

Further consideration of underlying principles are found in the various chapters of the volume edited by Drs. Alexander Leighton and F. C. Redlich entitled *Explorations in Social Psychiatry*.[4] Chapter 3 considers whether destructive social and economic processes influence *(a)* the incidence of the universal neurotic potential itself, or *(b)* the course of the universal yet variable neurotic process, or *(c)* the timing, nature, form, and intensity of the neurotic state as it crystallizes out of the neurotic process,[5] or *(d)* the precipitation of psychotic disorganization out of the neurotic process.[3]

This leads directly to a discussion of the changes which are needed to create a social order which will be preventive as well as therapeutic. An article published in *Daedalus* in 1959 entitled "Is Preventive Psychiatry Possible?"[6] considers some of the vested interests which oppose those changes without which a benign social alchemy cannot occur.

More recent publications on "territoriality"[7] also are relevant, since they bring up the effects of the population explosion and of population density. Yet one looks in vain through the current literature on community psychiatry for any consideration of what to do about real-estate greed, which manifests itself by piling too many people on too little land. This is a violation of public health more infamous than it would be to pour typhoid bacillus into the city water supply, but it receives no consideration in our literature.

ESSENTIAL REQUIREMENTS OF A REALISTIC PROGRAM OF COMMUNITY PSYCHIATRY

A Clear Definition of Goals and Concepts. Serious difficulties arise out of the ambiguous and contradictory implications of the concept of community psychiatry as it is currently used.

The drive for community psychiatry comes in part from those who are rightly distressed over the number of human beings who have latent or manifest neuroses or latent or manifest psychoses or a mixture. They feel that the numbers are so vast that neither individual nor group therapy can meet this challenge and that any effort to solve this problem will have to come from seeking for something other than the treatment of sick individuals, perhaps by using the community as a whole in some undefined way as a therapeutic instrument. This feeling is usually linked to a more precise realization that there are many psychonoxious social forces in our society and that through some alchemy the communities themselves can and must be changed if any progress is to be made. No one can dissent from the hope of making communities into sources of health, freer from neuroses; but whether this is to be done by general education or by changing the social mores in the face of deeply entrenched biases remains unclear. The one clear inference is that for this group, at least, the goal is not to be sought by better and earlier treatment. In general they feel that the only path to health is by changing fundamentally our economic and social processes and the structure of society and of the family.

Another concept which is advanced sometimes as a complementary plan and sometimes in opposition puts the emphasis on the reduction of the load of neurotic and psychotic illness by earlier diagnosis leading to earlier treatment.

Here again it is unclear whether this is to be done through individual treatment, group treatment, or some form of mass treatment.

One sympathizes with the warmth of feeling and the human concern which underlie all of these attitudes. Yet one has to ask whether they are sufficiently tough-minded. However that may be, everyone will agree that if psychiatry is to become a social force it must be represented by a certain number of psychiatrists who leave the ivory tower of exclusive concern with intensive individual psychotherapy. Yet one seeks in vain for precise discussions of the dangers which are inherent in this move, such as the danger of jeopardizing the psychiatrist's therapeutic leverage with his own patients and also the danger of jeopardizing the clarity and precision of his theoretical and practical thinking. The problem of how to protect the psychiatrist's theoretical precision and his therapeutic skill and leverage while leading him out of isolation needs more consideration than it has been given.[8]

If the psychiatrist is to be able to characterize with greater precision those social inequities which contribute to the neurotic process and influence both its development and its consequences, he will need long training in economics, sociology, social engineering, and social work as well as in the psychopathology of the neurotic process. He must clarify, deepen, and not oversimplify those basic concepts concerning the neurotic process which make of it an inclusive human discipline, ie, one of the fundamental humanities. Wishful oversimplifications about this can distort the approach to community psychiatry itself. Is all of this being planned realistically?

Of equal importance is the need to identify more clearly the role of the community itself as a complex constellation of psychonoxious or healing forces, and the processes by which a benign alchemy can be achieved which will move the community from one end of this spectrum toward the other. Any effort to effect such changes will confront many entrenched and tenacious community forces which will oppose change, however health-giving such change might be. These are areas in which greater clarity and detail is needed than any of the literature in this field presents.

We Must Break the Personnel Bottleneck. Earlier diagnosis and earlier therapy for more people are not all there is to the prevention of psychopathology nor all that is needed to bring psychiatry to the community. Yet they are indispensable ingredients in any community mental health program, since a lessening of prejudice against psychiatry has brought an increase in the articulate demand for help from all elements in our society. If the campaign for community psychiatry fails to provide enough trained men to serve these articulate needs, people will feel double-crossed by psychiatry, as they have frequently felt in the past. Resentment against psychiatry will boomerang, because again we will have raised hopes only to fail to meet them. In this the National Committee for Mental Hygiene was a prime offender.[1] We are in danger of repeating that mistake by pushing the slogan of community psychiatry without providing the manpower to implement its programs.

When patients and their families turn for help to the new community mental health centers, they will not care whether this help takes the form of drug therapy, individual psychotherapy, group therapy, psychological support from a therapeutic milieu, or social and economic readjustments. Each of these and any combination of them will require the services of men of matured clinical, therapeutic, and psychosocial judgment and technique. The limiting factor is and has always been the lack of enough trained personnel.[9] Therefore, one would anticipate that the first step in any campaign for community mental health would be a plan to provide enough experienced teachers and training centers to provide better training in social and individual pathology and in diagnosis and therapy not only to more medically-trained psychiatrists but also to non-medical behavioral scientists. Note that the emphasis would be on *better* training for more men, not quicker, briefer training. Therefore, the proponents of community psychiatry might also be expected to acknowledge the self-evident fact that they will need more men than the medical profession alone will ever be able to supply.[10-13] Around this issue has centered the long struggle over whether, in addition to training physicians in psychodiagnosis and psychotherapy, we must create a new doctorate in medical psychology for behavioral scientists who are not physicians but whose graduates would be licensed to work as partners to the medically-trained psychiatrists. The official position of the American Medical Association, the American Psychiatric Association, and the American Psychoanalytic Association as well is that one who is not a physician should not receive such training, no matter how fully schooled and experienced he may be in basic sciences, in experimental and statistical methods, in human biology, in clinical psychology and psychiatric social work, and in the behavioral sciences in general. As long as this remains the official position of the organizations which dominate the field, we will make propaganda for community psychiatry but no real progress toward it. Realistic plans for community psychiatry must provide for and finance additional years of longer and more intensive training. It is not enough merely to use more partially trained clinical psychologists and psychiatric social workers. Community psychiatry must spell out in detail the plans for recruiting, further training, financing, accrediting, and licensing. The current campaign for community psychiatry does not contemplate these goals in sufficient detail.

Community Psychiatry, Opportunism, and Space. At the moment, money for community psychiatry is so easily available that some leaders are seduced by it. Several department heads have stated frankly that they are glad to take federal money (or any other money that comes their way) in order to build facilities which they need. They admit that in today's climate, if they are to get this money, they are forced to call their new facilities "community mental health centers." They do not hesitate to add that within a dozen years the words will have dropped into innocuous desuetude, leaving the department in possession of the additional space it needs. There is no reason to object to such benevolent profiteering on the current fad, as long as basic thinking about psychiatry is not distorted by it, and as long as the training of future psychiatrists is not endangered by bad psychiatric practices (see below).

THE INFLUENCE OF EXPERIENCE IN COMMUNITY MENTAL HEALTH CENTERS

On the Learning Process in Psychiatry. Without mature psychiatrists there can be no psychiatry for any-

one to know about. Yet learning *about* psychiatry is not the same as becoming a psychiatrist. The latter is more than an indoctrination: it is a continuously evolving life-long therapeutic experience for the psychiatrist which gradually releases him from bondage to his own childhood, thus making possible a process of cognitive, purposive, and emotional maturation.[14] Today the scientific growth of psychiatry is seriously hampered by the fact that so many more people know *about* psychiatry than have gone through this searching, humbling, maturing process of *becoming*. Consequently, any movement which threatens to limit the maturation of psychiatrists threatens to destroy the future of psychiatry. To truncate the development of generations of future psychiatrists is too high a price to pay for any immediate gains. Yet there is a grave danger that this may be one of the destructive consequences of what today is called community psychiatry.

The reason for this is clear. One becomes a psychiatrist by working as a participant observer with a few patients at a time, intensively and over long periods, identifying closely with each patient as he moves through varying phases of his illness. This prolonged and intimate exposure to the struggles of the individual patient is the sine qua non of the student's evolution toward human and clinical maturity. Such experience can be gained in many settings, eg, private practice, individual or group psychotherapy, hospital or outpatient services, schools, courts, or social agencies, but only when these make possible intensive and long-sustained relationships to the illnesses of a few patients at a time. These considerations apply not only to individual face-to-face psychotherapy, but also to dual[15] and group therapies as well.[16] (Of course, other types of experience make subsidiary contributions to the process of becoming a psychiatrist.) Each setting has certain limitations, certain special advantages and disadvantages, and certain values as a learning experience. The setting of private practice challenges the therapist to independence and strength. The clinic and hospital provide invaluable opportunities for mutual scrutiny, comparison, and criticism which are not available in the isolation of private practice.

These rather obvious points are worth spelling out only to make it clear that this is not a special plea for private practice, but rather because it is important to understand how long it takes to acquire clinical maturity as a psychiatrist and how necessary it is to provide for this through the opportunity to work intensively for a long period with only a few patients at any one time in many and diverse settings.[14,17]

Young physicians are wise to start their psychiatric residencies in facilities through which patients move slowly, where the resident will have an opportunity to work with the same patients through many plases of improvement and relapse. In later stages of training, after this intensive experience, they are equally wise to work in large public hospitals, provided only that these hospitals allow the young psychiatrist time enough to study his patients. There are only two settings in which the process of growth cannot occur, namely in any setting which provides only an assembly-line approach to patients and in any setting which aims for and even prides itself on a rapid turnover of patients. The institutions which have no educational value whatsoever are those which overload their doctors with too many patients, and which hope to impress legislators or boards of trustees by rushing their patients through, under the influence of the prevailing fantasy that quick turnover is desirable and economical. (The influence of this on the content of training will be discussed below.) Obversely, facilities which are less vulnerable to such pressures and which go slowly provide a better training experience.

Yet the experience of intensive involvement with patients is emotionally painful. In most residents it tends to reactivate their every unsolved personal and familial problem. Consequently, no matter how ardent their interest in psychiatry, most residents go through periods in which they want to withdraw to a safe distance from patients. Sometimes they do this by teaching, by doing research, or by administering the work of others. Any of these seems preferable to the more painful work with the patients themselves. Recruitment policies which sometimes are used in the organization of community mental health centers tend to play into this need of the resident to escape. For instance, to staff the new center by offering young residents administrative posts with high sounding titles and large salaries is, in reality, seducing them away from the most important yet most painful part of their psychiatric learning experience.

In all of this there is no conscious and deliberate fraud. A few young men turn to community psychiatry for the sake of early prestige and higher salaries, but only a few. More turn to it out of their concern about destructive forces in the structure of our society. Not frequently they harbor the Russian fantasy that all psychiatric illnesses are due to social inequities and can be both cured and prevented by curing the ills of our social order.[18] Quite rightly they want to see psychiatry made available to more people earlier and irrespective of income. Yet if these young men do not allow themselves time enough to learn the inner nature of psychological illnesses, time enough to understand the processes of falling ill and of falling well, if they do not take time to learn how to deal with one patient at a time by learning to recognize those unsolved inner problems which the psychiatric patient can stir in the therapist, then despite their good will they cannot expect to improve the lot of any. Their hopes to be able to help a thousand patients before they can help even one will remain naive, and their good intentions will suffer the fate of all good intentions which are not guided by mature knowledge and experience. Instead of making psychiatry widely available, they will destroy it by truncating their own maturation as psychiatrists and that of countless others.

At this point I want to state explicitly that none of my fears for the current trends in community psychiatry is equally valid for every person or for every center which is involved in this campaign. Some men have turned to community psychiatry after sufficiently long experience with patients to enable them to understand what it takes to become a psychiatrist. But many other highly vocal advocates have turned to community psychiatry before they themselves had achieved any degree of clinical maturity, not realizing the extent to which they themselves were using community psychiatry as a way of escaping the pain of involvement with individual patients. They do not realize that by limiting their own psychiatric experience to social rather than intrapsychic forces, they are viewing patients from a safe but obscuring distance.

UNDERLYING FALLACIES

The idea of community psychiatry has many merits. Therefore, it is regrettable that the campaign for community psychiatry is being presented on the basis of so many fallacies. Without pretending to be exhaustive, I will cite a few of these.

Treatment Should be Launched and Carried on at Home or Near Home. Some protagonists write and talk as if they believe that the best place in which to treat mental illness is in the patient's home or at least in his home community, where (to quote one of them) there will be "the least possible break in 'normal' contacts with family, friends, job, and school." This assumption ignores elementary common sense and familiar clinical experience. The very words "normal contacts" are surprising. The patient became ill in the midst of these normal contacts with home, job, and community, among family and friends, among work and school associates! Why assume that this is where to help him find the road back to health? Would it be wise to launch the treatment of a malarial patient in the very malarial swamp in which he had contracted his illness? Are these words normal contacts just naive sentimentalisms? Those who use these words cannot be unaware that especially in the launching of treatment, whether of the neuroses or of the psychoses, it is almost the rule that it is not merely helpful but actually essential to lift the patient out of all of his familiar settings. They must know that for the successful launching of any psychiatric treatment, irrespective of the apparent severity of the illness, the patient frequently needs an equivalent to Thomas Mann's "Magic Mountain." This is one of the several vital functions of the residential psychiatric treatment center, admirably served for the neuroses by the Austen Riggs Center under the late Dr. Knight.[19] Practical circumstances may compel us to launch and conduct psychiatric treatment with the patient residing in his own home and community, but only rarely is this advisable. Ultimately, of course, the security of any "cure" must be tested by exposing the patient to his former activities and associations, but not at the start.

In fact, even when a patient has progressed well in treatment and is approaching its termination, the last place to which he should be exposed will usually be his home, his job, his community. Sometimes in response to family pressures, sometimes for financial reasons, sometimes out of the sentimentality of inexperienced residents, hospitals may allow their convalescent patients to visit their homes too early. This results consistently in episodes of upset or of relapse. The physical aspects of the home, its familiar inanimate objects, and the well-known feeling of the community can stir so many upsetting associations that exposure to them should usually be held in reserve until the patient is far along the road to health. Actually, when a gradual resumption of outside contacts is indicated during convalescence, it is wise to allow patients to have their first contacts with their families or friends in unfamiliar physical settings away from home. Visits to the home itself should be encouraged only after repeated reunions away from home have proved successful. When this is financially difficult, some wise hospitals provide simple motel-like accommodations in pleasant surroundings, but away from home, to be used as settings for weekend reunions. Alert hospitals are coming to realize this, and even when a patient is fully ready to leave the hospital, he will often be sent to halfway houses, to surrogate "friendly homes," or to recreational centers. It may be weeks or months before he is encouraged to return to his own home.

This is not new wisdom; it is so old that it seems to have been forgotten. Every parent knows that a disturbed child may do well away from home, only to slip back into his upset as soon as he comes home for a vacation. The same thing often happens to adult patients.

The Fallacy That Such Treatment Facilities Should be Located in General Hospitals in the Center of Large Urban Populations. These same facts should not be overlooked when we consider where it is best to locate psychiatric facilities for residential treatment, whether brief or lengthy. For many years psychiatry has battled against the ignorance, fear, and prejudice which, together with the relative cheapness of land which was distant from cities, led our predecessors to build psychiatric hospitals far from centers of population. This, however, does not mean that it is necessarily helpful to patients to construct psychiatric intreatment facilities in large urban centers. To do this may demonstrate that we are no longer afraid, ignorant, or prejudiced; also, it may make it easier to integrate the psychiatric hospital with medical schools and general medical centers. Nevertheless, the harsh fact remains that proximity to homes is not necessarily good for patients and may be actively noxious. Some statistics on the care of alcoholics and others addicts suggest that psychiatric services which are incorporated into general hospitals in large centers have higher escape and relapse rates than those which are located in the remote country. This is another area in which we must guard ourselves against sentimentality about the dubious values of being close to home.

The Fallacy That the Shorter the Hospitalization the Better. Closely linked to the fallacy that therapy should be launched with the patient in his home and community is the equally fallacious notion that because bad hospitals are bad for patients, any hospitalization is bad for them and should be avoided if possible or made as short as possible. (The obvious flaws in this position have been discussed in detail in a recent discussion of the future of the private psychiatric hospital.[20])

Because of the belief that hospitalization per se is bad for patients and that shortening the length of hospitalization is advantageous, many hospitals are discharging their patients too soon. Some unattached psychiatric hospitals and also some in medical schools set arbitrary limits to the duration of hospital stay, such as 30 days or 60 days. They even boast about this clinically unrealistic policy, under the illusion that the arbitrarily weighted statistics which this policy yields indicate a great advance in psychiatry and also that this practice will save money for taxpayers and families. (Those of us who knew the situation in the care of pulmonary tuberculosis before the days of chemotherapy for tuberculosis will recall a period of similar error, when as soon as their acute symptoms subsided, patients were sent home as cured. Families and communities paid heavily for this error, in the spread of infection and in an enormous increase in the ultimate economic burden both to the state and to families.)

This practice has two profoundly unfortunate consequences for the present state and future progress of psychiatry.

It eliminates automatically the study of one of psychiatry's most important unsolved problems; the problem of chronicity, as exemplified by the long term patient.

In some hospitals it had led to a total destruction of training programs. While on teaching visits to hospitals of all kinds all over the country, I have found that with increasing frequency young residents individually and in groups have sought me out in recent years to voice their desperation. The gist of their protest is that because of the pressures to which they are subjected by hospital administrations, they are being forced to do many destructive things: (1) They are forced to rush patients through all routine examinations in such a hurry that the tests themselves become disturbing to patients, and, therefore, inaccurate. (2) They are compelled to flood their patients with masking chemotherapies, sometimes from the day of admission, long before the nature of their illnesses has been established and before basic tests can be administered, thus further invalidating the tests. (3) They are forced to rush the patients out of the hospital in the shortest time possible, sometimes even before the reports have reached them from psychological and physiological tests and laboratory examinations or the social workers' reports on home visits. The residents complain that as a consequence they do not have time to learn anything about their patients, that in fact they see their patients so little during these brief bouts of hospitalization that they do not have time to study them. (The best of these young residents complain, "We are learning nothing here. Where can we go?") (4) Finally, they note that as a result of sending patients out to their homes prematurely and while they are still disturbingly upset, the families of these patients are becoming so bitterly resentful that they refuse to cooperate in any follow-up studies.

Such practices are a bad model to present to young psychiatrists. They yield misleading statistics on a quick turnover which may impress politicians but should not influence scientists. If these hurry-up and hurry-out hospitals continue in this way, they will destroy both their therapeutic and their educational value; the consequence, unfortunately, will be the stunting of an entire generation of future psychiatrists.

The Fallacy That This Attack on the Hospital Will Save Money. Behind the tendency to downgrade the hospital and to upgrade the home is the illusion that this will save money and taxes. Even if it is true that some money can be saved in this way and even if there are occasions when we must allow financial considerations to determine medical policies for a time, such considerations should never be confused with scientific, medical, and sociological values. Too often this turns out to be a penny-wise, pound-foolish policy which will cost future generations enormous amounts of human suffering and money. Every disturbed patient who is sent back to his home before he is well (perhaps in an illusory state of pseudo-health while saturated with drugs) will create new patients for the hospitals which our children's generations will have to support.

In view of these considerations it is a sad commentary that the name of one journal published by the American Psychiatric Association has been changed from *Mental Hospitals* to *Community Psychiatry*. Is this not a short-sighted abdication to political pressures, to fashion, and to an illusion of economy?

The Fallacy of Minor Psychiatry. Community psychiatry is not a minor psychiatry which can be carried out by beginners. There is no analogy here to minor surgery. Indeed, there is no such thing as minor psychiatry, and especially not in early psychiatry. It takes long training, long experience, and both personal and clinical maturity merely to recognize, and even more to deal effectively with, the subtle manifestations of early illness, its initial step-by-step development, the feedback of secondary distortions in human life, and the long chain of tertiary consequences. Such major psychiatry demands mature men of exceptionally mature experience with the neurotic process from childhood on, as well as with the psychosis at the end of the line. Therefore, it is unrealistic to set up a community mental health center under the leadership of a young psychiatrist who may have served in a psychiatric hospital for two or three years at the most, sometimes but not always with brief experience in an outpatient clinic. The appointment of such a

beginner as "medical director" of one of the community mental health centers is a betrayal of our responsibility not only to the patients who come to these centers but also for the training of that young doctor, because it enables him to escape into the snug harbor of administration from the clinical challenge of psychiatry.

In these centers psychiatry could easily regress to something that it took many years to eradicate from military psychiatry. In the early days of World War I and again between the two wars and at the beginning of World War II, military psychiatrists were primarily distributing agents. They "disposed of" patients by discharging them to a round of agencies, in none of which did they receive adequate treatment. This is precisely what can happen to civilian psychiatry if we continue to set up community mental health centers which we cannot staff at all, or else staff inadequately, as, for example, by one inexperienced young psychiatrist, one full-time social worker, and one part-time clinical psychologist. It is dismaying to hear this backward step touted as a great new forward step in psychiatry. There is nothing new about it. It is as old as the hills, and it was always bad. Doing it over again does not make it any better.

The Fallacy That All Psychopathology Is Due to Having Either Too Much or Too Little. Poupular prejudices sometimes influence psychiatric thinking. This is always disturbing, especially when it reproduces in American psychiatry some of the distortions of Russian psychiatry. I have in mind the prevalent oversimplifications about the effects of wealth and poverty on the neurotic process.[18] These fallacies lead to prejudices against the use of any form of treatment which takes a great deal of time and which can reach only a few people. This bias overlooks the fact that every field of medicine has had to learn from the slow, intensive study of a few patients how to treat masses of people by quicker and shorter methods. The pressure of widespread human need for a cure and prevention of cancer does not justify scorning the slow efforts of the investigator to clarify the nature of the cancer process in a few sufferers. Nor is it sound to scorn the psychiatrist whose gift is for that slow, microscopic study of individual lives out of which so much basic knowledge has come. (The fact that this knowledge has had its inevitable infusion of error does not lessen its importance.)

Nor does impatience for quicker techniques of treatment justify a show of contempt for patients, whether these are rich or poor. Nor does a critical attitude toward the slow treatment of the privileged few take into account the fact that medicine has always begun its attack on its problems by using many professionals in the intensive study of the few. Premature efforts to launch mass treatment or mass prevention before the nature of individual illness has been solved can only result in disappointments. This has been true in the history of infectious and metabolic diseases as well as in the history of psychiatry. There is danger that community psychiatry may be heading toward the same misuse of effort and money.

Furthermore, it is a basic principle in science that the design of research must limit as far as is possible the number and range of simultaneous variables. The nature of any somatic disease can be solved only if it can be isolated for the study of one illness at a time. In psychiatric illness many complex variables coexist not merely in the intrapsychic and psychophysiological processes of illness, but in additional groups of complex socioeconomic variables as well. In fact, so many variables have to be taken into consideration that it is possible to clarify the pure essence of the neurotic process itself only where the externals of life are relatively constant and not melodramatically complicated and unusual. Inevitably this is found only in privileged circumstances. Consequently, one can study only in the relatively privileged few that destruction of inner peace which man can cause himself, even under the best of circumstances, through the interaction of stormy unconscious intrapsychic conflicts. These subtle intrapsychic variables must be isolated from or at least studied apart from external variables before we can begin to understand the interaction between intrapsychic conflicts and the variables among external stresses. In the current enthusiasm for community psychiatry we are in danger of losing sight of this scientific perspective. The process of becoming mature and wise in psychiatry requires first of all an understanding of the intrapsychic variables. This again is the scientific reason why we must become mature practitioners of individual psychiatry before we attempt to become practitioners of community psychiatry.

SUMMARY

Let me now state again what I consider to be the major danger of this campaign: ie, the seduction and betrayal of the resident student of psychiatry. As I have said, there is a profound difference between learning *about* psychiatry and *becoming* a psychiatrist. Anyone may learn something *about* psychiatry, ie, its language, the evolution of its changing concepts and of its changing efforts to define meaningful nosological entities, the history of its therapeutic struggles and of its attempts to clarify the relationship of somatic to experiential variables. Much of this can even be learned from books and lectures. If the student who has mastered the text books then works in an assembly-line hospital where he will see many patients briefly, he may learn to use traditionally entrenched concepts, but he will not learn how to test and evaluate them with patients. There is only one way in which he can learn to *become* a psychiatrist—namely, by slow, patient work with a few patients at a time as a participant observer in the patient's struggles back and forth between illness and health. A young man achieves personal maturity through the repeated experiences of trial and error in his own life. He grows into professional psychiatric maturity by sharing with his patients their experiences of getting better and worse over and over and over again. He grows up by living through this experience. Clearly both for the psychiatrist and for the patient this involves a reexperiencing of the growth process itself, with an undoing and redoing of a lot of unhealthy growing. This is why[14] the rate at which the student of psychiatry can reach clinical maturity as a psychiatrist is limited not by his intelligence, diligence, or even by his psychological sensitivity, but by the rate at which patients change. There is no substitute for the time which such changes require.

Drugs have their place, but not all the drugs in the world can accelerate this. They can take the edge off of painful symptoms and painful affects, thereby making it possible to establish a therapeutic relationship with a patient who without drugs is walled off by illness and pain. But the ultimate therapeutic task is to facilitate change in the man behind the illness. This is what psychotherapy is really about. Without psychotherapy drugs may even mask symptoms, thus allowing the human being to become sicker. The end of that story is something for which our children will pay heavily in decades to come. Thus the misleading ballyhoo about community psychiatry is linked to premature and exaggerated claims for chemotherapy in psychiatry. Chemotherapy has an essential place as an aid to psychotherapy, to facilitate it and sometimes to make it possible, but not as an alternative to it. So again we are brought back to the importance of slow, long, sustained work with patients as indispensable both for the patient and for the clinical maturation of the psychiatrist.

Working with patients is painful. On preconscious and unconscious levels it stirs in most young psychiatrists distorted reflections of their own family relationships and of their own personal problems in general. It is as natural to shrink away from this, as it is to pull a hand away from a hot stove. Yet if the student allows himself to draw away, no matter how much he learns *about* psychiatry, he will never become a psychiatrist. And if we who are supposed to be his teachers seduce him from the daily struggle with patients, by offering him less painful jobs at higher salaries with high-sounding titles (such as "medical director") plus opportunities for community contacts, the novelty of newspaper interviews and of speech-making, we are creating propagandists and administrators but stunting the development of a whole generation of future psychiatrists. This is not an honest way to bring psychiatry to the community or to make psychiatry a potent force in the maturation of our immature culture.

References

1. Williams, F.: Is There a Mental Hygiene?, *Psychoanal Quart 1*:113–120, 1932.

2. Zilboorg, G., and Henry, G.: *The History of Medical Psychology,* New York: W. W. Norton & Co., Inc., Publishers, 1941.

3. Kubie, L. S.: A Research Project in Community Mental Hygiene: A Fantasy, *Ment Hyg 36*: 220–226 (April) 1952.

4. Kubie, L. S.: "Social Forces and the Neurotic Process," in Leighton, A. H., and Redlich, F. C. (eds.): *Explorations in Social Psychiatry,* New York: Basic Books, Inc., Publishers, 1957, pp. 77–99; *J Nerv Ment Dis 128*:65–80 (Jan) 1959.

5. Kubie, L. S.: The Neurotic Potential, the Neurotic Process, and the Neurotic State, *US Armed Forces Med J 2*:1–12 (Jan) 1951.

6. Kubie, L. S.: Is Preventive Psychiatry Possible?, *Daedalus: J Amer Acad Arts Sciences 88*: 646–668, 1959.

7. Ardrey, R.: *The Territorial Imperative,* New York: Atheneum Publishers, 1966.

8. Kubie, L. S.: The Dilemma of the Analyst in a Troubled World, *Bull Amer Psychoanal Assoc 6*:1–4 (Dec) 1950.

9. Kubie, L. S.: A Program of Training in Psychiatry to Break the Bottleneck in Rehabilitation, *Amer J Orthopsychiat 16*:447–454 (July) 1946.

10. Kubie, L. S.: The Need for a New Subdiscipline in the Medical Profession, *Arch Neurol Psychiat 78*:283–293 (Sept) 1957.

11. Kubie, L. S.: A School of Psychological Medicine Within the Framework of a Medical School and University, *J Med Educ 39*:476–480 (May) 1964.

12. Kubie, L. S.: *Transactions of the Gould House Conference,* R. Holt (ed.), New York: International Universities Press, Inc.1972.

13. Kubie, L. S.: The Over-All Manpower Problem in Mental Health Personnel, *J Nerv Ment Dis 144*:466–470 (June) 1967.

14. Kubie, L. S.: The Maturation of Psychiatrists or The Time That Changes Take, *J Nerv Ment Dis 136*:286–288 (Oct) 1962.

15. Flescher, J.: "The 'Dual Method' in Analytic Psychotherapy," in Jewish Board of Guardians, *New Frontiers in Child Guidance,* New York: International Universities Press, Inc., 1958, pp. 44–76.

16. Kubie, L. S.: Some Theoretical Concepts Underlying the Relationship Between Individual and Group Psychotherapies, *Int J Group Psychother 8*:3–19 (Jan) 1958.

17. Kubie, L. S.: The Problem of Maturity in Psychiatric Research, *J Med Educ 28*:11–27 (Oct) 1953.

18. Kubie, L. S.: Pavlov, Freud and Soviet Psychiatry, *Behav Sci 4*:29–34 (Jan) 1959.

19. Kubie, L. S.: *The Riggs Story,* New York: Paul B. Hoeber, Inc., Medical Book Dept. of Harper & Row, 1960.

20. Kubie, L. S.: "The Future of the Private Psychiatric Hospital," in Gibson, R. W. (ed.): *Crosscurrents in Psychiatry and Psychoanalysis,* Philadelphia: J. B. Lippincott Co., 1967, pp. 179–203, 241–242.

Part VI

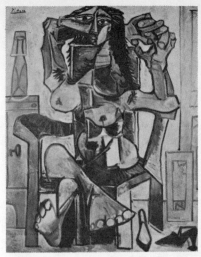

Integrative Theories

Pablo Picasso—*Seated Woman* (1959).

INTRODUCTION

As will become evident in the four papers that comprise this final section, there are those who contend that the major traditions of psychology and psychiatry have, for too long now, been doctrinaire in their assumptions. These critics claim that theories which focus their attention on only one level of data cannot help but generate formulations that are limited by their narrow preconceptions; moreover, their findings must, inevitably, be incompatible with the simple fact that psychological processes are multidetermined and multidimensional in expression. In rebuttal, those who endorse a single-level approach assert that theories which seek to encompass this totality will sink in a sea of data that can be neither charted conceptually nor navigated methodologically. Clearly, those who undertake to propose "integrative theories" are faced with the formidable task, not only of exposing the inadequacies of single-level theories, but of providing a convincing alternative that is both comprehensive and systematic. It is for the reader to judge whether integra-

tive theorists possess the intellectual skills and analytic powers necessary, not only to penetrate the vast labyrinths of man's mind and behavior, but to chart these intricate pathways in a manner that is both conceptually clear and methodologically testable.

Adolf Meyer, originator of the "psychobiologic" school at the turn of this century, spoke out vigorously for the principle of man's intrinsic biological and psychological unity. Writing at a time when this principle was persistently obscured or overlooked, Meyer's remained a voice in the wilderness. Bringing the accumulated knowledge of six decades to bear, Roy Grinker revives and extends the integrative thesis in his broadranging and erudite presentation. Paul Meehl, in his incisive and brilliantly speculative article, illustrates the fruits of this orientation in a theory of schizophrenia. Theodore Millon, formulating a deductive model for personality pathology, outlines the central themes of his biosocial-learning theory.

465

51. The Role of the Mental Factors in Psychiatry

ADOLF MEYER

Nearly forty years ago John P. Gray made a plea for the view that mind cannot become diseased itself, and that there cannot be any *mental* diseases, but only diseases of the brain. To prove this, he eradicated as a superstition the idea that mental or moral causes could figure in the etiology of mental disorders. He published a table of the causes in the cases admitted during the years 1843-1870 and in these he gave the following ratio in percentages (selection from the complete table):

	1843	1851	1860	1865	1866	1867	1868
Moral causes	46.38	30.05	13.95	5.41	3.09		
Physical causes	33.70	62.57	70.33	73.35	67.78	80.05	77.49
Unascertained causes	19.93	7.37	15.73	21.24	29.12	19.95	22.51

He achieved his practical aim to harmonize the theory and the wise aspiration to obtain the supremacy of physicians in the care of the insane. But he went from one extreme—the tendency to systematic ignoring of the somatic factors in the lay public—to another extreme, the disregard of the mental factors.

Pathology also had to pass through extremes. From witchcraft and humoral pathology, it had become a study of *lesions* and their consequences. Lesions of the brain figured as the only possible explanations of disorders of its functions. So numerous were the anatomical and histological discoveries that they absorbed all the attention; and what was not known yet was nevertheless put down in terms of some kind of "lesion" and the *knowledge of the lesion* was the pathology.

In the meantime a revolution has taken place. The theory of immunity brought pathology to experimental terms. The great fact had to be accepted that an organism which had had smallpox was protected for a period. The capacity of *resistance* to degrees of virulence of anthrax became an issue greater than that of a mere knowledge of the tissue changes. The mere histologist has given way to the experimentalist; or rather, a *combination* of all the available facts, causal, functional and structural, in terms of experiments, has become the central thought of pathology.

The finest histological demonstration of the posterior column lesions of tabes—by many thought to be "the pathology of the disease"—would not tell us that if you wish to avoid tabes you must avoid syphilis. The knowledge of lesions is but *one* of the resources of the formula of real pathology, and this formula is : (1) What is the condition under study (the disturbance expressed functionally or anatomically, but at least sufficiently to distinguish it from other similar conditions)? (2) What are the conditions under which it arises? and (3) To what extent are the conditions and the developments modifiable?

We know now that the lesion itself, if we know it, is only one of the *symptoms* (although to be sure one of the type which "keep" and can be bottled up and demonstrated longer than the functional symptoms), and that the whole condition must be expressed in a lucid equation of an experiment of nature before it gives us the satisfaction of knowing the "pathology."

Hence the mere *assumption* of a hypothetical lesion is no solution and not even necessarily the most stimulating hypothesis. Thus we come to hear again of "psychogenetic developments" of cases of dementia praecox and of depressions, hysterical tantrums, etc. What can this mean?

Take the case of a woman of somewhat restricted capacity who was forced by circumstances to move on two occasions, and each time and on no other occasion worked herself into a depression; she did not see how she could do the work and, instead of doing the best she could, she dropped into a state of evil anticipation, lamentation, perplexity—a typical depression of several months' duration. Her sister too had a depression of a rather different character, but also on provocation. We do well to point to the constitutional peculiarity—a lack of immunity. Since there *are* cases in which we cannot find any precipitating factors, we are apt to spread ourselves on a statement of

From *American Journal of Insanity*, LXV (1908), 39–52.

heredity and possibly degeneracy of make-up, of possible lesions, etc., and to overemphasize these issues. What we actually know is that this patient is apt to react with a peculiar depressive reaction where others get along with fair balance. The etiology thus involves (1) constitutional make-up, and (2) a precipitating factor; and in our eagerness we cut out the latter and only speak of the heredity or constitutional make-up. It is my contention that we must use *both* facts and that of the two, for *prevention* and for the special characterization of the make-up, the precipitating factor is of the greater importance, because *it* alone gives us an idea of the actual defect and a suggestion as to how to strengthen the person that he may become resistive. It is a problem of index of resistance with regard to *certain difficulties of mental adjustment*.

Take another case: a girl taken advantage of by a neighbor's boy at six. She did not dare tell any one for shame; and without knowing what it all meant, she imagined things about it, that she had become different from others. It is difficult to know how much children can elaborate such feelings and how much they can become entangled and twisted by amplifying dreams and talk of others and what not, if once started on a track without the normal corrections. At eleven, the patient had a slight accident and limped for six months. A plain ovarialgia with typical hysterical convulsions and paraplegia followed her nursing her sister through an illness at eighteen; recovery in one year. Then, at twenty-one, after nursing and losing her grandmother, she experienced a new collapse, again with recovery. At twenty-five, there came a hysterical psychosis which was mismanaged and drifted into stupor, then excitement and then a classical catatonic dementia. For every step there are adequate causes; usually causes which would not have upset you or me, but which upset the patient. Now what makes the difference between her and you and me? A different make-up, yes; but what kind? Can we expect a full answer in some general term? Do we not, to explain it usefully and practically, have to express it in the very facts of the history? Every step is like an experiment telling us the story, and giving us the concrete facts to be minded; while to speak merely of "hysteria" or later of "dementia praecox" gives us no good clue as

to what to prevent, and what sore spots to protect and what weak sides to strengthen, but only a general characterization of the possible mischief and the probable *absence* of a palpable lesion, and the fact that the disorder consists of a faulty hanging together of the mental reactions or adjustments, shown by and promoted by previous maladjustments.

Some of you are probably familiar with my explanation of many of the conditions now lumped together as dementia praecox. I started from the realization that in some diseases we are continually promising ourselves lesions, and over that we neglect facts which are even now at hand and ready to be sized up and the very things we must learn to handle. Some persons are immune and readily balanced, others get wrecked. The main question is, What makes the difference? Some talk of degeneracy, others of autointoxications and still others of glia overgrowth—but these statements are often enough mere conjectures or refer to merely incidental facts and do not give us much to go by.

Take a case of catatonic stupor. There are evidently many factors involved. All I want to know is whether I can best clinch the facts actually known about the patient by using what is accessible (usually a characteristic string of habit developments and experiences and maladjustments), or by *inventing* some poisons or what not.

It has been my experience to find in many a case of dementia praecox far more forerunners of actual mischief than the average psychiatrist gets at by his examination when he avoids these facts or does not know how to use them. And it has become my conviction that the developments in some mental diseases are rather the results of peculiar mental tangles than the result of any coarsely appreciable and demonstrable brain lesion or poisoning—the natural further development of inefficient reaction types; and that I would rather look at the bird in the hand, and act on the available facts, while I can still live in hope that some day I might find an organ or poison which is more involved than another, and which might be given a prop.

I should consider it preposterously absurd to try to explain an alcoholic delirium merely on fears and psychogenetic factors, leaving out of sight the stomach condition and lack of food and sleep; and I consider it as equally absurd to disregard the experience with the moving and all it implied, the twist of the hysterical woman along the line of a supposed internal injury, and its being used in the development of a catatonia, or the weight of habitual indecision and lack of completion in psychasthenia, the habit conflicts and deterioration of sane instincts in dementia praecox, etc. Where these facts *exist,* we should use *them* rather than wholly hypothetical poisons. Where we *do* find somatic disorders we use them; where we should have to invent them first in order to get anything to work with, we had better use the facts at hand for what they are worth to reconstruct the disorder in terms of an experiment of nature.

Why the dissatisfaction with explanations of a psychogenetic character?

(1) Because the facts are difficult to get at, and difficult to control critically, and often used for stupid inferences, for instance, a notion that a psychogenetic origin, i.e. a development out of natural mental activities which need not harm you and me, could not explain occasional lasting and frequently progressive disorders (in the face of the fact that nothing is more difficult to change than a political or religious or other deeply rooted conviction or tendency and nothing more difficult to stem than an unbalanced tendency to mysticism, lying, etc.).

(2) Because there prevail misleading dogmatic ideas about mind.

It is unfortunate that science still adheres to an effete and impossible contrast between mental and physical. More and more we realize that what figures to our mind as *matter* is much better expressed in terms of combinations of electrons, if not simply of energies, which throw off many of the forbidding and restrictive features of those masses which form the starting point of our concept of inert matter, which is practically sufficient for most demands of ordinary physics, but a hindrance to a better conception of the more complex happenings of biochemistry. Mind, on the other hand, is a *sufficiently organized living being in action*; and not a peculiar form of mind-stuff. A sufficiently organized brain is the main central link, but mental activity is really best understood in its full meaning as the adaptation and adjustment of the individual as a whole, in contrast to the simple activity of single organs such as those of circulation, respiration, digestion, elimination, or simple reflex activity.

We know, of course, that in these reactions which we know as mental, the brain forms the central link at work, although we know but little of the detail working. Sensorimotor adjustments form an essential part and as soon as we pass from the simple representative reactions such as sensations and thoughts, to the affective reactions, emotions and actions, we get a distinct participation of the work of glands, of circulation, of respiration and muscular adjustments, so that organs serving *as such* more limited "infrapsychic" purposes enter as intrinsic parts into emotions, appetites, instincts and actions, so as to form the concrete *conduct and behavior,* which is the main thing deranged in our patients.

Thus we do not contrast mental activity with physical activity, which can be shown to be an artificial contrast with untenable and not truly scientific foundation, but mental activity and non-mental activity; activity of the person as a whole as mental activity, contrasted with the activity of the individual organs when working without mental links (as the heart does when removed from the body, or the various organs in the mere vegetative regulations and functions).

We do not know all the details of the modes of collaboration, but the main lines. We study their differences of various reaction types and of modifiability in various individuals and determine their chances of adjustment, and their ability to work themselves through the conflicts, tangles and temptations of usual and unusual demands. The extent to which the individual is capable of elaborating an efficient reaction determines the person's level. Our comparative measure of the various disabilities (of a patient getting through the difficulty of moving, the difficulty of getting square with an infantile trauma and its imaginary elaborations, the difficulty and twist resulting from habitual indecision and substitution of ruminations and panics and all that) is the normal complete reaction or adjustment to and of the situation. Why the tantrum? How can it be forestalled? Such would be the questions and problems uppermost in my mind.

The common reasoning is that if the patient gets through one tangle or one delusion, the disease still remains and other delusions will form. This I think is very often not correct, unless we bow dogmatically to an unwarrantedly broad notion of "disease." Mere disposition is not the disease. In practice that assumption is certainly very often *proved* to be false if we handle the conditions correctly. Very often the supposed disease back of it all is a myth and merely a self-protective term for an insufficient knowledge of the conditions of reaction and inadequacy of our present remedial skill.

Unfortunately our habits of diction lead us to call mental only the most specialized central reaction, the "thought," or at least the more essentially subjective part of the reaction. Yet as practical persons you do not take the word of an unknown person, but the act, as the real event. If you do that in psychopathology, and not before that, you also deal with conclusive factors. The act, not merely the possible step to it, counts; the *reaction* of the person as a whole, not merely one "thought," or part-step. We can under no circumstances afford to ignore the mental facts in the development of a large group of mental disorders. They *can* be the only expression of the facts to be heeded and to be worked with. But the mental facts we speak of are not mere thoughts but actual attitudes, affects, volitions and activities and possibly disorders of discrimination (which are oftener due to infrapsychic disturbances, as is shown by the psychosensory deliria).

Every mental adjustment must be in keeping with the laws of anabolism and catabolism; it has its somatic components. It is, therefore, intelligible that it *may* be easier to precipitate harm than to correct it, and that some disorders or conflicts may permanently damage the processes of anabolism.

I should like to illustrate further the influence of such an event as an upsetting shame and its setting in a depression, or an anxiety—but I have used too much of your time already. I only want to say one more word and that with regard to the *test* of the whole proposition: the existence or non-existence of psychotherapeutic helps.

If mental factors meant nothing, psychotherapy would be a snare and a delusion. Is it so? What is psychotherapy? Lately I heard two papers on this question—one an excellent sketch of the history and not without an occasional

emphasis on the queer and on the yellow streak in what is commonly known as psychotherapy and suggestion. The other was a simple discussion of the treatment of constipation by establishing an unshakable habit. It was psychologically interesting to watch the distinguished audience. The first paper expressed what in the main has been the general practice and the foundations of some of the more recent developments, with many sidelights but no urgent appeal to any special reform in the attitude of the physician. It elicited full appreciation as a fair and conservative general statement.

The report of the cures of even the most obstinate constipations with the simple method of Dubois and good sense and establishment of a habit met with smiles. Why? Because many men believe they *have* tried that method and have failed; and they do not realize that usually it is because they did not insist on the chief principle of psychotherapy, viz., that it is not talk or "thought" alone, but *the doing of things,* that is wanted. A physician will ask a patient whether he took his pill; but when he gives a sometimes somewhat elaborate regime of how to do things —i.e., the best psychotherapy by help and education—he often does not take correspondingly elaborate pains to control the carrying out of the plan to the dot—and he fails.

Psychotherapy is regulation of action, and only complete when action is reached. This is why we all use it in the form of occupation or rest, where it is an efficient and controllable form of regulation. This is why we teach patients actually to take different attitudes to things. Habit training is the backbone of psychotherapy; suggestion merely a step to the end, and of use only to the one who knows that the end can and *must* be *attained.* Action with flesh and bone is the only safe criterion of efficient mental activity; and actions and attitude and their adaptation is the issue in psychotherapy.

To sum up: There are conditions in which disorders of function (possibly with definite lesions) of special organs are the essential explanation of a mental disorder—a perversion of metabolism by poison, a digestive upset, a syphilitic reaction or an antisyphilitic reaction of the nervous system, an arteriosclerosis, and, in *these,* the *mental* facts are the *incidental* facts of the experimental chain.

But there *are* cases in which the apparent disorder of individual organs is merely an incident in a development which we could not understand correctly except by comparing it with the normal and efficient reaction of the individual as a whole, and for that we must use terms of psychology—not of mysterious events, but *actions* and *reactions* of which we know that they *do* things, a truly dynamic psychology. There we find the irrepressible instincts and habits at work, and finally the characteristic mental reaction type constituting the obviously pathological aberrations, and while it may be too late in many cases to stem the stream of destructive action—action beyond correction and in conflict with the laws of balance of anabolism and catabolism—seeing the facts in the right way will help us set aright what *can* be set aright, prevent what *can* be prevented and do what *can* be done to secure gymnastics and orthopaedics of mind—i.e., of the conduct and efficiency of the person as a whole.

Modern pathology sees in most "diseases" nature's way of righting inadequate balance. They are crude ways of *repair,* not the enemy itself; reactions to be guided, not to be suppressed; and to understand the whole process you can no longer get along by dreaming of lesions when your facts are too meagre; but you see the facts as they are, the reaction of the patient;—and *he* is a psychopathologist who can help nature strike the balance with the least expense to the patient. Much psychopathology and psychotherapy will depend on the bracing of weak organs; but its work is not concluded before the patient is shown the level of his mental metabolism, the level of efficient anabolism and catabolism in terms of conduct and behavior and efficient meeting of the difficulties worth meeting, and avoidance of what otherwise would be a foolish attempt.

This is a progress beyond John P. Gray, and I feel that had he seen the recent developments, man of action as he was, he would himself have subscribed to the rule that the real aim of psychiatry is to attain balance of the metabolism of conduct, obtained, according to the accessibility of the facts, from the adjustment of the individual organs, or from adjustment of the activities and attitudes which we can only size up in terms of a psychology of "activity of the individual as a whole." And, last but not least, we see that there is a deep reason for our interest in the adjustment of the *tasks* of adaptation, a straightening out of the situation outside of the patient, the family and other problems of adjustment which may be too much for the patient. These have always been the practical ways; and by dropping some unnecessary shells and traditions, we can see a psychopathology develop without absurd contrasts between mental and physical, and rather a division into adjustments of the person as a whole and adjustments of individual organs.

52. "Open-System" Psychiatry

ROY R. GRINKER, SR.

I

The broad term, bio-psycho-social, encompasses all aspects of the living organism. It indicates the inseparability of environment from organic life and the relationship between human existence and its social and cultural products. The term

Abridged and reprinted by permission of the Editor of *The American Journal of Psychoanalysis.* 1966, Vol. 26, No. 2, pp. 115–128.

is not easy to grasp theoretically and difficult to implement operationally. With its holistic concepts it is often used to deny the significance of particular frames of reference and the importance of one or another variable in health or illness. I have little use for the futile plea to utilize holistic approaches operationally. The scientist has to focus, with a particular frame of reference and from a specified position, on a part of the world of man. Yet unified or holistic concepts in general are important as organizing principles for the understanding of general processes. For example, information theory applied in genetics as an explanatory device for the role of DNA and RNA in protein synthesis, may be applied to intrapsychic processes in the synthesis of perception, feeling and thinking for behavior.

The same criticism can be applied to the term psychosomatic, which connotes more than a kind of illness. It is indeed a comprehensive approach to the totality of an integrated process of transactions among the somatic, psychic and cultural systems. It likewise deals with a living process that is born, matures and develops through differentiation and successive stages of new forms of integration of parts, and transactions with other wholes. It deals with stresses, strains and adjustments, with acute emergency mechanisms, disintegrations and current defensive states. In fact, as I stated in 1953, "psychosomatic refers not to physiology or pathophysiology, not to psychology or psychopathology but to a concept of process among all living systems and their social and cultural collaborations. The totality is referred to as the bio-psycho-social system."

In 1951, in my presidential address before the American Psychosomatic Society, I stated that "we would fare better if we used the term *behavioral science,* which implies psychosomatic or comprehensive approaches. It considers man as a biological organism, striving as part of his animal, human and physical environment for continuity and for self-fulfillment as an individual, as he integrates into varying sized groups. It deals with the vicissitudes of his struggle between his inner pressures, their quantitative and economic aspects and the forces conducive and antagonistic to their discharge or satisfactions. The evolution of these forces and their internal signs, with their satisfactions and dangers, into socially communicable symbols and the evolution of irritability into vigilance and consciously experienced anxiety has led to the process of symbolic internalization of danger and intrapsychic defenses. As a result, the acute emergency responses to external dangers are less disturbing to man than the long continuous reactions to stresses that have become internalized and cannot be avoided or abandoned."

The intertwining of processes in current transaction with the end-results of previous experiences make a great deal of difficulty for the investigator who tries to maintain a holistic point of view. In fact, the so-called psychosomatic unity is faintly observable only at birth at which time differentiation and part-functions have already appeared and subsequent processes of maturation accelerate differentiation with tremendous speed.

The infant is born with specific inherited potentials within its visceral, motoric and ego systems, but despite genic derivation they require potentiation, and are modified, through stimulation and deprivations stemming from the social and physical environment. Although the neonatal organism is already somewhat differentiated at birth, it tends to react diffusely in response to all forms of stress and in this earlier phase learning probably occurs through the process of imprinting which is not yet fully understood.

Subsequent maturation is associated with differentiation into part-functions, which orient the infant towards the part-objects necessary for gratification. These communicate by means of signs and major learning at this period seems to occur through conditioning and reinforcement.

In a later phase the actions and subsequent reactions between the infant and mother establish a transactional feedback relationship within the open system which they constitute, first as a symbiotic unit and later as separate organisms. The mother is influenced by her own developmental personality derivatives, her ethnic tradition and the current cultural values, and she has her own problems in maintaining an integrative capacity in relation to her child. The infant's requirements influence the mother towards the role of mothering, although it may be insufficient for the particular infant.

As the ego functions which are concerned with cognition of communication with the environment develop, the human attributes of symbolic transformation mature. At this period greater capacity for reverberating transactions occur replacing the linear effect of child or mother on each other in simple interactions. At this time human symbolic learning increases in quantity and refinement and, as the neocortical systems mature, object relationships are possible with the formation of word symbols which in themselves screen or react against the imprints of earlier experiences, memory traces and primary affects. Finally, although still not yet well understood, learning through identification becomes an important factor in adaptation.

Thus, we see that the mental or psychological system is not only an evolutionary, but is also an ontological process culminating in functions which reside in a hypothetical space between biological functions and outer environments. This system receives, stores and retrieves information as does any biological system and also can start, stop or delay action. As a system associated with verbal behavior, it has the function of symbolic transformation of signs, the capacity to identify a self and the ability to project this self into the future.

II

The highly acclaimed "breakthrough" into the understanding of the course of a variety of degenerative diseases, by ascribing a specific emotional etiology to each, has been disappointing. As a result, psychosomatic research focusing on specific syndromes has been superceded by psychophysiological investigations, utilizing modern instrumentation, into the phenomena of relationship between mind and body, concentrating mainly on emotions for the mental and on autonomic and endocrine functions for the somatic.

Unfortunately, these relationships cannot be reduced to the desired simplicity by considering somatic processes to be in the service of internal regulation and maintenance of homeostatic boundaries, and by considering the mental to be concerned with outer adaptation of total behavior to events, things and other living objects. There are several reasons for this major difficulty: the inner-outer dichotomy breaks down operationally; the temporal characteristics of and within each system are widely different; and the mental is not examinable as a form of energy. Let me be more explicit.

1. Inner regulations do not consist only of reactions to outer stimuli, but also of responses to inner pressures leading to goal-seeking behavior. In addition, tension states are restlessly *sought* and facilitate *goal-changing behavior* which in turn requires a shift in internal regulation. *In* and *out* are inseparable as are man and his environment at every level of interaction from genes to behavior.

2. The temporal characteristics of mental operations are as rapid as neural conduction, while other somatic processes such as the endocrine secretions and peripheral sympathetic activities are far slower and dependent on chains or summations of effects involving autonomic, metabolic and chemical processes. Correspondingly some of these processes occur later than those on which their sequence depends. Obviously many somatic events may become evident long after the mental stimulus has apparently been dissipated making correlations difficult if not impossible.

3. Mentation is a function which transcends space-time characteristics of bodily processes even though it is dependent on them. As Sherrington stated, energy concepts cannot bridge the chasm between physiology and psychology. Nevertheless, the history of American psychology has been replete with attempts to use the neural models of reflex activity relating stimulus and response, ultimately minimizing the mental.

Beginning with our war experiences during which severe physiological and psychological disturbances were frequently observed as a result of long continued anxiety, we have been involved in a program of research on stress. Stress and anxiety are focal points of interest for psychiatry since theoretically the anxiety component of stress responses evoke psychological defenses which constitute all of the categories of illness known as psychiatric: phobias, compulsions, depression, withdrawals, etc. As a focal point of interest, stressors, anxiety and resultant psychophysiological processes have opened up vast unknown areas significant for theory, for research methods and for the practice of medicine and psychiatry.

Questions arise as to what constitutes stressors; are the emotional stress-responses discrete or multiple; are they and the physiological concomitants stimulus-response or individual-response specific; what are the components of stress-response as sequences of mechanisms and what purposes do they serve; and finally, how are the long-term processes as part of chronic stress conditions related to the development of degenerative diseases?

Although we do not completely understand how psychological stimuli act as stressors, we can generalize by stating that those that are most effective threaten survival of human subjects through threats of bodily or psychological harm, or by partial or total excommunication from other humans by degrees of sensory or social isolation. Within this general area are countless individual variations depending on past experiences and residual sensitivities.

Research in the field is handicapped by the fact that technical difficulties are present under all conditions: in studying stress responses in life situations, in special field conditions such as war or training in dangerous skills, or in experimental and contrived situations. Efforts at teasing out the relative significance of general laws (nomothetic) and the special reactions or events (ideographic) require much greater control and quantification of the stimuli employed than heretofore applied.

The multiplicity of variables requiring simultaneous observations demands the use of multidisciplinary research teams which we were one of the first to develop in psychiatry. Our methodological general innovations—without specifying details —consisted of:

1. Simultaneous (as close as possible) measurement of variables studied.
2. The development of reliable rating estimates of aroused anger, anxiety and depression as well as defenses.
3. The use of a transactional probing interview to stir up emotional responses through meaningful stimuli communicated to prone individuals.
4. Measurements of hormonal changes, autonomic responses (heart-rate and amplitude, respiratory rate, blood pressure, etc.), somatic voluntary muscle tension, affective responses and total behavior.

Thereby we tapped within known social conditions after the application of natural, contrived and laboratory stressors, changes in the endocrine, autonomic and voluntary nervous systems, personality and behavior.

The general results indicate that adrenocortical responses accompany any affective arousal and are not specific for anxiety although quantitative variations occur with shame, harm or disintegrative anxiety. For the economy of the organism these responses may have significance for adaptation to physical stress by potentiating the activity of the sympathetic nervous system revealed in part by elevation of heart rate and blood pressure. Yet, their utility in psychological stress seems minimal. As an hereditary anachronism— stupidity rather than wisdom of the body —they place a subsequent burden on the detoxifying functions of the liver as measured by the hippuric acid test.

We have found that the neuromuscular system exhibits individual response-specificity as does the autonomic nervous system. It was expected that these should be related to personality traits—not diagnostic entities. We have developed an EMB score comprising traits evoked by psychological tests which indicates that character strength, inner ideation and clear sense of body boundaries are associated with high muscle tension. These people with active inner-fantasy lives at the same time have restraints against action, hence their muscle tension is increased. Likewise we have developed rating scales for psychological defenses against emotional arousal within 5 categories: situation interest and attention, defense intensity, defense primitivity, defense against awareness and general coping devices.

We have taken a simple theoretical concept of a specific emotional reaction to a specific physiological response and helped make it a highly complicated and puzzling field in which there is a complex transactional pattern of stressors, stress-responses, defenses and personality involving, in various combinations, multiple chains of events from the central nervous system to its various peripheral outflows. This complicated picture hardly seems to indicate progress.

Perhaps it is progress to assume that there can be no psychogenesis, sociogenesis, or somatogenesis alone. All systems by virtue of their past—genic or genetic—are prepared for variable responses which are both patterned or structuralized as well as novel and adaptive to new situations. Secondly, crude linearity has to be abandoned, since in nature most transactions are curvilinear. Thirdly, causality as a goal is superceded by concepts of threshold, temporal and quantitative properties of a wide number of responses whose end point may vary by virtue of changing conditions or whose final state may be the end-point of a variety of intermediate processes (equifinality). The common final pathway may be reached through a number of diverse processes. Science today requires the transactional approach especially when multiple biological systems, as in the psychosomatic approach, are under scrutiny.

In sum: depending on the drives and needs of the organism and the changing environment, stimuli constantly entering the central nervous system derived from meaningful environmental cues set off responses in appropriately sensitive individuals. Depending upon the somatic and psychological sensitivity of the individual, the nature and intensity of the stimulus, the quality of the protective devices, and the defenses psychologically available, greater quantities of disturbance lasting for long periods of time (sometimes shorter as in bereavement) may end in so-called diseases. The ultimate application of this research is to determine the pathways to this end-point of illness.

From these investigations and theoretical statements it would seem clear that severe stressors or strains in later life would evoke, in addition to various specific stress responses or defensive maneuvers, what we call regression or what can be termed disintegration. Then the total system begins to break down into its parts which have been important in the development of the more mature integrative states. It is then that the various parts reveal in their own way the impact of the earliest experiences which have impinged upon the organism while still undifferentiated.

This hypothesis states that the differentiated mental and physiological systems respond in correlated patterns revealing the imprinting experienced by both during an undifferentiated phase. These patterns are maintained by each system after differentiation, and stimulation of one can cue off the other. For example, Kepecs in the Institute was able to test patients with asthma, neurodermatitis and arthritis with three types of sensory stimulation: cutaneous, muscular and olfactory. The subjects later drew spontaneously and associated to their drawings. Cutaneous stimulation produced the strongest emotional responses in patients with dermatitis, muscle stimulation in arthritics and olfactory stimulation in asthmatics. Likewise, appropriate emotional arousal evoked responses in the corresponding organ system.

III

When progress in psychoanalysis reached the point where libido theory (closed system) was superceded by adaptational theory (open system), biology and sociology were brought back into focus. The dual-drive theory, consisting of life and death instincts, is being replaced by a monolithic theory of motivation not too different from the ancients' ideas of life. About life we can only speculate, since it is a process that is there and given. Avoiding speculations, philosophy, or religion we can state as Herrick did, "life is a system of forces maintained by energy exchanged between a system and its environment correlated to conserve the identity of the system as an individual and to propagate it as a species." What is gradually replacing concepts of psychological energy, libido and specific drives is modern information theory. In a rapidly changing society, man becomes involved in various quantities of information exchanges—too little, too much, or incongruous qualities. Such qualities and quantities of information act upon all levels of the organism at all times. It is the task of the specialist in child development to investigate the qualities of communication between the child and his human environment that determine specific patterns of personality, character and susceptibility to serious stress responses.

In each phase of life we can observe the phenomena of goal-seeking and goal-changing behavior and the question is becoming increasingly urgent as to what is healthy. Therapists certainly should have some idea as to the value of various types of adaptive behavior. I have recently become interested in so-called health or normality when I encountered such a population at a local college. I called these subjects Homoclites because they tended to follow the common rule, that is to adapt to the expectations of their environment. These subjects, whose aspirations were to do well, to do good, and to be liked, were the product of a consistent life pattern happily furnished by the continuity of certain cultural conditions. They certainly could not be understood apart from the culture in which they were reared.

Parental emphasis on early work habits, sound religious training and the ideals associated with doing good were associated with the genuine parental concern with the child's welfare. Their value systems constitute aspects of Protestant virtues and ethics which were acceptable without rebellion because of the sincere manifestations of parental love and a consistency in attitudes. Identifications seem therefore to be favored.

The character structure of these young men included slight compulsivity, hard work, neatness, orderliness and concern about school and avoidance of failure. They had been termed by others "upright young men." They were more interested in avoiding failure than attaining great success and "doing the best one can" became a virtue as a way of life. It is impossible to determine what would happen to these youngsters if they were uprooted from their environment to which they were well adapted, and forced to exist in a highly competitive situation. Their identifications had prepared them for a limited number of social roles which constitutes the cost of their particular form of adaptation. Certainly, there are many other forms of health and normality but one cannot understand them apart from the social environment in which they developed.

IV

Psychoanalysis, which has come to dominate the field of psychiatry, has seriously interfered with clinical research oriented toward a study of behavior. Internal conflicts, defenses and energic concepts have attracted attention away from the social matrix, culture and behaviors in specific environmental settings. This is a fact which Horney spoke vigorously against. As a result, psychiatric formulations became stereotypes replacing observations and descriptions which were depreciated. Not only were the old diagnostic entities accepted as unchangeable, but new clinical entities, such as the borderline, appearing with rapid social changes, are poorly described and their sub-categories are not investigated.

In this current era of psychoanalytic or psychodynamic psychiatry, clinical observations and descriptions which constitute the core of clinical medicine and produce its data from which hypotheses may be developed, have been derogated until recently. The practical questions concerning the results of treatment of various kinds seemed to have presented no concern to clinicians until the advent of the new tranquilizing and antidepressive drugs. Each psychiatrist usually diagnosed, treated and evaluated his results on few patients—hardly a scientific project. When the new drugs appeared, a rash of rating scales were developed; controls, double-blind techniques and statistical methods were hurriedly devised. The dynamic psychiatrist or psychoanalyst has little interest in diagnosis or classification of various types of behavior. Concerned with the individual, he is more interested in his patient's problems and dynamics. He cannot be expected to contribute to a practical nosological classification. When he does, such abortions as "passive-aggressive personality" have been induced.

An unfortunate concomitant of dynamic psychiatry has been the underemphasis on sound observation, and descriptions which are considered obsolete and old-fashioned. Even the GAP committee on "Training the Psychiatrist to Meet Changing Needs" published in 1963 considers observation, description and classification as a biological technique in which the patient is treated as an object and as the first phase of the development of psychiatry as a science. The second phase is called psychodynamic and the third, which we are apparently about to enter, is termed social or community psychiatry.

I affirm that behavior, both verbal and non-verbal, is the basic data of psychiatry as a science. It represents in actuality functions allocated to a hypothetical ego which filters perceptions on the one hand and actions on the other, which express reportable motivations, affects, defenses and compromises, which employ symptoms and sublimations and demonstrates integrative capacities and disintegrative trends. Behavior is the final common pathway of all these processes. In brief, I believe that behavioral transactional researches constitute a valuable bridge between internal psychological and biological processes on the one hand, and social, cultural and economic (ecological) factors on the other hand.

In using the term "ego," I designate a process or an allocated function which has "structure" in the sense of an enduring pattern over time. Behavior as I use it has no connection with behaviorism as a theoretical position à la Watson and Skinner which depreciates the mental as an object of scientific investigation. Instead, behavior becomes a process for scientific investigation for which objective data are necessary to be acquired by special methods. From this hard data, speculations, inferences, hypothesis-building may *follow* ad lib. Behavior can be observed, described, classified, quantified, modified and analyzed within the matrix of scientific inquiry. All of the derived data are public and therefore can be coded, rated, repeated, replicated and tracked through time.

The approach to behavior need not be contaminated by therapeutic interferences which modify behavior in an uncontrolled fashion and restrict the extent of observations by virtue of the supposed ethics of therapists. Behavior as the final common pathway of a wide variety of processes, actions and reactions demonstrates not only liabilities or "illness," but also assets. As I have stated many times, we need to observe not only goal-seeking behavior as the repetitive neurotic trends or at the worst the symptoms of illness, but also the goal-changing activities of adaptation and creativity indicative of autonomy of the ego and freedom to change the human situation. Such goal-changing activities may be adaptive and creative but place a burden on internal homeostasis. It may be developmental and related to crises in growth, or it may be disruptive to the environment.

If the so-called third phase of psychiatry suggested by the GAP report is to develop, its data must be from behavior as it is influenced by and influences the social community. Humans are not accepted or rejected by their society because they feel badly nor does the common man indicate his need for help because he is not happy enough. He becomes aberrant and feels differently because his behavior is not adaptive within a particular socio-cultural environment.

All this indicates to me that psychiatrists should again learn how to observe and describe. The scientifically curious will classify behavior into types and correlate them with a variety of biological, psychological and environmental factors in the field within which behaviors transact with other behaviors.

We attempted to employ, in the study of depressions, a technique which would enable us to describe the feelings and concerns of depressed patients during the process of several uncovering interviews. At the same time we employed the techniques of observation and description, focussing on the behavior of these patients living in a nursing unit. From these two frames of reference employed on 120 patients, we were able to develop by statistical analysis, factors for feelings and concerns, as well as behaviors. Combining these, we elicited four factor-patterns of combinations of feelings and behaviors which are now available for appropriate sociological psychodynamic and biological correlation.

From these data, we were able to formulate hypotheses indicating the meaning of the various factors which we had elicited. For the feelings and concerns, the first factor described characteristics of hopelessness, helplessness, failure, sadness, unworthiness, and internal suffering, with no appeal to the outside world and no conviction that receiving anything from the environment would change how the patient felt. This factor is the essence of depression and hence its strength indicates the depth of the affective disturbance. The fourth factor described all the characteristics of free anxiety and seemed to be an indicator of activity in the process and a signal of increasing or decreasing affective arousal. In fact, other work indicates this clearly in that the quantity of free anxiety is correlated with the level of adrenocortical activity and is correlated with an increased drive towards suicide. The other factors indicate varying attempts at defense and resolution of the depression. So, for example, factor two described characteristics of concern over material loss and the conviction that suffering could be changed if only the outside world would provide something. This we called a projective defense. On the other hand, factor three indicates that the patient feels guilty over wrongdoing and wishes to make restitution since the illness was brought on by himself and is well deserved. This we may call the restitutional resolution. Factor five describes characteristics of envy, loneliness, martyred affliction, gratification from illness and attempts to force the world into making redress. This factor indicates an attempt by slavery of external object to deny anger and secondarily to regain love.

Following the success of our operational behavioral research with depressed patients, we began a study of the so-called borderline states using, however, more observations and descriptions by a wide group of professionals. The borderline is a fairly new label in clinical psychiatry, unfortunately utilized with increasing frequency as a wastebasket entity to describe a variety of patients whose condition cannot be clearly diagnosed as either psychotic or neurotic. Yet, from the experience of practitioners as well as from the literature, there seems to be little general understanding of the term, or of criteria which would lead to accurate, consistent or reliable diagnoses. In whatever ways there are disagreements about the borderline patients, there is agreement that certain functions are impaired based on the fact that these patients have little depth or consistency in their feelings toward other humans. Aside from this central fact, the clinical symptomatology is variable.

Our present behavioral approach assumes that a large enough time sample of the behavior of a patient is an adequate index of his psychological structure. We therefore study hospital patients because we can get a time sample around the clock over days and weeks. We can through the eyes and ears of the staff that serves the patient see him as he actually lives in his daily life and as he experiences and uses his hospital stay. Thereby, we observe his assets as well as his liabilities in his spontaneous and natural behavior. There may be fifteen of twenty professional and subprofessional observers who by their numbers wash out the possible distortion of one or two biased persons. The trans-cribed tape recordings of each observer are then rated by professionals who do not see the subjects and discrepant ratings are reconciled by another rating.

We then translate the protocols of behavior into clinical terms by means of about 225 questions, developed within a logical framework of ego functions. These are divided into five major categories: 1) Outward behavior; 2) Perception; 3) Communications; 4) Affects and Defenses and 5) Synthesis. We then used clinical judgment to arrive at answers in quantitative terms to: "How much?" "To what degree?" We characterized this study as one designed to simulate a diagnostic practice model, based on behavior. That is, our basic data is naturalistic which is then translated into a clinical framework via a clinical judgment and finally ending up through speculation into the setting up of discrete hypotheses.

For some time it has been observed by clinical psychiatrists that the characteristic histrionic and dramatic neuroses which could be fitted into the classical nosological categories have changed. Instead, we see rigid, constricted, inhibited, unfeeling characters who have been called character neuroses. Lately, however, they have been receiving the diagnostic appellation of borderline cases. In their behaviors they resemble very closely Harlow's monkeys who have been deprived of their natural mothers and who seem to thrive physically, but at adolescence reveal difficulty in playing with their peers and inability to have sexual relations with either sex. The impairments in the borderline humans and monkeys seem to stem from damage far earlier than the time ascribed to the oedipus complex. They are the result of much earlier deficiencies in child-mother relationships at a critical period which cannot yet be pinpointed.

Philosophers like Susanne Langer put the blame for the current character neuroses and borderline conditions on the rapid developments in science as the source and pacemaker of modern civilization which is sweeping away the role of cultural values in life. In her opinion the seeds of civilization are in every culture but it is city life which brings them to fruition, and which in turn drains from life the cultural values that engender and support it. Susanne Langer believes that a shift of balance between conservative and progressive elements may tip the scales of feelings toward the personalistic pole and away from piety and decorum. This shift of balance, she believes, occurs with flagrant exhibits of complete imbalance such as lives culturally lost and degenerated, the familiar criminal elements and irresponsible drifters of every big city in the world. Here we have a philosopher who views the borderline and all it represents from a broader frame of reference. As psychiatrists we tend to attribute the fault or direct cause to child-rearing practices. Even if this be true the primary causes are involved in the rapid shifts of civilization away from its cultural foundations.

V

Once classical psychoanalysis moved from its earliest position as an open system to a closed system ignoring the biological and sociological, then the social and cultural determinants of personality and the neuroses became minimized. Correspondingly, in psychoanalytic therapy the analyst and patient formed a closed transference and countertransference system excluding contact or information from all other human informants. As a closed system, psychoanalysis ignored the other behavioral disciplines and their findings. Organized psychoanalysis has never moved far from this position, even though Freud himself did later when the structural frame of reference and adaptation came to be considered an important aspect of ego psychology.

Each therapeutic discipline operates within the framework of some theory which becomes even more important when the process involves the use of words only. For example, theory determines when, what and how the therapist communicates to his patient and how he utilizes the information he receives. Although this theory is at a low level of abstraction not utilizing metapsychology, it does influence the therapeutic process decidedly. When we consider that the patient and the therapist comprise an open system, then we become interested in the patient's real life and in his behavior in the world, as well as our own real persons in relationship to our patients. It is in this sense that meaning or the nature of existence becomes important. Horney became involved in problems of alienation, responsibility and social attitudes of compliance, aggression and detachment long before psychoanalysts recognized that these were problems of adaptation. Neurotic conflicts are more than internal drive derivatives but include a consideration of the social, physical and cultural environment in the processes of living.

When the focus of analysis seemed to be on the oedipus complex, it was natural to consider that its resolution was the main work to be done in analysis and any flight from it was supposedly regressive. This led Alexander to practice modifications of technique to block regression, forcing his patient to avoid flight and to focus on oedipal and competitive problems. Unfortunately, this did not take into consideration that the majority of patients whom we see today have failed in achieving an identity. Their general pessimistic attitude toward life, poor object relationships, and the failure of affectional consistency all indicate that the crucial failure and development began much earlier during the phase of important information input when there are defects such as overloading, insufficient or distorted information, and learning from signs to the phase of symbolic transformation is impaired. These patients need to experience new satisfactions, leading to a better degree of mastery. It is for these patients, especially, and their number is increasing, that the social situation in the therapeutic dyad must become real, gratifying, and applicable to other external phases of existence and needs to be emphasized and re-emphasized in relation to the therapy. It is here, I think, where the so-called neo-Freudians have taken the lead.

In my opinion there is no sharp division between psychoanalysis and psychotherapy. This is a wide spectrum which constitutes a continuum. Whether one uses the interpersonal approach of Sullivan or the methods of Horney, we are involved in a form of therapy oriented toward changing the behavior of our patients. Some of these changes may follow internal reorganization or insight and, on the other hand, change of behavior may be *followed by* intrapsychic shifts in the balance of various forces involved in conflict. I once stated that one has to be a fairly normal person to profit by psychoanalysis. If this be true, then, most of our patients are at the other end of the spectrum and should be involved in psychotherapy, which contains large amounts of control, direction, reassurance, support, and education, as well as insight.

VI

In the course of this brief presentation, I have given you some extracts of my work in various fields. These include psychosomatic research, stress research, and investigations on normality, depression and borderline cases. Finally, I have briefly discussed some aspects of therapy. In all the work which I have been engaged in over the years, I have utilized what is euphemistically called "field theory" and attempted to place in proper perspective the various phenomena which can be subsumed under the biological, psychological and social foci in total field. Modern psychoanalysts have subscribed to structural and adaptational theory which enables psychology as a study of the mental system to be investigated in open relationship with other systems and investigated in terms of the relationships of its parts to one another in the whole.

There are concentrated efforts to define psychoanalytic terms clearly, to clear out semantic confusions and to specify levels of discourse. This requires a form of scientific rigor applied to conceptual thinking and to methodology, without creating a fear of throwing away intuition which can itself be investigated by new approaches to countertransference.

It becomes obvious that investigations which I have conducted are not directly psychoanalytic. They are, in fact, researches which utilize the functions of the ego in behavior. They are indirectly psychoanalytic because behavior expresses as a final common pathway a wide variety of internal biological and psychological processes and two-way involvement with society, culture and civilization.

This broad frame of reference has been derogated because it was instituted by people outside the field of classical analysis, or by those who once were within the field and then withdrew to form their own groups. The best examples, of course, are Sullivan on the one hand and Horney on the other. The term "neo-Freudian," however, in my mind is no derogation; it has been applied several

times to me although I am not a member of any of the societies other than the Academy. But I am a neo-Freudian in the sense that every progressive investigator and every curious modern analyst is, because to be a Freudian has come to mean that we accept in a religious sense the words of Freud as scriptures that must be followed directly. As progressive analysts or psychiatrists or what not, we make use of what Freud started and developed to a high degree, but when we maintain adherence to a spoken or written word we become not only unprogressive but regressive. To be called a neo-Freudian then means to be approved as someone who has progressed beyond the 19th-century concepts of Freud.

If we agree that psychiatry is in part one of the behavioral sciences and in part includes several other scientific disciplines, it needs a unified theory. For several years, under the auspices of the Carnegie Foundation, we assembled a multidisciplinary conference group to discuss this problem, later publishing a book entitled *Toward a Unified Theory of Human Behavior*.

This beginning attempt was not very successful in achieving its goal. Nevertheless, it did emphasize information, communication and transactional theory which had a profound effect on the participants of our conferences. Like language, which is the organizer of conceptual processes, unified theories may serve as models for scientists' thinking and transcend the narrowness and isolation of their involvement in a particular discipline. In fact, one pressing 20th-century problem is how to relate sciences with each other and to develop a universal or bridging and dynamic language. This is so essential in psychiatry because of its many participant sciences.

The time will soon come, however, when the total field can no longer be continued to be viewed and amplified by independent disciplines or by a multiplicity of institutes serving as training centers for the development of parts of the field. If we really believe in a unified theory or in a total field concept then all the aspects of psychiatry, including psychoanalysis both classical and progressive, need to be investigated and to be taught within an academic environment. It is for this reason that I am convinced that psychiatry, which includes all that I have enumerated, will eventually be advanced in the universities and not in independent institutes. It is high time that those parts which have drawn away from the whole again be brought into the total field, under the control of scientific leadership. To my way of thinking this can only be done in an academic setting where the spirit of investigation, of tolerance for aberrant ideas, and for skepticism and scrutiny of what seems to be correct can be achieved.

53. Schizotaxia, Schizotypy, Schizophrenia

PAUL E. MEEHL

In the course of the last decade, while spending several thousand hours in the practice of intensive psychotherapy, I have treated—sometimes unknowingly except in retrospect—a considerable number of schizoid and schizophrenic patients. Like all clinicians, I have formed some theoretical opinions as a result of these experiences. While I have not until recently begun any systematic research efforts on this baffling disorder, I felt that to share with you some of my thoughts, based though they are upon clinical impressions in the context of selected research by others, might be an acceptable use of this occasion.

Let me begin by putting a question which I find is almost never answered correctly by our clinical students on PhD orals, and the answer which they seem to dislike when it is offered. Suppose that you were required to write down a procedure for selecting an individual from the population who would be diagnosed as schizophrenic by a psychiatric staff; you have to wager $1,000 on being right; you may not include in your selection procedure any behavioral fact, such as a symptom or trait, manifested by the individual. What would you write down? So far as I have been able to ascertain, there is only one thing you could write down that would give you a better than even chance of winning such a bet—namely, "Find an individual X who has a schizophrenic

identical twin." Admittedly, there are many other facts which would raise your odds somewhat above the low base of schizophrenia. You might, for example, identify X by first finding mothers who have certain unhealthy child-rearing attitudes; you might enter a subpopulation defined jointly by such demographic variables as age, size of community, religion, ethnic background, or social class. But these would leave you with a pretty unfair wager, as would the rule, "Find an X who has a fraternal twin, of the same sex, diagnosed as schizophrenic" (Fuller & Thompson, 1960, pp. 272–283; Stern, 1960, pp. 581–584).

Now the twin studies leave a good deal to be desired methodologically (Rosenthal, 1962); but there seems to be a kind of "double standard of methodological morals" in our profession, in that we place a good deal of faith in our knowledge of schizophrenic dynamics, and we make theoretical inferences about social learning factors from the establishment of group trends which may be statistically significant and replicable although of small or moderate size; but when we come to the genetic studies, our standards of rigor suddenly increase. I would argue that the concordance rates in the twin studies need not be accepted uncritically as highly precise parameter estimates in order for us to say that their magnitudes represent the most important piece of etiological information we possess about schizophrenia.

It is worthwhile, I think, to pause here over a question in the sociology of

From the *Amer. Psychol.* 17:827–838, 1962, by permission of the American Psychological Association and the author.

knowledge, namely, why do psychologists exhibit an aversive response to the twin data? I have no wish to argue *ad hominem* here—I raise this question in a constructive and irenic spirit, because I think that a substantive confusion often lies at the bottom of this resistance, and one which can be easily dispelled. Everybody readily assents to such vague dicta as "heredity and environment interact," "there need be no conflict between organic and functional concepts," "we always deal with the total organism," etc. But it almost seems that clinicians do not fully believe these principles in any concrete sense, because they show signs of thinking that *if* a genetic basis were found for schizophrenia, the psychodynamics of the disorder (especially in relation to intrafamilial social learnings) would be somehow negated or, at least, greatly demoted in importance. To what extent, if at all, is this true?

Here we run into some widespread misconceptions as to what is meant by *specific etiology* in nonpsychiatric medicine. By postulating a "specific etiology" one does *not* imply any of the following:

1. The etiological factor always, or even usually, produces clinical illness.
2. If illness occurs, the particular form and content of symptoms is derivable by reference to the specific etiology alone.
3. The course of the illness can be materially influenced only by procedures directed against the specific etiology.
4. All persons who share the specific etiology will have closely similar histories, symptoms, and course.
5. The largest single contributor to symptom variance is the specific etiology.

In medicine, not one of these is part of the concept of specific etiology, yet they are repeatedly invoked as arguments against a genetic interpretation of schizophrenia. I am not trying to impose the causal model of medicine by analogy; I merely wish to emphasize that *if* one postulates a genetic mutation as the specific etiology of schizophrenia, he is not thereby committed to any of the above as implications. Consequently such familiar objections as, "Schizophrenics differ widely from one another" or "Many schizophrenics can be helped by purely psychological methods" should not disturb one who opts for a genetic hypothesis. In medicine, the concept of

specific etiology means the *sine qua non*—the causal condition which is necessary, but not sufficient, for the disorder to occur. A genetic theory of schizophrenia would, in this sense, be stronger than that of "one contributor to variance"; but weaker than that of "largest contributor to variance." In analysis of variance terms, it means an interaction effect such that no other variables can exert a main effect when the specific etiology is lacking.

Now it goes without saying that "clinical schizophrenia" as such cannot be inherited, because it has behavioral and phenomenal contents which are learned. As Bleuler says, in order to have a delusion involving Jesuits one must first have learned about Jesuits. It seems inappropriate to apply the geneticist's concept of "penetrance" to the crude statistics of formal diagnosis—if a specific genetic etiology exists, its phenotypic expression in *psychological* categories would be a quantitative aberration in some parameter of a behavioral acquisition function. What could possibly be a genetically determined functional parameter capable of generating such diverse behavioral outcomes, including the preservation of normal function in certain domains?

The theoretical puzzle is exaggerated when we fail to conceptualize at different levels of molarity. For instance, there is a tendency among organically minded theorists to analogize between catatonic phenomena and various neurological or chemically induced states in animals. But Bleuler's masterly *Theory of Schizophrenic Negativism* (1912) shows how the whole range of catatonic behavior, including diametrically opposite modes of relating to the interpersonal environment, can be satisfactorily explained as instrumental acts; thus even a convinced organicist, postulating a biochemical defect as specific etiology, should recognize that the causal linkage between this etiology and catatonia is indirect, requiring for the latter's derivation a lengthy chain of statements which are not even formulable except in molar psychological language.

What kind of behavioral fact about the patient leads us to diagnose schizophrenia? There are a number of traits and symptoms which get a high weight, and the weights differ among clinicians. But thought disorder continues to hold its own in spite of today's greater clinical interest in motivational (especially interpersonal) variables. If you are inclined to doubt this for yourself, consider the following indicators: Patient experiences intense ambivalence, readily reports conscious hatred of family figures, is pananxious, subjects therapist to a long series of testing operations, is withdrawn, and says, "Naturally, I am growing my father's hair."

While all of these are schizophrenic indicators, the last one is the diagnostic bell ringer. In this respect we are still Bleulerians, although we know a lot more about the schizophrenic's psychodynamics than Bleuler did. The significance of thought disorder, associative dyscontrol (or, as I prefer to call it so as to include the very mildest forms it may take, "cognitive slippage"), in schizophrenia has been somewhat de-emphasized in recent years. Partly this is due to the greater interest in interpersonal dynamics, but partly also to the realization that much of our earlier psychometric assessment of the thought disorder was mainly reflecting the schizophrenic's tendency to underperform because uninterested, preoccupied, resentful, or frightened. I suggest that this realization has been overgeneralized and led us to swing too far the other way, as if we had shown that there really *is* no cognitive slippage factor present. One rather common assumption seems to be that if one can demonstrate the potentiating effect of a motivational state upon cognitive slippage, light has thereby been shed upon the etiology of schizophrenia. Why are we entitled to think this? Clinically, we see a degree of cognitive slippage not found to a comparable degree among non-schizophrenic persons. Some patients (e.g., pseudoneurotics) are highly anxious and exhibit minimal slippage; others (e.g., burnt-out cases) are minimally anxious with marked slippage. The demonstration that we can intensify a particular patient's cognitive dysfunction by manipulating his affects is not really very illuminating. After all, even ordinary neurological diseases can often be tremendously influenced symptomatically via emotional stimuli; but if a psychologist demonstrates that the spasticity or tremor of a multiple sclerotic is affected by rage or fear, we would not thereby have learned anything about the etiology of multiple sclerosis.

Consequent upon our general assimilation of the insights given us by psychoanalysis, there is today a widespread and largely unquestioned assumption that when we can trace out the motivational forces linked to the content of aberrant behavior, then we understand why the person has fallen ill. There is no compelling reason to assume this, when the evidence is mainly our dynamic understanding of the patient, however valid that may be. The phrase "why the person has fallen ill" may, of course, be legitimately taken to include these things; an account of how and when he falls ill will certainly include them. But they may be quite inadequate to answer the question, "Why does X fall ill and not Y, granted that we can understand both of them?" I like the analogy of a color psychosis, which might be developed by certain individuals in a society entirely oriented around the making of fine color discriminations. Social, sexual, economic signals are color mediated; to misuse a color word is strictly taboo; compulsive mothers are horribly ashamed of a child who is retarded in color development, and so forth. Some color-blind individuals (not all, perhaps not most) develop a color psychosis in this culture; as adults, they are found on the couches of color therapists, where a great deal of *valid* understanding is achieved about color dynamics. Some of them make a social recovery. Nonetheless, if we ask, "What was basically the matter with these patients?" meaning, "What is the specific etiology of the color psychosis?" the answer is that mutated gene on the X chromosome. This is why my own therapeutic experience with schizophrenic patients has not yet convinced me of the schizophrenogenic mother as a specific etiology, even though the picture I get of my patients' mothers is pretty much in accord with the familiar one. There is no question here of accepting the patient's account; my point is that *given* the account, and taking it quite at face value, does not tell me why the patient is a patient and not just a fellow who had a bad mother.

Another theoretical lead is the one given greatest current emphasis, namely, *interpersonal aversiveness*. The schizophrene suffers a degree of social fear, distrust, expectation of rejection, and conviction of his own unlovability which cannot be matched in its depth, pervasity, and resistance to corrective experience by any other diagnostic group.

Then there is a quasi-pathognomonic sign, emphasized by Rado (1956; Rado & Daniels, 1956) but largely ignored in psychologists' diagnostic usage, namely, *anhedonia*—a marked, widespread, and refractory defect in pleasure capacity which, once you learn how to examine for it, is one of the most consistent and dramatic behavioral signs of the disease.

Finally, I include *ambivalence* from Bleuler's cardinal four (1950). His other two, "autism" and "dereism," I consider derivative from the combination of slippage, anhedonia, and aversiveness. Crudely put, if a person cannot think straight, gets little pleasure, and is afraid of everyone, he will of course learn to be autistic and dereistic.

If these clinical characterizations are correct, and we combine them with the hypothesis of a genetic specific etiology, do they give us any lead on theoretical possibilities?

Granting its initial vagueness as a construct, requiring to be filled in by neurophysiological research, I believe we should take seriously the old European notion of an "integrative neural defect" as the only direct phenotypic consequence produced by the genic mutation. This is an aberration in some parameter of single cell function, which may or may not be manifested in the functioning of more molar CNS systems, depending upon the organization of the mutual feedback controls and upon the stochastic parameters of the reinforcement regime. This neural integrative defect, which I shall christen *schizotaxia,* is all that can properly be spoken of as inherited. The imposition of a social learning history upon schizotaxic individuals results in a personality organization which I shall call, following Rado, the *schizotype.* The four core behavior traits are obviously not innate; but I postulate that they are universally learned by schizotaxic individuals, given any of the actually existing social reinforcement regimes, from the best to the worst. If the interpersonal regime is favorable, and the schizotaxic person also has the good fortune to inherit a low anxiety readiness, physical vigor, general resistance to stress and the like, he will remain a well-compensated "normal" schizotype, never manifesting symptoms of mental disease.

He will be like the gout-prone male whose genes determine him to have an elevated blood uric acid titer, but who never develops clinical gout.

Only a subset of schizotypic personalities decompensate into clinical schizophrenia. It seems likely that the most important causal influence pushing the schizotype toward schizophrenic decompensation is the schizophrenogenic mother.

I hope it is clear that this view does not conflict with what has been established about the mother-child interaction. If this interaction were totally free of material ambivalence and aversive inputs to the schizotaxic child, even compensated schizotypy might be avoided; at most, we might expect to find only the faintest signs of cognitive slippage and other minimal neurological aberrations, possibly including body image and other proprioceptive deviations, but not the interpersonal aversiveness which is central to the clinical picture.

Nevertheless, while assuming the etiological importance of mother in determining the course of aversive social learnings, it is worthwhile to speculate about the modification our genetic equations might take on this hypothesis. Many schizophrenogenic mothers are themselves schizotypes in varying degrees of compensation. Their etiological contribution then consists jointly in their passing on the gene, *and* in the fact that being schizotypic, they provide the kind of ambivalent regime which potentiates the schizotypy of the child and raises the odds of his decompensating. Hence the incidence of the several parental genotypes among parent pairs of diagnosed proband cases is not calculable from the usual genetic formulas. For example, given a schizophrenic proband, the odds that mother is homozygous (or, if the gene were dominant, that it is mother who carries it) are different from those for father; since we have begun by selecting a decompensated case, and formal diagnosis as the phenotype involves a potentiating factor for mother which is psychodynamically greater than that for a schizotypic father. Another important influence would be the likelihood that the lower fertility of schizophrenics is also present, but to an unknown degree, among compensated schizotypes. Clinical experience suggests that in the semicompensated range, this lowering of fertility is greater among males, since many schizotypic women relate to men in an exploited or exploitive sexual way, whereas the male schizotype usually displays a marked deficit in heterosexual aggressiveness. Such a sex difference in fertility among decompensated cases has been reported by Meyers and Goldfarb (1962).

Since the extent of aversive learnings is a critical factor in decompensation, the inherited anxiety readiness is presumably greater among diagnosed cases. Since the more fertile mothers are likely to be compensated, hence themselves to be relatively low anxiety if schizotaxic, a frequent parent pattern should be a compensated schizotypic mother married to a neurotic father, the latter being the source of the proband's high-anxiety genes (plus providing a poor paternal model for identification in male patients, and a weak defender of the child against mother's schizotypic hostility).

These considerations make ordinary family concordance studies, based upon formal diagnosis, impossible to interpret. The most important research need here is development of high-validity indicators for compensated schizotypy. I see some evidence for these conceptions in the report of Lidz and co-workers, who in studying intensively the parents of 15 schizophrenic patients were surprised to find that "minimally, 9 of the 15 patients had at least one parent who could be called schizophrenic, or ambulatory schizophrenic, or clearly paranoid in behavior and attitudes" (Lidz, Cornelison, Terry, and Fleck, 1958, p. 308). As I read the brief personality sketches presented, I would judge that all but two of the probands had a clearly schizotypic parent. These authors, while favoring a "learned irrationality" interpretation of their data, also recognize the alternative genetic interpretation. Such facts do not permit a decision, obviously; my main point is the striking difference between the high incidence of parental schizotypes, mostly quite decompensated (some to the point of diagnosable psychosis), and the zero incidence which a conventional study would have yielded for this group.

Another line of evidence, based upon a very small sample but exciting because of its uniformity, is McConaghy's report (1959) that among nondiagnosed parent pairs of 10 schizophrenics, subclinical thought disorder was psychometrically detectable in at least one parent of every pair. Rosenthal (1962) reports that he can add five tallies to this parent-pair count, and suggests that such results might indicate that the specific heredity is dominant, and completely penetrant, rather than recessive. The attempt to replicate these findings, and other psychometric efforts to tap subclinical cognitive slippage in the "normal" relatives of schizophrenics, should receive top priority in our research efforts.

Summarizing, I hypothesize that the statistical relation between schizotaxia, schizotypy, and schizophrenia is class inclusion: All schizotaxics become, *on all actually existing social learning regimes,* schizotypic in personality organization; but most of these remain compensated. A minority, disadvantaged by other (largely polygenically determined) constitutional weaknesses, and put on a bad regime by schizophrenogenic mothers (most of whom are themselves schizotypes) are thereby potentiated into clinical schizophrenia. What makes schizotaxia etiologically specific is its role as a *necessary* condition. I postulate that a nonschizotaxic individual, whatever his other genetic makeup and whatever his learning history, would at most develop a character disorder or a psychoneurosis; but he would not become a schizotype and therefore could never manifest its decompensated form, schizophrenia.

What sort of quantitative aberration in the structural or functional parameters of the nervous system can we conceive to be directly determined by a mutated gene, and to so alter initial dispositions that affected individuals will, in the course of their childhood learning history, develop the four schizotypal source traits: cognitive slippage, anhedonia, ambivalence, and interpersonal aversiveness? To me, the most baffling thing about the disorder is the phenotypic heterogeneity of this tetrad. If one sets himself to the task of doing a theoretical Vigotsky job on this list of psychological dispositions, he may manage part of it by invoking a sufficiently vague kind of descriptive unity between ambivalence and interpersonal aversiveness; and perhaps even anhedonia could be somehow subsumed. But the cognitive slippage presents a real roadblock. Since I consider cognitive slippage to be a core element in schizophrenia, any characterization of schizophrenic or schizotypic behavior which purports to abstract its essence but does not include the cognitive slippage must be deemed unsatisfactory. I believe that an adequate theoretical account will necessitate moving downward in the pyramid of the sciences to invoke explanatory constructs not found in social, psychodynamic, or even learning theory language, but instead at the neurophysiological level.

Perhaps we don't know enough about "how the brain works" to theorize profitably at that level; and I daresay that the more a psychologist knows about the latest research on brain function, the more reluctant he would be to engage in etiological speculation. Let me entreat my physiologically expert listeners to be charitable toward this clinician's premature speculations about how the schizotaxic brain might work. I feel partially justified in such speculating because there are some well-attested general truths about mammalian learned behavior which could almost have been set down from the armchair, in the way engineers draw block diagrams indicating what kinds of parts or subsystems a physical system *must* have, and what their interconnections *must* be, in order to function "appropriately." Brain research of the last decade provides a direct neurophysiological substrate for such cardinal behavior requirements as avoidance, escape, reward, drive differentiation, general and specific arousal or activation, and the like (see Delafresnaye, 1961; Ramey & O'Doherty, 1960). The discovery in the limbic system of specific positive reinforcement centers by Olds and Milner in 1954, and of aversive centers in the same year by Delgado, Roberts, and Miller (1954), seems to me to have an importance that can scarcely be exaggerated; and while the ensuing lines of research on the laws of intracranial stimulation as a mode of behavior control present some puzzles and paradoxes, what *has* been shown up to now may already suffice to provide a theoretical framework. As a general kind of brain model let us take a broadly Hebbian conception in combination with the findings on intracranial stimulation.

To avoid repetition I shall list some basic assumptions first but introduce others in context and only implicitly when the implication is obvious. I shall assume that:

When a presynaptic cell participates in firing a postsynaptic cell, the former gains an increment in firing control over the latter. Coactivation of anatomically connected cell assemblies or assembly systems therefore increases their stochastic control linkage, and the frequency of discharges by neurons of a system may be taken as an intensity variable influencing the growth rate of intersystem control linkage as well as the momentary activity level induced in the other systems. (I shall dichotomize acquired cortical systems into "perceptual-cognitive," including central representations of goal objects; and "instrumental," including overarching monitor systems which select and guide specific effector patterns.)

Most learning in mature organisms involves altering control linkages between systems which themselves have been consolidated by previous learnings, sometimes requiring thousands of activations and not necessarily related to the reinforcement operation to the extent that perceptual-to-instrumental linkage growth functions are.

Control linkage increments from coactivation depend heavily, if not entirely, upon a period of reverberatory activity facilitating consolidation.

Feedback from positive limbic centers is facilitative to concurrent perceptual-cognitive or instrumental sequences, whereas negative center feedback exerts an inhibitory influence. (These statements refer to initial features of the direct wiring diagram, not to all long-term results of learning.) Aversive input also has excitatory effects via the arousal system, which maintain activity permitting escape learning to occur because the organism is alerted and keeps doing things. But I postulate that this overall influence is working along with an opposite effect, quite clear from both molar and intracranial experiments, that a major biological function of aversive-center activation is to produce "stoppage" of whatever the organism is currently doing.

Perceptual-cognitive systems and limbic motivational control centers develop two-way mutual controls (e.g., discriminative stimuli acquire the reinforcing property; "thoughts" become pleasantly toned; drive-relevant perceptual components are "souped-up.")

What kind of heritable parametric

aberration could underlie the schizotaxic's readiness to acquire the schizotypic tetrad? It would seem, first of all, that the defect is much more likely to reside in the neurone's synaptic control function than in its storage function. It is hard to conceive of a general defect in storage which would on the one hand permit so many perceptual-cognitive functions, such as tapped by intelligence tests, school learning, or the high order cognitive powers displayed by some schizotypes, and yet have the diffuse motivational and emotional effects found in these same individuals. I am not saying that a storage deficit is clearly excludable, but it hardly seems the best place to look. So we direct our attention to parameters of control.

One possibility is to take the anhedonia as fundamental. What is *phenomenologically* a radical pleasure deficiency may be roughly identified *behaviorally* with a quantitative deficit in the positive reinforcement growth constant, and each of these—the "inner" and "outer" aspects of the organism's appetitive control system—reflect a quantitative deficit in the limbic "positive" centers. The anhedonia would then be a direct consequence of the genetic defect in wiring. Ambivalence and interpersonal aversiveness would be quantitative deviations in the balance of appetitive-aversive controls. Most perceptual-cognitive and instrumental learnings occur under mixed positive and negative schedules, so the normal consequence is a collection of habits and expectancies varying widely in the intensity of their positive and negative components, but mostly "mixed" in character. Crudely put, everybody has *some* ambivalence about almost everything, and everybody has *some* capacity for "social fear." Now if the brain centers which mediate phenomenal pleasure and behavioral reward are numerically sparse or functionally feeble, the aversive centers meanwhile functioning normally, the long-term result would be a general shift toward the aversive end, appearing clinically as ambivalence and exaggerated interpersonal fear. If, as Brady believes, there is a wired-in reciprocal inhibiting relation between positive and negative centers, the long-term aversive drift would be further potentiated (i.e., what we see at the molar level as a sort of "softening" or "soothing" effect of feeding or petting upon anxiety elicitors would be reduced).

Cognitive slippage is not as easy to fit in, but if we assume that normal ego function is acquired by a combination of social reinforcements and the self-reinforcements which become available to the child via identification; then we might say roughly that "everybody has to learn *how* to think straight." Rationality is socially acquired; the secondary process and the reality principle are slowly and imperfectly learned, by even the most clear headed. Insofar as slippage is manifested in the social sphere, such an explanation has some plausibility. An overall aversive drift would account for the paradoxical schizotypic combination of interpersonal distortions and acute perceptiveness of others' unconscious, since the latter is really a hypersensitivity to aversive signals rather than an overall superiority in realistically discriminating social cues. On the output side, we might view the cognitive slippage of mildly schizoid speech as originating from poorly consolidated second-order "monitor" assembly systems which function in an editing role, their momentary regnancy constituting the "set to communicate." At this level, selection among competing verbal operants involves slight differences in appropriateness for which a washed-out social reinforcement history provides an insufficiently refined monitor system. However, if one is impressed with the presence of a pervasive and primary slippage, showing up in a diversity of tests (cf. Payne, 1961) and also on occasions when the patient is desperately trying to communicate, an explanation on the basis of deficient positive center activity is not too convincing.

This hypothesis has some other troubles which I shall merely indicate. Schizoid anhedonia is mainly interpersonal, i.e., schizotypes seem to derive adequate pleasure from esthetic and cognitive rewards. Secondly, some successful psychotherapeutic results include what appears to be a genuine normality of hedonic capacity. Thirdly, regressive electroshock sometimes has the same effect, and the animal evidence suggests that shock works by knocking out the aversive control system rather than by souping up appetitive centers. Finally, if the anhedonia is really general in extent, it is hard to conceive of any simple genetic basis for weakening the different positive centers, whose reactivity has been shown by Olds and others to be chemically drive specific.

A second neurological hypothesis takes the slippage factor as primary. Suppose that the immediate consequence of whatever biochemical aberration the gene directly controls were a specific alteration in the neurone's membrane stability, such that the distribution of optional transmission probabilities is more widely dispersed over the synaptic signal space than in normals. That is, presynaptic input signals whose spatio-temporal configuration locates them peripherally in the neurone's signal space yield transmission probabilities which are relatively closer to those at the maximum point, thereby producing a kind of dedifferentiation or flattening of the cell's selectivity. Under suitable parametric assumptions, this synaptic slippage would lead to a corresponding dedifferentiation of competing interassembly controls, because the elements in the less frequently or intensely coactivated control assembly would be accumulating control increments more rapidly than normal. Consider a perceptual-cognitive system whose regnancy is preponderantly associated with positive-center coactivation but sometimes with aversive. The cumulation of control increments will draw these apart; but if synaptic slippage exists, their difference, at least during intermediate stages of control development, will be attenuated. The intensity of aversive-center activation by a given level of perceptual-cognitive system activity will be exaggerated relative to that induced in the positive centers. For a preponderantly aversive control this will be reversed. But now the different algebraic sign of the feedbacks introduces an important asymmetry. Exaggerated negative feedback will tend to lower activity level in the predominantly appetitive case, retarding the growth of the control linkage; whereas exaggerated positive feedback in the predominantly aversive case will tend to heighten activity levels, accelerating the linkage growth. The long-term tendency will be that movement in the negative direction which I call *aversive drift*. In addition to the asymmetry generated by the difference in feedback signs, certain other features in the mixed-regime setup contribute to aversive drift. One factor is the characteristic difference between positive and negative reinforcers in their role as strengtheners. It seems a

fairly safe generalization to say that positive centers function only weakly as strengtheners when "on" continuously, and mainly when they are turned on as terminators of a cognitive or instrumental sequence; by contrast, negative centers work mainly as "off" signals, tending to inhibit elements while steadily "on." We may suppose that the former strengthen mainly by facilitating postactivity reverberation (and hence consolidation) in successful systems, the latter mainly by holding down such reverberation in unsuccessful ones. Now a slippage-heightened aversive steady state during predominantly appetitive control sequences reduces their activity level, leaves fewer recently active elements available for a subsequent Olds-plus "on" signal to consolidate. Whereas a slippage-heightened Olds-plus steady state during predominantly aversive control sequences (a) increases their negative control *during* the "on" period and (b) leaves relatively more of their elements recently active and hence further consolidated by the negative "off" signal when it occurs. Another factor is exaggerated competition by aversively controlled sequences, whereby the appetitive chains do not continue to the stage of receiving socially mediated positive reinforcement, because avoidant chains (e.g., phobic behavior, withdrawal, intellectualization) are getting in the way. It is worth mentioning that the schizophrenogenic mother's regime is presumably "mixed" not only in the sense of the frequent and unpredictable aversive inputs she provides in response to the child's need signals, but also in her greater tendency to present such aversive inputs *concurrently* with drive reducers—thereby facilitating the "scrambling" of appetitive-and-aversive controls so typical of schizophrenia.

The schizotype's dependency guilt and aversive overreaction to offers of help are here seen as residues of the early knitting together of his cortical representations of appetitive goals with punishment-expectancy assembly systems. Roughly speaking, he has learned that to want anything interpersonally provided is to be endangered.

The cognitive slippage is here conceived as a direct molar consequence of synaptic slippage, potentiated by the disruptive effects of aversive control and inadequate development of interpersonal communication sets. Cognitive and instrumental linkages based upon sufficiently massive and consistent regimes, such as reaching for a seen pencil, will coverge to asymptotes hardly distinguishable from the normal. But systems involving closely competing strengths and automatized selection among alternatives, especially when the main basis of acquisition and control is social reward, will exhibit evidences of malfunction.

My third speculative model revives a notion with a long history, namely, that the primary schizotaxic defect is a quantitative deficiency of inhibition. (In the light of Milner's revision of Hebb, in which the inhibitory action of Golgi Type II cells is crucial even for the formation of functionally differentiated cell assemblies, a defective inhibitory parameter could be an alternative basis for a kind of slippage similar in its consequences to the one we have just finished discussing.) There are two things about this somewhat moth-eaten "defective inhibition" idea which I find appealing. First, it is the most direct and uncomplicated neurologizing of the schizoid cognitive slippage. Schizoid cognitive slippage is neither an incapacity to link, nor is it an unhealthy overcapacity to link; rather it seems to be a defective *control* over associations which are also accessible to the healthy (as in dreams, wit, psychoanalytic free association, and certain types of creative work) but are normally "edited out" or "automatically suppressed" by those super-ordinate monitoring assembly systems we lump together under the term "set." Secondly, in working with pseudoneurotic cases one sees a phenomenon to which insufficient theoretical attention has been paid: Namely, these patients cannot turn off painful thoughts. They suffer constantly and intensely from painful thoughts about themselves, about possible adverse outcomes, about the past, about the attitudes and intentions of others. The "weak ego" of schizophrenia means a number of things, one of which is failure of defense; the schizophrenic has too ready access to his own id, and is too perceptive of the unconscious of others. It is tempting to read "failure of defense" as "quantitatively deficient inhibitory feedback." As mentioned earlier, aversive signals (whether exteroceptive or internally originated) must exert both an exciting effect via the arousal system and a quick-

stoppage effect upon cortical sequences which fail to terminate the ongoing aversive signal, leading the organism to shift to another. Suppose the gene resulted in an insufficient production (or too rapid inactivation) of the specific inhibitory transmitter substance, rendering all inhibitory neurones quantitatively weaker than normal. When aversively linked cognitive sequences activate negative limbic centers, these in turn soup up the arousal system normally but provide a subnormal inhibitory feedback, thereby permitting their elicitor to persist for a longer time and at higher intensity than normal. This further activates the negative control center, and so on, until an equilibrium level is reached which is above normal in intensity all around, and which meanwhile permits an excessive linkage growth in the aversive chain. (In this respect the semicompensated case would differ from the late-stage deteriorated schizophrenic, whose aversive drift has gradually proliferated so widely that almost any cognitive or instrumental chain elicits an overlearned defensive "stoppage," whereby even the inner life undergoes a profound and diffuse impoverishment.)

The mammalian brain is so wired that aversive signals tend to produce stoppage of regnant cognitive or instrumental sequences without the aversive signal having been specifically connected to their controlling cues or motivational systems. E.g., lever pressing under thirst or hunger can be inhibited by shock-associated buzzer, even though the latter has not been previously connected with hunger, paired with the discriminative stimulus, nor presented as punishment for the operant. A deficient capacity to inhibit concurrent activity of fringe elements (aversively connected to ambiguous social inputs from ambivalent mother) would accelerate the growth of linkages between them and appetitive systems not hitherto punished. Sequential effects are here especially important, and combine with the schizophrenogenic mother's tendency not to provide differential cues of high consistency as predictors of whether aversive or appetitive consequences will follow upon the child's indications of demand.

Consider two cortical systems having shared "fringe" subsystems (e.g., part percepts of mother's face). When exteroceptive inputs are the elicitors, negative feedback from aversive centers cannot usually produce stoppage; in the absence of such overdetermining external controls, the relative activity levels are determined by the balance of facilitative and inhibitory feedbacks. "Fringe" assemblies which have already acquired more aversive control, if they begin to be activated by regnant perceptual-cognitive sequences, will increase inhibitory feedback; and being "fringe" they can thereby be held down. The schizotaxic, whose aversive-feedback stoppage of fringe-element activity is weakened, accumulates excessive intertrial Hebbian increments toward the aversive side, the predominantly aversive fringe elements being more active and becoming more knit into the system than normally. On subsequent exteroceptively controlled trials, whenever the overdetermining stimulus input activates predominantly aversive perceptual-cognitive assemblies, their driving of the negative centers will be heightened. The resulting negative feedback may now be strong enough that, when imposed upon "fringe" assemblies weakly activated and toward the appetitive side, it can produce stoppage. On such occasions the more appetitive fringe elements will be retarded in their linkage growth, receiving fewer Hebbian increments. And those which do get over threshold will become further linked during such trials to the concurrent negative center activity. The result is twofold: a retarded growth of appetitive perceptual-cognitive linkages; and a progressive drawing of fringe elements into the aversive ambit.

"Ambiguous regimes," where the pairing of S+ and S− inputs occurs very unpredictably, will have a larger number of fringe elements. Also, if the external schedule is dependent upon regnant appetitive drive states as manifested in the child's instrumental social acts, so that these are often met with mixed S+ (drive-relevant) and S− (anxiety-eliciting) inputs, the appetitive and aversive assemblies will tend to become linked, and to activate positive and negative centers concurrently. The anhedonia and ambivalence would be consequences of this plus-minus "scrambling," especially if the positive and negative limbic centers are mutually inhibitory but here deficiently so. We would then expect schizotypic anhedonia to be basically interpersonal, and only derivatively present, if at all, in other contexts. This would in part explain the schizotype's preservation of relatively normal function in a large body of instrumental domains. For example, the acquisition of basic motor and cognitive skills would be relatively less geared to a mixed input, since "successful" mastery is both mechanically rewarded (e.g., how to open a door) and also interpersonally rewarded as "school success," etc. The hypercathexis of intellect, often found even among nonbright schizotypes, might arise from the fact that these performances are rewarded rather "impersonally" and make minimal demands on the reinforcing others. Also, the same cognitive and mechanical instrumental acts can often be employed both to turn on positive center feedback and to turn off negative, an equivalence much less true of purely social signals linked to interpersonal needs.

Having briefly sketched three neurological possibilities for the postulated schizotaxic aberration, let me emphasize that while each has sufficient merit to be worth pursuing, they are mainly meant to be illustrative of the vague concept "integrative neural defect." I shall myself not be surprised if all three are refuted, whereas I shall be astounded if future research shows no fundamental aberration in nerve-cell function in the schizotype. Postulating schizotaxia as an open concept seems at first to pose a search problem of needle-in-haystack proportions, but I suggest that the plausible alternatives are really somewhat limited. After all, what does a neuron do to another neuron? It excites, or it inhibits! The schizotypic preservation of relatively normal function in selected domains directs our search toward some minimal deviation in a synaptic control parameter, as opposed to, say, a gross defect in cell distribution or structure, or the kind of biochemical anomaly that yields mental deficiency. Anything which would give rise to defective storage, grossly impaired transmission, or sizable limitations on functional complexity can be pretty well excluded on present evidence. What we are looking for is a quantitative aberration in synaptic control—a deviation in amount or patterning of excitatory or inhibitory action—capable of yielding cumulative departures from normal control linkages under mixed appetitive-aversive regimes; but slight enough to permit convergence to quasi-normal asymptotes under more consistent schedules (or when massive repetition with motive-incentive factors unimportant is the chief basis for consolidation). The defect must generate aversive drift on mixed social reinforcement regimes, and must yield a primary cognitive slippage which, however, may be extremely small in magnitude except as potentiated by the cumulative effects of aversive drift. Taken together these molar constraints limit our degrees of freedom considerably when it comes to filling in the neurophysiology of schizotaxia.

Leaving aside the specific nature of schizotaxia, we must now raise the familiar question whether such a basic neurological defect, however subtle and nonstructural it might be, should not have been demonstrated hitherto? In reply to this objection I shall content myself with pointing out that there are several lines of evidence which, while not strongly arguing *for* a neurological theory, are rebuttals of an argument presupposing clear and consistent *negative* findings. For example: Ignoring several early European reports with inadequate controls, the literature contains a half-dozen quantitative studies showing marked vestibular system dysfunction in schizophrenics (Angyal & Blackman, 1940, 1941; Angyal & Sherman, 1942; Colbert & Koegler, 1959; Freeman & Rodnick, 1942; Leach, 1960; Payne & Hewlett, 1960; Pollock & Krieger, 1958). Hoskins (1946) concluded that a neurological defect in the vestibular system was one of the few clear-cut biological findings in the Worcester studios. It is of prime importance to replicate these findings among compensated and pseudoneurotic cases, where the diffuse withdrawal and deactivation factor would not provide the explanation it does in the chronic, burnt-out case (cf. Collins, Crampton, & Posner, 1961). Another line of evidence is in the work of King (1954) on psychomotor deficit, noteworthy for its careful use of task simplicity, asymptote performance, concern for patient cooperation, and inclusion of an outpatient pseudoneurotic sample. King himself regards his data as indicative of a rather basic behavior defect, although he does not hold it to be schizophrenia-specific. Then we have such research as that of Barbara Fish (1961) indicating the occurrence of varying signs of perceptual-motor

maldevelopment among infants and children who subsequently manifest clinical schizophrenia. The earlier work of Schilder and Bender along these lines is of course well known, and there has always been a strong minority report in clinical psychiatry that many schizophrenics provide subtle and fluctuating neurological signs of the "soft" variety, if one keeps alert to notice or elicit them. I have myself been struck by the frequent occurrence, even among pseudoneurotic patients, of transitory neurologic-like complaints (e.g., diplopia, localized weakness, one-sided tremor, temperature dyscontrol, dizziness, disorientation) which seem to lack dynamic meaning or secondary gain and whose main effect upon the patient is to produce bafflement and anxiety. I have seen preliminary findings by J. McVicker Hunt and his students in which a rather dramatic quantitative deficiency in spatial cognizing is detectable in schizophrenics of above-normal verbal intelligence. Research by Cleveland (1960; Cleveland, Fisher, Reitman, & Rothaus, 1962) and by Arnhoff and Damianopoulos (1964) on the clinically well-known body-image anomalies in schizophrenia suggests that this domain yields quantitative departures from the norm of such magnitude that with further instrumental and statistical refinement it might be used as a quasi-pathognomonic sign of the disease. It is interesting to note a certain thread of unity running through this evidence, which perhaps lends support to Rado's hypothesis that a kinesthetic integrative defect is even more characteristic of schizotypy than is the radical anhedonia.

All these kinds of data are capable of a psychodynamic interpretation. "Soft" neurological signs are admittedly ambiguous, especially when found in the severely decompensated case. The only point I wish to make here is that *since* they exist and are at present unclear in etiology, an otherwise plausible neurological view cannot be refuted on the ground that there is a *lack* of any sign of neurological dysfunction in schizophrenia; there is no such lack.

Time forces me to leave detailed research strategy for another place, but the main directions are obvious and may be stated briefly: The clinician's Mental Status ratings on anhedonia, ambivalence, and interpersonal aversiveness should be objectified and preferably replaced by psychometric measures. The research findings on cognitive slippage, psychomotor dyscontrol, vestibular malfunction, body image, and other spatial aberrations should be thoroughly replicated and extended into the pseudoneurotic and semicompensated ranges. If these efforts succeed, it will be possible to set up a multiple sign pattern, using optimal cuts on phenotypically diverse indicators, for identifying compensated schizotypes in the nonclinical population. Statistics used must be appropriate to the theoretical model of a dichotomous latent taxonomy reflecting itself in otherwise independent quantitative indicators. Finally concordance studies should then be run relating proband schizophrenia to schizotypy as identified by this multiple indicator pattern. Meanwhile we should carry on an active and varied search for more direct neurological signs of schizotaxia, concentrating our hunches on novel stimulus inputs (e.g., the stabilized retinal image situation) which may provide a better context for basic neural dysfunction to show up instead of being masked by learned compensations or imitated by psychopathology.

In closing, I should like to take this unusual propaganda opportunity to play the prophet. It is my strong personal conviction that such a research strategy will enable psychologists to make a unique contribution in the near future, using psychological techniques to establish that schizophrenia, while its content is learned, is fundamentally a neurological disease of genetic origin.

References

Angyal, A., and Blackman, N. Vestibular reactivity in schizophrenia. *Arch. Neurol. Psychiat.*, 1940, *44*, 611–620.

Angyal, A., and Blackman, N. Paradoxical reactions in schizophrenia under the influence of alcohol, hyperpnea, and CO_2 inhalation. *Amer. J. Psychiat.*, 1941, *97*, 893–903.

Angyal, A., and Sherman, N. Postural reactions to vestibular stimulation in schizophrenic and normal subjects. *Amer. J. Psychiat.*, 1942, *98*, 857–862.

Arnhoff, F., and Damianopoulos, E. Self-body recognition and schizophrenia: An exploratory study. *J. Gen. Psychol.*, 1964, *70*, 353–61.

Bleuler, E. *Theory of schizophrenic negativism.* New York: Nervous and Mental Disease Publishing, 1912.

Bleuler, E. *Dementia praecox.* New York: International Universities Press, 1950.

Cleveland, S. E. Judgment of body size in a schizo-phrenic and a control group. *Psychol. Rep.*, 1960, *7*, 304.

Cleveland, S. E., Fisher, S., Reitman, E. E., and Rothaus, P. Perception of body size in schizophrenia. *Arch. gen. Psychiat.*, 1962, *7*, 277–285.

Colbert, G., and Koegler, R. Vestibular dysfunction in childhood schizophrenia. *AMA Arch. gen. Psychiat.*, 1959, *1*, 600–617.

Collins, W. E., Crampton, G. H., and Posner, J. B. The effect of mental set upon vestibular nystagmus and the EEG. *USA Med. Res. Lab. Rep.*, 1961, No. 439.

Delafresnaye, J. F. (Ed.) *Brain mechanisms and learning.* Springfield, Ill.: Charles C Thomas, 1961.

Delgado, J. M. R., Roberts, W. W., and Miller, N. E. Learning motivated by electrical stimulation of the brain. *Amer. J. Physiol.*, 1954, *179*, 587–593.

Fish, Barbara. The study of motor development in infancy and its relationship to psychological functioning. *Amer. J. Psychiat.*, 1961, *117*, 1113–1118.

Freeman, H., and Rodnick, E. H. Effect of rotation on postural steadiness in normal and schizophrenic subjects. *Arch. Neurol. Psychiat.*, 1942, *48*, 47–53.

Fuller, J. L., and Thompson, W. R. *Behavior genetics.* New York: Wiley, 1960. pp. 272–283.

Hoskins, R. G. *The biology of schizophrenia.* New York: Norton, 1946.

King, H. E. *Psychomotor aspects of mental disease.* Cambridge: Harvard Univer. Press, 1954.

Leach, W. W. Nystagmus: An integrative neural deficit in schizophrenia. *J. abnorm. soc. Psychol.*, 1960, *60*, 305–309.

Lidz, T., Cornelison, A., Terry, D., and Fleck, S. Intrafamilial environment of the schizophrenic patient: VI. The transmission of irrationality. *AMA Arch. Neurol. Psychiat.*, 1958, *79*, 305–316.

McConaghy, N. The use of an object sorting test in elucidating the hereditary factor in schizophrenia. *J. Neurol. Neurosurg. Psychiat.*, 1959, *22*, 243–246.

Meyers, D., and Goldfarb, W. Psychiatric appraisals of parents and siblings of schizophrenic children. *Amer. J. Psychiat.*, 1962, *118*, 902–908.

Olds, J., and Milner, P. Positive reinforcement produced by electrical stimulation of septal area and other regions of rat brain. *J. comp. physiol. Psychol.*, 1954, *47*, 419–427.

Payne, R. W. Cognitive abnormalities. In H. J. Eysenck (Ed.), *Handbook of abnormal psychology.* New York: Basic Books, 1961. pp. 248–250.

Payne, R. S., and Hewlett, J. H. G. Thought disorder in psychotic patients. In H. J. Eysenck (Ed.), *Experiments in personality.* Vol. 2. London: Routledge, Kegan, Paul, 1960. pp. 3–106.

Pollack, M., and Krieger, H. P. Oculomotor and postural patterns in schizophrenic children. *AMA Arch. Neurol. Psychiat.*, 1958, *79*, 720–726.

Rado, S. *Psychoanalysis of behavior.* New York: Grune & Stratton, 1956.

Rado, S., and Daniels, G. *Changing concepts of psychoanalytic medicine.* New York: Grune & Stratton, 1956.

Ramey, E. R., and O'Doherty, D. S. (Ed.) *Electrical studies on the unanesthetized brain.* New York: Hoeber, 1960.

Rosenthal, D. Problems of sampling and diagnosis in the major twin studies of schizophrenia. *J. psychiat. Res.*, 1962, *1*, 16–34.

Stern, K. *Principles of human genetics.* San Francisco: Freeman, 1960. pp. 581–584.

54. A Biosocial-Learning Approach

THEODORE MILLON

As the title of this paper suggests, an attempt will be made to formulate a schema that is neither doctrinaire nor loosely eclectic in its approach; rather, the theory presented is intended to be both broad in scope and sufficiently systematic in its application of principles to enable the major varieties of psychopathology to be derived logically and coherently. In the following sections a few of the major themes of the model will be provided in condensed form.

ETIOLOGY: AN INTERACTIONAL VIEW

A. For pedagogical purposes, it is often necessary to separate biogenic from psychogenic factors as influences in personality development; this bifurcation does not exist in reality. Biological and experiential determinants combine and interact in a reciprocal interplay throughout life. This sequence of biogenic-psychogenic interaction evolves through a never-ending spiral; each step in the interplay builds upon prior interactions and creates, in turn, new potentialities for future reactivity and experience. *Etiology in psychopathology may be viewed, then, as a developmental process in which intraorganismic and environmental forces display not only a reciprocity and circularity of influence but an orderly and sequential continuity throughout the life of the individual.*

The circular feedback and serially unfolding character of the developmental process defy simplification, and must constantly be kept in mind when analyzing the etiological background of personality. There are few unidirectional effects in development; it is a multideterminant transaction in which a unique pattern of biogenic potentials and a distinctive constellation of psychogenic influences mold each other in a reciprocal and successively more intricate fashion.

B. Each individual is endowed at conception with a unique set of chromosomes that shapes the course of his physical maturation and psychological develop-

ment. The physical and psychological characteristics of children are in large measure similar to their parents because they possess many of the same genetic units. Children are genetically disposed to be similar to their parents not only physically but also in stamina, energy, emotional sensitivity and intelligence.

Each infant displays a distinctive pattern of behaviors from the first moments after birth. These characteristics are attributed usually to the infant's "nature," that is, his constitutional makeup, since it is displayed prior to the effects of postnatal influences.

It is erroneous to assume that children of the same chronological age are comparable with respect to the level and character of their biological capacities. Not only does each infant start life with a distinctive pattern of neurological, physiochemical and sensory equipment, but he progresses at his own maturational rate toward some ultimate but unknown level of potential. Thus, above and beyond initial differences and their not insignificant consequences, are differences in the rate with which the typical sequence of maturation unfolds. Furthermore, different regions in the complex nervous system within a single child may mature at different rates. To top it all, the potential or ultimate level of development of each of these neurological capacities will vary widely, not only among children but within each child.

C. The maturation of the biological substrate for psychological capacities is anchored initially to genetic processes, but its development is substantially dependent on environmental stimulation. The concept of *stimulus nutriment* may be introduced to represent the belief that the quantity of environmental experience activates chemical processes requisite to the maturation of neural collaterals. Stimulus impoverishment may lead to irrevocable deficiencies in neural development and their associated psychological functions; stimulus enrichment may prove equally deleterious by producing pathological overdevelopments or imbalances among these functions.

D. The notion of sensitive develop-

Abridged from *Modern Psychopathology*. Philadelphia: W. B. Saunders Co., 1969.

mental periods may be proposed to convey the belief that stimuli produce different effects at different ages, that is, there are limited time periods during maturation when particular stimuli have pronounced effects which they do not have either before or after these periods. It may be suggested, further, that these peak periods occur at points in maturation when the potential is greatest for growth and expansion of neural collaterals.

Three neuropsychological stages of development, representing peak periods in neurological maturation, may be proposed. Each developmental stage reflects transactions between constitutional and experiential influences which combine to set a foundation for subsequent stages; if the interactions at one stage are deficient or distorted, all subsequent stages will be affected since they rest on a defective base.

The first stage, termed *sensory-attachment,* predominates from birth to approximately 18 months of age. This period is characterized by a rapid maturation of neurological substrates for sensory processes, and by the infant's attachment and dependency on others.

The second stage, referred to as *sensorimotor-autonomy,* begins roughly at 12 months and extends in its peak development through the sixth year. It is characterized by a rapid differentiation of motor capacities which coordinate with established sensory functions; this coalescence enables the young child to locomote, manipulate and verbalize in increasingly skillful ways.

The third stage, called the period of *intracortical-initiative,* is primary from about the fourth year through adolescence. There is a rapid growth potential among the higher cortical centers during this stage, enabling the child to reflect, plan and act independent of parental supervision. Integrations developed during earlier phases of this period undergo substantial reorganization as a product of the biological and social effects of puberty.

Maladaptive consequences can arise as a result of either stimulus impoverishment or stimulus enrichment at each of the three stages.

From experimental animal research and naturalistic studies with human infants, it appears that marked stimulus impoverishment during the sensory-attachment period will produce deficiencies in sensory capacities and a marked diminution of interpersonal sensitivity and behavior. There is little evidence available with regard to the effects of stimulus enrichment during this stage; it may be proposed, however, that excessive stimulation results in hypersensitivities, stimulus seeking behaviors and abnormal interpersonal dependencies.

Deprived of adequate stimulation during the sensorimotor stage, the child will be deficient in skills for behavioral autonomy, will display a lack of exploratory and competitive activity and be characterized by timidity and submissiveness. In contrast, excessive enrichment and indulgence of sensorimotor capacities may result in uncontrolled self-expression, narcissism and social irresponsibility.

Among the consequences of understimulation during the intracortical-initiative stage is an identity diffusion, an inability to fashion an integrated and consistent purpose for one's existence and an inefficiency in channeling and directing one's energies, capacities and impulses. Excessive stimulation, in the form of overtraining and overguidance, results in the loss of several functions, notably spontaneity, flexibility and creativity.

E. There has been little systematic attention to the child's own contribution to the course of his development. Environmental theorists of psychopathology have viewed disorders to be the result of detrimental experiences that the individual has had no part in producing himself. This is a gross simplification. Each infant possesses a biologically based pattern of reaction sensitivities and behavioral dispositions which shape the nature of his experiences and may contribute directly to the creation of environmental difficulties.

The biological dispositions of the maturing child are important because they strengthen the probability that certain kinds of behavior will be learned.

Highly active and responsive children relate to and learn about their environment quickly. Their liveliness, zest and power may lead them to a high measure of personal gratification. Conversely, their energy and exploratory behavior may result in excess frustration if they overaspire or run into insuperable barriers; unable to gratify their activity needs effectively, they may grope and strike out in erratic and maladaptive ways.

Adaptive learning in constitutionally passive children also is shaped by their biological equipment. Ill-disposed to deal with their environment assertively and little inclined to discharge their tensions physically, they may learn to avoid conflicts and step aside when difficulties arise. They are less likely to develop guilt feelings about misbehavior than active youngsters who more frequently get into trouble, receive more punishment and are therefore inclined to develop aggressive feelings toward others. But in their passivity, these youngsters may deprive themselves of rewarding experiences and relationships; they may feel "left out of things" and become dependent on others to fight their battles and to protect them from experiences they are ill-equipped to handle on their own.

It appears clear from studies of early patterns of reactivity that *constitutional tendencies evoke counterreactions from others which accentuate these initial dispositions*. The child's biological endowment shapes not only his behavior but that of his parents as well.

If the child's primary disposition is cheerful and adaptable and has made his care easy, the mother will tend quickly to display a positive reciprocal attitude; conversely, if the child is tense and wound up, or if his care is difficult and time consuming, the mother will react with dismay, fatigue or hostility. Through his own behavioral disposition then, the child elicits a series of parental behaviors which reinforce his initial pattern.

Unfortunately, the reciprocal interplay of primary patterns and parental reactions has not been sufficiently explored. It may prove to be one of the most fruitful spheres of research concerning the etiology of psychopathology and merits the serious attention of investigators. The *biosocial-learning approach* presented in this paper stems largely from the thesis that the child's constitutional pattern shapes and interacts with his social reinforcement experiences.

F. The fact that early experiences are likely to contribute a disproportionate share to learned behavior is attributable in part to the fact that their effects are difficult to extinguish. This resistance to extinction stems largely from the fact that

learning in early life is presymbolic, random and highly generalized.

Additional factors which contribute to the persistence and continuity of early learnings are social factors such as the repetitive nature of experience, the tendency for interpersonal relations to be reciprocally reinforcing and the perseverance of early character stereotypes.

Beyond these are a number of self-perpetuating processes which derive from the individual's own actions. Among them are protective efforts which constrict the person's awareness and experience, the tendency to perceptually and cognitively distort events in line with expectancies, the inappropriate generalization to new events of old behavior patterns and the repetitive compulsion to create conditions which parallel the past.

Children learn complicated sequences of attitudes, reactions and expectancies in response to the experiences to which they were exposed. Initially, these responses are specific to the particular events which prompted them; they are piecemeal, scattered and changeable. Over the course of time, however, through learning what responses are successful in obtaining rewards and avoiding punishments, the child begins to crystallize a stable pattern of instrumental behaviors for handling the events of everyday life. These coping and adaptive strategies come to characterize his way of relating to others, and comprise one of the most important facets of what we may term his personality pattern.

CONCEPT OF PERSONALITY PATTERNS

A. As noted above, in the first years of life children engage in a wide variety of spontaneous behaviors. Although they display certain characteristics consonant with their innate or constitutional dispositions, their way of reacting to others and coping with their environment tends, at first, to be capricious and unpredictable; flexibility and changeability characterize their moods, attitudes and behaviors. This seemingly random behavior serves an exploratory function; each child is "trying out" and testing during this period alternative modes for coping with his environment. As time progresses, the child learns which techniques "work," that is, which of these varied behaviors enable him to achieve his desires and avoid discomforts. Endowed with a distinctive pattern of capacities, energies and temperaments, which serve as base, he learns specific preferences among activities and goals and, perhaps of greater importance, learns that certain types of behaviors and strategies are especially successful for him in obtaining these goals. In his interaction with parents, siblings and peers, he learns to discriminate which goals are permissible, which are rewarded and which are not.

Throughout these years, then, a shaping process has taken place in which the range of initially diverse behaviors becomes narrowed, selective and, finally, crystallized into particular preferred modes of seeking and achieving. In time, these behaviors persist and become accentuated; not only are they highly resistant to extinction but they are reinforced by the restrictions and repetitions of a limited social environment, and are perpetuated and intensified by the child's own perceptions, needs and actions. Thus, given a continuity in basic biological equipment, and a narrow band of experiences for learning behavioral alternatives, the child develops a distinctive pattern of characteristics that are deeply etched, cannot be eradicated easily and pervade every facet of his functioning. In short, these characteristics *are* the essence and sum of his personality, his automatic way of perceiving, feeling, thinking and behaving.

When we speak of a personality pattern, then, we are referring to those intrinsic and pervasive modes of functioning which emerge from the entire matrix of the individual's developmental history, and which now characterize his perceptions and ways of dealing with his environment. We have chosen the term pattern for two reasons: first, to focus on the fact that these behaviors and attitudes derive from the constant and pervasive interaction of both biological dispositions and learned experience; and second, to denote the fact that these personality characteristics are not just a potpourri of unrelated behavior tendencies, but a tightly knit organization of needs, attitudes and behaviors. People may start out in life with random and diverse reactions, but the repetitive sequence of reinforcing experiences to which they are exposed gradually narrows their repertoire to certain habitual strategies, perceptions and behaviors which become prepotent, and come to characterize their distinctive way of relating to the world.

B. We stress the centrality of personality patterns in our formulations in order to break the long entrenched habit of thinking that all forms of psychopathology are diseases, that is, identifiable foreign entities or intruders which attach themselves insidiously to the person, and destroy his "normal" functions. The archaic notion that all forms of illness are a product of external intruders can be traced back to such prescientific ideas as demons, spirits and witches, which ostensibly "possessed" the person and cast spells upon him. The recognition in modern medicine of the role of infectious agents has reawakened this archaic view; no longer do we see "demons," but we still think, using current medical jargon, that alien, malevolent and insidious forces undermine the patient's otherwise healthy status. This view is a comforting and appealing simplification to the layman; he can attribute his discomforts, pains and irrationalities to the intrusive influence of some external agent, something he ate or caught or some foreign object he can blame that has assaulted his normal and "true" self. This simplification of "alien disease bodies" has its appeal to the physician as well; it enables him to believe that he can find a malevolent intruder, some tangible factor he can hunt down and destroy.

The disease model carries little weight among informed and sophisticated psychiatrists and psychologists today. Increasingly, both in medicine and psychiatry, disorders and disturbances are conceptualized in terms of the patient's *total capacity to cope* with the stress he faces. In medicine, it is the patient's overall constitution—his vitality and stamina—which determine his proclivity to, or resistance against, ill health. Likewise, in psychiatry, it is the patient's personality pattern, his coping skills, outlook and objectivity, which determines whether or not he will be characterized as mentally ill. Physical ill health, then, is less a matter of some alien disease than it is an imbalance or dysfunction in the overall capacity to deal effectively with one's physical environment. In the same manner, psychological ill health is less the product of an intrusive psychic strain or problem than it is an imbalance or dysfunction in the overall capacity to deal effectively with one's psychological environment. Viewed this way, the individual's personality pattern becomes the foundation for his capacity to function in a mentally healthy or ill way.

C. Normality and pathology are relative concepts; they represent arbitrary points on a continuum or gradient. Psychopathology is shaped according to the same processes and principles as those involved in normal development and learning; however, because of differences in the character, timing, intensity or persistence of certain influences, some individuals acquire maladaptive habits and attitudes whereas others do not.

When an individual displays an ability to cope with his environment in a flexible and adaptive manner and when his characteristic perceptions and behaviors foster increments in personal gratification, then he may be said to possess a normal and healthy personality pattern. Conversely, when average responsibilities and everyday relationships are responded to inflexibly or defectively, or when the individual's characteristic perceptions and behaviors foster increments in personal discomfort or curtail his opportunities to learn and grow, then a pathological personality pattern may be said to exist. Of course, no sharp line divides normality and pathology; not only are personality patterns so complex that certain spheres of functioning may operate ''normally'' while others do not, but environmental circumstances may change such that certain behaviors and strategies prove ''healthy'' one time but not another.

Despite the tenuous and fluctuating nature of the normality-pathology distinction, it may be useful to note three criteria by which it may be made: *adaptive inflexibility*, that is, the rigid use of a limited repertoire of strategies for coping with different and varied experiences; *vicious circles*, that is, possessing attitudes and behaviors which intensify old difficulties, and which set into motion new self-defeating consequences; and *tenuous stability*, that is, a susceptibility and lack of resilience to conditions of stress.

Together, these three features perpetuate problems and make life increasingly difficult for the unfortunate individual.

COPING STRATEGIES AND PATHOLOGICAL PERSONALITIES

A. Coping strategies may be viewed as complex forms of instrumental behavior, that is, ways of achieving positive reinforcements and avoiding negative reinforcements. These strategies reflect what reinforcements the individual has learned to seek or avoid, where he looks to obtain these reinforcements and how he performs in order to elicit or escape them.

It would be extremely useful if a consistent theoretical framework were provided to coordinate the various syndromes into a coherent classification system. Toward this end, we will describe briefly how eight coping strategies that are conducive to pathological personality functioning can be derived essentially from a 4×2 matrix combining two basic variables: (a) the patient's interpersonal style; and (b) the nature and source of the reinforcements he seeks, and the instrumental acts he utilizes to achieve them.

a. Interpersonal behaviors are considered important for several reasons. Most notably, they alert the clinician to significant relationships in the patient's developmental history, and provide suggestive leads for treatment. Moreover, interpersonal factors are especially relevant in the case of the mild personality patterns since these patients maintain active contact with others, meeting and interacting with people in normal everyday life. The character of the interpersonal behaviors they exhibit in these relationships will shape the kinds of reactions they evoke from others, and these reactions, in turn, will influence whether the patient's present degree of pathology will remain stable, improve or become worse.

b. The other major feature guiding our analysis relates to: the kinds of reinforcements the patient seeks (positive or negative); where he looks to find them (self or others); and how he behaves instrumentally to acquire them (active or passive).

Those patients who fail to seek positive reinforcements are referred to as *detached;* within this category are those who seek neither to gain positive reinforcements nor to avoid negative reinforcements (passive-detached or asocial personality), and those who do not seek positive reinforcements but do seek to avoid negative ones (active-detached or avoidant personality). All the other personality syndromes seek both to gain positive reinforcements and to avoid negative reinforcements.

Those who experience reinforcements primarily from sources other than themselves are referred to as *dependent;* within this group are those who wait for others to provide these reinforcements (passive-dependent or submissive personality), and those who manipulate and seduce others to provide reinforcements for them (active-dependent or gregarious personality).

Patients who experience reinforcements primarily from themselves are referred to as *independent;* within this category are those who are self-satisfied and content to leave matters as they are (passive-independent or narcissistic personality), and those who seek to arrogate more power to themselves (active-independent or aggressive-personality).

The fourth major category, referred to as *ambivalent,* is composed of patients who have conflicting attitudes about dependence or independence; some submerge their desire for independence and behave in an overly acquiescent manner (passive-ambivalent or conforming personality) whereas others vacillate erratically from one position to another (active-ambivalent or negativistic personality).

B. Before we outline the principal personality syndromes, let us be mindful that the classification schema is merely a theory-derived synthesis, a set of "armchair" prototypes drawn from diverse sources such as hospital psychiatry, multivariate cluster studies, learning research and psychoanalytic theory. It is a typology documented only in part by systematic empirical research; it is a theory, a provisional tool which hopefully will aid us in organizing our subject more clearly and with greater understanding, a convenient format designed to focus and systematize our thinking about psychopathology.

1. The *passive-detached* strategy is characterized by social impassivity; affectionate needs and emotional feelings are minimal, and the individual functions as a passive observer detached from the rewards and affections, as well as from the dangers of human relationships.

2. The *active-detached* strategy represents an intense mistrust of others. The individual maintains a constant vigil lest his impulses and longing for affection result in a repetition of the pain and anguish he has experienced previously; distance must be kept between himself and others. Only by an active detachment and suspiciousness can he protect himself from others. Despite desires to relate to others, he has learned that it is best to deny these desires and withdraw from interpersonal relationships.

3. The *passive-dependent* strategy is characterized by a search for relationships in which one can lean upon others for affection, security and leadership. This patient displays a lack of both initiative and autonomy. As a function of early experience, he has learned to assume a passive role in interpersonal relations, accepting whatever kindness and support he may find, and willingly submitting to the wishes of others in order to maintain their affection.

4. In the *active-dependent* strategy we observe an insatiable and indiscriminate search for stimulation and affection. The patient's gregarious and capricious behavior gives the appearance of considerable independence of others, but beneath this guise lies a fear of autonomy and an intense need for signs of social approval and affection. Affection must be replenished constantly and must be obtained from every source of interpersonal experience.

5. The *passive-independent* strategy is noted by narcissism and self-involvement. As a function of early experience the individual has learned to overvalue his self-worth; however, his confidence in his superiority may be based on false premises. Nevertheless, he assumes that others will recognize his worth, and he maintains a self-assured distance from those whom he views to be inferior to himself.

6. The *active-independent* strategy reflects a mistrust of others and a desire to assert one's autonomy; the result is an indiscriminate striving for power. Rejection of others is justified because they cannot be trusted; autonomy and initiative are

claimed to be the only means of heading off betrayal by others.

7. The *passive-ambivalent* strategy is based on a combination of hostility toward others and a fear of social rejection and disapproval. The patient resolves this conflict by repressing his resentment. He overconforms and overcomplies on the surface; however, lurking behind this front of propriety and restraint are intense contrary feelings which, on rare occasion, seep through his controls.

8. The *active-ambivalent* strategy represents an inability to resolve conflicts similar to those of the passive-ambivalent; however, these conflicts remain close to consciousness and intrude into everyday life. The individual gets himself into endless wrangles and disappointments as he vacillates between deference and conformity, at one time, and aggressive negativism, the next. His behavior displays an erratic pattern of explosive anger or stubbornness intermingled with moments of hopeless dependency, guilt and shame.

C. A major theme stressed in the theory is the intrinsic continuity of personality development. Granting the validity of this assertion, it is proposed that the more severe forms of psychopathology are elaborations and extensions of a patient's basic personality style, and that a successful analysis of his decompensated state rests on a thorough understanding of his basic personality. Severe states are viewed, then, as logical outgrowths of one of the basic eight styles of coping seen under the pressure of intense or unrelieved adversity. No matter how dramatic or maladaptive a patient's behavior may be, it is best understood as an accentuation or distortion that derives from, and is fully consonant with, his personality coping pattern.

A MILD PATHOLOGICAL PERSONALITY PATTERN

One of the eight basic personality patterns (active-ambivalent) will be described in detail in the following sections to provide the reader with an in-depth view of the theory-generated syndromes.

The *active-ambivalent pattern* or negativistic personality is perhaps the most frequent of the milder forms of pathological coping; it arises in large measure as a consequence of inconsis-

tency in parental attitudes and training methods, a feature of experience that is not uncommon in our complex and everchanging society. What distinguishes life for the active-ambivalent child is the fact that he is subject to appreciably more than his share of contradictory parental attitudes and behaviors. His erraticism and vacillation, his tendency to shift capriciously from one mood to another, may be viewed as mirroring the varied and inconsistent models and reinforcements to which he was exposed.

There are two diagnostic syndromes in the DSM-II that relate to the principal clinical features of the active-ambivalent pattern: the *explosive personality* and the *passive-aggressive personality*. The characteristics described under these separate labels represent, we believe, the same basic coping pattern, and should be combined, therefore, into one syndrome. Excerpts from the DSM-II are quoted below; the first paragraph describes the "explosive" type, and the second that of the "passive-aggressive." Together, they provide a brief portrait of the typical behavior of the active-ambivalent pattern as we have conceived it.

This behavior pattern is characterized by gross outbursts of rage or of verbal and physical aggressiveness. These outbursts are strikingly different from the patient's usual behavior, and he may be regretful and repentant for them. These patients are generally considered excitable, aggressive and over-responsive to environmental pressures. It is the intensity of the outbursts and the individual's inability to control them that distinguishes this group.

The aggressiveness may be expressed passively, for example by obstructionism, pouting, procrastination, intentional inefficiency or stubbornness. This behavior commonly reflects hostility which the individual feels he dare not express openly. Often the behavior is one expression of the patient's resentment at failing to find gratification in a relationship with an individual or institution upon which he is overdependent.

As we perceive it, the active-ambivalent displays an everyday "passive-aggressive" style, punctuated periodically by "explosive" outbursts, for which he is subsequently regretful and repentant.

Clinical Picture

A. The negativistic person displays a rapid succession of moods and seems restless, unstable and erratic in his feelings. These persons are easily nettled, offended by trifles and can readily be provoked into being sullen and contrary. There is a low tolerance for frustration; they seem impatient much of the time and are irritable and fidgety unless things go their way. They vacillate from being distraught and despondent, at one time, to being petty, spiteful, stubborn and contentious, another. At times they may appear enthusiastic and cheerful, but this mood is short lived. In no time, they again become disgruntled, critical and envious of others. They begrudge the good fortunes of others and are jealous, quarrelsome and easily piqued by indifference and minor slights. Their emotions are "worn on their sleeves"; they are excitable and impulsive and may suddenly burst into tears and guilt or anger and abuse.

The impulsive, unpredictable and often explosive reactions of the negativist make it difficult for others to feel comfortable in his presence, or to establish reciprocally rewarding and enduring relationships. Although there are periods of pleasant sociability, most acquaintances of these personalities feel "on edge," waiting for them to display a sullen and hurt look or become obstinate and nasty.

B.   The active-ambivalent can be quite articulate in describing his subjective discomfort, but rarely does he display insight into its roots. In speaking of his sensitivities and difficulties, he does not recognize that they reflect, in largest measure, his own inner conflicts and ambivalence.

Self-reports alternate between preoccupations with their own personal inadequacies, bodily ailments and guilt feelings, on the one hand, and resentments, frustrations and disillusionments with others, on the other. They voice their dismay about the sorry state of their lives, their worries, their sadness, their disappointments, their "nervousness" and so on; they express a desire to be rid of distress and difficulty, but seem unable, or perhaps unwilling, to find any solution to them.

Cognitive ambivalence characterizes the thinking of negativistic persons; no sooner do they "see" the merits of solving their problems one way than they find themselves saying, "but . . . ." Fearful of committing themselves and unsure of

their own competencies or the loyalties of others, they find their thoughts shifting erratically from one solution to another. Because of their intense ambivalences, they often end up acting precipitously, on the spur of the moment; for them, any other course would lead only to hesitation, vacillation and immobility.

The negative personality often asserts that he has been trapped by fate, that nothing ever "works out" for him and that whatever he desires runs aground. These persons express envy and resentment over the "easy life" of others; they are critical and cynical with regard to what others have attained, yet covet these achievements themselves. Life has been unkind to them, they claim. They feel discontent, cheated and unappreciated; their efforts have been for naught; they have been misunderstood and are disillusioned.

The obstructiveness, pessimism and immaturity which others attribute to them are only a reflection, they feel, of their "sensitivity," the pain they have suffered from persistent physical illness or the inconsiderateness that others have shown toward them. But here again, the negativist's ambivalence intrudes; perhaps, they say, it is their own unworthiness, their own failures and their own "bad temper" which is the cause of their misery and the pain they bring to others. This struggle between feelings of guilt and resentment permeates every facet of the patient's thoughts and feelings.

C.   A distinguishing clinical feature of the active-ambivalent is his paucity of intrapsychic controls and mechanisms. His moods, thoughts and desires rarely are worked out internally; few unconscious processes and maneuvers are employed to handle the upsurge of feelings; as a consequence, these emotions come directly to the surface, untransformed and unmoderated. Thus, negativistic personalities are like children in that they react spontaneously and impulsively to events on the passing scene; each new stimulus seems to elicit a separate and different emotion; there is no damping down, no consistency and no predictability to their reactions.

D.   Negativistic personalities do not exhibit a distinctive or characteristic level of biological activation or energy. However, there is some reason to believe that they may possess an intrinsic irritability or hyper-reactivity to stimulation. These patients seem easily aroused, testy, high-strung, thin-skinned and quick-tempered. All sorts of minor events provoke and chafe them; they get inflamed and aggrieved by the most incidental and insignificant behaviors on the part of others. Be mindful, however, that this hypersensitivity may result from adverse experiences as well as constitutional proclivities.

Note should be made here of the high frequency of psychophysiological disorders found among these personalities. In addition to specific ailments, many negativistic individuals complain of ill-defined physical discomforts and generalized states of fatigue.

In summary, four major characteristics distinguish the personality type under review. Several of these have been described in the "clinical picture"; others will be developed in later sections. These characteristics have been labeled as follows: *irritable affectivity* (is moody, high-strung and quick-tempered), *cognitive ambivalence* (holds incompatible ideas and shifts erratically among them), *discontented self-image* (feels misunderstood, disillusioned, a failure) and *interpersonal vacillation* (is impatient and unpredictable with others; switches from resentment to guilt).

Etiology and Development

A.   Fretful and "nervous" youngsters are good candidates for the negativistic pattern because they are likely to provoke bewilderment, confusion and vacillation in parental training methods. Such "irregular" children may set into motion erratic and contradictory reactions from their parents which then serve, in circular fashion, to reinforce their initial tendency to be spasmodic and variable.

Children who mature in an unbalanced progression, or at an uneven rate, are more likely to evoke inconsistent reactions from their parents than normally developing children. Thus, a "very bright" but "emotionally immature" youngster may precipitate anger in response to the "childish" dimensions of his behavior, but commendation in response to the "cleverness" he displayed while behaving childishly. Such a child will be confused whether to continue or to inhibit his behavior since the reactions

it prompted were contradictory. Additionally, such children may possess "mature" desires and aspirations but lack the equipment to achieve these goals; this can lead only to feelings of discontent and disappointment, features associated with the active-ambivalent pattern.

Conceivably, the affective excitability of the negativistic personality may arise in part from a high level of reticular activity or a dominance of the sympathetic division of the autonomic nervous system.

Equally speculative, but plausible, are hypotheses which implicate segments of the limbic system. Anatomically dense or well-branched centers subserving several different, and irreconcilable, emotions such as "anger," "sadness" and "fear" could account for the ambivalent behavioral proclivities seen in this pattern. Of interest in this regard is the recently uncovered "ambivalence" center in the limbic region; hypotheses concerning this area may also be considered as plausible.

Active-ambivalent personalities develop with appreciably greater frequency among women than men. Conceivably, many negativistic women may be subject to extreme hormonal changes during their menstrual cycles, thereby precipitating marked, short-lived and variable moods. Such rapid mood changes may set into motion sequences of erratic behavior and associated interpersonal reactions conducive to the acquisition and perpetuation of this pattern. Let us caution the reader that these hypotheses are merely unconfirmed speculations.

B.   The central role of inconsistent parental attitudes and contradictory training methods in the development of the negativistic personality has been referred to repeatedly in our discussions. Although every child experiences some degree of parental inconstancy, the active-ambivalent youngster is likely to have been exposed to appreciably more than his share. His parents may have swayed from hostility and rejection, at one time, to affection and love another; and this erratic pattern has probably been capricious, frequent, pronounced and lifelong.

These children constantly are forced into what are termed approach-avoidance conflicts. Furthermore, they never are sure what their parents really desire, and no matter what course they take, they find that they cannot do right. This latter form of entrapment has been referred to as a double-bind; thus, the child is unable not only to find a clear direction for his behavior but to extricate himself from the irreconcilable demands that have been made of him. The double-bind difficulty is often compounded by the fact that the contradictions in the parental message are subtle or concealed. Thus, he cannot readily accuse his parents of failing to mean what they overtly say since the evidence for such accusations is rather tenuous; moreover, the consequences of making an accusation of parental dishonesty or deception may be rather severe. Unable to discriminate, and fearful of misinterpreting, the intent of these communications, the child becomes anxious, and may learn to become ambivalent in his thinking and erratic in his own behavior.

Paradoxical and contradictory parental behaviors often are found in "schismatic" families, that is, in families where the parents are manifestly in conflict with each other. Here, there is constant bickering, and an undermining of one parent by the other through disqualifying and contradicting statements. A child raised in this setting not only suffers the constant threat of family dissolution, but, in addition, often is forced to serve as a mediator to moderate tensions generated by his parents. He constantly switches sides and divides his loyalties; he cannot be "himself" for he must shift his attitudes and emotions to satisfy changing and antagonistic parental desires and expectations. The different roles he must assume to placate his parents and to salvage a measure of family stability are markedly divergent; as long as his parents remain at odds, he must persist with behavior and thoughts that are intrinsically irreconcilable.

This state of affairs prevents the child from identifying consistently with one parent; as a consequence, he ends up modeling himself after two intrinsically antagonistic figures, with the result that he forms opposing sets of attitudes, emotions and behaviors. As is evident, schismatic families are perfect training grounds for the development of an ambivalent pattern.

We may summarize as follows. *First,* the child learns vicariously to imitate the erratic and capricious behavior of his parents. *Second,* he fails to learn what "pays off" instrumentally; he never acquires a reliable strategy that achieves the reinforcements he seeks. *Third,* he internalizes a series of conflicting attitudes toward himself and others; for example, he does not know whether he is competent or incompetent; he is unsure whether he loves or hates those upon whom he depends. *Fourth,* unable to predict the consequences of his behaviors, he gets "tied up in emotional knots," and behaves irrationally and impulsively.

Coping Strategies

It would appear from first impressions that the erratic course of the active-ambivalent pattern would fail to provide the individual with reinforcements; if this were the case, we would expect these persons to quickly decompensate into severe forms of pathology. Obviously, most do not, and we are forced to inquire, then, as to what gains, supports and rewards an individual can achieve in the course of behaving in the erratic and vacillating active-ambivalent pattern.

The strategy of negativism, of being discontent and unpredictable, of being both seductive and rejecting and of being demanding and then dissatisfied, is an effective weapon not only with the intimidated or pliant but with people in general. Switching back and forth among the roles of the martyr, the affronted, the aggrieved, the misunderstood, the contrite, the guilt-ridden, the sickly and the overworked, is a clever tactic of interpersonal behavior which gains the active-ambivalent the attention, reassurance and dependency he craves, while at the same time, it allows him to subtly vent his angers and resentments. Thus, for all the seeming ineffectuality of vacillation, it recruits affection and support, on the one hand, and provides a means of discharging the tensions of frustration and hostility, on the other. Interspersed with periods of self-deprecation and contrition, acts which relieve unconscious guilt and serve to solicit forgiveness and reassuring comments from others, this strategy proves *not* to be a total instrumental failure.

In an earlier section we noted the paucity of controls which characterize the active-ambivalent personality. The muddle and confusion of feelings that active-ambivalents experience prompt a variety of erratic and contradictory intrapsychic mechanisms. Thus, sometimes the negativist will turn his externally directed, hostile feelings back toward himself, a mechanism termed by some theorists as introjection, the converse of projection. For example, hatred felt toward others is directed toward the self, taking the form of guilt or self-condemnation. But, true to form, the active-ambivalent often alternates between introjection and projection. Thus, at one time, by projection, he ascribes his own destructive impulses to others, accusing them, unjustly, of being malicious and unkind to him. At other times, by introjection, he reverses the sequence, and accuses himself of faults which, justifiably, should be ascribed to others.

Thus, even in the use of unconscious mechanisms, the active-ambivalent behaves in an erratic and contradictory manner. Those at the receiving end of these bizarre intrapsychic processes cannot help but observe their irrationality, uncalled for outbursts and peculiar inconsistency.

Self-Perpetuation

The mere process of behaving erratically, of vacillating from one course of action to another, is a sheer waste of energy. By attempting to secure his incompatible goals, the negativistic personality scatters his efforts and dilutes his effectiveness. Caught in his own cross currents, he fails to commit himself to one clear direction; he swings indecisively back and forth, performs ineffectually and experiences a paralyzing sense of inertia or exhaustion.

In addition to the wasteful nature of ambivalence, the negativistic person may actively impede his own progress toward conflict resolution and goal attainment. Thus, active-ambivalents often undo what good they previously have done. Driven by contrary feelings, they may retract their own "kind words" to others and replace them with harshness, or contaminate and undermine achievements they struggled so hard to attain. In short, their ambivalence may rob them of the few steps they secured toward progress.

The inconstant "blowing hot and cold" behavior of the active-ambivalent precipitates other persons into reacting in a parallel capricious and inconsistent manner; thus, by prompting these reactions he recreates the same conditions of his childhood that initially fostered the development of his unstable behavior.

People weary quickly of the moping, sulking, manipulative, stubborn and unpredictable explosive behaviors of the active-ambivalent. They are goaded into exasperation and into feelings of confusion and futility when their persistent efforts to placate the negativist invariably meet with failure. Eventually, these persons express hostility and disaffiliation, reactions which then serve to intensify the dismay and anxiety of the negativistic personality.

Not only does the active-ambivalent precipitate real difficulties through his negativistic behaviors, but he often perceives and anticipates difficulties where none in fact exist. He has learned from past experience that "good things don't last," that the pleasant and affectionate attitudes of those from whom he seeks love will abruptly and capriciously come to an end, and be followed by disappointment, anger and rejection.

Rather than be embittered again, rather than allowing himself to be led down the "primrose path" and to suffer the humiliation and pain of having one's high hopes dashed, it would be better to put a halt to illusory gratifications, to the futility, deception and heartache of short-lived pleasures. Protectively, then, he refuses to wait for others to make the turnabout; he "jumps the gun," pulls back when things are going well and thereby cuts off experiences which may have proved gratifying, had they been completed. His anticipation of being frustrated and of being set back and left in the lurch prompts him into creating a self-fulfilling prophecy. Thus, by his own hand, he defeats his own chances to experience events which may promote change and growth.

These crushing experiences recur repeatedly, and with each recurrence, the negativist further reinforces his pessimistic anticipations. And in his effort to overcome past disillusionments, he throws himself blindly into new ventures that lead inevitably to further disillusion.